THE DIABETES
ANNUAL/3

THE DIABETES ANNUAL/3

Edited by

K.G.M.M. ALBERTI
Department of Medicine, The University of Newcastle upon Tyne,
Newcastle upon Tyne, U.K.

L.P. KRALL
Joslin Diabetes Center, Harvard Medical School,
Boston, Massachusetts, U.S.A.

ELSEVIER
Amsterdam — New York — Oxford

ISBN 0 444 90427 1
ISSN 0168-9282

Notice   The editors and publishers of this work have made every effort to ensure that the drug dosage schedules herein are accurate and in accord with the standards accepted at the time of publication. Readers are advised, however, to check the product information sheet included in the package of each drug prior to administration to be certain that changes have not been made in either the recommended dose or contra-indications. Such verification is especially important with regard to new or infrequently used drugs.

Published by:
Elsevier Science Publishers B.V.
P.O. Box 1527
1000 BM Amsterdam

Sole distributors for the USA and Canada:
Elsevier Science Publishing Co. Inc.
52 Vanderbilt Avenue
New York, NY 10017

Printed in The Netherlands by Casparie — Amsterdam

List of contributors

N.N. ABUMRAD
Department of Surgery
Vanderbilt University Medical School
Nashville, TN 37232
U.S.A.

K.G.M.M. ALBERTI
Department of Medicine
Medical School
Framlington Place
Newcastle upon Tyne NE2 4HH
U.K.

G.M. ARGOUD
Division of Endocrinology
   and Metabolism
Department of Medicine
The University of New Mexico
School of Medicine
Albuquerque, NM 87131
U.S.A.

D.W. BEAVEN
Department of Medicine
Christchurch Clinical School
   of Medicine
The Princess Margaret Hospital
Christchurch 2
New Zealand

C. BINDER
Steno Memorial Hospital
DK-2820 Gentofte
Denmark

G.F. BOTTAZZO
Department of Immunology
The Middlesex Hospital
   Medical School
London W1 9PG
U.K.

M.F. CARDOSI
Bioelectronics Division
Biotechnology Centre
Cranfield Institute of
   Technology
Cranfield
Bedfordshire MK43 OAL
U.K.

A.D. CHERRINGTON
Department of Molecular Physiology
   and Biophysics
Vanderbilt University
Nashville, TN 37232
U.S.A.

J.A. COLWELL
Veterans Administration
   Medical Center and
   Department of Medicine
Medical University of South Carolina
Charleston, SC 29425
U.S.A.

R.M. DENTON
Department of Biochemistry
University of Bristol Medical
   School
University Walk
Bristol BS8 1TD
U.K.

S.M. DUNN
Department of Medicine
University of Sydney
Sydney, N.S.W. 2006
Australia

O.K. FABER
Niels Steensens Hospital
DK-2820 Gentofte
Denmark

J.S. FLIER
Diabetes Unit
Beth Israel Hospital
330 Brookline Avenue
Boston, MA 02215
U.S.A.

E.A.M. GALE
Department of Immunology
The Middlesex Hospital
    Medical School
London W1 9PG
U.K.

S.G. HARTLING
Niels Steensens Hospital
DK-2820 Gentofte
Denmark

M.W. HAYMOND
Endocrine Research Unit
Department of Pediatrics
Mayo Graduate School of Medicine
Mayo Clinic and Foundation
Rochester, MN 55905
U.S.A.

P.D. HOME
Department of Medicine
Medical School
Framlington Place
Newcastle upon Tyne NE2 4HH
U.K.

D.J. HOSKING
City Hospital
Queen's Medical Centre
Nottingham NG7 2UHG
U.K.

G.L. KING
Research Division
Joslin Diabetes Center
Department of Medicine
Brigham and Women's Hospital
Harvard Medical School
One Joslin Place
Boston, MA 02215
U.S.A.

H. KING
Research Unit
Department of Community Health
University of Tasmania
Hobart
Australia

E.M. KOHNER
Department of Medicine
Hammersmith Hospital
Du Cane Road
London W12 OHS
U.K.

C. KÜHL
Medical Department &
    Drug Regulatory Affairs
Novo Industri A/S
Novo Alle
DK-2880 Bagsvaerd
Denmark

P.E. LACY
Department of Pathology
Washington University
School of Medicine
St. Louis, MO 63110
U.S.A.

M.F. LAKER
Department of Clinical Biochemistry
    and Metabolic Medicine
Royal Victoria Infirmary
Newcastle upon Tyne NE1 4LP
U.K.

H.E. LEBOVITZ
Endocrinology & Diabetes
SUNY Health Science Centre
450 Clarkson Avenue
Brooklyn, NY 11203
U.S.A.

R.D.G. LESLIE
Diabetes Clinic
King's College Hospital
Denmark Hill
London SE5 9RS
U.K.

J.I. MANN
Department of Community
 Medicine and General Practice
Gibson Laboratory Building
Radcliffe Infirmary
Oxford OX2 6HE
U.K.

S.M. MARSHALL
Department of Medicine
The Medical School
Framlington Place
Newcastle upon Tyne NE2 4HH
U.K.

O.P. McGUINNESS
Department of Molecular Physiology
 and Biophysics and Surgery
Vanderbilt University
Nashville, TN 37232
U.S.A.

D.E. McMILLAN
Hal B. Wallis Research Facility
Eisenhower Medical Center
39000 Bob Hope Drive
Rancho Mirage, CA 92270
U.S.A.

C.E. MOGENSEN
Second University Clinic of
 Internal Medicine
Kommunehospitalet
DK-8000 Aarhus C
Denmark

L. MØLSTED-PEDERSEN
Diabetes Centre
Department of Obstetrics and
 Gynaecology Y
Rigshospitalet
University of Copenhagen and
 Hvidøre Hospital
Blegdamsvej 9
DK-2100 Copenhagen
Denmark

A.C. MOSES
Diabetes Unit
Beth Israel Hospital
330 Brookline Avenue
Boston, MA 02215
U.S.A.

T.J. NELSON
Endocrine Research Unit
Department of Pediatrics
Mayo Graduate School of Medicine
Mayo Clinic and Foundation
Rochester, MN 55905
U.S.A.

I. PEACOCK
Department of Medicine
Derby Royal Infirmary
London Road
Derby
U.K.

R. PUJOL-BORRELL
Department of Immunology
The Middlesex Hospital
 Medical School
London W1 9PG
U.K.

D.A. PYKE
Diabetic Clinic
King's College Hospital
Denmark Hill
London SE5 9RS
U.K.

S. REDDY
Research Division
Joslin Diabetes Center
Department of Medicine
Brigham and Women's Hospital
Harvard Medical School
One Joslin Place
Boston, MA 02215
U.S.A.

A.L. ROSENBLOOM
University of Florida
    College of Medicine
Division of Endocrinology
Department of Pediatrics
Gainesville, FL 32610
U.S.A.

D.S. SCHADE
Division of Endocrinology
    and Metabolism
Department of Medicine
The University of New Mexico
School of Medicine
Albuquerque, NM 87131
U.S.A.

R.S. SCOTT
Department of Medicine
Christchurch Clinical School
    of Medicine
The Princess Margaret Hospital
Christchurch 2
New Zealand

G.W.G. SHARP
Department of Pharmacology
College of Veterinary Medicine
and
Division of Biological Sciences
Cornell University
Ithaca, NY 14853
U.S.A.

P.S. SHARP
Royal Postgraduate Medical
    School
Hammersmith Hospital
Du Cane Road
London W12 OHS
U.K.

K.E. STEINER
Department of Molecular
    Physiology and Biophysics
Vanderbilt University Medical School
Nashville, TN 37232
U.S.A.

D.E.R. SUTHERLAND
Department of Surgery
Medical School
University of Minnesota
Phillips Wangensteen Building
516 Delaware Street S.E.
Minneapolis, MN 55455
U.S.A.

R. TATTERSALL
Department of Medicine, Ward C54
University Hospital
Queen's Medical Center
Nottingham NG7 2UH
U.K.

J.M. TAVARÉ
Department of Biochemistry
University of Bristol
    Medical School
University Walk
Bristol BS8 1TD
U.K.

A.P.F. TURNER
Bioelectronics Division
Biotechnology Centre
Cranfield Institute of
    Technology
Cranfield
Bedfordshire MK43 OAL
U.K.

J.R.TURTLE
Department of Medicine
University of Sydney
Sydney, N.S.W. 2006
Australia

M. VRANIC
Flat 1
56 Holywell Street
Oxford OX1
U.K.

D.H. WASSERMAN
Department of Molecular
   Physiology and Biophysics
Vanderbilt University School
   of Medicine
Nashville, TN 37203
U.S.A.

P. ZIMMET
Lions International Diabetes
   Institute
Royal Southern Memorial Hospital
260 Kooyong Road, Caulfield 3162
Melbourne
Australia

Preface

Another year has swiftly passed us by, since Volume 2 of the Annual has appeared. There has been a very positive reply from those who have read (or at least acquired or browsed through) the first two volumes. This encouraging response means that we shall continue to add yet another book to the saturated market each year or so. Volume 3 is indeed a bumper issue — due partly to the enthusiasm of all our authors — and partly to the natural verbosity of some of us! There have, however, been major developments in many areas and these are reflected by several of the chapters.

Several topics appear for the first time, including classification, autonomic neuropathy, insulin action, protein metabolism, glucose sensors and keto-acidosis. Others have reappeared after a gap of one volume. In yet others, new authors have joined the team in line with our overall policy to give fresh views on important areas. There is inevitably overlap between some chapters — for this we apologise, but to eliminate it all would have destroyed the flavour of some of the contributions.

Our aim continues to be rapid, but comprehensive, and timely coverage of important areas of diabetes. It is up to you now to determine whether we have achieved this goal (please let us know if you feel we have not!).

K.G.M.M. Alberti
L.P. Krall

Contents

The Diabetes Annual/3
K.G.M.M. Alberti and L.P. Krall, editors
© 1987 Elsevier Science Publishers, B.V.

1   Classification and diagnosis of diabetes mellitus

P. ZIMMET AND H. KING

Historical aspects

Pertinent to the whole issue of epidemiological and clinical research, as well as management of diabetes mellitus, is the question of the appropriate diagnostic criteria for, and classification of, this heterogeneous disorder. The failure to acknowledge this heterogeneity until recently has been a major handicap to research into aetiological aspects of the various forms of diabetes.

As early as 1936, Himsworth proposed that there were at least two clinical types of diabetes, one of which was caused by true insulin deficiency (1). It was not until the development of a bioassay for insulin in 1949 (2) that scientific credibility could be lent to his suggestion. Further confirmation, a decade later, came with the development of the insulin radioimmunoassay (3) and the widespread use of the terms 'juvenile-onset' and 'maturity-onset' diabetes became a testament to the acceptance of the concept of at least two major forms of diabetes.

Perhaps a much more controversial issue was the question of the appropriate levels of glycaemia needed to make a diagnosis of diabetes. A plethora of sets of diagnostic criteria for diabetes were published with wide variation both between and within countries (4-7). In 1978, a survey was conducted on methods and diagnostic criteria for the oral glucose tolerance test (OGTT) as practised throughout Australasia. Over 100 hospital and private laboratories responded to the questionnaire and a wide variety of differing glucose loads and biochemical methods was apparent. Not only this, but at least 15 different sets of diagnostic criteria were being used, so that, given the same test result, a 'normal' report could be issued by one laboratory and diabetes could be diagnosed by another (7). Thus, it was possible to be a diabetic in Sydney and, by the simple act of moving to Melbourne, a person could be classified as having normal glucose tolerance. In addition, a survey by West of 20 American and overseas diabetologists showed widely differing opinions on the same set of results for an OGTT (8). Under certain circumstances, some diabetologists classified as normal more than half of the 1- and 2-hour glucose values considered to be abnormal by other well-qualified diabetologists.

It became increasingly clear that international consensus was needed on diagnostic criteria for diabetes. In addition, with increasing knowledge of immunology and genetics in relation to the diabetes syndrome, and with new epidemiological perspectives, a review of the classification of diabetes mellitus became a necessity.

During 1978-1979, working parties in three countries — the United States, the United Kingdom, and Australia — prepared reports on standardisation and diagnostic criteria for the OGTT. Although the reports were prepared independently, the three groups emerged with very similar proposals. The American report, prepared by the National Diabetes Data Group (NDDG) and published in 1979, also provided recommendations for the classification of diabetes and other categories of glucose intolerance (9).

The stage was set for international consensus on diagnostic criteria for diabetes and for a uniform framework in which to conduct clinical and epidemiological studies to provide comparable data on the scope and impact of diabetes and other categories of glucose intolerance. A WHO Expert Committee on Diabetes Mellitus was convened in September 1979 and their report, published in 1980 (10) and following upon that of the NDDG (9), set new ground rules for standardization of both the classification of, and criteria for, abnormal glucose tolerance.

In a scholarly fashion, and with the wisdom of Solomon, the WHO Expert Committee proposed an 'interim' classification recognizing that there were still areas of uncertainty but that it was most important for scientific and comparative purposes that investigators used standardized descriptive terminology and diagnostic criteria (10).

Another important feature of the report was the recommendation for a category of impaired glucose tolerance (IGT). The introduction of this term followed recognition that a zone of diagnostic uncertainty existed in the interpretation of the OGTT result between what was clearly normal or diabetic. These subjects were formerly regarded as suffering from 'borderline' diabetes, an epithet considered inappropriate as many such subjects were unlikely to develop overt diabetes (9, 10).

The WHO Expert Committee challenged diabetologists to pursue research into these aspects with the eventual hope of further improving the classification and confirming or improving on the sensitivity and specificity of the diagnostic criteria they recommended.

This review will focus on recent studies that have taken up this challenge.

Classification of diabetes mellitus

IDDM/NIDDM or Type I/Type II or both?

Few people have enlivened and contributed to the debate on classification more than the international diabetologist, Professor Harry Keen. His recent elegant review of the subject (11) highlights the continuing controversy and outlines the inconsistencies of the NDDG and WHO classification. The terms IDDM (insulin-dependent diabetes) and NIDDM (non-insulin dependent diabetes) are basically descriptive clinical terms and have become synonymous with Type I and Type II diabetes, respectively. This has created some confusion as some workers have used the term 'Type I diabetes' in a pathogenetic sense to describe the form of IDDM associated with certain genetic markers and with characteristics of an autoimmune disease.

One of the reasons for the NDDG and WHO recommendation to dispense with the terms 'juvenile-onset' and 'maturity-onset' was because the onset of IDDM in subjects over the age of 40 years is not uncommon (12). In Minnesota, U.S.A., Melton et al (13) found that 32% of subjects with IDDM had been diagnosed after the age of 30 years. Laakso and Pyörälä (14) found 32% of IDDM subjects in Finland fitted into this category. Moreover, it is now clear that IDDM can occur after a prolonged period of what is clinically and conventionally accepted as NIDDM (12, 15).

Clearly there is a group of subjects who present as NIDDM and can be treated with diet alone or with diet and oral hypoglycaemic agents (OHA) for up to several years, but who eventually progress to insulin dependency. Can this subgroup be separated *a priori* from the majority of NIDDM subjects? Groop et al (16) studied 154 unselected subjects with nonketotic diabetes diagnosed between the ages of 35 and 75 years who were treated with diet or OHA for at least 1 year and they obtained baseline information on the following parameters: glycaemic control (weight loss, blood glucose and glycosylated haemoglobin concentrations), islet cell function (fasting and glucagon-stimulated C-peptide concentrations) and immunological markers of insulitis and autoimmunity. These parameters were all repeated in 9 of 22 islet cell antibody (ICA)-positive patients after 2 years and data were correlated with secondary OHA failure. Patients with ICA had lower initial C-peptide levels and showed little rise after glucagon stimulation. B cell function deteriorated significantly during the 2 years in 9 of the 22 ICA-positive patients and more ICA-positive patients required insulin. Groop and co-workers suggested that these 'latent' insulin-dependent subjects could be characterized by persistent ICA, progressive loss of B cells, and a high frequency of thyrogastric autoimmunity. Furthermore, they found an excess frequency of HLA-DR3 and -DR4 in these subjects, confirming an earlier report by Di Mario et al (17).

4 *P. Zimmet and H. King*

These findings have confirmed the clinical impression of 'blurring' between IDDM and NIDDM. It has been suggested that these cases should represent a category that has been labelled as 'Type 1½' diabetes (12)! The plot (or confusion) thickens, as Keen has correctly pointed out, as the Type II designation implies a mechanism responsible for all non-Type I diabetes with the exception of gestational and other types of diabetes which are secondary to a known cause or associated with other defined syndromes.

Thus, the recently convened WHO Study Group on Diabetes (18) recommended that in order to avoid confusion, the terms Type I and Type II should be regarded as completely synonymous with IDDM and NIDDM, respectively (i.e. that the former two terms should be free of aetiopathogenic implications).

TABLE 1. *Classification of diabetes mellitus and allied categories of glucose intolerance*

A. *Clinical classes*

Diabetes mellitus (DM)
   Insulin-dependent diabetes mellitus (IDDM)

Non-insulin-dependent diabetes mellitus (NIDDM)
   (a)   Non-obese
   (b)   Obese

Malnutrition-related diabetes mellitus (MRDM)

Other types of diabetes associated with certain conditions and syndromes:
(1) pancreatic disease; (2) disease of hormonal etiology; (3) drug-induced or chemical-induced conditions: (4) abnormalities of insulin or its receptors; (5) certain genetic syndromes; (6) miscellaneous

Impaired glucose tolerance (IGT)
   (a)   Non-obese
   (b)   Obese
   (c)   Associated with certain conditions and syndromes

Gestational diabetes mellitus (GDM)

B. *Statistical risk classes (subjects with normal glucose tolerance but substantially increased risk of developing diabetes)*

Previous abnormality of glucose tolerance

Potential abnormality of glucose tolerance

From WHO Study Group on Diabetes Mellitus (18).

Tropical diabetes or malnutrition related diabetes?

The wisdom of the WHO Study Group in its recommendation on the terminology IDDM and NIDDM gave few grounds for controversy. However, another of the recommendations on classification (see Table 1) was more contentious. The heterogenous syndrome known as 'tropical diabetes' (reviewed by Mohan et al (19)) was elevated from the 'Other Types' category to a single entity, 'malnutrition related diabetes mellitus' (MRDM), automatically legitimizing what Abu-Bakare et al (20) have claimed may yet prove to be 'a child or children of indeterminate origin'. Recently, Abu-Bakare et al (20) and Mohan et al (19) have reviewed the literature relating to tropical diabetes with respect to the clinical and biochemical variants. Although malnutrition is a plausible unifying factor, these workers felt that a good case existed for retaining the term 'tropical diabetes' (as opposed to MRDM) until there was more information on clinical and biochemical features and on aetiology. There is also a strong case for more detailed epidemiological studies on the prevalence, incidence and global distribution of this syndrome in order to assess its true magnitude (18).

Bajaj has contributed extensively to the literature on this subject and in a recent comprehensive review (21) on the interfacing of epidemiological and biochemical aspects highlighted the apparent magnitude of the problem, while calling for a comprehensive international collaborative effort that might define its true status. He has proposed at least two subclasses — protein-deficient and fibrocalculous pancreatic diabetes — which were accepted by the WHO Study Group (18).

The debate as to the true status of MRDM will undoubtedly continue and it will surely stimulate the type of studies necessary to resolve it.

Classification — new proposals

Turner et al (22) have joined the debate on diabetes nomenclature and definition by pointing out that the WHO classification provides only arbitrary descriptions of the severity of diabetes and not diagnostic categories. They have suggested that it might be more appropriate to differentiate the forms of diabetes by: (a) the *diagnosis* in terms of basic aetiology and pathology; (b) a *descriptive grading* of the main disease components.

They noted that it is more appropriate to classify diseases according to aetiological, pathological and pathophysiological aspects rather than by the treatment regimen. Table 2 illustrates the approach they have proposed for the classification of diabetes, along with comparisons of other disease states, namely renal disease and anaemia.

Turner and colleagues argue for the use of the terms Type I and Type II diabetes as they might represent the beginnings of an aetiological classification.

TABLE 2   *Current classification of diabetes and analogous approximate equivalents for renal disease and anaemia*

Official names		Non-diabetic	IGT	NIDD	IDD
Approximate criteria	Fasting plasma glucose (mmol/l)	<5.5	5.5-8.0	<8.0 ± symptoms	Ketosis 'Requires insulin'
Analogous categories for renal disease and anaemia					
Renal disease	creatinine (µmol/l)	<150	150-220	<220 ± uraemic symptoms	'End-stage renal failure'
Anaemia	haemoglobin (g/100 ml)	>12.0	10.0-12.0	<10 ± symptoms	'Blood-transfusion-dependent anaemia'

IGT = impaired glucose tolerance; NIDD = non-insulin-dependent diabetes; IDD = insulin-dependent diabetes.
Reprinted from Turner et al (22) by courtesy of the Editor of *Diabetic Medicine*.

They propose the addition of an accepted method for grading the severity of diabetes such as the use of fasting plasma glucose concentration (see Table 2) as it provides a simple, precise and repeatable measure of glycaemia in those subjects treated with diet and OHA (23). They further recommend the determination of the degree of impairment of B cell function by measurement of C-peptide concentration.

Welborn and co-workers have suggested that the basal serum C-peptide concentration is a useful test for discriminating between Type I and Type II diabetes (24), particularly in subjects who have been taking insulin for many years. The fasting C-peptide level clearly discriminated between Type I and Type II diabetes in all but a small minority of diabetics (5.5%). In these latter subjects, 73% were receiving insulin therapy, and they may well represent the group who can be categorized as 'Type 1½' diabetes (12).

A study of 10 Caucasoid Type I diabetic and 10 Pima Indians with Type II diabetes by Katzeff and co-workers supported this concept (25). Thus, the addition of the C-peptide estimation to the recommendations of Turner et al (22) perhaps provides a further approach to a more precise classification of the two major forms of diabetes.

The debate on the appropriate classification of subjects with diabetes will continue and it is quite possible that new subgroups will emerge. In the meantime, it is vital for comparability of data and results that the studies on the epidemiology and aetiopathogenesis of diabetes are reported in a consistent manner.

Criteria for diagnosis of diabetes — NDDG vs WHO

General considerations

A major achievement of the NDDG (9, 26) and WHO (10, 18) reports has been the standardization of methodology and diagnostic criteria for the diagnosis of diabetes. There are subtle differences in the recommendations of these groups (27, 28), as shown in Table 3, but the overall thrust of their deliberations has been a global move to standardization and this had led to a more realistic comparison of the magnitude of the problem of diabetes within and between countries.

The rationale for the new diagnostic criteria has been reviewed in the respective original reports (9, 10). Although the NDDG and WHO criteria are almost identical, those of NDDG require that a mid-test blood sample be taken after the 75 gram oral glucose challenge and that the venous plasma glucose level be

TABLE 3. *Comparison of NDDG and WHO diagnostic criteria*

	Plasma glucose mg/100 ml (mmol/l)*					
			Oral glucose tolerance test			
Class	Fasting		Mid-test		2-Hour test	
NDDG						
Normal	<115 (<6.4)	and	<200 (<11.1)	and	<140 (<7.8)	
IGT	<140 (<7.8)	and	≥200 (≥11.1)	and	140-199 (7.8-11.1)	
Diabetes**	≥140 (≥7.8)	or	≥200 (≥11.1)	and	≥200 (≥11.1)	
Non-diagnostic	all other combinations of fasting, mid-test and 2-h values					
WHO						
Normal***	<140 (<7.8)		—	and	<140 (<7.8)	
IGT	<140 (<7.8)		—	and	140-199 (7.8-11.1)	
Diabetes**	≥140 (≥7.8)		—	or	≥200 (≥11.1)	

*The mmol/l values were computed by dividing mg/100 ml values by 18.016 (the number of mg of glucose in 100 ml of a 1-mM solution) and rounding to the nearest 0.1 mmol/l. WHO obtained mmol/l values by dividing mg/100 ml values by 18 and rounding to the nearest 1 mmol/l.
**NDDG and WHO require both the fasting and 2-h values to classify a subject, except when the fasting is ≥ 140 mg/100 ml, which by itself is diagnostic of diabetes.
***Although WHO does not define a 'normal' OGTT, the term is used here to include subjects who do not meet criteria for diabetes or IGT.

Reprinted from Harris et al (28) by courtesy of the Editor of *Diabetes Care*.

$\geqq 11.1$ mmol/l (200 mg/100 ml) (27). As Harris et al (28) have shown, the omission of the mid-test value only makes a small difference: of the 3.6% of persons in a national probability sample of subjects with no medical history of diabetes in the United States population who were diagnosed as having diabetes by WHO criteria, 94% (180/191) also had diabetes according to NDDG criteria.

However, the NDDG requirement for the mid-test value resulted in 11.3% of OGTTs being non-diagnostic, whereas all were classifiable according to WHO criteria. In the absence of specific advantages, this observation weighs against the NDDG system.

With regard to the respective merits of the fasting and 2-hour blood glucose concentration for the diagnosis of diabetes, both the study of Harris et al (28) in the United States and that of Taylor and Zimmet (29) in the Pacific have demonstrated the greater sensitivity of the 2-hour value and have shown that results using the 2-hour value alone are almost identical to those using the two values. This is now the recommendation of WHO (18) and the European Diabetes Epidemiology Study Group (30). Clearly, in an epidemiological setting where a large number of subjects are to be examined and voluntary cooperation is to be maximised, single testing is much to be preferred. The only argument in favour of retaining the fasting blood test under such circumstances would appear to relate to the examination of related biochemical measures which may be influenced by the glucose load.

The NDDG/WHO difference may be more real and have more relevance with respect to the diagnosis and prevalence of impaired glucose tolerance (IGT), the latter being generally lower with the NDDG criteria due to a substantial proportion being non-diagnostic due to the lack of an elevated mid-test value (28). On the other hand, IGT is rarely diagnosed in the clinical situation because of lack of knowledge of its clinical significance. IGT is still the subject of research to determine its mechanisms and prognostic implications (18).

It is also important to recognize that the greatest use of the OGTT today is for epidemiological studies. The OGTT is rarely required in clinical practice except in pregnancy (31, 32). In addition, criticisms are now focused primarily on NDDG criteria while, globally, it is the WHO criteria that are used more commonly.

Implications and significance of the new criteria

An important aspect to consider, in relation to changing the diagnostic criteria for diabetes, is the impact of these on studies of the natural history of diabetes. Melton et al (33) have examined this by applying the new NDDG criteria as opposed to an age-related venous whole blood glucose concentration of 110-160 mg/100 ml 2 hours after a 1 g/kg oral glucose load to the incidence of diabetes in a population-based cohort (1945-1969) in Rochester, U.S.A. The incidence of diabetes in this cohort was reduced by about 20% and the clinical spectrum, at diagnosis, was shifted towards more severe disease, a reduction in relative survival and an increase in the risk of developing macro- or microvascular complications. They found, however, that changes in the natural history of diabetes were modest in magnitude and should have little practical impact on comparisons of diabetes prognosis under the two different sets of diagnostic criteria they used. Their findings will be reassuring to the many workers who may have been concerned that data from studies predating the new NDDG and WHO criteria could not be used for comparison with future studies which utilize those new criteria.

Massari et al (34) found that the application of the new criteria compared with 7 other previous sets showed a major redistribution of asymptomatic subjects in the 3 categories of glucose tolerance with a lower percentage of 'diabetic' and 'normal' subjects and a higher percentage of 'IGT' subjects. An important percentage (33%) of their population could not be classified into the 3 categories of glucose tolerance using NDDG criteria — 20% were 'non-diagnostic' and 13% could not be classified. Providing workers use the WHO criteria, their criticisms have little practical significance within the context of correct usage of the OGTT.

Riccardi et al (35) have called for a re-evaluation of the diagnostic criteria for IGT. They found poor reproducibility of the OGTT for diagnosing IGT. Only 56% of subjects found to have IGT at the first test showed glucose intolerance on a second OGTT. They suggest that if an initial OGTT demonstrates IGT, then the OGTT should be repeated.

Diabetes in pregnancy

In the main, remarkable consensus exists between the NDDG (9) and WHO (10, 18) reports for the diagnosis of diabetes in non-pregnant subjects. However, the classification of glucose tolerance in pregnancy has been handled differently by these groups. The 1980 WHO Expert Committee (10) recommended that the diagnostic procedures and criteria for pregnant women should be the same as those proposed for all adults — a decision recently confirmed by the 1985 WHO Study Group (18). An important point in the WHO recommendations is that during pregnancy, the treatment for IGT should be the same as for diabetes. On the other hand, in 1979 NDDG (9) proposed a 50 g OGTT using the diagnostic criteria proposed by O'Sullivan and Mahan (36), and this has recently been reaffirmed (26).

A recent position statement by the American Diabetes Association (37) has added to the confusion by recommending a random 50 g OGTT for screening in pregnancy with a full 3 hour OGTT after a 100 g load to confirm the diagnosis.

If experts cannot make up their minds, what is the clinician meant to think or do in relation to the diagnosis of diabetes in pregnancy? There are insufficient studies comparing the two sets of criteria and their relationship to pregnancy outcome for mother and foetus. As Hadden (38) has pointed out: 'If it becomes accepted that plasma glucose in pregnancy that is within the upper part of the normal distribution is not pathologic to mother or foetus, then either the WHO or NDDG criteria will be acceptable. Furthermore, in relation to the different glucose loads, there is probably no difference in the populations they will determine.'

Impaired glucose tolerance

Studies that support the recognition of IGT as an independent category of glucose tolerance were reviewed in *The Diabetes Annual/1* (p. 8) (39). There have been few publications that have shed new light on the possible significance of this category since this earlier review.

Stern et al (40) may have brought us one step closer to understanding this elusive entity by defining 3 groups of subjects included under the common heading of IGT: subjects in the upper range of normality, those in the lower range of hyperglycaemia, and a minority who are in transition between normal and abnormal glucose tolerance.

This concept has some important implications for the conclusions of earlier studies which took the excess in cardiovascular risk which has been demonstrated by prospective studies of subjects with IGT as evidence in favour of the IGT category as a discrete entity (9, 10). However, an alternative hypothesis must now be entertained, namely that this observed excess risk is due to the misclassification of a small number of diabetics who subsequently develop cardiovascular disease in the course of their illness.

Two recent cross-sectional studies from the Pacific (41, 42) showed a discrepancy between associations with IGT in subjects of different ethnicity. In a study of Micronesian subjects in the Republic of Kiribati (41), IGT subjects were found to be intermediate between those with normal glucose tolerance and those with diabetes with respect to certain biological characteristics known to be associated with abnormal glucose tolerance. However, in both Melanesian and Indian subjects in Fiji (42), those with IGT were found to lie closer to the diabetic than to the normal population with respect to the same characteristics, the survey methods being carefully standardized.

These discrepancies support Stern and his colleagues' theory, in that they may be explained by postulating that the group with IGT in Kiribati contained an approximately equal proportion of misclassified normal and diabetic objects, whereas those in Fiji contained a greater proportion of misclassified diabetics. One possible implication of this proposal is that an appropriate cut-off point separating normality from abnormality may vary between populations of different ethnic origin.

Clearly, there is much scope for further research into the true nature of IGT.

Glycosylated haemoglobin in the diagnosis of diabetes

There is general consensus on the usefulness of glycosylated haemoglobin with respect to assessment of the control of diabetes (43, 44). Despite a number of earlier studies which indicated its lack of specificity in the diagnosis of diabetes (44-47), and recommendations by expert groups that it should not be used for this purpose, some workers have persevered with investigating the possibility that it might be useful.

In a recent review, Duncan and Heiss (48) suggested that glycosylated haemoglobin was a useful test for screening for diabetes. The hope here, of course, was that for epidemiological purposes a single blood sample might save the need for the OGTT, and that glycosylated haemoglobin might be a more specific test.

Two recent studies have compared the value of glycosylated haemoglobin with the OGTT criteria based on the WHO recommendations. Cederholm et al (49) found that HbA_1 was of little clinical value for the detection of diabetes when used as a screening test in a health survey of 819 residents of Uppsala, Sweden. Albutt et al (50) found, as have other workers (44-47), that the HbA_1 level was within the normal reference range in many persons with newly diagnosed diabetes or other minor abnormalities of glucose tolerance and stated that the OGTT must remain the test of choice. In relation to the diagnosis of diabetes, glycosylated haemoglobin has a high specificity but low sensitivity.

Duncan and Heiss (48) have highlighted the potential for error when using either fasting blood glucose concentration or OGTT as surrogate indices of cumulative glycaemia over time and that the non-enzymatic glycosylated proteins do offer the potential to quantify the latter, and to improve the investigation of the operative hypothesis that cumulative hyperglycaemia plays a causal role in the pathogenesis of chronic disease.

However, Ferrell et al (51) in assessing the specificity and sensitivity of glycosylated haemoglobin and fasting and casual blood glucose as screening devices in a survey of diabetes prevalence revealed that glycosylated haemoglobin was only superior to the casual blood glucose and, with a glycosylated Hb cutoff point of 8%, close to the sensitivity and specificity of the fasting blood glucose concentration.

Modan et al (52) studied the effectiveness of glycosylated haemoglobin, fasting plasma glucose and 1- and 2-hour post-load plasma glucose concentrations in population screening for glucose intolerance. They found that glycosylated haemoglobin was inefficient and considerably inferior to fasting plasma glucose. The 2-hour post-load plasma glucose proved to be the best single screening test for the detection of diabetes. Their results indicated that effective screening for diabetes has to rely on the OGTT. It seems that, for the present, there is insufficient evidence to recommend glycosylated haemoglobin as a diagnostic test for diabetes, but also insufficient evidence to completely discount the use of such agents in future epidemiological investigations.

Conclusions

This review has highlighted important advances in the classification and diagnosis of diabetes, including both development and the critical evaluation of the new NDDG and WHO criteria, the introduction and examination of the intermediate IGT category, and the identification of the 2-hour postprandial blood glucose concentration as the preferred benchmark for the epidemiological definition for glucose intolerance.

We have also identified several areas of continuing uncertainty and controversy, including the classification of tropical diabetes, the true status of 'Type 1½' diabetes, the diagnosis of diabetes in pregnancy, the extent to which excess morbidity in IGT subjects may be a consequence of the misclassification of a small number of diabetics, and the continuing lack of a valid index of cumulative glycaemia for diagnostic purposes.

Much has already been achieved. Much yet remains to be done in the field of classification and diagnosis of diabetes mellitus, an area in which the needs of patients, clinicians, epidemiologists and all those involved with health care delivery are so clearly united.

References

1. Himsworth HP (1936): Diabetes mellitus: its differentiation into insulin-sensitive and insulin-insensitive types. *Lancet, 1,* 117.
2. Bornstein J, Lawrence RD (1951): Plasma insulin in human diabetes mellitus. *Br. Med. J., 2,* 1541.
3. Yalow RS, Berson SA (1960): Immunoassay of endogenous plasma insulin in man. *J. Clin. Invest., 39,* 1157.
4. Committee on Statistics of the American Diabetes Association (1969): Standardization of the oral glucose tolerance test. *Diabetes, 18,* 299.
5. WHO Expert Committee (1965): Diabetes mellitus. *WHO Techn. Rep. Ser., 310,* 5.
6. Fitzgerald MG, Keen H (1964): Diagnostic classification of diabetes. *Lancet, 1,* 1325.
7. Zimmet P (1980): When is diabetes? A new look at diagnostic criteria for diabetes mellitus. *Aust. NZ J. Med., 10,* 346.

8. West KM (1975): Substantial differences in the diagnostic criteria used by diabetes experts. *Diabetes, 24,* 641.

9. National Diabetes Data Group (1979): Classification and diagnosis of diabetes mellitus and other categories of glucose intolerance. *Diabetes, 28,* 1039.

10. WHO Expert Committee on Diabetes Mellitus (1980): Second Report. *WHO Techn. Rep. Ser.,* 656.

11. Keen H (1986): What's in a name? IDDM/NIDDM, Type 1/Type 2. *Diabetic Med., 3,* 11.

12. Editorial (1985): Insulin dependent? *Lancet, 2,* 89.

13. Melton LJ, Palumbo PJ, Chu-pin C (1983): Incidence of diabetes mellitus by clinical type. *Diabetes Care, 6,* 75.

14. Laakso M, Pyörälä K (1985): Age of onset and type of diabetes. *Diabetes Care, 8,* 114.

15. Lyons TJ, Kennedy L, Atkinson AB et al (1984): Predicting the need for insulin therapy in late onset (40-69 years) diabetes mellitus. *Diabetic Med., 1,* 105.

16. Groop LC, Bottazzo GF, Doniach D (1986): Islet cell antibodies identify latent type 1 diabetes in patients aged 35-75 years at diagnosis. *Diabetes, 25,* 237.

17. Di Mario U, Irvine WJ, Borsey DO et al J, (1983): Immune abnormalities in diabetic patients not requiring insulin at diagnosis. *Diabetologia, 25,* 392.

18. WHO Study Group on Diabetes Mellitus (1985): Diabetes mellitus. *WHO Techn. Rep. Ser., 727,* 32.

19. Mohan V, Ramachandran A, Viswanathan M (1986): Tropical diabetes. In: Alberti KGMM, Krall LP (Eds), *Diabetes Annual/2,* p. 30. Elsevier, Amsterdam.

20. Abu-Bakare A, Gill GV, Taylor R, Alberti KGMM (1986): Tropical or malnutrition-related diabetes: a real syndrome? *Lancet, 1,* 1136.

21. Bajaj JS (1986: Malnutrition-related fibrocalculous pancreatic diabetes. In: Serrano-Rios M, LeFebvre PJ (Eds), *Diabetes 1985,* p. 1055. Excerpta Medica, Amsterdam.

22. Turner RC, Holman RR, Mathews DR et al (1986): Diabetes nomenclature: classification or grading of severity. *Diabetic Med., 3,* 216.

23. Holman RR, Turner RC (1980): The basal plasma glucose: a simple, relevant index of maturity-onset diabetes. *Clin. Endocrinol., 14,* 279.

24. Welborn TA, Garcia-Webb P, Bonser AM (1981): Basal C-peptide in the discrimination of Type I from Type II diabetes. *Diabetes Care, 4,* 616.

25. Katzeff HL, Savage PJ, Barclay-White B et al (1985): C-peptide measurement in the differentiation of Type I (insulin-dependent) diabetes mellitus. *Diabetologia, 28,* 264.

26. National Diabetes Data Group (1985): Report of an Expert Committee on Diabetes. Administrative document, National Institutes of Health, Bethesda, MD.

27. Harris M (1985): Classification and diagnostic criteria for diabetes and other categories of glucose intolerance. In: Harris MI, Hamman RF (Eds), *Diabetes in America,* p. 11.1. Publ. No. 85-1468, US Department of Health and Human Services, NIH, Washington, DC.

28. Harris MI, Hadden WC, Knowler WC, Bennet PH (1985): International criteria for the diagnosis of diabetes and impaired glucose tolerance. *Diabetes Care, 8,* 562.

29. Taylor R, Zimmet (1981): Limitation of fasting plasma glucose for the diagnosis of diabetes mellitus. *Diabetes Care, 4,* 556.

30. Teuscher A, Jarrett RJ (1984): Diabetes mellitus: diagnostic criteria. *Diabetic Med., 1,* 305.

31. Alberti KGMM (1983): Diagnostic criteria. *Diabetologia, 25,* 451.

32. Zimmet P (1986): The diagnosis of diabetes mellitus. *Med. J. Aust., 145,* 88.

33. Melton LJ, Palumbo PJ, Dwyer MS, Chu-Pin C (1983: Impact of recent changes in diagnostic criteria on the apparent natural history of diabetes mellitus. *Am. J. Epidemiol., 117,* 559.

34. Massari V, Eschwege E, Valleron AJ (1983): Imprecision of new criteria for the oral glucose tolerance test. *Diabetologia, 24,* 100.

35. Riccardi G, Vaccaro O, Rivellese A et al (1985): Reproducibility of the new diagnostic criteria for impaired glucose tolerance. *Am. J. Epidemiol., 121,* 422.

36. O'Sullivan JM, Mahan CM (1964): Criteria for the oral glucose tolerance test in pregnancy. *Diabetes, 13,* 278.
37. American Diabetes Association (1986): Position statement: gestational diabetes mellitus. *Diabetes Care, 9,* 430.
38. Hadden DR (1985): Geographic, ethnic and racial variations in the incidence of gestational diabetes mellitus. *Diabetes, 34, Suppl. 2,* 8.
39. Zimmet P, King H (1986): The epidemiology of diabetes mellitus. In: Alberti KGMM, Krall LP (Eds), *Diabetes Annual/2,* p 1. Elsevier, Amsterdam.
40. Stern MP, Rosenthal M, Haffner SM (1985): A new concept of impaired glucose tolerance: relation to cardiovascular risk. *Atherosclerosis, 5,* 311.
41. Collins V, Taylor R, Zimmet P et al (1984): Impaired glucose tolerance in Kiribati. *NZ J. Med., 97,* 809.
42. Coventry J, King H, Zimmet P et al (1986): Impaired glucose tolerance in the biethnic (Melanesian and Indian) populations of Fiji. *Diabetes Res., 3,* 427.
43. National Diabetes Data Group (1984): Report of an Expert Committee on Glucosylated Haemoglobin. *Diabetes Care, 7,* 602.
44. Nathan DM, Singer DE, Hurxthal K, Goodson JD (1984): The clinical information value of the glycosylated hemoglobin assay. *N. Engl. J. Med., 310,* 341.
45. Dunn PJ, Cole RA, Soeldner JS, Gleason RE (1979): Reproducibility of haemoglobin A_{1c} and sensitivity to various degrees for glucose tolerance. *Ann. Int. Med., 91,* 390.
46. Verrillo A, De Teresa A, Golia R et al (1983): The relationship between glycosylated haemoglobin levels and various degrees of glucose intolerance. *Diabetologia, 24,* 391.
47. Santiago JD, Davis JE, Fisher F (1978): Haemoglobin A_{1c} levels in a diabetes detection program. *J. Clin. Endocrinol. Metab., 47,* 578.
48. Duncan BB, Heiss G (1984): Nonenzymatic glycosylations of proteins — a new tool for assessment of cumulative hyperglycaemia in epidemiologic studies, past and future. *Am. J. Epidemiol., 120,* 169.
49. Cederholm J, Ronquist G, Wibell L (1984): Comparison of glycosylated haemoglobin with the oral glucose tolerance test. *Diabète Métabl., 10,* 224.
50. Albutt EC, Nattrass M, Northan BE (1985): Glucose tolerance test and glycosylated haemoglobin measurement for diagnosis of diabetes mellitus — an assessment of the criteria of the WHO Expert Committee on Diabetes Mellitus 1980. *Ann. Clin. Biochem., 22,* 67.
51. Ferrell Re, Hanis CL, Aguilar L et al (1984): Glycosylated hemoglobin determination from capillary blood samples: utility in an epidemiology survey of diabetes. *Am. J. Epidemiol., 119,* 159.
52. Modan M, Halkin H, Karasik A, Lusky A (1984): Effectiveness of glycosylated hemoglobin, fasting plasma glucose, and a single post-load plasma glucose level in population screening for glucose intolerance. *Am. J. Epidemiol., 119,* 431.

The Diabetes Annual/3
K.G.M.M. Alberti and L.P. Krall, editors
© 1987 Elsevier Science Publishers, B.V.

2   Autoimmunity and Type I diabetes: bringing the story up to date

GIAN FRANCO BOTTAZZO, RICARDO PUJOL-BORRELL AND EDWIN A.M. GALE

Introduction

Since we wrote the last chapter in this series in July, 1985 (1), our knowledge in this field has progressed in a number of international diabetes meetings, workshops and symposia. A full report appeared following a workshop held in Miami in spring, 1985 (2); the First International Workshop on the Standardisation of Cytoplasmic Islet Cell Antibodies was held in Monte Carlo in October, 1985 (3); and in 1986 the 8th International Symposium on 'Immunology of Diabetes' was held in Edmonton (4). In addition, some interesting (5-7) and unorthodox (8) reviews have appeared, and an international debate on the pathogenesis of diabetes will shortly be published (9).

The prediabetic period

There is general agreement that Type I diabetes develops against a background of genetic susceptibility, and has a long preclinical prodrome characterised by the presence of circulating islet cell antibodies (ICA) and other autoimmune phenomena and, at a later stage, by loss of the first-phase insulin response to intravenous glucose. Beyond this point there is considerable uncertainty. The main reason for this is that clinical experience of the prediabetic period is limited. Most experience has been gained with identical twins discordant for diabetes and with first-degree relatives of a child with diabetes, although other predisposed groups exist such as children with the congenital rubella syndrome and older patients with features of multiple organ-specific endocrine autoimmunity (see below).

Twin studies have yielded a wealth of information, but is this model always relevant to the sporadic presentation that typifies most cases of diabetes? Even family studies are open to this doubt since only 1 in 8 of new cases is familial. In general, only the Pittsburgh and Bart's-Windsor (now Bart's-Oxford) family

15

studies have aimed at systematic follow-up of large cohorts over many years. In studies such as these the yield of high-titre ICA or complement-fixing (CF) ICA-positive individuals is limited to 2-3% of the non-diabetic population, and only a proportion of these have undergone adequate prospective study up to the period at which diabetes has developed. Depending upon the criteria of adequacy applied the world literature probably does not contain more than 20-30 carefully studied cases. This situation is likely to be remedied in the next few years as new population studies develop in the United States, Scandinavia and other parts of Europe. It is to be hoped that these populations will be studied using comparable protocols and that in time some sort of central register can be established.

One recent observation of considerable clinical importance is that the clinical onset of Type I diabetes is typically not abrupt. An early hint of this finding came from the work of Rosenbloom (10) who tested a group of siblings of diabetic children who had had an oral glucose tolerance test 10-12 years previously. Of the 105 children they traced, 6 had developed diabetes, and all of these came from a subgroup of 44 with borderline or abnormal glucose tolerance (admittedly by very stringent criteria) at the time of the first study.

A second line of evidence came more recently from the study of growth in identical twins preceding the onset of diabetes in the first to be affected. The mean duration of symptoms was 6 weeks, but many affected twins showed growth delay in the period before diagnosis, with a mean equivalent to 35 weeks (11).

We ourselves have had the opportunity to study family members prospectively and found that 10 of 13 had progressive or intermittent hyperglycaemia for many months prior to clinical presentation. Nine showed random blood glucose levels above the 97.5th percentile (6.3 mmol/l; 114 mg/100 ml) 6-34 months before diagnosis (12). The interest of these observations does not only rest on the possible usefulness of a raised random blood glucose or abnormal glucose tolerance test as a marker of future diabetes. If individuals typically drift into clinical diabetes, the observed natural history and progression of the condition will obviously differ if the diagnosis happens to be made early. Could the 'remission' phase simply reflect earlier detection and a milder (because earlier) clinical course, and not a period of true B-cell recovery and regeneration?

ICA retain their unchallenged position as the best available marker of future diabetes. Most of the debate over past years has been methodological (see below), and the eventual introduction of International Units to express results should allow direct comparability of studies for the first time. Equally fierce methodological argument has surrounded the measurement and interpretation of insulin autoantibodies (IAA) in the prediabetic period (see below). The literature is divided as to whether IAA have predictive value for the onset of diabetes (13-15, 76). One study in identical twins (13) found insulin autoantibodies in almost half, even after a long period of discordance (and hence a low risk of progression to diabetes). The inference was that they represented a marker of susceptibility that might or might not progress to clinical expression. On the other hand, two recent studies have found that the coexistence of ICA and insulin autoantibodies appears to offer better prediction of diabetes than ICA alone. In the study of Srikanta et al (14) 38 ICA-positive individuals were studied. Of 12 who additionally had insulin autoantibodies, 7 developed diabetes, as against 7 of 26 who had ICA alone. Closely similar findings emerged from the report of Dean et al (15): 8 of 11 with both antibodies went on to develop diabetes as against 3 of 9 with ICA alone.

In the latter study the majority of IAA when measured with enzyme-linked immunosorbent assay (ELISA) were of IgG specificity and IgM IAA were of less predictive value. Interestingly, when a series of children with viral infections and no symptoms of diabetes were tested for the same specificities IgM IAA predominated and IgG IAA were less frequent (16). During follow-up the former tended to persist, but none converted to IgG IAA and no children developed features of glucose intolerance. This might indicate an unexpectedly wide range of cross-reactivity between antigens expressed on common viruses and endogenous hormone molecules.

Does the appearance of ICA in a non-diabetic individual represent a point of no return? Here again twin studies and family studies tend to reach different conclusions. The group at King's College Hospital has reported ICA, activated T lymphocytes and impaired glucose tolerance in almost all their short-term discordant twins, although only a proportion are expected to progress to diabetes (17). If their interpretation is correct, and can be generalised to other groups, it would imply that susceptible individuals may undergo a limited immune onslaught on their B cell population which does not progress to the clinical disease. Our own experience suggests the opposite: of 24 CF-ICA-positive individuals only one has lost this specificity whereas 15 have progressed to diabetes. This discrepancy will only be resolved by continuing and enlarging prospective clinical studies.

Metabolic testing has also been widely applied in the prediabetic period since the observation of a progressive fall in the first-phase insulin response to intravenous glucose (18). This report raised the hope that progression to diabetes could be predicted — and even timed — in terms of a progressive fall in the first-phase response within the normal range. Although this report has not been challenged, our experience has been that the first-phase response is too variable within a given individual to form the basis of any confident prediction. On the other hand, *loss* of the first-phase response probably does represent a point of no return, although by this stage glucose tolerance itself is often abnormal.

In summary, much remains to be learned about the prediabetic period. The initial trigger remains obscure, and it is uncertain whether aborted attacks on

the B cells are common or unusual in susceptible individuals. A better understanding is needed of the natural history of the prediabetic period, as is a reliable means of predicting progression to diabetes. Only when these precondi-
tions are satisfied will controlled trials of preventive strategies be possible at a
time when viable B cells are still present in adequate numbers to guarantee a life
without diabetes.

The concept of heterogeneity

Histological evidence

Our knowledge of the histopathology of Type I diabetes has grown steadily
over the past 20 years, due almost exclusively to the inspiration and pioneering
work of Willy Gepts. A book with contributions from many friends will shortly
be published in his honour (19). The major obstacle in this field has always been
a lack of pancreatic specimens for detailed study, especially from patients who
died shortly after diagnosis. Pancreatic blocks from patients with long-standing
diabetes are usually unrevealing because local immune changes such as insulitis
disappear rapidly, sometimes within a few months of presentation. A similar
and equally unexplained change occurs in the peripheral blood with disappearance of ICA and normalization of T-cell subsets, numbers and function.

   Foulis has reopened the topic over the past few years. He has now studied 119
pancreatic blocks from patients with Type I diabetes who died shortly after
onset of the disease. Before his report (20) the number of cases studied at a
histological level totalled 73 in 5 separate papers (21-24), including his own preliminary observations (25). Of 60 patients who died in the first year of the disease 47 (78%) showed the expected classical pattern of insulitis, but this was
also seen in 3 of 35 more long-standing cases, one after 6 years. This suggests
that the immune attack not only begins years before the metabolic disorder becomes manifest, but may also have a very protracted course. In the latter cases
the observation that lymphocytic infiltration is only seen around islets which still
contain B cells was confirmed, and in all the blocks studied insulitis was observed in 23% of these islets.

   A detailed analysis of the PP rich lobe showed virtually no B cells in islets
localised in this part of the gland. This, and the absence of local inflammation,
strongly suggests that destruction of B cells is completed earlier in this region
than in the glucagon-rich portion of the pancreas, confirming an earlier observation in a single case-report (26). There were also 4 patients who developed
diabetes either at birth (1 case) or in early neonatal life, and who died before the
age of 18 months. In this group, florid insulitis was not observed and the great
majority of islets looked quite normal. This once again raises the possibility that

the disease has a different pathogenesis in infants and may explain why the prevalence of ICA seems to be lower in children diagnosed under the age of 10 (27), and may be lower still in the very young (personal observation).

Three patients had Down's syndrome, and the histological picture here once again supported the concept of heterogeneity in the disease process. One resembled the neonatal cases just described, one had typical insulitis, and the third (who had had diabetes for several years) showed a curious pattern of extensive lymphocytic infiltration organised in germinal centres. These were mainly located in the exocrine pancreas, a pattern rarely observed even at the onset of the disease. It may be relevant to recall that patients with trisomy of the 21st chromosome have a high prevalence of clinical and subclinical organ-specific autoimmunity (28).

HLA associations

Several large populations of newly diagnosed diabetics have now been described. In one multicentre study of 745 cases HLA-DR3 characterised patients with a milder form of the disease, even when HLA-DR4 was also present (29). The usual age and seasonal variations at onset were absent in this group, as previously reported in patients with associated organ-specific immune disorders (30). Although there was no mention of this in the report, we wonder if there was an increase in clinical or subclinical autoimmune disease in the HLA-DR3-positive patients. In contrast those with DR4, especially females, had more severe symptoms at presentation, confirming an observation in a smaller group of patients from Pittsburgh (31). Patients with DR4 were more likely to have evidence of a preceding viral infection, especially with Coxsackie B viruses. Comparable findings emerged from another study (32), but significant correlations were only found when patients with HLA-DR3, -DR4, or both were analysed as a single group. This difference was probably due to smaller numbers. The C-peptide response was more impaired in patients with raised antibody titres to Coxsackie B viruses and a similar observation was made in Finland (33), but only in patients with the heterozygous status Dw3/Dw4. It remains to be established whether these differences were due to typing techniques, since cellular technology was used in the latter study rather than conventional HLA serology.

The overall message is that HLA-DR(w)4-associated genes appear to confer susceptibility to more rapid B-cell failure, with a reduced likelihood of a prolonged remission or 'honeymoon' period following diagnosis. This might be explained by a number of conjectures; B cells may be more susceptible to direct viral attack or less able to regenerate following injury, or DR4-positive individuals may be less capable of clearing viral infections, especially in the more virulent forms found in epidemics (34). It might turn out that invading viruses have a higher affinity for receptors located on their B cells, resulting in a very efficient yet dangerous presentation to immunocompetent cells which will in turn set about clearing the infected (i.e. B) cells in large numbers.

A major and recurrent problem is that HLA-DR3 and -DR4 are common in Caucasoid populations, yet only a minute proportion develop diabetes. Attempts to dissect out the basis of this genetic susceptibility are clearly of great importance. Alloreactive T-cell clones have been raised and tested by a prime lymphocyte-typing technique (35), and a new subset of the HLA-DR4 antigen has been defined in some 80% of DR4-positive diabetic patients as compared to 47% of DR4-positive controls (36). This substantiates earlier work in Ashkenazy Jews with diabetes (37) and the combined data might now indicate that an important role is played by specific functional cell-surface epitopes in conferring susceptibility to certain diseases. We are anxious for these data to be correlated with the growing yield of information from restriction-fragment length polymorphism (RFLP) analysis, which has shown that DQ beta (38, 39) and possibly DX (40) polymorphisms give closer susceptibility to Type I diabetes. The technique has also demonstrated further heterogeneity within the DR4 complex. Thus, even though there are more and more sophisticated genetic markers, these have still failed to demonstrate a specific set of genes in the HLA region conferring the ultimate basis for susceptibility to diabetes.

The large studies referred to above have confirmed the protective role of DR2, and it has also been shown that HLA-DR5 is rarely detected in diabetic patients (38). The dogma that DR2 is virtually absent in Type I patients is however untenable, although the total number is small. DR2 has now been reported in patients who are negative for DR3 and DR4 (29), and an ICA-positive sibling has been described who shared DR2 with the diabetic proband and was negative for DR3 and DR4 (41). RFLP analysis may clarify this apparent paradox by identifying heterogeneity at the level of DR2 (42).

ICA testing

It has long been suggested that ICA might also be used to help define heterogeneity within Type I diabetes. The subclassification originally proposed (43) was based on differences observed when persistence of ICA following diagnosis was examined in large populations. The common pattern in young patients (Type IA) was for ICA to disappear in the first few years from diagnosis; there was the expected slight male preponderance in this group. In contrast, a second and much smaller group referred to as 'Type IB' was characterised by later onset of diabetes, female preponderance, milder clinical onset, persistence of ICA and features of the polyendocrine endocrine autoimmunity syndrome (44). Study of patients with non-insulin-dependent diabetes mellitus (NIDDM) strengthened this concept. In one study the majority of patients who showed secondary failure on treatment with oral agents were ICA-positive, and almost all were affected by other features of autoimmune disorder (45). More recently, late-onset patients with ICA were shown to be more likely to carry HLA-DR3 and/or -DR4 and to progress to insulin treatment (46). In another study, patients with NIDDM positive for CF-ICA showed a lower C-peptide response to arginine infusion, female preponderance, and an increased prevalence of thyroid and gastric antibodies (47). In practical terms, measurement of ICA in late-onset patients may help clinicians to identify those who are likely to go on to need insulin.

The 'honeymoon' or remission period following diagnosis is still poorly understood, but high-titre ICA (48) or CF-ICA (32, 49) at diagnosis is predictive of a shorter remission period and a lower C-peptide response than in those who are negative or show only a low titre. In apparent contrast with this, ICA does not correlate with rate of remission in patients on immunosuppressive therapy with cyclosporin A (27). Possible explanations are either that cyclosporin A is not acting at the level of the B lymphocyte, or that its immunosuppressive effect cannot be disentangled from its cytotoxic action on the B cell itself, as demonstrated in vitro (50, 51) or in experimental systems (52). Nevertheless, the findings described above in conventionally treated patients suggest that ICA may, in combination with other immunological factors, still have a decisive role in the pathogenesis of cell damage. Deposits of immunoglobulin and complement have after all been found in diabetic islets (26).

Progress towards standardization of the cytoplasmic ICA test

It is more than a decade since cytoplasmic ICA were described in diabetic patients with associated autoimmune endocrine abnormalities (53) and subsequently identified in a high proportion of uncomplicated juvenile patients (54), and these markers have increasingly been applied to the study of diabetes. The ICA test has been used to classify diabetes (43), to define heterogeneity within Type I diabetes (55), and to predict progressive B-cell failure in susceptible predisposed individuals (56, 57). The test has also been correlated with impaired B-cell function in established diabetic patients (58-60), and has been used to assess the therapeutic effect of islet (61) or segmental pancreatic grafts (62). As indicated, however, it does not help to monitor the progress of diabetic patients on immunosuppressive therapy (27). All potential applications serve to emphasise the need for international agreement on standardization of this test.

The First International Workshop on standardization of cytoplasmic ICA involved 26 laboratories (3). Before the meeting 13 coded samples were sent to each participant who was asked to test them according to a protocol previously circulated. All sera were titred to end-point and all groups (apart from two which employed monkey pancreas) used human group O pancreas. Sera included known ICA-positive and -negative samples together with other 'tricky' specimens which contained autoantibodies known to interfere with the reading of ICA on pancreatic sections, whether alone or when mixed with ICA, i.e. antinuclear (ANA) and antimitochondrial (AMA) antibodies. To avoid unnecessary complications, each laboratory was free to test sera on their own pancreas sections and to stain with their routine antihuman fluoresceinated (FITC) conjugated antisera. Because many modifications have flourished since the technique was originally described (63), each laboratory was asked to try them for comparison before the results were analysed and discussed.

Analysis of data collected with the standard protocol showed an inter-laboratory concordance greater than 90% with high-titre-positive samples, and of 52-79% with lower titres. The use of different FITC-labelled conjugates did not appear to influence the final result greatly. Most laboratories recognised ANA and AMA; ANA (which clearly stain the large nuclei in the islet) were recognised more easily, but AMA created more problems since they produce a fine granular diffuse staining in the cytoplasm of islets and exocrine cells with additional intense staining of 'oncocytes'. These are large cuboidal cells known to be rich in mitochondria, which are normally scattered, isolated or in clumps, in the exocrine portion of the gland where they sometimes resemble islet structure (64, 65).

Acetone fixation of pancreatic sections did not change the end-point titres from those obtained by the standard method in the majority of determinations. Brief immersion in this reagent before staining helps adhesion to the slide during the extensive washing steps or during the multiple-layer two-colour immunofluorescence procedure. With the latter assay (66, 67) little variation in ICA titres was observed, and this modification aids rapid identification of 'ghosts' (negative islets scattered in sections with a surrounding intense dark background). This method is apparently particularly suited to 'beginners' setting up the test, and to large population-screening programmes, although high background staining can still create problems.

Prolonged incubation in the presence of aprotinin (68) improved the sensitivity of the test without apparent loss of substrate specificity. Although promising, modification with proteinase inhibitors requires further development before it can be incorporated in routine assays.

Few laboratories employed the histochemical technique using glucose oxidase (69), but improvement of this modification is needed if we are to eliminate the interference of high background staining on sections. There was also limited experience with monkey pancreas, but this indicated a possible increase in sensitivity. Discrepancies were however also reported, raising the possibility that the cytoplasmic autoantigen content may vary between different monkey pancreases. A decreased ICA titre was found after heat inactivation of the test samples, after use of FITC-labelled protein A as revealing reagent (67), and when testing the samples for CF-ICA (70). It was confirmed that CF-ICA were present in about 50% of ICA-positive samples originally identified with anti-IgG conjugate, and they were predominantly detected in sera with high-titre ICA (71).

Epidemiological data to date seem to indicate that decreasing the sensitivity of the test (e.g. by use of CF-ICA or protein A) improves identification of the population at risk for future development to Type I diabetes. It remains to be confirmed that high-titre ICA (detected by conventional anti-IgG antisera) retain this degree of specificity without increasing the number of 'false positive' reactions. Prolonged follow-up studies of predisposed individuals with weakly positive or fluctuating reactions (72) may help discover how the humoral response against the islets is first initiated and subsequently sustained. Later appearance of high-titre ICA, as detected by the CF-ICA or protein A test, would indicate that an individual had moved into the high-risk category. From the practical point of view the ultimate method of choice will probably be selected on the grounds of speed and precision, particularly if it eliminates the need for the tedious procedure of titring all positive samples identified with undiluted sera to end-point.

Despite all these considerations, the crucial question remains: which of the tests so far available offers the best sensitivity and specificity in terms of susceptibility to the disease? To overcome the differing characteristics of the assays proposed, calibrated standard curves were presented for each participating laboratory. The approach to data analysis was derived from experience built up during a recent international standardization programme for the immunofluorescence test for ANA. Most laboratories produced linear standard curves, but quantitative inter-laboratory differences between sera were also observed. It remains to be established whether this reflected poor precision or true variation, but it is of interest that when titres from two sera were converted into units derived from the standard curve the inter-laboratory variation decreased, illustrating that the use of standard sera and standard curves may improve concordance. Thus, from these preliminary results, it emerges that availability of reference sera should allow standard curves to be established and ultimately used to define ICA in terms of common units.

Despite recent scepticism expressed concerning the ICA test (73) it remains the best marker of autoimmune aggression directed against the B cell and the best predictor of future progressive B-cell destruction. Furthermore, it seems likely to maintain this role until the cytoplasmic autoantigen can finally be isolated from human tissue, purified and characterised on a molecular basis. The ultimate aim of the standardization programme is to establish precision and accuracy so that results can be compared with confidence. Presentation in terms of units may also allow us to define the threshold value for future insulin dependency and may even give an indication of the rate at which the damage is progressing.

The nature of the islet autoantigens — any progress?

With the demonstration of spontaneous antibodies to insulin in newly diagnosed diabetic patients (74) and in individuals predisposed to develop the disease (14, 15, 75), there is now at least one well-defined autoantigen — the B-cell hormone itself. An International Workshop for the standardization of anti-insulin autoantibodies is underway. Among several contentious issues, discussion will concentrate on comparison between the various assays in current use (ELISA or RIA), on how species-specific the reaction is, on definition of the precise antigenic determinant(s), and on comparison with the binding characteristics of antibodies produced after insulin administration. In addition, better knowledge of the heterogeneity of the autoantibody response is required in terms of its specific reactivity with various parts of the hormone and related molecules (C-peptide and proinsulin). The definition of the Ig class specificity of the reaction itself is needed, including the possibility of identifying restricted clonality (Wilkin, personal communication) resembling that observed in other autoantibody responses, as with thyroid-stimulating antibodies in Graves' disease (76). Certainly the most important question is whether the test be used to identify individuals at risk of future diabetes (75, 77, 78).

Monoclonal antibodies to insulin now available (79) are useful tools for the clarification of some of these problems. They can be used to map epitopes in competitive blocking studies using sera containing insulin autoantibodies, or the size of resulting circulating immune complexes may be compared with that produced by the monoclonal reagents after reacting with insulin.

Characterization of the cellular autoantigens is proceeding slowly, due to the chronic shortage of human islets in sufficient numbers for biochemical purification of the target antigen. The latest findings concerning the autoantigenic protein component of the ICA reaction (originally defined as the 64K band) seem to indicate that the molecule is localised in the cytoplasm rather than on the cell surface as originally postulated (80). This conclusion has been reached after experiments in which sera containing ICA were not able to precipitate a 64K protein after human islets were surface-labelled with radioactive iodine (Harrison, personal communication). On the other hand, the same authors have been able to confirm the presence of the 64K protein after biosynthetically labelling the islets with ^{35}S-methionine, indicating its presence in the cell cytoplasm. These results were obtained after careful preabsorption of the sera with bovine serum albumin (BSA), whose presence in the culture medium constituted an early major point of controversy (see *The Diabetes Annual/2*). Although anti-BSA antibodies present in some of the sera originally employed in the precipitation methods created most of the early problems, the same Australian team has also been able to show that a high proportion of normal human sera also contain anti-BSA antibodies. Consequently, their presence is less useful than another potential serological marker in individuals predisposed to diabetes (Harrison, personal communication).

More information has emerged concerning the glycolipid component of the islet autoantigen. It has been shown by pretreatment of pancreatic sections with appropriate biochemical procedures that sialic acid residues were a potential target of the ICA reaction (81). By comparing similar results with those obtained using monoclonal antibodies to gangliosides, it has been possible to conclude that this particular cell component is also part of the autoantigen complex (82). It must however be emphasised that most of the monoclonal antibodies which react with islets by direct immunofluorescence were originally raised against other tissue gangliosides and therefore crossreact widely with different organs. It is therefore difficult to interpret these data in the light of the known exquisite organ-specific reactivity of autoantibodies present in patients with endocrine autoimmune diseases such as Type I diabetes. Only by extending these biochemical experiments with monoclonal antibodies which react specifically with the ganglioside present in B cells (83) and by proper competitive inhibition assays using ICA obtained from patients will it be possible to clarify this important issue.

Producing monoclonal antibodies with the same specificity as that shown by spontaneous antibodies from patients remains an insurmountable task. Clearly, their availability is still essential as part of the programme for attempting the final characterisation of the putative B-cell autoantigen(s).

It is only recently that IgG monoclonals against insulin and thyroglobulin have been produced by fusing human lymphocytes with human myeloma cell partners (84). Most of the monoclonal antibodies raised from patients' lymphocytes by conventional techniques react with cytoplasmic components, are of IgM class and crossreact with several organs. This applies to those raised after the immunisation of mice with islet preparations (85). They thus resemble the monoclonal antibodies raised from normal individuals and classified as 'natural' autoantibodies (1).

It has been argued that these latter specificities may be part of the complex immune defence homeostatic mechanism and do not exert a pathological effect. It has been suggested that naturally occurring autoantibodies may be regulated by a tight anti-idiotypic response (86) or that their function could be simply that of acting by 'blinding' a physiological immune response against potentially dangerous epitopes expressed on micro-organisms and crossreactive with similar structures widely expressed on normal cells in the body (87). We have also speculated on their significance and we argue that perhaps they could be much less relevant than has been envisaged until now (88). They could represent an 'artifact' of the monoclonal technology, as there is no evidence that natural autoantibodies react with cell surface components (if so, the 'blinding' concept would make much more sense), and there is no proof that they could be absorbed out by a variety of viable preparations obtained from common environmental agents. In addition, they are below the threshold of detection by conventional tests for the determination of 'true' autoantibodies with pathological significance.

The special status of HLA expression on the islets

HLA molecules are cell membrane glycoproteins which act as restriction elements in the recognition of antigens by T lymphocytes. They are responsible for the rejection of transplanted tissue, but also influence all types of immune response. At least schematically, Class I products (HLA-A,B,C,) are recognised by CD8+ T cells (belonging to the cytotoxic population), and Class II molecules (HLA-DR, DP, DQ) are recognised by CD4+ T cells (belonging to helper/inducer and delayed type of hypersensitivity populations).

It is therefore not surprising that in recent years there has been growing interest in the expression of HLA proteins on different cell types, including those in the islets. Transplantation research has been aimed at reducing the immunogenicity of the islets by extracting Class II positive passenger lymphocytes which are, according to one hypothesis, the main stimulators of the final rejection process (89). In the first place, it has been necessary to study the expression of transplantation antigens in the islets of different species used for experimental transplantation as well as in human islets. Recent work combining immune histochemistry techniques with both light and electron microscopy, and further experiments in our own laboratory have shown quite convincingly that in human islets the endocrine cells normally express low levels of Class I products, and that Class II is not at all expressed (90). On the other hand, there is, as in mice (91), a small population of Class II positive cells made up of endothelial and macrophage-like cells which are normal constituents of the islets.

Endothelial cells in rat and dog islets do not normally express Class II antigens, and this may explain the ease with which Class II positive cells may be removed (by culturing them for a few days), and the repeated successes in grafting these islets across histocompatibility barriers without immunosuppression. The feasibility of applying this principle to human islets is more in question, especially since a proportion of capillary endothelial cells around and inside islets normally express Class II products.

The study of HLA expression in endocrine islet cells has also been of interest to researchers trying to understand the origins of the autoimmune response which ultimately destroys the B cells in Type I diabetes. When 'aberrant' Class II expression was observed in the thyrocytes of patients with Graves' and

Hashimoto's diseases (92), it was proposed that Class II positive endocrine cells might play a major part in directing the autoimmune response against themselves (93). The selective detection of Class II positive B-cells in the pancreas of a single patient with Type I diabetes suggested that the hypothesis could also be applied to this disease (26).

Foulis and Farquharson (94) have recently extended this observation in a study of 14 pancreases fixed in formalin, using immunoperoxidase staining and monoclonal antibodies which recognise Class II determinants which are resistant to fixatives (95). The results are remarkable in several ways: (a) only islets containing insulin showed aberrant Class II expression; (b) double staining proved that Class II expression was confined to B cells; (c) Class II expression was often seen in islets free of lymphocytic infiltration; (d) Class II expression was also markedly increased in islet capillary cells; (e) islets which had lost their B cells showed neither Class II expression nor lymphocytic infiltration.

These overlapping observations have suggested the following sequence of events. Class II expression is selectively induced on the B cells, with an accompanying increase in Class II expression on endothelial cells. This is followed at a later stage by infiltration of the islets by modest numbers of lymphocytes, with predominance of the T cytotoxic subset CD8+ (26). There follows progressive destruction of the B cells. As the process burns itself out, the lymphocytic infiltration remits and aberrant expression of HLA products diminishes, and only a few scattered B cells persist in the islets. Since islets at a similar stage of the process appear to be anatomically grouped according to the lobular structure of the pancreas, with marked variations between adjacent lobes, it is possible to see islets displaying all of the pathological features described above within a single pancreatic section (Foulis, personal communication).

Aberrant Class II expression is characteristic of Type I diabetes and is not found in other inflammatory processes of the pancreas such as Type II diabetes and cystic fibrosis (94) or chronic pancreatitis (94, 96). In some of the specimens with chronic pancreatitis, islets were seen to be immersed in a heavy inflammatory infiltrate, presumably rich in interferons and other lymphokines. In spite of this, the islets remained negative for Class II. It is of great interest that islet cells in pancreatic grafts transplanted to diabetic patients did not express Class II. The same phenomenon was observed in pancreatic isografts transplanted from unaffected individuals to their monozygotic diabetic co-twins (62). These grafts were not rejected, but the islets were rapidly destroyed, most probably by a reactivation of the autoimmune cellular response (CD8+ cells predominated in the infiltrate). These observations suggest that the effector mechanisms of the immune system are not themselves responsible for the induction of inappropriate Class II expression on pancreatic B cells.

The absence of Class II expression in conditions other than early Type I diabetes suggests the existence of a 'special' mechanism influencing HLA expression on the islets in vivo. Early attempts to reproduce the phenomenon in vitro using rodent and human islets incubated with interferons were repeatedly unsuccessful (97-100), although Class II was induced in the ductal and exocrine cells (100). This is in sharp contrast with the ease with which Class II expression may be induced in human thyroid cells in vitro using a variety of modulators (101, 102, and reviewed in 103). Class II expression in cultured human islet cells was eventually achieved using the combinations of interferon-γ + tumour necrosis factor (TNF) and interferon-γ + lymphotoxin (104). However, the *de novo* Class II expression was induced simultaneously in B cells and in glucagon cells, and was both time-related and dose-dependent. It has recently been observed that interferon-γ synergises with TNF or lymphotoxin to retard viral replication in infected cells (105). Thus, local release of these mediators in response to viral infection may be one of the mechanisms underlying inappropriate Class II expression in B cells; the possibility that latent viral infections of the B cells are the underlying cause of Type I diabetes has been suggested repeatedly (106-108).

One problem is that the synergistic action of interferon-γ with TNF or lymphotoxin is not B-cell-specific, in contrast with the histopathological findings described above (reviewed in 109). These differences might in part be explained by localised release of these mediators in vivo where their short half-life would inevitably limit their sphere of action. It is difficult, however, to reconcile the observation that two lymphokines are required to induce Class II expression on the islets with the reported absence of lymphocytes or macrophages in islets with strong inappropriate Class II expression. Although more extensive histopathological studies using fresh pancreatic material might help, other possible explanations should be explored. Latent viral infection is once again a possibility. It has recently been shown that some viruses may induce Class II expression directly in certain types of cells such as astrocytes (110). Thus, in Type I diabetes a virus could provide the first stimulus to Class II expression, later amplified by local release of interferon-γ with TNF and/or lymphotoxin. Another possibility is that, whatever the factor involved, the first effect it produces is upon the endothelial cells of the islets. These have been observed to be swollen and expressing increased amounts of Class II in diabetic islets which are otherwise entirely normal (26, 94). These endothelial cells might in turn secrete additional factors causing selective expression of Class II by the B cells (103).

If human islets require a two-mediator signal, mouse islet cells have been reported to become inducible only when very high doses of interferon-γ (6000 U/ml) or conditioned media are used (111). In contrast, the B cells of diabetes-prone BB rats expressed Class II products after culture with only moderate doses of interferon-γ (100 U/ml) (112). One possible explanation is that these islets had already been exposed in vivo to other lymphokines such as TNF and thus made more responsive to interferon-γ. However, these latter findings must be critically compared with those obtained in normal islets of certain strains of rats where there is the suggestion that Class II molecules might be spontaneously expressed, though at very low levels (113). It may be concluded that islet cells are particularly unresponsive to the induction of HLA expression, in contrast to most cell types which respond promptly to interferon-γ. In this respect, they resemble neurones and oligodendrocytes which are also refractory to the action of lymphokines or combinations of them (114). Owing to their irreplaceable biological function, human B cells may have developed this lack of response as a way of remaining excluded from dangerous immunological pathways.

What are the effectors of B-cell destruction?

Only antibodies or T cells possess the recognition mechanisms capable of directing the selective destruction of B cells that occurs in Type I diabetes. The 'coup de grace' could however be administered in many ways. Apart from the classic antigen-specific mechanisms such as complement-dependent antibody-mediated cytotoxicity (115), antibody-dependent cell cytotoxicity and classic T-cell-mediated cytotoxicity (116), much attention has recently been devoted to non-specific mechanisms. Free radicals, cytotoxins and natural killer (NK) cells have been studied. Islet cells seem to be particularly susceptible to peroxide compounds (117), and indeed free radical scavenger substances and nicotinamide (118) can prevent diabetes in NOD mice. Interleukin-1 but not TNF has been found to inhibit insulin release when exposed to islets in vitro, so it has been proposed as one candidate among the lymphokines likely to be involved in B-cell destruction (119, 120). It is worth emphasising that interleukin-1 at different concentrations can also stimulate insulin secretion (121) and its selective action on the B cell is not completely proven. Finally, non-T lymphocytes from diabetic patients, in spite of a decrease in general NK activity, have been shown to have increased NK cytotoxicity to rat B cells in vitro (122).

The cell specificity of the destructive process is hard to explain in all these models, in which much of the damage is attributed to non-specific mechanisms and macrophage products such as interleukin-1 and free radicals. Even invoking the fact that most of these factors are only efficient at very close range, how else can the macrophages or NK cells be directed to the B cells except via the action of T cells or antibodies?

Lessons from the immunotherapy trials

Over the past year and a half we have witnessed a proliferation of immunotherapy trials following the initial encouraging results reported by the group from London, Ontario (123) and subsequently from Paris (124) in open trials. After the first double-blind trials (125), at present more than 800 patients are taking part in cyclosporin trials around the world. To this number may be added those using other forms of immunotherapy including azathioprine (126), prednisone (127), lymphocyte transfusion (128), plasmapheresis (129), and ciamexone (130). This intense activity raises a very real risk of unnecessary duplication of studies involving potential risk to the patient. In an attempt to minimise this problem, a number of leading researchers have recently formed the International Diabetes Study Group (ISGD) whose aim is to 'encourage the exchange of information and discussion of experimental protocols and results'. The founders of this group point out that the initial findings have great importance for our understanding of the pathogenesis of diabetes, and raise a real possibility that its natural history may be altered either by preventive treatment or by immunotherapy following clinical presentation. At the same time, they are at pains to point out that immunosuppression is a research tool and not as yet a prescription for clinical management (131).

The first lesson that can be derived from these studies is a very positive one — final confirmation that immunologically mediated processes are involved in B-cell destruction. The various forms of therapy employed so far all seem able to produce a temporary slowing in the rate of B-cell loss in man. These observations find a parallel in the BB rat (132) and NOD mouse (133) models in which a variety of interventions can prevent (if not cure) the development of the disease.

The ways in which these differing forms of immunotherapy impinge on the immune system in human and animal models vary, but all are relatively non-specific. Their effect is transient and does not persist following withdrawal of the agent. These observations all suggest that the balance in the immunoregulatory system is merely being tipped without in any way influencing or reversing the original causal mechanism. Cyclosporin, the most promising agent, seems to derive its action from inhibition of the release of interleukin-1 and -2, both of which are involved in the generation of helper T cells while sparing the T suppressor subset. Prevention of diabetes in the BB rat by dietary measures (134) may be due to major shifts in the T-cell repertoire resulting from changes in exposure to dietary antigens. Or, to take another example, lymphocyte transfusion (128) may constitute such a powerful allogenic stimulus to the immune system of a diabetic that temporary paralysis of autoimmune mechanisms may result. These latter interpretations are purely speculative. We are entering a period of empirical non-specific immunotherapy, and some of the observed effects may remain unexplained for some time. This, of course, in no way invalidates the attempts themselves. By comparison, years of empirical trials have allowed workers to develop protocols which are successful in inducing remission in systemic lupus erythematosus, Wegener's granulomatosis and kidney rejection, and thereby have improved the survival and quality of life of many patients. Is such an outcome likely in Type I diabetes?

The answer is a qualified 'yes'. New regimens will be tried in the quest for a magic combination of immunosuppressive drugs which can be given in the 'window' period following onset of Type I diabetes, in which some B-cell regeneration might occur, and thus induce a lasting remission. There is, however, a major drawback to this approach. Whereas the rheumatologist is happy to obtain a temporary remission because he has no alternative therapy, the diabetologist can offer the safe and well-tried alternative of carefully supervised insulin therapy to this patients. As things stand, it is uncertain whether the risk of long-term complications of diabetes is greater than the risks of the immunotherapy on offer. Thus, quite apart from the known complications of cyclosporin therapy, it has recently been shown in experimental graft-versus-host disease that withdrawal of the drug precipitated autoimmune manifestations in the animals (135).

The real answer must ultimately come from specific immune intervention, resulting in selective obliteration of the sector of the immune system involved in the autoimmune reaction. Specific immuno-intervention is still in its infancy, but its promise is firm. Basic immunologists are providing the information and tools to dissect normal and abnormal immune reactions, and at an ever-faster rate. We have entered the era of immunotherapy for diabetes by using the tools available, but it can safely be predicted that better ones are on the way. Only then will immunological treatment of Type I diabetes and other organ-specific immune diseases become a clinical reality.

Acknowledgements

We thank our colleagues and close collaborators for much stimulating discussion and many new ideas.

References

1. Bottazzo GF, Pujol-Borrell R, Gale E (1986): Autoimmunity and diabetes: progress, consolidation and controversy. In: Alberti KGMM, Krall LP (Eds), *The Diabetes Annual/2*, pp 13-29. Elsevier, Amsterdam.
2. Janeway C (1985): The immune destruction of pancreatic B cells. *Immunol. Today*, 6, 229.
3. Bottazzo GF, Gleichmann H (1986): Immunology and Diabetes Workshops: Report of the First International Workshop on the Standardization of Cytoplasmic Islet Cell Antibodies. *Diabetologia, 29*, 125.
4. Jaworski MA, Molnar GD, Rajotte RV, Singh B (Eds) (1986): *The Immunology of Diabetes Mellitus*. International Congress Series No. 717, Excerpta Medica, Amsterdam.
5. Eisenbarth GS (1986): Type I diabetes mellitus: a chronic autoimmune disease. *N. Engl. J. Med., 314*, 1360.

6. Doniach D, Spencer KM, Bottazzo GF (1985): Immunology of insulin-dependent diabetes. In: Rose NR, Mackay I (Eds), *The Autoimmune Diseases,* pp 227-242. Academic Press, Orlando, FL.

7. Vergani D (1986): Complement. *Diabetic Med., 3,* 306.

8. Bottazzo GF (1986): Death of a beta cell: homicide or suicide? *Diabetic Med., 3,* 119.

9. Bach JF (Ed.) (1986): Forum: Effector mechanisms in Type I diabetes. *Ann. Inst. Pasteur Immunol., 137D,* 451; *138* (1987), 117.

10. Rosenbloom AL, Hunt SS, Rosenbloom EK, MacLaren NK (1982): Ten year prognosis of impaired glucose tolerance in siblings of patients with insulin-dependent diabetes. *Diabetes, 31,* 385.

11. Hoskins PJ, Leslie RDG, Pyke DA (1985): Height at diagnosis of diabetes in children: a study in identical twins. *Br. Med. J., 1,* 278.

12. Tarn AC, Smith CP, Spencer KM et al (1987): Type I (insulin-dependent) diabetes: a disease of slow clinical onset? *Br. Med. J., 294,* 342.

13. Wilkin TJ, Hoskins PJ, Armitage M et al (1985): Value of insulin autoantibodies as serum markers for insulin dependent diabetes mellitus. *Lancet, 1,* 480.

14. Srikanta S, Ricker AT, McCulloch DK et al (1986): Autoimmunity to insulin, beta cell dysfunction, and development of insulin dependent diabetes mellitus. *Diabetes, 35,* 139.

15. Dean BM, Becker F, McNally JM et al (1986): Insulin autoantibodies in the prediabetic period: correlation with islet cell antibodies and development of diabetes. *Diabetologia, 29,* 339.

16. Bodansky HJ, Grant PJ, Dean BM et al (1986): Islet-cell antibodies and insulin auto-antibodies in association with common viral infections. *Lancet, 2,* 1351-1353.

17. Millward BA, Alviggi L, Hoskins PJ et al (1986): Immune changes associated with insulin-dependent diabetes may remit without causing the disease: a study in identical twins. *Br. Med. J., 292,* 793.

18. Srikanta S, Ganda OP, Eisenbarth GS, Soeldner JS (1983): Islet cell antibodies and beta cell function in monozygotic triplets and twins initially discordant for Type I diabetes. *N. Engl. J. Med., 308,* 322.

19. Lefebvre PJ, Pipeleers D (Eds) (1987): *The Pathology of the Endocrine Pancreas in Diabetes.* Springer-Verlag, Berlin. In press.

20. Foulis AK, Liddle CN, Farquharson MA et al (1986): The histopathology of the pancreas in Type I (insulin-dependent) diabetes mellitus: a 25 year review of deaths in patients under 20 years of age in the United Kingdom. *Diabetologia, 29,* 267.

21. Maclean N, Ogilvie RF (1959): Observations on the pancreatic islet tissue of young diabetic subjects. *Diabetes, 8,* 83.

22. Gepts W (1965): Pathologic anatomy of the pancreas in juvenile diabetes mellitus. *Diabetes, 14,* 619.

23. Doniach I, Morgan AG (1973): Islets of Langerhans in juvenile diabetes mellitus. *Clin. Endocrinol., 2,* 233.

24. Junker K, Egeberg J, Kromann H, Nerup J (1977): An autopsy study of the islets of Langerhans in acute-onset juvenile diabetes mellitus. *Acta Pathol. Microbiol. Scand., Sect. A, 85,* 699.

25. Foulis AK, Stewart JA (1984): The pancreas in recent-onset Type I (insulin-dependent) diabetes mellitus: insulin content of islets, insulitis and associated changes in the exocrine acinar tissue. *Diabetologia, 26,* 456.

26. Bottazzo GF, Dean BM, McNally J et al (1985): In situ characterization of autoimmune phenomena and expression of HLA molecules in the pancreas in diabetic insulitis. *N. Engl. J. Med., 313,* 353.

27. Mandrup-Poulsen T, Nerup J, Stiller CR et al (1985): Disappearance and reappearance of

islet cell cytoplasmic antibodies in cyclosporin-treated insulin-dependent diabetics. *Lancet,* *1*, 599.

28. Doniach D, Roitt IM, Polani PE (1968): Thyroid antibodies and sex-chromosome anomalies. *Proc. R. Soc. Med., 61*, 278.
29. Ludvigsson J, Samuelsson U, Beauforts C et al (1986): HLA-DR3 is associated with a more slowly progressive form of Type I (insulin-dependent) diabetes. *Diabetologia, 29*, 207.
30. Irvine WJ, Gray RS, Steel JM (1980): Islet cell antibody as a marker for early stage Type I diabetes mellitus. In: Irvine WJ (Ed.), *Immunology of Diabetes*, pp 117-154. Teviot Scientific Publications, Edinburgh.
31. Eberhardt MS, Wagener DK, Orchard TJ et al (1985): HLA heterogeneity of insulin-dependent diabetes mellitus at diagnosis. *Diabetes, 34*, 1247.
32. Schernthaner G, Banatvala JE, Scherbaum W et al (1985): Coxsackie-B-virus-specific IgM responses, complement-fixing islet cell antibodies, HLA DR antigens, and C-peptide secretion in insulin-dependent diabetes mellitus. *Lancet, 1*, 630.
33. Knip M, Ilonen J, Mustanen A, Akerblom HK (1986): Evidence of an accelerated B-cell destruction in HLA-Dw3/Dw4 heterozygous children with Type I (insulin-dependent) diabetes. *Diabetologia, 29*, 347.
34. Frisk G, Fohlman J, Kobban M et al (1985): High frequency of Coxsackie-B-virus-specific IgM in children developing Type I diabetes during a period of high diabetes morbidity. *J. Med. Virol., 17*, 219.
35. Sheehy MJ, Sondel PM, Bach ML et al (1975): HL-D LD typing: a rapid assay using primed lymphocytes. *Science, 188*, 1308.
36. Sheehy MJ, Rowe JR, MacDonald MJ (1985): A particular subset of HLA-DR4 accounts for all or most of the DR4 association in Type I diabetes. *Diabetes, 34*, 942.
37. Sheehy MJ, Quintieri FB, Yang SY et al (1984): HLA antigens of insulin-dependent diabetics. I. PLT colonies detecting Dw10 and a new Class II determinant distinct from HLA-D, DR, MB (DC), MT and SB. *Tissue Antigens, 23*, 290.
38. Henson V, MacLaren N, Winter E et al (1986): Molecular genetics of insulin-dependent diabetes mellitus. *Mol. Biol. Med., 3*, 129.
39. Michelsen B, Lernmark A (1986): HLA-DQ gene polymorphism in insulin-dependent diabetes. In: Jaworski MA, Molnaar GD, Rasotte RV, Singh B (Eds), *The Immunology of Diabetes Mellitus*, pp 3-8. International Congress Series, No. 717, Excerpta Medica, Amsterdam.
40. Hitman GA, Sachs J, Cassell P et al (1986): A DR3 related DX gene polymorphism strongly associated with insulin-dependent mellitus. *J. Immunogenet., 23*, 47.
41. Eisenbarth GS, Srikanta S, Fleischnick E et al (1985): Progressive autoimmune beta cell insufficiency: occurrence in the absence of high-risk HLA alleles DR3, DR4. *Diabetes Care, 8*, 477.
42. Cohen D, Cohen O, Marcadet A et al (1984): Class II HLA-DC B-chain restriction fragments differentiate among HLA-DR2 individuals in insulin-dependent diabetes and multiple sclerosis. *Proc. Natl Acad. Sci. USA, 81*, 1774.
43. Bottazzo GF, Doniach D (1976): Pancreatic autoimmunity and HLA-antigens (Letter to Editor). *Lancet, 2*, 800.
44. Becker F, Tarn AC, Gale EAM et al (1986): Polyendocrine autoimmune disease and diabetes. In: Laron Z, Karp M, Tikua P (Eds), *Future Trends in Juvenile Diabetes: Therapy and Research*, pp. 95-194. Karger, Basel.
45. Gray RS, Irvine WJ, Cameron EHD, Duncan LJP (1980): Glucose and insulin responses to oral glucose in overt non-insulin-dependent diabetics with and without the islet cell antibody. *Diabetes, 29*, 312.
46. Gleichman H, Zorcher B, Greutlich B et al (1984): Correlation of islet cell antibodies and

HLA-DR phenotypes with diabetes mellitus in adults. *Diabetologia, 27,* 90.

47. Groop LC, Bottazzo GF, Doniach D (1986): Islet cell antibodies identify latent Type I diabetes in patients aged 35-75 years at diagnosis. *Diabetes, 35,* 237.

48. Marner B, Agner T, Binder C et al (1985): Increased reduction in fasting C-peptide is associated with islet cell antibodies in Type I (insulin-dependent) diabetic patients. *Diabetologia, 28,* 875.

49. Peig M, Pujol-Borrell R, Gomis R et al (1986): High titre complement fixing islet cell antibodies predict B cell function loss in Type I (insulin-dependent) diabetes. *Diabetologia, 29,* 581A.

50. Nielsen JH, Mandrup-Poulsen T, Nerup J (1986): Direct effects of cyclosporin A on human pancreatic B-cells. *Diabetes, 35,* 1049.

51. Robertson RP (1986): Cyclosporin induced inhibition of insulin secretion in isolated rat islets and HIT cells. *Diabetes, 35,* 1016.

52. Iwakiri R, Nagafuchi S, Kounoue E et al (1986): Cyclosporin A enhances streptozotocin-induced diabetes in CD-1 mice. In: Jaworski MA, Molnaar GD, Rajotte RV, Singh B (Eds), *The Immunology of Diabetes Mellitus,* pp 393-397. International Congress Series, No 717, Excerpta Medica, Amsterdam.

53. Bottazzo GF, Florin-Christensen A, Doniach D (1974): Islet cell antibodies in diabetes mellitus with autoimmune polyendocrine deficiences. *Lancet, 2,* 1279.

54. Lendrum R, Walker G, Gamble DR (1975): Islet cell antibodies in juvenile diabetes mellitus of recent onset. *Lancet, 1,* 880.

55. Bottazzo GF, Mirakian R, Dean BM et al (1982): How immunology helps to define heterogeneity in diabetes mellitus. In: Kobberling J, Tattersal R (Eds), *The Genetics of Diabetes Mellitus,* pp 79-90. Academic Press, New York.

56. Gorsuch AN, Spencer KM, Lister J et al (1981): Evidence for a long prediabetic period in Type I (insulin-dependent) diabetes mellitus. *Lancet, 2,* 1363.

57. Srikanta S, Ganda OMP, Rabizadeh A et al (1985): First degree relatives of patients with Type I diabetes: islet cell antibodies and abnormal insulin secretion. *N. Engl. J. Med., 313,* 461.

58. Steel JM, Irvine WJ, Clarke BF (1980): The significance of pancreatic islet cell antibody and abnormal glucose tolerance during pregnancy. *J. Clin. Lab. Immunol., 4,* 83.

59. Madsbad S, Bottazzo GF, Cudworth AG et al (1980): Islet cell antibodies and beta cell function in insulin-dependent diabetics. *Diabetologia, 18,* 45.

60. Mustonen A, Knip M, Akerholm HK (1983): An association between complement-fixing cytoplasmic islet cell antibodies and endogenous insulin secretion in children with insulin-dependent diabetes mellitus. *Diabetes, 32,* 743.

61. Gunnarson R, Bottazzo GF, Freedman ZR et al (1982): Does specific immunity to islet cell tissue develop in diabetics receiving pancreatic grafts? *Horm. Metab. Res., Suppl. 12,* 108.

62. Sibley DK, Sutherland DFR, Goetz FC, Michael AF (1985): Recurrent diabetes mellitus in the pancreas iso- and allograft: a light and electron microscopic and immunohistochemical analysis. *Lab. Invest., 53,* 132.

63. Gleichmann H, Bottazzo GF (1987): Progress towards standardization of the cytoplasmic islet-cell antibody assay: analysis of the data presented at the First International Workshop. *Diabetes, April.*

64. Swana GT, Swana MR, Bottazzo GF, Doniach D (1977): A human mitochondrial antibody (HAMA): its importance in the identification of organ-specific reaction. *Clin. Exp. Immunol., 28,* 517.

65. Betterle C, Caretto A, Zeviani M et al (1985): Demonstration and characterization of anti-human mitochondria autoantibodies in idiopathic hypoparathyroidism and in other conditions. *Clin. Exp. Immunol., 62,* 353.

66. Madsen OD, Landrin Olsson M, Bille G et al (1986): A two-colour immunofluorescence test with a monoclonal human proinsulin antibody improves the assay for islet cell antibodies. *Diabetologia, 29,* 115.
67. Srikanta S, Rabizaden A, Omar MAK, Eisenbarth GS (1985): Assay for islet cell antibodies: protein A monoclonal antibody method. *Diabetes, 34,* 300.
68. Pilcher C, Elliott RB (1984): Improved sensitivity of islet cell cytoplasmic antibody assay in diabetics (Letter to Editor). *Lancet, 1,* 1352.
69. Krell J, Rabin BS (1984): Comparison of an immunohistochemical and immunofluorescence procedure to detect antibody to pancreatic islet cells. *Diabetes, 33,* 709.
70. Bottazzo GF, Dean BM, Gorsuch AN et al (1980): Complement-fixing islet cell antibodies in Type I diabetes: possible monitors of active beta cell damage. *Lancet, 1,* 668.
71. Bruining GJ, Molenaar J, Tuk CW et al (1984): Clinical time course and characteristics of islet cell cytoplasmic antibodies in childhood diabetes. *Diabetologia, 26,* 24.
72. Spencer KH, Tarn AC, Dean BM et al (1984): Family studies in Type I (insulin-dependent) diabetes: evidence of fluctuating islet cell autoimmunity in unaffected relatives. *Lancet, 1,* 764.
73. Wilkin TJ, Armitage M (1986): Markers for insulin dependent diabetes: towards early detection. *Br. Med. J., 293,* 1323.
74. Palmer JP, Asplin CM, Clemons P et al (1983): Insulin antibodies in insulin-dependent diabetics before insulin treatment. *Science, 222,* 1337.
75. Wilkin TJ, Armitage M, Casey C et al (1985): Value of insulin autoantibodies as serum markers for insulin-dependent diabetes mellitus. *Lancet, 2,* 480.
76. Atkinson MA, McLaren NK, Riley WJ et al (1986) Are insulin autoantibodies markers for insulin-dependent diabetes mellitus? *Diabetes, 35,* 139.
77. Wilkin TJ, Armitage M (1986): Insulin antibody during the pre-diabetic period (Letter to Editor). *Diabetologia, 10,* 752.
78. Dean BM, Gale E, Bottazzo GF (1986): Insulin antibody during the pre-diabetic period: an answer (Letter to Editor). *Diabetologia, 10,* 753.
79. Storch MJ, Petersen K, Licht T, Kerp L (1985): Recognition of human insulin and proinsulin by monoclonal antibodies. *Diabetes, 34,* 808.
80. Baekkeskov S, Nielsen JH, Marner B et al (1982): Autoantibodies in newly diagnosed diabetic children: immunoprecipitate human pancreatic islet cell proteins. *Nature (London), 298,* 167.
81. Nayak RC, Omar MAK, Rabizaden A et al (1985): Cytoplasmic islet cell antibodies: evidence that the target antigen is a sialoglycoprotein. *Diabetes, 34,* 617.
82. Nayak RC, Colman PG, Eisenbarth GS (1987): How are monoclonal antibodies related to autoimmune serology? In: *Baillière's Clinical Immunology and Allergy, Vol. 1.* In press.
83. Alejandro R, Shienvold FL, Hajek SAV et al (1984): A ganglioside antigen on the rat pancreatic B cell surface identified by monoclonal antibody R2D6. *J. Clin. Invest., 74,* 25.
84. Casali CP, Inghirami G, Nakamura M et al (1986): Human monoclonals from antigen specific selection of B lymphocytes and transformation by EBV. *Science, 234,* 476.
85. Srikanta S, Krisch K, Eisenbarth GS (1986): Islet cell proteins defined by monoclonal islet cell antibody HISL-19. *Diabetes, 35,* 300.
86. Holmberg D, Coutinho A (1985): Natural antibodies and autoimmunity. *Immunol. Today, 6,* 356.
87. Cohen IR, Cooke A (1986): Natural autoantibodies might prevent autoimmune disease. *Immunol. Today, 7,* 363.
88. Todd I, Pujol-Borrell R, Bottazzo GF et al (1986): Autoantigen presentation by target cells: its possible role in determining autoantibody specificity. *Ann. Inst. Pasteur Immunol., 137D,* 149.

89. Lafferty KJ, Prowse SJ, Simeonovic CJ, Warren HS (1983): Immunobiology of tissue transplantation: a return to the passenger leukocyte concept. *Ann. Rev. Immunol., 1,* 143.

90. Shienvold FL, Alejandro R, Mintz DH (1986): Identification of Ia-bearing cells in rat, dog, pig and human islets of Langerhans. *Transplantation, 41,* 364.

91. Farr AG, Anderson SK (1985): In situ ultrastructural demonstration of cells bearing Ia antigens in the murine pancreas. *Diabetes, 34,* 987.

92. Hanafusa T, Pujol-Borrell R, Chiovato L et al (1983): Aberrant expression of HLA-DR antigen on thyrocytes in Graves' disease: relevance for autoimmunity. *Lancet, 2,* 1111.

93. Bottazzo GF, Pujol-Borrell R, Hanafusa T, Feldmann M (1983): Role of aberrant HLA-DR expression and antigen presentation in the induction of endocrine autoimmunity. *Lancet, 2,* 1115.

94. Foulis AK, Farquharson MA (1986): Aberrant expression of HLA-DR antigens by insulin-containing B cells in recent-onset type I diabetes mellitus. *Diabetes, 35,* 1215.

95. Epenetos AA, Bobrow LG, Adams TE et al (1985): A monoclonal antibody that detects HLA-D region antigen in routinely fixed, wax embedded sections of normal and neoplastic lymphoid tissues. *J. Clin. Pathol., 38,* 12.

96. Bovo P, Mirakian R, Medigo F et al (1987): Chronic pancreatitis: is there a role for auto-immunity? *Pancreas,* in press.

97. Campbell IL, Wong GHW, Schrader JW, Harrison LC (1985): Interferon-gamma enhances the expression of the major histocompatibility Class I antigens on mouse pancreatic B cells. *Diabetes, 34,* 1205.

98. Campbell IL, Harrison LC, Colman PG et al (1985): Expression of Class I MHC proteins on RIN-m5F cells is increased by interferon-gamma and lymphokine-conditioned medium. *Diabetes, 35,* 1225.

99. Campbell I, Bizilj K, Colman PG et al (1986): Interferon-gamma induces the expression of HLA-A,B,C but not HLA-DR on human pancreatic B-cells. *J. Clin. Endocrinol. Metab., 62,* 1102.

100. Pujol-Borrell R, Todd I, Doshi M et al (1986): Differential expression and regulation of MHC products in the endocrine and exocrine cells of the human pancreas. *Clin. Exp. Immunol., 65,* 128.

101. Pujol-Borrell R, Hanafusa T, Chiovato L, Bottazzo GF (1983): Lectin-induced expression of DR antigen on human cultured follicular thyroid cells. *Nature (London), 303,* 71.

102. Todd I, Pujol-Borrell R, Hammond LJ et al (1985): Interferon-gamma induces HLA-DR expression by thyroid epithelium. *Clin. Exp. Immunol., 61,* 265.

103. Bottazzo GF, Todd I, Mirakian R et al (1986): Organ-specific autoimmunity — a 1986 review. *Immunol. Rev., 94,* 137.

104. Pujol-Borrell R, Todd I, Doshi M et al (1987): HLA Class II induction in human islet cells by interferon-gamma and tumour necrosis factor or lymphotoxin. *Nature (London), 326,* 304.

105. Wong GHW, Goeddel DU (1986): Tumour necrosis factors alpha and beta inhibit virus replication and synergize with interferons. *Nature (London), 323,* 819.

106. Oldstone MBA, Southern P, Rodriguez M, Lampert P (1985): Virus persist in beta cells associated with chemical manifestations of diabetes. *Science, 224,* 1440.

107. Leiter EH, Fewell JW, Kuff EL (1986): Glucose induces intracisternal Type A retroviral gene transcription and translation in pancreatic B cells. *J. Exp. Med., 163,* 87.

108. Yoon JW, Rayfield EJ (1986): Two possible pathogenic mechanisms for virus induced diabetes. In: Jaworsky MA, Molnaar GD, Rajotte RV, Singh B (Eds), *The Immunology of Diabetes Mellitus,* pp 287-289. International Congress Series, No. 717, Excerpta Medica, Amsterdam.

109. Pujol-Borrell R, Todd I (1987): Inappropriate Class II in autoimmunity: is it the primary event? In: *Ballières Clinical Immunology and Allergy, Vol. 1.* In press.

110. Massa PT, Dorries R, Ter Meulen V (1986): Viral particles induce Ia antigen expression on astrocytes. *Nature (London), 320,* 543.

111. Wright JR, Lacy PE, Unanue ER et al (1986): Interferon-gamma mediated induction of Ia antigen expression on isolated murine whole islets and dispersed islet cells. *Diabetes, 35,* 1174.

112. Walker R, Cooke A, Bone AJ et al (1986): Induction of Class II MHC antigens on pancreatic B cells isolated from BB/E rats. *Diabetologia, 29,* 749.

113. Ulrichs K, Nothling R, Keller R et al (1987): Genetically determined variation of constitutive MHC Class II antigen expression in various rat strains and cell types. *Transplant. Proc.,* in press.

114. Mauerhoff T, Pujol-Borrell R, Mirakian R, Bottazzo GF (1987): Differential expression and regulation of MHC products in neural and glial cells of human fetal brain. Submitted for publication.

115. Toguchi Y, Ginsberg-Fellner F, Rubinstein P (1985): Cytotoxic islet cell surface antibodies (ICSA) in patients with Type I diabetes and their first-degree relatives. *Diabetes, 234,* 855.

116. Lohmann D, Krug J, Lampeter EF et al (1986): Cell mediated immune reactions against B cells and defect of suppressor cell activity in Type I (insulin-dependent) diabetes mellitus. *Diabetologia, 29,* 421.

117. Okamoto H, Yamamoto H, Yamagami T, Takasawa S (1986): Mechanism of B cell injury and its prevention in IDDM — a molecular approach. In: Serrano-Rios M, Lefebvre PJ (Eds), *Diabetes 1985,* pp 509-512. International Congress Series, No. 700, Excerpta Medica, Amsterdam.

118. Yamada K, Nonaka K, Hanafusa T et al (1982): Prevention and therapeutic effects of large dose nicotinamide injections on diabetes associated with insulitis. *Diabetes, 32,* 749.

119. Bendtzen K, Mandrup-Poulsen T, Nerup J et al (1986): Cytotoxicity of human P17 interleuking-1 for pancreatic islets of Langerhans. *Science, 232,* 1545.

120. Zawalich WS, Diaz VA (1986): Interleukin-1 inhibits insulin secretion from isolated perifused rat islets. *Diabetes, 35,* 1119.

121. Nielsen JH, Mandrup-Poulsen T, Spinas GA et al (1986): Possible role of interleukin-1 (IL-1) in the pathogenesis of insulin-dependent diabetes mellitus (IDDM). In: Jaworski MA, Molnaar GD, Rajotte RV, Singh B (Eds), *The Immunology of Diabetes Mellitus,* pp 95-103. International Congress Series, No. 717, Excerpta Medica, Amsterdam.

122. Negishi K, Waldeck N, Chandy G et al (1986): Natural killer cell and islet killer cell activities in Type I (insulin-dependent) diabetes. *Diabetologia, 29,* 352.

123. Stiller CR, Dupre J, Gent M et al (1984): Effects of cyclosporin immunosuppression in insulin-dependent diabetes mellitus of recent onset. *Science, 223,* 1362.

124. Assan R, Debray-Sachs M, Laborie C et al (1985): Metabolic and immunological effects of cyclosporin in recently diagnosed Type I diabetes mellitus. *Lancet, 2,* 67.

125. Feutren G, Assan R, Karsenty G et al (1986): Cyclosporin increases the rate and length of remissions in insulin-dependent diabetes of recent onset. *Lancet, 2,* 119.

126. Harrison LC, Colman PG, Dean B et al (1985): Increase in remission rate in newly diagnosed Type I diabetic subjects treated with azathioprine. *Diabetes, 34,* 1306.

127. Silverstein J, MacLaren N, Riley W et al (1986): Prednisone and imuran treatment of insulin dependent diabetes. In: Jaworski MA, Molnaar GD, Rajotte RV, Singh B (Eds), *The Immunology of Diabetes Mellitus,* pp 351-357. International Congress Series, No. 717, Excerpta Medica, Amsterdam.

128. Lohmann D, Bierwolf B, Lampeter E, Verlohren HJ (1986): Inhibition of cell mediated immune reactions against B cells in Type I (insulin-dependent) diabetes by transfusion of lymphocytes. *Diabetologia, 29,* 566A.

129. Marner B, Lernmark A, Ludvigsson J et al (1985): Islet cell antibodies in insulin-dependent (Type I) diabetic children treated with plasmapheresis. *Diabetes Res., 2,* 231.
130. Usadel KH, Teuber J, Schmeidl R et al (1986): Management of Type I diabetes with ciamexone (Letter to Editor). *Lancet, 2,* 567.
131. Assan R, Bach JF, Czernichow P et al (1986): Immunosuppressive drugs in diabetes (Letter to Editor). *Lancet, 2,* 1097.
132. Mordes JP, Rossini AA (1987): Keys to understanding autoimmune diabetes mellitus: the animal models of insulin-dependent diabetes mellitus. In: *Baillières Clinical Immunology and Allergy, Vol. 1.* In press.
133. Tarui S, Tochino Y, Nonaka K (Eds) (1986): *Insulitis and Type I Diabetes: Lessons from the NOD Mouse.* Academic Press, Tokyo.
134. Scott FW, Mongaeu R, Kardish M et al (1985): Diet can prevent diabetes in the BB rat. *Diabetes, 34,* 1059.
135. Sorkin R, Kimura H, Schroden K et al (1986): Cyclosporin induced autoimmunity: conditions for expressing disease, requirement for intact thymus and potency estimates of autoimmune lymphocytes in drug treated rats. *J. Exp. Med., 164,* 1615.

The Diabetes Annual/3
K.G M.M. Alberti and L.P. Krall, editors
© 1987 Elsevier Science Publishers, B.V.

3   Genetics of diabetes

R.D.G. LESLIE AND D.A. PYKE

Our understanding of the genetics of diabetes has been revolutionized in the last decade by studies in identical twins and of HLA genes. These studies have proved that the two clinical types of the disorder — insulin-dependent diabetes (IDDM or Type I diabetes) and non-insulin-dependent diabetes (NIDDM or Type II) — are genetically distinct. IDDM is associated with genes in the HLA region of Chromosome 6, while NIDDM is not.

In this Chapter we shall bring up to date our review in *The Diabetes Annual/1*, but although there has been new work in the 2 years since that volume was published, much of what we wrote then remains true.

Insulin-dependent diabetes (IDDM)

Genetic influences are powerful in IDDM, but the disease is in part determined by non-genetic factors. Studies of identical twins have shown that in over half of those with IDDM the co-twin is not diabetic; as identical twins share the same germ-like genes, such differences must be due to environmental factors (1). It remains possible, however, that certain genes have undergone rearrangements leading to genetic differences in, for example, immunoglobulin and T-cell receptor genes, thus leading to genetic differences even between identical twins. Nevertheless, environmental agents or chance cannot entirely account for the development of IDDM since even those IDDM twins with a non-diabetic co-twin are themselves genetically susceptible to the disease through genes in the HLA region (2). The nature of an environmental agent which could be implicated is unclear; both viruses and toxins have been proposed, but the evidence remains incomplete.

The HLA association with IDDM is principally through alleles of the HLA-D locus. Until the discovery of the association with the HLA-DQ region the strongest positive association was between HLA-D/DR3 and D/DR4 and the strongest negative association was with HLA-D/DR2 (3). The positive associations with HLA-B8, Bl5 and Bl8 are due to linkage disequilibrium of these genes with D/DR3 and D/DR4; and in the same way the negative association with HLA-B7 is due to this gene being in linkage disequilibrium with D/DR2.

Population studies demonstrate that HLA-DR4 is positively and HLA-DR2 is negatively associated with IDDM in all ethnic groups. HLA-DR3 is associated with IDDM only in American black and Caucasian populations. The strength of these associations is expressed as a relative risk (RR), which is the factor by which disease risk is increased in those with as compared to those without a genetic marker. Thus, an increased relative risk is carried by individuals with HLA-DR4 (RR = 7) and DR3 (RR = 5) and a decreased risk by HLA-DR2 (RR = 0.12). The most powerful evidence that IDDM is associated with an HLA-haplotype is provided by family studies. If IDDM is linked with an HLA-haplotype, then the disease and the haplotype should segregate together in families such that similarly affected sibs will tend to share one or two haplotypes. This is indeed the case; about 95% of subjects with IDDM share an HLA-haplotype with an affected sib (4). However, it remains to be established that HLA-D/DR2 has a protective effect since the only segregation analysis of DR2 indicated that the transmission deficit was due merely to the increase of other DR genes (5).

One or two HLA genes?

The mode of inheritance of IDDM remains controversial. Current genetic models employ HLA-DR data and it is unlikely that any further information can be culled from such models until details are available regarding the associations between the disease and HLA-DQ and HLA-DR subtypes. Autosomal dominant inheritance is unlikely. A simple autosomal recessive model can be rejected using a method devised by Rotter et al (6). This model rejects simple recessive inheritance when the number of DR3/DR4 heterozygotes exceeds the combined sum of DR3/3 and DR4/4 homozygotes in a diabetic population. The method does not depend on ratios of data from non-diabetic populations. Recessive inheritance was rejected since of 193 patients with IDDM the number of heterozygotes was 68 compared with a maximum number of 22 homozygotes (P< 0.0001).

This method does not reject two alleles at a single locus acting in addition to increase gene penetrance. However, this single-locus gene dosage model can also be rejected since it cannot account for the consistent increase observed in the relative risk of DR3/DR4 heterozygotes (RR = 14) compared with DR3 or DR4 homozygotes. More strikingly it cannot account for the increased disease expression in identical co-twins of IDDMs heterozygous for HLA-DR3/DR4 as compared with co-twins of IDDMs with either DR3 or DR4 alone (2). A total of 106 pairs of identical twins were typed for HLA-DR of whom 56 were concordant and 50 discordant for IDDM. The heterozygote phenotype DR3/DR4 was more prevalent in concordant than discordant pairs (59 and 28%, respectively). The discordant pairs were likely to remain discordant as at least 5 years had elapsed since the affected twin had been diagnosed. Phenotypes, not genotypes, were studied, so the rate of homozygosity could not be established. However, if we assume that those twins in whom the second DR antigen could not be identified were actually homozygous for HLA-DR3 or DR4, then 70% of HLA-DR3/DR4 heterozygotes were concordant for diabetes as compared with at the most 38% of both DR3 and DR4 homozygotes.

This increase in disease expression in heterozygotes as compared with homozygotes has been confirmed in family studies (7) and is incompatible with a single-gene two-allele model in which there is a gene dosage effect. Current evidence therefore favours two susceptibility genes associated with HLA-DR3 and DR4, respectively.

Heterogeneity

If there are two or more genes causing diabetes, then each gene might be associated with a different disease pathogenesis. Hence, IDDM has been divided into an autoimmune and a viral-induced type (8). There is no evidence, however, to support the existence of the latter type. Several recent studies have sought a clinical difference between diabetics with HLA-D/DR3 and D/DR4 at the time of diagnosis. The results are not conclusive; nevertheless, there is a tendency for patients with HLA-DR4 to have more ketonuria at diagnosis while those with HLA-DR3/DR4 have lower C-peptide levels 21 months after diagnosis (9, 10). Evidence that diabetic subjects with HLA-D/DR3 are more likely to show a seasonal variation in time of diagnosis has not been confirmed.

More strikingly, in support of genetic heterogeneity, patients in whom islet cell antibodies persist have an increased prevalence of HLA-B8 and DR3 as compared with patients in whom the antibody does not persist (11). Genetic control of autoantibody production has been confirmed in a family study for complement-fixing but not non-complement-fixing islet cell antibodies (12). Of 323 sibs of 193 diabetics 42 had islet cell antibodies and these antibodies were distributed in a random fashion between HLA non-identical, haplo-identical and identical sibs. The distribution of those 13 with complement-fixing islet cell antibodies, on the other hand, favored an HLA association since none was found in HLA-non-identical sibs as against 7 in haplo-identical and 6 in HLA-identical sibs. Since the non-HLA identical sibs are unlikely to develop IDDM, these observations imply that islet cell antibodies might not be good markers of the disease. In addition, it would appear that activation of B lymphocytes producing islet cell antibodies can occur independently of the HLA susceptibility to IDDM. It has been suggested that those diabetic subjects with persistent islet cell antibodies have a strong autoimmune basis to their diabetes which often appears in middle age (11). However, there is no evidence that the frequency of HLA-DR3 increases with age at diagnosis of diabetes. In this it differs from

HLA-DR4 which is found in some 77% of IDDMs diagnosed under the age of 10 but only 27% diagnosed over the age of 30 (8th International Tissue Typing Workshop). Nevertheless, HLA-DR4 remains a high-risk antigen in Caucasians diagnosed in middle age (13). In 54 insulin-requiring, ketosis-prone, lean diabetic patients diagnosed after the age of 40 the frequency of HLA-DR4 was increased (RR = 4.6) and that of HLA-DR2 was decreased (RR = 0.18) even after correction for the number of antigens tested.

Susceptibility axes

The question arises whether the tendency for genes to coexist in IDDM in the HLA-B, C, D, DR and Bf and complement region of Chromosome 6 is due to linkage disequilibrium with HLA-D/DR genes or whether these other genes themselves play a role in the pathogenesis of the disease through gene interaction. There is no evidence that either complement or Bf genes confer genetic susceptibility independently of the HLA system. Thus, in a study of HLA and Bf genotypes in 75 families with an IDDM proband the frequency of the rare allele BfFl was increased but only in association with HLA-B18 and Cw5 (14). All HLA-B8 subjects and 15 of 16 Bw62 subjects had the BfS allele.

If the association between IDDM and complement and Bf alleles is through linkage disequilibrium with the HLA-DR region, then the alleles associated with HLA-DR3 and DR4 should be the same in diabetics and non-diabetics. A study of genetic markers in 60 patients with IDDM and 169 control subjects indicated that the association between IDDM and HLA-DR3 is accounted for by the haplotype of the susceptibility axis HLA-B8 BfS C4AQO C4B1 DR3 (RR = 1.9) and B18 BfF1 C4A3 C4BQO DR3 (RR = 7.6) but not by other DR3 axes such as B8 BfS C4QO C4A1 DR3 (RR = 1) (15). Similarly the association between HLA-DR4 and IDDM is accounted by the axis HLA-B15 BfS C4A3 C4B2 DR4 (RR = 17.7) but not by other axes such as B4 BfS C4A3 C4QO DR4 (RR = 0.6). Several studies have confirmed these associations; in one the estimated risk of IDDM in subjects homozygous for B18 C4A3 C4BQO BfF1 DR3 was approximately 0.5 (16, 17). Thus, certain susceptibility axes in some IDDM patients carry a greater risk than the HLA-DR allele alone, suggesting that gene interaction is important because linkage disequilibrium cannot of itself explain the association with complement and Bf alleles.

This assumes that both HLA-DR3 and DR4 are single alleles each linked to a susceptibility gene. Recent evidence indicates that they are not. The human HLA-D region encodes Class 2 antigens each of which consists of two polypeptide chains (a and b) inserted into the plasma membrane. The B-chain is coded by several genes which show marked polymorphism. Differences may exist in hybridization patterns of DNA coding for the B-chain in patients positive for HLA-DR4 with and without IDDM (18). A B-chain cDNA probe, pDR-B-1, has been prepared which contains DNA sequences complementary to both the coding region and 3′-non-translated sequences of Class 2 antigen B-chain messenger RNA. DNA from HLA-DR4 subjects was digested with endonucleases BamH1, EcorR1 and PstI. A 3.7 kb fragment following BamH1 digestion was absent in 29 diabetics but present in 3 of 9 HLA-DR4 non-diabetics. An 18 kb fragment following PstI digestion was found in all 15 diabetics with HLA-DR4 but only 6 of 9 non-diabetics with HLA-DR4. These genetic differences in the HLA-D region between diabetics and non-diabetics who are HLA-DR4-positive suggests that certain genes in the HLA/D/DR region may carry a particular disease risk which the usual immunological typing techniques cannot at present demonstrate.

The human HLA-D region contains over 14 genes and can be broadly divided into three subregions: HLA-DR, HLA-DQ and HLA-DP. Genomic probes are available for most of these genes and there has been considerable interest in possible restriction fragment length polymorphism of these genes which might be associated with IDDM. Preliminary data suggest that IDDM is more closely associated with gene polymorphisms of the HLA-DQ than of the HLA-DR region. Thus, an HLA-DQ chain gene polymorphism (designated DX) identified by the restriction enzyme Taq1 is found in more patients with IDDM who have HLA-DR3 than in those who do not have DR3 (19). Another DQ B-chain gene polymorphism revealed by the restriction enzyme Taq1 and designated HLA-DQR4 is positively associated with DR4 and appears to be more closely associated with the disease than DR4 (20, 21). Finally a polymorphism of DQ, designated DQR1, is found in HLA-DR2 patients with IDDM while the DQR2 polymorphism tends to be found in HLA-DR2 patients with multiple sclerosis (22, 23).

In summary, genes in the HLA-DQ region are more closely associated with IDDM than genes in the DR region. Linkage of these genes with the disease remains to be established. The strength of the association is relatively weak since these genes are also commonly found in non-diabetics. These differences between diabetic and non-diabetic HLA genes may yet enable us to explain the association with complement and Bf alleles through linkage disequilibrium.

Non-HLA genes

Approximately 50% of non-diabetics are HLA-DR3 or DR4 and yet only about 0.1% of the population develops IDDM. How can so many people carry the susceptibility gene when only a few develop the disease? Non-genetic factors must in part explain this discrepancy. Further studies of HLA-DR subtypes, complement and Bf alleles should enable us to define further the difference between HLA-DR3 and DR4 persons with and without IDDM. Since a large number of autoimmune disorders are associated with HLA-DR3, the question arises as to which factor, genetic or non-genetic, confers that specificity which produces IDDM rather than, for example, chronic active hepatitis.

There is evidence for a second non-HLA-linked gene which predisposes to IDDM. The insulin gene on the short arm of Chromosome 11 is flanked by a polymorphic region with three major alleles: a common small Class 1 allele averaging 570 base pairs, a rare intermediate Class 2 allele of 1320 base pairs, and a large Class 3 allele which averages 2470 base pairs. In a study of 113 unrelated IDDM subjects and 83 non-diabetic subjects there was a significantly higher frequency of both Class 1 alleles and genotypes containing two Class 1 alleles in the diabetic group (24). This important observation has been confirmed in a family study, although analysis of 17 pedigrees including 34 diabetic and 69 non-diabetic subjects failed to demonstrate linkage with IDDM (25). In addition, there was no co-inheritance between HLA-DR3 or DR4 and the insulin gene polymorphism. In summary, the insulin gene polymorphism shows an association with IDDM but no linkage to the disease and it therefore may have no role to play in the pathogenesis of the disease.

The search for other non-HLA markers has been less fruitful. A preliminary observation indicated an association between the Kidd (Jk) red blood cell marker located on Chromosome 2 and IDDM (26). This observation has not been confirmed by the same authors in an extended study of 103 patients with IDDM (27). In another study of 133 families with IDDM there was strong evidence that Kidd and IDDM were not linked (28). Assuming three genetic models (autosomal recessive, additive and dominant), the lod scores at zero recombination were -18.51, -11.62 and -6.03 for each model, respectively (a positive lod score would suggest linkage).

An interesting but very preliminary observation has suggested linkage between IDDM and an immunoglobulin gene allotype on Chromosome 2, which codes for the constant region of kappa light-chain antibodies (29). Since constant-region genes are closely linked to variable-region genes, the suggestion is that the linkage is between IDDM and variable-region genes. A study of 4 patients with Graves' disease and 6 with IDDM and Graves' disease showed that all 10 patients shared the same kappa light-chain allotype with a similarly affected sibling. This observation indicates linkage between Graves' disease and this light-chain allotype. Two further families were studied in whom the proband had IDDM and a similarly affected sibling. In both the diabetic probands shared the same kappa light-chain allotype. The results from these two families were pooled with those from the 6 families with IDDM and Graves' disease and the authors concluded that IDDM also showed linkage with certain light-chain allotypes. This conclusion is not valid since it ignores the established linkage between Graves' disease and these allotypes and is based on only two observations. Further data should be available soon since gene probes which characterise variable and constant immunoglobulin gene regions have been developed.

Acetylator status is another possible genetic marker for IDDM. However, all the recently reported studies have been designed to assess a relationship between acetylator status and diabetic neuropathy. Fast acetylators were found in 74% of 116 IDDM patients, 54% of non-insulin-dependent diabetics and 48% of non-diabetics in one study (30) and in 49% of IDDM subjects and 37% of non-diabetics in another (31). It remains to be determined whether acetylator status is influenced by metabolic changes and whether this association is found in an unbiased population study.

Non-insulin-dependent diabetes (NIDDM)

The genetics of NIDDM is distinct from that of IDDM. The two types breed true. NIDDM, being much the commoner type in all communities, is often found in relatives of IDDM subjects but no more often than in the general population (32). There is a strong inherited component in the etiology of NIDDM which is unassociated with HLA types. This is proved by twin studies.

Twin studies in NIDDM

Concordance in identical (monozygotic) twins with respect to diabetes (or any other disease) does not prove that it is genetically determined; co-twins usually share the same environment, at least in early life, and will therefore be concordant (both twins affected) for diseases such as measles or tuberculosis, because they are both exposed to the infecting organism. However, if twin pairs are concordant for a disease with onset in later life, when co-twins are living apart and thus exposed to different environments, the evidence becomes more persuasive.

In the case of NIDDM concordance among identical twins is high; more so than for IDDM (1). Among 53 pairs of identical twins 48 were concordant for NIDDM, only 5 discordant. Furthermore, in the 5 discordant pairs the affected twins had been discovered to be diabetic only within the previous 5 years and the unaffected twins might therefore be expected to become diabetic themselves.

When the 5 unaffected twins were tested by glucose challenge, mean glucose values were raised, insulin secretion was diminished and metabolite values were also abnormal (33). It might be concluded from this that most or all of these 'unaffected' twins are destined to become diabetic, but it remains to be established whether this will be so.

Later results (unpublished) have shown a larger number of discordant pairs of twins, highlighting the risks of biased ascertainment in studies of this kind in which diabetic twins are reported, not through population surveys, but by their physicians because they happen to have been diagnosed as such. Nevertheless, it remains true that of 37 pairs in which NIDDM was diagnosed in one twin before 1970 the other has become diabetic in every case, 75% of them within 6 years.

This high degree of concordance for NIDDM is seen despite the fact that co-twins are almost always living apart when diabetes is diagnosed in the index twin and, perhaps more important and surprising, when neither twin is obese and when their weights are widely different. Co-twins differed from each other at the time of diagnosis by 5 kg or more in 75% of cases and by more than 15 kg in about 30% and it was as often that the diagnosis was made first in the lighter twin as it was in the heavier.

These results, whilst not refuting the well-known association of NIDDM with obesity, cast doubt upon its etiological significance. Furthermore, they suggest that other environmental or non-genetic factors, such as diet or occupation, are also unlikely to play important roles in the production of NIDDM, at least in these twin pairs.

An interesting observation, which might have bearing on the association of NIDDM and obesity, is that obesity itself seems to depend on genetic influences. Evidence for this has come from a study of children who were adopted. When they grew up, their weights closely resembled those of their biological parents, especially their mothers, not those of their adoptive parents (34).

Is NIDDM a single entity?

We have spoken as if NIDDM were a single disease, but there is little direct evidence for this belief and considerable reason to doubt it.

NIDDM usually appears in late life, but it has been recognized for many years that it may be diagnosed in childhood. It may then be referred to as maturity-onset diabetes (a term now no longer used) of youth, or MODY. This is a useful but purely descriptive term. It is probable that MODY itself is not a single disorder; indeed, some cases of MODY turn out, on follow-up, to be insulin-dependent diabetes of unusually slow development.

However, the majority of cases are probably due to the apparently discrete disorder which we prefer to call by the neutral term Mason-type diabetes — after the proposita (35). A further description was given in *The Diabetes Annual/1*. This type of diabetes is not linked with HLA (36) or to variations of the flanking region of the insulin gene (37) (see next section).

Insulin and insulin receptor variants

Proinsulin is the precursor of insulin and C-peptide. Proinsulin has a low insulin-like biological activity, but it cross-reacts with the insulin antibody used in the radioimmunoassay of serum insulin. Normally less than 10% of insulin immunoreactivity is due to proinsulin. A rare syndrome of familial hyperproinsulinaemia has been described, in which affected patients have very high levels of proinsulin, presumably due to deficient breakdown of the parent molecule to insulin and C-peptide (38). The defect is transmitted through families as an autosomal dominant trait. Affected individuals have in addition normal circulating insulin, which probably accounts for their normal glucose tolerance. However, in a few subjects the level of normal insulin may be inadequate and patients with NIDDM and hyperproinsulinaemia have been described (38). When a hormone with reduced biological activity is produced, it may be secreted to excess. Therefore the search for other insulin variants has centered on those patients with hyperglycaemia and hyperinsulinaemia typical of insulin resistance but in whom the response to exogenous insulin is normal. Three mutant insulins from such individuals have been described (39). One, designated insulin Chicago, has been identified as normal insulin except for the 25-position on the β-chain where leucine has been substituted for phenylalanine. In two of these three patients it has been possible to demonstrate mutation at a site corresponding to B24 or B25 in one insulin gene allele. Insulin extracted from pancreatic tissue of the patient with a B25 substitution contained both normal insulin and the variant insulin, suggesting co-dominant expression of both insulin alleles. The importance of these observations and their relevance, if any, to the aetiology of NIDDM in general remains to be determined.

A further patient with mild diabetes, fasting hyperinsulinaemia and normal sensitivity to exogenous insulin had a serine for phenylalanine substitution at position 24 on the insulin β-chain (40).

A genetic deficiency of insulin receptors causing insulin resistance and severe diabetes has been described in a 14-year-old girl (41). The patient had normal circulating insulin and no detectable insulin receptor antibodies. However, insulin binding to erythrocytes, monocytes, adipocytes and cultured fibroblasts was markedly reduced. Insulin-stimulated glucose transport both in vivo, using a euglycaemic clamp, and in isolated adipocytes was decreased. The patient's mother and two sisters were also insulin-resistant with hyperinsulinaemia.

Insulin gene

In *The Diabetes Annual/1* we described the uncertain position with regard to the association of NIDDM with a variable locus near the insulin gene on the 11th chromosome.

This locus is thought to have at least three classes of alleles and an association between two Class 1 alleles and IDDM, and a weaker association with NIDDM, has been reported in one study but not in another; a third study reported an increase in genotypes containing two Class 3 alleles in NIDDM (42, 43). Another confusing factor was the possible association of Class 3 alleles with atherosclerosis, a common condition in patients with NIDDM, many of whom are elderly. Finally, it has been claimed that there is an association between Class 3 alleles and hypertriglyceridaemia (44).

It now seems that a link between the polymorphic locus near the insulin gene and NIDDM or IDDM has been excluded. None was found in family studies of young patients with NIDDM apparently inherited in a dominant fashion ('Mason-type' diabetes). The lack of family studies in cases of NIDDM in older patients, the common form, left unsettled the question of a significant association in that condition. A family study has now been reported (45).

The frequency of the two alleles of 6.0 and 7.6 kb in the 5′ flanking region were studied in 7 pedigrees (5 white and 2 black) with a high frequency of NIDDM. The 7.6 kb allele was found in slightly over half of all persons whether diabetic or non-diabetic. In these cases the polymorphism flanking the insulin gene was inherited in a mendelian fashion but was not associated with diabetes (insulin-dependent or non-insulin-dependent).

Whether maturity-onset diabetes of the young (Mason-type diabetes) is a variant of NIDDM or a separate entity is not clear and studies of insulin gene polymorphism have not helped to settle the question. A study of a family with many members affected with this condition (46) has confirmed the findings in two earlier reports (37, 47) in *The Diabetes Annual/1* of a lack of association between Mason-type diabetes and insulin gene polymorphism.

It seems likely, therefore, that the polymorphism, which was always difficult to explain in terms of the aetiology of NIDDM (and still more of IDDM), is irrelevant to it.

Chlorpropamide alcohol flushing (CPAF)

Facial flushing after alcohol in diabetics taking chlorpropamide was first reported soon after chlorpropamide was introduced more than 25 years ago. The suggestion that this harmless drug side effect might be inherited and linked to some cases of NIDDM came from the observation of CPAF in two cases of Mason-type diabetes. It soon became apparent that CPAF commonly occured in other, more common types of NIDDM, in IDDMs, and in non-diabetic subjects (see *The Diabetes Annual/1*).

The significance of CPAF is confused largely because of difficulty in its assessment — the reaction is subjective (although associated with objective evidence of facial temperature rise) and is to some extent dependent upon chlorpropamide dosage. There is still no generally accepted technique for testing for CPAF although a dose which leads to a blood level of over 40 mg/l and an assessment which combines subjective sensation of flushing with a rise of facial temperature, from a resting temperature of no more than 32°C, of 1.5°C or more provide a good separation of 'flushers' from 'non-flushers', with only a few 'intermediates'.

The original suggestion was that CPAF is inherited as a simple autosomal dominant (48). Evidence of its genetic character comes from studies in identical twins who are in all, or nearly all, cases concordant for CPAF even when discordant for diabetes and from the fact that in those 'flushers' whose parents have been tested one has been found to be positive, as have half of their siblings.

In view of the technical difficulties of CPAF testing and doubts about its frequency and association with diabetes these observations should be treated with caution, but it still remains probable that CPAF is, in some families at least, an inherited phenomenon.

Since our previous review (*The Diabetes Annual/1,* p. 53) uncertainty concerning the significance of CPAF has continued. The importance of alcohol and chlorpropamide dosage and of body weight have been re-emphasised (49). Making allowance for these variables, a study of 160 patients with NIDDM (50) showed that the 38% who were classed as CPAF-positive more often had a first degree family history of diabetes and the authors concluded that the phenomenon was genetically determined but were sceptical about whether it acted as a marker for diabetes. On the other hand, a study of 53 Jewish Israeli diabetics found an association of CPAF and NIDDM (51).

With improved techniques of CPAF assessment, measurements of serum levels of acetaldehyde (higher in 'flushers' than in 'non-flushers') and perhaps of liver aldehyde dehydrogenase and of serum levels of metenkephalin (increased by chlorpropamide and alcohol in both flushers and non-flushers), we may learn more about the pathogenesis of the reaction, its mode of inheritance and its association and relevance, if any, to NIDDM.

Microvascular complications of diabetes

Complications affecting especially the retina and glomerulus are common in diabetes. The prevailing view is that the better the control, the less the frequency and severity of the complications.

There is certainly much clinical evidence to support this view, but is it the whole truth? Could other, perhaps genetic, factors play a role? An immediate objection to accepting the view that complications result exclusively from poor control is the frequent case of the badly controlled diabetic patient who escapes all complications. Extensive background retinopathy may be seen at the time of diagnosis, especially in subjects with NIDDM. On the other hand, series of diabetic patients studied after 40 years or more include a high proportion (as much as one third) who are free of all detectable complications (52). These incongruities have raised the suspicion that constitutional factors are involved in the appearance and non-appearance of diabetic complications.

Some support for this comes from identical twin studies. In a series of 85 pairs, 48 IDDM and 37 NIDDM, the co-twins resembled each other in respect of the presence and severity of retinopathy, especially in the NIDDM pairs (53). Classifying retinopathy as nil, background or severe co-twins in 35 of the 37 NIDDM pairs, all of whom had been diabetic for at least 9 years, were in the same category. Among the IDDM pairs, however, the similarity was much less marked; of 10 pairs in which the co-twins had been diabetic for the same time, 5 showed striking differences between co-twins. It seems from this study, therefore, that a genetic element in the pathogenesis of diabetic microvascular disease may be strong in NIDDM but less so in IDDM. Nevertheless, whatever the genetic background, the presence of diabetes seems to be necessary before microvascular disease appears; none of the unaffected co-twins showed any retinopathy. When studies were performed of the basement membrane thickness of muscle capillaries, thickening was found in some of the diabetic twins but in none of the unaffected co-twins. (54, 55).

Microvascular complications are rare in Mason-type diabetes and, when present, nearly always mild (56). This might be due to the mildness of the diabetes itself, but that does not seem to protect against complications in other forms of NIDDM and the relative freedom from complications may be part of the inherited picture.

In a few families with apparently dominant inheritance of early-onset, non-insulin requiring diabetes severe complications are found. It is probable, therefore, that Mason-type diabetes is itself a mixed syndrome consisting of a common complication-free type and a less common complication-prone variant. Whether these are separate entities or merely variants of one pattern is uncertain.

There have been suggestions that another diabetic complication — neuropathy — may be linked to an inherited factor — acetylator status — fast acetylators being less prone to develop peripheral neuropathy. Even in the early studies the association was weak (57) and in a later, small, but well controlled study no difference was found in acetylator status between diabetics with and without neuropathy (58). There has been much interest and controversy concerning a possible relationship between HLA type and the long-term complications of diabetes. Several reports have been published which have geven conflicting results and they are reviewed by Barbosa and Saner (59). There are as many reports failing to find an association as there are which do and it seems reasonable, therefore, to conclude that there is little, if any, association between HLA-DR3 and DR4 molecules and the appearance or severity of retinopathy, nephropathy or neuropathy (60).

However, a new and promising approach has emerged from studies of Class III molecules, the complement loci. Subjects with IDDM show a deficiency of the fourth component of complement (C4), which is genetically determined as it is found in non-diabetic co-twins of insulin-dependent diabetic patients. There are two C4 genes (C4A and C4B) which are highly polymorphic with a large number of allotypes at each locus, including null genes which lead to a reduced production of complement. These null genes are rare in the general population (less than 1%) but relatively common (13-17%) in IDDM and, in particular, the C4B3 allotype is commoner in those patients with retinopathy (61, 62). Low C4 plasma concentration may be found in some (although not in all) cases of microangiopathy (63). If this observation is substantiated, it suggests that defective complement function — the clearing of immune complexes — might be relevant to the development of microangiopathy; on the other hand, the association might be secondary to that with another gene(s) which might act singly or in combination.

Other immunogenetic mechanisms may be involved in microangiopathy which are not linked to the HLA loci, in particular genes in the immunoglobulin heavy-chain constant region of Chromosome 14. There are several subtypes of these Gm markers and one (Gm zafnbg) has been found more frequently than expected in cases of retinopathy, conferring a relative risk of retinopathy of about 5 (64). The complement and immunoglobulin phenotypes seem to be independent in conferring risk of retinopathy; the relative risk of C4B3 *and* Gm zafnbg is 14. These results need confirmation and amplification; this should be possible within a short time as new populations are studied and new techniques developed

The importance of these reports is not only in identifying risk factors for retinopathy but in the evidence they provide that immunogenetic factors are involved in its aetiology (60).

We have perhaps been too preoccupied in the past with the importance of control of blood glucose in relation to diabetic complications, an understandable but ultimately inconclusive approach. Now we may have the chance of a different approach to this intractable problem.

References

1. Barnett AH, Eff C, Leslie RDG, Pyke DA (1981): Diabetes in identical twins: a study of 200 pairs. *Diabetologia, 20*, 87.
2. Johnston C, Pyke DA, Cudworth AG, Wolf E (1983): HLA-DR typing in identical twins with insulin-dependent diabetes: a difference between concordant and discordant pairs. *Br. Med. J., 286*, 253.
3 Platz P, Jakobsen BK, Morling N et al (1981): HLA-D and -DR antigens in genetic analysis of insulin dependent diabetes mellitus. *Diabetologia, 21*, 108.
4. Wolf E, Spencer KM, Cudworth AG (1983): The genetic susceptibility to Type 1 (insulin-dependent) diabetes, analysis of the HLA-DR association. *Diabetologia, 24*, 224.

5. Deschamps I, Goderel I, Lestradet H et al (1984): Segregation of HLA-DR2 among affected and non-affected offspring of 66 families with Type I (insulin-dependent) diabetes. *Diabetologia, 27, Suppl. 1*, 80.
6. Rotter JI, Anderson CE, Rubin R et al (1983): HLA genotype study of insulin-dependent diabetes: the excess of DR3/DR4 heterozygotes allows rejection of the recessive hypothesis. *Diabetes, 32*, 169.
7. Cudworth AG (1983): Type I diabetes mellitus. *Diabetologia, 24*, 281.
8. Irvine WJ (1977): Classification of idiopathic diabetes. *Lancet, 1*, 638.
9. Eberhardt MS, Wagener DK, Orchard TJ et al (1985): HLA heterogeneity of insulin-dependent diabetes mellitus at diagnosis: the Pittsburg IDDM study. *Diabetes, 34*, 1247.
10. Knip M, Ilonen J, Mustonen A, Akerbloom HK (1986): Evidence of an accelerated B-cell destruction in HLA DW3/DW4 heterozygous children with Type I (insulin-dependent) diabetes. *Diabetologia, 29*, 347.
11. Bottazzo G, Cudworth AG, Moul D et al (1978): Evidence for a primary autoimmune type of diabetes mellitus. *Br. Med. J., 2*, 1253.
12. Spencer KM, Tarn A, Dean BM et al (1984): Fluctuating islet cell autoimmunity in unaffected relatives of patients with insulin dependent diabetes. *Lancet, 1*, 764.
13. Pittman WB, Acton RT, Berger BD et al (1982): HLA-A, -B, and -DR associations in type I diabetes mellitus with onset after age forty. *Diabetes, 31*, 122.
14. Wolf E, Cudworth AG, Markwick JR et al (1982): The Bf system in diabetes-gene interaction or linkage disequilibrium. *Diabetologia, 22*, 85.
15. McCluskey J, McCann WJ, Kay PH et al (1983): HLA and complement allotypes in type I (insulin-dependent) diabetes. *Diabetologia, 24*, 162.
16. Raum D, Awdeh Z, Yams EJ et al (1984): Extended major histocompatibility complex haplotypes in Type I diabetes mellitus. *Clin. Invest., 74*, 449.
17. Rich SS, Weitkamp LR, Barbosa J (1984): Genetic heterogeneity of insulin-dependent (type I) diabetes mellitus: evidence from a study of extended haplotypes. *Am. J. Hum. Genet., 36*, 1015.
18. Owerbach D, Lernmark A, Platz P et al (1983): HLA-D region B chain DNA endonuclease fragments differ between HLA-DR identical healthy and insulin-dependent diabetic individuals. *Nature (London), 303*, 815.
19. Hitman GA, Sachs J, Cassell P et al (1986): A DR related DX gene polymorphism strongly associates with insulin-dependent diabetes mellitus. *Immunogenetics, 23*, 47.
20. Cohen-Hughnenauer O, Robbins E, Massart C et al (1985): A systematic study of the HLA Class II B DNA restriction fragments in insulin dependent diabetes mellitus. *Proc. Natl. Acad. Sci. USA, 83*, 3335.
21. Festenstein H, Awad J, Hitman GA et al (1986): New HLA-DQ associations with rheumatoid arthritis and insulin dependent diabetes mellitus. *Nature (London), 322*, 64.
22. Marcadet A, Massart C, Semana G et al (1985): Association of Class II HLA-DQ (beta) chain DNA restriction fragments with multiple sclerosis. *Immunogenetics, 22*, 93.
23. Cohen N, Brantbar C, Font M-P et al (1985): HLA-DR2 associated DW subtypes correlate with RFLP clusters: most DR2 IDDM patients belong to one of these clusters. *Immunogenetics, 23*, 84.
24. Bell GI, Horita S, Karam JH (1984): A polymorphic locus near the human insulin gene in association with insulin-dependent diabetes mellitus. *Diabetes, 33*, 176.
25. Hitman GA, Tam AC, Winter RM et al (1985): Type I (insulin-dependent) diabetes and a highly variable locus close to the insulin gene on chromosome 11. *Diabetologia, 28*, 218.
26. Hodge SE, Anderson CE, Weiswanger K et al (1981): A second genetic locus for insulin-dependent diabetes mellitus (IDDM): evidence for close linkage between IDDM and Kidd blood group. *Lancet, 2*, 893.

27. Hodge SE, Anderson CE, Weiswanger K et al (1983): Association studies between type I (insulin-dependent) diabetes and 27 genetic markers: lack of association between type 1 diabetes and Kidd blood group. *Diabetologia, 25,* 343.
28. Dunsworth TS, Rich SS, Swenson J, Barbosa J (1982): No evidence for linkage between diabetes and the Kidd marker. *Diabetes, 31,* 991.
29. Adams DD, Adams YJ, Knight TG et al (1984): A solution to the genetic and environmental puzzles of insulin-dependent diabetes mellitus. *Lancet, 1,* 420.
30. Shenfield GM, McCann VJ, Tjokresetio R et al (1982): Acetylator status and diabetic neuropathy. *Diabetologia, 22,* 441.
31. Bodansky HJ, Wolf E, Cudworth AG et al (1982): Genetic and immunologic factors in microvascular disease in type I insulin-dependent diabetes. *Diabetes, 31,* 70.
32. Irvine WJ, Toft AD, Holton DE et al (1977): Familial studies of type I and type II idiopathic diabetes mellitus. *Lancet, 2,* 325.
33. Barnett AH, Spiliopoulos AJ, Pyke DA et al (1981) Metabolic studies in unaffected co-twins of non-insulin dependent diabetics. *Br. Med. J., 1,* 1656.
34. Stunkard AJ, Sorensen TIA, Harris C et al (1986): An adoption study of human obesity. *N. Engl. J. Med., 314,* 193.
35. Tattersall RB (1974): Mild familial diabetes with dominant inheritance. *Q. J. Med., 43,* 339.
36. Nelson PG, Pyke DA (1976): Genetic diabetes not linked to the HLA locus. *Br. Med. J., 1,* 196.
37. Bell JI, Wainscoat JS, Old JM et al (1983): Maturity onset diabetes of the young is not linked to the insulin gene. *Br. Med. J., 1,* 590.
38. Robbins DC, Shoelson SE, Rubenstein AH, Tager HS (1984): Familial hyperproinsulinaemia: two cohorts secreting indistinguishable Type II intermediates of proinsulin conversion. *J. Clin. Invest., 73,* 714.
39. Shoelson S, Haneda M, Blix P et al (1983): Three mutant insulins in man. *Nature (London), 302,* 540.
40. Haneda M, Polansky KS, Berganstal RM et al (1984): Familial hyperinsulinaemia due to a structurally abnormal insulin: definition of an emerging new clinical syndrome. *N. Engl. J. Med., 310,* 1288.
41. Scarlett JA, Kolterman OG, Moore P et al (1982): Insulin resistance and diabetes due to a genetic defect in insulin receptors. *J. Clin. Endocrinol. Metab., 55,* 123.
42. Rotwein P, Chergwin J, Province M et al (1983): Polymorphism in the 5'-flanking region of the human insulin gene: a genetic marker for non-insulin dependent diabetes. *N. Engl. J. Med., 308,* 65.
43. Owerbach D, Nerup J (1982): Restriction fragment length polymorphism of the insulin gene in diabetes mellitus. *Diabetes, 31,* 275.
44. Owerbach D, Billesbolle P, Schroll M et al (1982): Possible association between DNA sequences flanking the insulin gene and atherosclerosis. *Lancet, 2,* 1291.
45. Dobs AS, Phillips JA, Mallonee RL et al (1986): Pedigree analysis of the 5' flanking region of the insulin gene in familial diabetes mellitus. *Metabolism, 35,* 13.
46. Andreone T, Fajans S, Rotwein P et al (1985): Insulin gene analysis in a family with maturity-onset diabetes of the young. *Diabetes, 34,* 108.
47. Owerbach D, Thomsen B, Johansen K et al (1983): DNA insertion sequences near the insulin gene are not associated with maturity-onset diabetes of young people. *Diabetologia, 25,* 18.
48. Leslie RDG, Pyke DA (1978): Chlorpropamide alcohol flushing: a dominantly inherited trait associated with diabetes. *Br. Med. J., 2,* 1519.
49. Groop L, Eriksson CJP, Huupponen R et al (1984): Roles of chlorpropamide, alcohol and acetaldehyde in determining the chlorpropamide alcohol flush. *Diabetologia, 26,* 34.

50. Groop L, Kiskimies S, Tolppanen EM (1984): Characterisation of patients with chlorpropamide alcohol flush. *Acta Med. Scand., 215,* 141.
51. Segal P, Brazu-Albu J, Almog S et al (1985): Prevalence of chlorpropamide alcohol flush in Jewish Israeli diabetics. *Isr. J. Med. Sci., 21,* 98.
52. Oakley WG, Pyke DA, Tattersall RB, Watkins PJ (1974): Long-term diabetes: a clinical study of 92 patients after 40 years. *Q. J. Med., 43,* 145.
53. Leslie RDG, Pyke DA (1982): Diabetic retinopathy in identical twins. *Diabetes, 31,* 19.
54. Ganda OM, Williamson JR, Soeldner JS et al (1983): Muscle capillary basement membrane width and its relationship to diabetes mellitus in monozygotic twins. *Diabetes, 32,* 549.
55. Barnett AH, Spiliopoulos AJ, Pyke DA et al (1983): Muscle capillary basement membrane in identical twins dicordant for insulin-dependent diabetes. *Diabetes, 32,* 557.
56. Fajans SS, Cloutier MC, Crowther RL (1978): Clinical and aetiological heterogeneity of idiopathic diabetes mellitus. *Diabetes, 27,* 1112.
57. Bodansky HJ, Drury PL, Cudworth AG et al (1981): Acetylator phenotypes and type I (insulin-dependent) diabetics with microvascular disease. *Diabetes, 30,* 907.
58. Boulton AJM, Worth RC, Drury J (1984): Genetic and metabolic studies in diabetic neuropathy. *Diabetologia, 26,* 15.
59. Barbosa J, Saner B (1984): Do genetic factors play a role in the pathogenesis of diabetic microangiopathy? *Diabetologia, 27,* 487.
60. Barnett AH, Pyke DA (1986): The genetics of diabetic complications. *Clin. Endocrinol., 15,* 715.
61. McCann VJ, McCluskey J, Kay PH (1983): HLA and complement genetic markers in diabetic retinopathy. *Diabetologia, 24,* 221.
62. Mijovic C, Fletcher J, Bradwell AR (1985): Relation of gene expression (allotypes) of the fourth component of complement to insulin dependent diabetes and its microangiopathic complications. *Br. Med. J., 291,* 9.
63. Fletcher J, Mijovic C, Bradwell AR et al (1985): HLA and C4 types in diabetic microangiopathy. *Diabetic Med., 2,* 508.
64. Mijovic C, Fletcher J, Bradwell et al (1986): Phenotypes of the heavy chains of immunoglobulins in patients with diabetic microangiopathy: evidence for an immunogenetic predisposition. *Br. Med. J., 292,* 433.

The Diabetes Annual/3
K.G.M.M. Alberti and L.P. Krall, editors
© 1987 Elsevier Science Publishers, B.V.

4   Diet and diabetes: some agreement, but controversies continue

J.I. MANN

Introduction

At least 7 national diabetes associations have revised and reissued their dietary recommendations during the past 8 years, in all cases with added emphasis on the importance of diet in the management of diabetes. Several aspects are common to these recommendations: (a) the importance of energy balance and achieving and maintaining ideal body weight; (b) reduction in intake of saturated fatty acids; (c) increase in intake of dietary fibre (especially gel-forming fibre) and unprocessed starchy foods; (d) the need for compatibility between meals and injected insulin in those taking insulin; and (e) the need for dietitians or other trained educators to teach the practical aspects of these dietary principles. The numerous studies which have led to these recommendations have been summarized in the publications describing these and other recent reviews including *The Diabetes Annual/2* (1-9) and they will therefore not be discussed again in detail here. This Chapter will consider some of the areas in which controversy continues.

Attitudes of doctors and patients towards the dietary management of diabetes

In 1975, Truswell and colleagues reported that more than 150 printed diet sheets were in use in diabetic clinics in Britain and dietary advice for people with diabetes was found to vary widely between individual consultants (10). Few similar studies have been undertaken and the findings of the recent survey of the management of diet in 26 diabetes centres in Europe are of particular interest since they reflect the attitudes of practising clinicians in centres of excellence, mostly in countries where recommendations have recently been made (11). There was universal agreement concerning 3 dietary principles: a high intake of dietary fibre for all diabetics, restriction and calculation of energy intake for the overweight and the importance of meal-timing for insulin-dependent diabetics. There was also strong support for the suggestion that carbohydrate should provide more than 50% of total daily energy in the diet of insulin-dependent diabetic patients, for restriction of alcohol in the obese, and for a general restriction of sucrose and food containing concentrated sugars. On several other issues opinions vary widely. There are no consistent recommendations concerning quantity and type of fat, the amount of protein, which carbohydrate exchange units should be used and whether sodium restriction should be recommended.

The disagreements and uncertainties of doctors are to some extent reflected in the behaviour of patients. In one study based on all diabetic patients in a geographically defined area of Oxford, England, compliance with dietary advice was regarded as the greatest single difficulty in the management of their diabetes (12). Nearly 40% reported moderate or great difficulty with the diet. On the other hand, newly diagnosed diabetic patients who were restudied 1 year after enthusiastic education concerning the new dietary recommendations were found to have maintained their substantial increase in dietary fibre at around 35 grams per day, compared with a level of around 20 grams per day amongst non-diabetic patients and those with diabetes who had not received detailed dietary advice (13). These patients were also given clear-cut advice concerning fat restriction, and fat intake as a percentage of total energy intake was reduced from 42 to 33%. Thus, it seems that when unequivocal and detailed dietary instructions are given, there is at least a reasonable likelihood that patients will respond. It therefore seems relevant to examine some of the areas of uncertainty to determine whether sufficient grounds exist for making firm recommendations.

Quantity and type of fat in the diabetic diet

The recommendation that saturated fatty acids (SFA) in the diabetic diet should be decreased is largely based on epidemiological evidence. In populations with low intakes of SFA, coronary heart disease (CHD) is uncommon in diabetic and non-diabetic people and there is no evidence of an untoward effect of low-fat diets. Decrease in intake of SFA can lower total and low-density lipoprotein (LDL) cholesterol and there is strong evidence that the abnormalities of lipoprotein metabolism play a role in the aetiology of CHD in diabetic and non-diabetic persons. Cholesterol-lowering in non-diabetic subjects is associated with a marked reduction in morbidity and mortality from CHD (14). No classical clinical trial has been conducted as to CHD in people with diabetes making this dietary change. However, the risk of CHD amongst diabetic patients in Western countries is so high and the circumstantial evidence so strong that this advice has been included in all sets of recommendations (see also Chapter 18).

Present debate centres around whether certain essential fatty acids and other long-chain polyunsaturated fatty acids (PUFA) may confer particular benefit on people with diabetes with regard to platelet function, lipid-lowering, and prevention of complications. There is also debate as to whether mono-unsaturated fatty acids (MUFA) may be equivalent to PUFA in terms of cholesterol-lowering effect.

The abnormalities of platelet function in diabetes have been extensively studied and reviewed (15-17). Increased platelet aggregation (especially second-phase aggregation), more rapid platelet turnover and decreased platelet survival have been repeatedly demonstrated. The metabolism of arachidonic acid in the platelet to thromboxane A_2 (TxA_2) and prostaglandin E_2 (PGE_2) is increased in patients with diabetes compared with control subjects. Those patients with vascular disease appear to have the greatest rates of synthesis. Some studies suggest an association between some of these abnormalities and degree of hyperglycaemia and reversal associated with an improvement in diabetic control, but these have not been universal findings. Several attempts have been made to examine the fatty acid composition of the platelets (which is at least to some extent influenced by diet) and to relate the findings to abnormalities of platelet function. The findings have not been consistent. Thus, some groups have found low levels of arachidonate in platelet phospholipid and others have found the proportion to be increased. The following have variously been reported to be inversely associated with some measure of increased platelet aggregability in diabetics: linolenate and eicosapentaenoate in platelet phospholipid; a high ratio between the fatty acids (20:3/20:4) in cholesteryl esters; and the ratio of PUFA to SFA (P/S) in triglycerides (18).

Several groups have given diabetic patients diets containing appreciable quantities of these unsaturated fatty acids. Houtsmuller and colleagues have shown that in addition to the cholesterol-lowering properties, a diet high in linoleic acid was able to reduce the rate of development of diabetic retinopathy in 102 patients followed for 6 years when compared with a diet high in saturated fat. A strong inverse association was found between progression of retinopathy and serum cholesteryl linoleate. Fewer patients in the experimental group showed features of myocardial ischaemia (19). Some support for these findings comes from a prospective study in Oxford in which 149 diabetic patients were ophthalmologically assessed 7 and 8 years after randomization to a low-carbohydrate (LC) or modified-fat (MF) diet which was rich in linoleic acid. A much lower intake of linoleic acid was achieved than in the Dutch study, but cholesterol levels were lower on MF than on LC. Poorly controlled diabetic patients with low levels of linoleic acid in cholesteryl ester had a significantly greater frequency of retinopathy than well-controlled patients or patients with similarly unsatisfactory control but higher levels of linoleic acid (20). The effects were particularly striking for exudative retinopathy. MF also induced changes in platelet-membrane fatty acids which might be expected to influence platelet function favourably (21).

Two studies have examined the effects of giving γ-linolenate. Chaintreuil and colleagues (22) gave 2 grams per day (Group 1) or 500 mg per day (Group 2) to 17 patients for 6 weeks. In Group 1 serum triglyceride, cholesterol and plasma β-thromboglobulin levels fell while the sum of the percentages of 18:3w6 and its chain elongated (20:3w6) and desaturated (20:4w6) metabolites increased in serum triglycerides, cholesteryl esters and phospholipids. No changes were observed in Group 2. Unfortunately platelet fatty acid composition was not studied (22).

In the second study, Mikhailides and colleagues compared the effects of substantial quantities of dihomogammalinolenate (DHLA) on platelet aggregation, prostaglandin release, red cell membrane fatty acids and serum lipids in healthy subjects and those with insulin-dependent diabetes mellitus (IDDM). In healthy subjects DHLA produced a significant inhibition of ADP-induced platelet aggregation and an increase in platelet PGE release. Those with IDDM did not show these changes. There were no differences, however, in platelet thromboxane A_2 or PGE_2 release between healthy subjects and those with IDDM before and after DHLA. Following DHLA, the arachidonate content of red cell membranes increased in healthy subjects but not in those with diabetes. DHLA produced a fall in serum non-esterified fatty acids in both groups without altering cholesterol or triglyceride concentrations. These data suggest that platelets in those with IDDM may have a specific defect of PGE_1 synthesis quite distinct from other desaturase deficiencies known to be associated with diabetes. This defect may contribute to the platelet hyperaggregability of diabetes and prevent DHLA from exerting a favourable effect on platelet function in diabetes. DHLA does however appear to have a potent antilipolytic effect in diabetic and non-diabetic subjects alike (23).

In non-diabetic people large supplements of the fatty acid eicosapentaenoate (C20:5), which is also usually present in the diet in only very small quantities, can lower triglycerides, cholesterol and blood pressure, prolong and may also reduce bleeding time. Very limited information is available concerning the effects of this fatty acid, found particularly in oily fish, in people with diabetes. Schinke and colleagues have examined the effect of an eicosapentaenoate-rich diet (provided as codliver oil) in patients with IDDM. There were increases in the eicosapentaenoic acid fractions in the serum triglyceride, cholesterol ester and phospholipid and inhibition of the 'platelet hyperaggregation'. However, the experimental period was very short (2 weeks) and a number of methodological issues preclude firm conclusions (24).

Another development which needs to be pursued in diabetic patients is the finding that in healthy subjects MUFA (previously regarded as neutral with regard to blood cholesterol) have a similiar effect on blood cholesterol to that of PUFA (25). Diets relatively high in MUFA have been taken for centuries by diabetic and non-diabetic individuals living in Mediterranean countries and are most unlikely to have any untoward effects. Because of various enzyme deficiencies results of studies concerning fatty acid feeding to non-diabetic people cannot be extrapolated to diabetics. Comparisons of MUFA and PUFA with SFA are urgently required in diabetic populations since being able to show beneficial effects in terms of lipid metabolism and platelet function would enable the recommendation of diets which might greatly enhance the variety and palatability of diabetic diets. Further studies of DHLA and C20:5 would also be of considerable interest since the present studies cannot be regarded as anything more than pilot investigations. However, if those fatty acids are shown to have beneficial effects, they would probably need to be given as dietary supplements since the quantities needed to produce detectable effects are too great to be readily incorporated into an ordinary diet.

It is obviously this uncertainty about the optimal nature of dietary fat which has resulted in so many doctors failing to give clear advice on any aspect of fat intake. Restriction of SFA is included in all dietary recommendations and is likely to be one of the most important therapeutic measures in reducing cardiovascular risk. While waiting for more data concerning the effects of the different fatty acids, the importance of reducing SFA to no more than 10% of total energy (and total fat to below 30% total energy) should be emphasized. This advice, perhaps applied even more stringently, is suitable also (with recommendations about optimal protein and carbohydrate which will be discussed later) for patients with the various forms of hyperlipidaemia associated with diabetes. The importance of specific dietary cholesterol restriction may have been overstated. Restriction of SFA is associated with a substantial reduction in dietary cholesterol. In non-diabetic people, including those with familial hyperlipidaemia, on diets low in SFA (when daily cholesterol intake is likely to be around 300 mg) further restriction appears to make no appreciable difference to total cholesterol or cholesterol in the various lipoprotein fractions (26). Obviously this needs further testing in diabetic patients, but removal of this further restriction would be of considerable practical help in planning a diabetic diet.

Simple sugars and diabetes

Avoiding simple sugars has been one of the few, almost universally accepted principles of treatment in diabetes. In addition, lay people, as well as some doctors throughout the world, regard a high intake of sucrose and other refined carbohydrates as being a major aetiological factor in diabetes. There is in fact no evidence that any nutrition-related factor apart from obesity is involved in the aetiology of non-insulin-dependent diabetes (NIDDM) (for review, see Ref. 27) and the acute metabolic effects of simple sugars as compared with complex carbohydrates were reviewed in *The Diabetes Annual/2*. The results of those acute experiments (where the carbohydrates were fed either as single foods or part of meals) appear to be unequivocal. Many simple sugars do not elicit a greater glycaemic response than a number of complex carbohydrates and fructose and sucrose may be associated with a smaller glycaemic response than several polysaccharides. Several authors have suggested that fructose may be a particularly useful sweetener for diabetic patients. There are two major reservations in interpreting the results of these acute studies. Firstly, the complex carbohydrate foods used for the comparisons have not been fibre-rich carbohydrates. A different result might emerge when using such foods. Secondly, while meal studies are preferable to single-food experiments, the results cannot be extrapolated to the longer-term situation when different effects may emerge as a result of use of simple sugars.

The first formal medium-term study was published by Brunzell and colleagues in 1971 (28). They compared 45% and 85% carbohydrate formula diets (each fed for 10 days) in mildly diabetic patients. Dextrose and maltose provided the carbohydrate. Glucose and insulin responses to a glucose load were lower on the high-carbohydrate formula than on the basal diet. Coulston and colleagues have compared high-carbohydrate and control diets providing 60% and 40% of energy respectively from carbohydrates, each diet being fed for 10 days (29). The diets had a high ratio of polyunsaturated to saturated fatty acids but were low in dietary fibre and contained 75 and 50 grams sucrose daily. Fasting triglycerides were higher and HDL cholesterol lower on the 60% carbohydrate diet. Triglyceride and insulin responses to meal tolerance tests were also higher on the 60% carbohydrate diet. These results in patients with NIDDM supported earlier results in healthy volunteers (30) and the authors consider that they provide evidence against the use of high-carbohydrate diets.

The first medium-term study specifically examining the question of acceptability of sucrose in the diabetic diet was published by Jellish et al (31). They studied diet-only treated hypertriglyceridaemic NIDDM patients on a control diet (50% energy from carbohydrate, 120 g sucrose) and after randomization to isocaloric high (220 g), intermediate (120 g) or low (3 g or less) sucrose diets for 4 weeks. The high-sucrose diet produced a significant increase in fasting triglyceride levels, but there were no differences in fasting or postprandial glucose or lipid levels on the intermediate- or low-sucrose diets. The authors conclude that isocaloric sucrose and carbohydrate restriction below usual daily levels (120 g/d) offers no consistent benefit in glycaemic or lipid control in this particular group of diabetic patients. Interpretation of the data is complicated by the fact that some weight changes occurred. The diets were all low in dietary fibre.

An important study has recently been published by Chantelau et al (32). Patients with IDDM treated by continuous subcutaneous insulin infusion were studied while using sodium cyclamate as a sweetener or while using an average of 25 grams of sucrose daily. Blood glucose levels and insulin requirements were identical during the 4-week study periods. The authors draw attention to the limitations of their data: the results apply only to very well-controlled patients with IDDM and cannot be extrapolated to people with diabetes in general. Secondly, the quantity of sucrose used is small. The only study which has examined medium-term sucrose intake in an unselected group of diabetic patients is that of Peterson and colleagues. They compared a high-carbohydrate/high-fibre/low-fat diet with no added sucrose (as recommended by the British Diabetic Association) with a diet in which approximately 45 grams of sucrose replaced an isocaloric amount of complex carbohydrate (mainly bread and potato) (33). Thus, the mean intake of total simple sugars (both refined and naturally occurring) increased from 49 grams daily on the control diet to 92 grams on the experimental diet. The study was based on a randomised cross-over design, each dietary period being continued for 6 weeks. As shown in Table 1, there was no deterioration in diabetic control (as measured by blood glucose profiles and HbA_{1c}) or blood lipid levels (either fasting or when measured throughout the day). This study included patients with NIDDM and IDDM with varying levels of glycaemic control.

TABLE 1. *Indices of glycaemic control from diurnal profiles for 12 Type I (insulin-dependent) diabetic patients**

Measure	Control diet	Sucrose diet
Plasma glucose (mmol/l)		
Fasting	10.5 (1.8)	10.3 (1.5)
Preprandial*	10.5 (1.3)	10.0 (1.3)
Incremental mean***	3.3 (0.7)	3.7 (0.8)
Mean daily	11.4 (1.0)	11.4 (1.2)
HbA_1 (%)	9.9 (0.3)	10.3 (0.6)

*Similar results were observed for Type II patients.
**Mean of 3 meals and 3 snacks.
***Mean of increments for 2 h after breakfast and lunch.
Values are expressed as mean ± SEM. Reprinted from Peterson et al (60) by courtesy of the Editors of *Diabetologia*.

In view of the widespread use of fructose as a sweetener by diabetic patients, it is surprising that there are not more long-term studies of fructose feeding. The two major studies were carried out more than 15 years ago. Pelkonen and colleagues studied the effects of replacing 75 grams of dietary starch by fructose in IDDM patients (34). Fructose feeding did not alter diurnal blood glucose or urinary output of glucose, but a tendency to an increase of plasma triglycerides and free fatty acids (FFA) was noted during the fructose period. In this study the experimental periods were only of 10 days duration. Akerblom and colleagues studied diabetic children (35). For 4 weeks they alternated between 1-week periods of diets which include fructose 1.5 g/kg/d and control weeks of their usual isocaloric sugar-free diets. Twent-four hour urinary glucose excretion was similar during the two diets. No changes in triglycerides were observed. Crapo et al (36) studied the effects of fructose over a 2-week period in healthy volunteers. During the experimental period fructose replaced virtually all the added sucrose taken during the control period so that total quantities eaten ranged between 60 and 100 grams per day. No adverse effects of the fructose-containing diet were found on triglycerides or on pyruvate, lactate or urate metabolism. Postprandial glucose and insulin levels were lower after fructose-containing mixed meals than meals containing sucrose; glucose tolerance tests on fructose and control diets were identical.

Two of the 3 medium-term studies of sucrose apply to a very limited group of diabetic patients. It would therefore be reassuring to see further studies along the lines of those conducted by Peterson et al (33), including diabetic patients with varying degrees of glycaemic control and comparing diets compatible with present dietary recommendations fed for relatively long periods of time. For the present, it seems that the following considerations should be borne in mind before making recommendations concerning sucrose. Firstly, the background diet may be particularly important. The findings of Peterson apply only to those eating a high-carbohydrate/high-fibre/low-fat diet and may not be applicable to those diabetic patients still following the old low-carbohydrate dietary advice. Secondly, moderate amounts of sucrose can only be taken as a replacement for some complex carbohydrate and not as additional carbohydrate. All the studies have compared sucrose with complex carbohydrate which has a relatively high glycaemic index like bread or potato. A different result might be observed were sucrose to be compared with low-glycaemic-index foods (i.e. those high in gel-forming fibre). However, this does not limit the practical applications of Peterson's findings since few diabetic patients are ever likely to follow a diet which consists entirely of low-glycaemic-index carbohydrates nor is there any evidence that this is necessary (9). Many diabetic patients, especially those with NIDDM, are overweight and for them restriction of all energy-dense foods (fat and sucrose) should be recommended.

It seems likely that for many diabetic patients permitting a modest amount of sucrose may enhance palatability and this may aid long-term compliance to a high-fibre/low-fat diet. Further long-term studies of sucrose and fructose feeding are urgently needed. For the present it would seem reasonable to permit the usc of sucrose in moderate quantities (up to 50 g/d) provided that an isocaloric quantity of carbohydrate is removed from the calculated daily energy requirement. The replacement carbohydrate should be taken from the high-glycaemic-index carbohydrate already in the diet and low-glycaemic-index foods should not be reduced. There is no evidence to suggest that in the context of a balanced diet the effects of refined sugar are different from sugars derived from 'natural' sources. Permitting up to 50 grams of added sucrose to the diet might mean an increase from 50 to 100 grams daily of total simple sugars (both refined and naturally occurring) for a diabetic having an energy intake of 2000 kcal/d. Fructose is currently permitted in amounts not exceeding 50 g/d. If sucrose is included, this allowance should probably be reduced. There is no evidence that simple sugars in these quantities and within the restrictions defined will produce deterioration of glycaemic control or blood lipids.

Dietary protein and the diabetic kidney *(see also Chapter 17)*

The review on diet and diabetes in *The Diabetes Annual/2* concludes that apart from patients with chronic renal failure, in whom protein intake should be judiciously restricted, there is no justification for restriction or modification of protein intake. Indeed, the importance of children having sufficient amounts of protein to assure normal growth and development is stressed and adults with diabetes are recommended to have 10-20% of their energy as protein. I would not wish to imply that there is now sufficient evidence to make firm recommendations concerning protein intake. However, a number of observations and more recent studies suggest that this may prove to be a particularly interesting and important area.

Diabetes may result in progressive glomerulosclerosis and renal failure in 40% of patients with IDDM (37). Albumin excretion rate (AER) and glomerular filtration rate (GFR) may be elevated before any clinically apparent signs of renal disease (38, 39) and both microalbuminuria and hyperfiltration are thought to be predictive of later clinically overt diabetic nephropathy (40, 41). The treatment of established diabetic nephropathy is disappointing. Radical improvement of blood glucose control using continuous subcutaneous insulin infusion (42), aggressive antihypertensive treatment (43) and reduction of total dietary protein (44) have not shown arrest or reversal of progression of renal failure, though early treatment of blood pressure can decrease albuminuria and slow the rate of GFR decline, delaying but not preventing the eventual onset of end-stage renal failure. A 20-30 gram protein diet has failed to show a change in disease progression in patients with end-stage renal failure, but symptoms are improved (44). In view of this therapeutic impotence in established diabetic nephropathy, attention has focussed on the treatment of early kidney abnormalities of diabetes in the hope that this might prevent or delay the later onset of clinical nephropathy. Preliminary data suggest that early antihypertensive treatment may reduce elevated AER and strict glycaemic control can reduce both elevated AER and GFR (45, 46), though kidney size is not changed by a year of improved glycaemia, and moderate relaxation of glycaemic control leads to an immediate return of GFR to elevated levels (46).

Few data are available concerning protein modification in the earliest stages of diabetic renal failure. Bognetti and colleagues have examined the effect of a 55% reduction in dietary protein (to approx. 45 g/d) on GFR in diabetic patients with hyperfiltration (47). After 3 weeks mean GFR fell from 148 ± 13 to 133 ± 16 ml/min/1.73 m^2 without any change in glucose or blood pressure. They also examined the response to eating 70-100 grams of grilled steak in both controls and diabetics with normal or increased glomerular filtration when they were moderately hyperglycaemic. Those with normal filtration and controls showed a 10-15% rise in GFR whereas those with hyperfiltration showed no change. Normoglycaemia restored a normal response in some of those with hyperfiltration, but only after 3 weeks of a low-protein diet did all these patients respond normally to protein with a GFR rise. AER increased 3-4-fold after a protein load in all subjects. In the healthy controls this rise remained within the normal range of urinary albumin excretion, but in the diabetic patients with microalbuminuria it reached levels of 'clinical' albuminuria. These findings are of interest in view of observations by the same group in non-diabetic vegetarians, vegans and meat eaters (48). AER, GFR and diastolic blood pressure were appreciably lower in vegans than meat eaters, and vegetarians (who eat dairy products but no meat) showed intermediate results. Total protein intake of vegans is only about 30% lower than meat eaters (approx. 59 g/d), so it would seem that type as well as quantity of dietary protein can have a profound effect on several variables (blood pressure, AER, GFR) known to influence risk of diabetic nephropathy. Further studies of dietary intervention involving protein type and quality in those with microalbuminuria and hyperfiltration would seem to be of particular interest in view of these findings.

Complex carbohydrates and dietary fibre

Does a high-carbohydrate/high-fibre diet confer long-term benefit?

The case for the benefits of a high-carbohydrate/ high-fibre diet is presented in some detail in *The Diabetes Annual/2*. On the basis of a substantial number of medium-term studies (4-16 weeks) as well as epidemiological data, there would seem to be little doubt that such a diet can produce an appreciable improvement in glycaemic control as well as reduction in LDL cholesterol as compared with a low-carbohydrate diet. Arky has drawn attention to the problem of extrapolating long-term effects from these relatively short-term studies. Two other issues are worth considering in this regard.

First, since the publication of the last review, McCulloch and colleagues have published the only controlled long-term study of a high-fibre/low-fat diet in practice (49). Forty patients with IDDM were randomised into 3 groups after a 3-month run-in period, during which their glycaemic control was optimized without specific reference to diet. After this, 14 patients acted as controls, receiving standard instructions from a dietitian. The remaining 26 patients received either videotape education or 'live' demonstrations to improve their dietary knowledge. Both intervention groups showed a significant improvement in overall glycaemic control, relative to controls. They were then randomised to an 'experimental' high-carbohydrate/high-fibre/low-fat diet or a 'standard' (low-carbohydrate) diabetic diet. On the experimental diet, control as judged by glycosylated haemoglobin deteriorated. After 4 months of intensive dietary follow-up, the patients were left alone and reassessed 6 months later. Mean glycosylated haemoglobin had fallen again in those on the standard diet, leading the authors to conclude that the experimental diet was detrimental. However, patients on a 'high' carbohydrate diet only achieved a 6.6% increase in carbohydrate intake, from 38.8 to 45.4% total energy. The standard-diet intervention group increased their fibre intake (although not instructed to do so) from 20.3 to 28.5 grams per day which was only 3.3 grams per day less than the high-carbohydrate group. Thus, the two diets being compared differed more in the amount of available carbohydrate than in fibre and the results are therefore perhaps not surprising. Subsequent correspondence also drew attention to the failure to measure anything other than glucose and glycosylated haemoglobin, especially the omission of lipids, the different lengths of study of the two intervention groups, and that several patients were lost to follow-up (50, 51).

The second issue which has perhaps not been sufficiently emphasized is that the great majority of studies which have shown a beneficial effect of a high-carbohydrate/high-fibre diet have contained 50 grams or more dietary fibre. The study by Geekie and colleagues quoted earlier suggest that well-motivated British patients might be able to achieve a daily intake of dietary fibre of around 40 grams (13) and yet none of the studies has examined the effects of this level of fibre intake.

Whilst the McCulloch study, because of the criticisms mentioned, in no way invalidates the recommendations concerning carbohydrate and fibre, there is clearly an urgent need for further long-term studies in which fibre should be given at a level where it is likely to be acceptable in the long term. There is no doubt that modification of dietary fat can produce cholesterol-lowering over a prolonged period (5 years) in patients with diabetes (20), so information is particularly required concerning the long-term effects of fibre on glycaemic control as well as metabolism of vitamins and minerals. This author believes strongly in the need for such a study, but ironically, in view of the widespread recommendations concerning the benefit of such a diet, many now seem to regard such a study as unethical. It may therefore never be carried out!

Optimal carbohydrate-containing foods for diabetic patients

Several concerns have been expressed regarding the role of the glycaemic index of foods as the best means of determining the optimal carbohydrate-containing foods for diabetic patients and some of these are discussed in *The Diabetes Annual/2*. One issue of particular concern is that use of the glycaemic index presumes that decreased postprandial glycaemia, reflecting delayed digestion and absorption, is the major mechanism by which certain high-carbohydrate/high-fibre foods exert their beneficial effect. It is certainly not the only mechanism. Long-term feeding studies carried out in Oxford and elsewhere suggest that the major effect of a high-carbohydrate/high-fibre diet is a downward shift of the entire blood glucose baseline (42, 53). Table 2, based on a study of relatively poorly controlled diabetic patients on maximum doses of oral therapy, shows that a considerable improvement of blood glucose occurs despite higher incremental blood glucose on a high-carbohydrate/high-fibre diet. Similarly, a

TABLE 2. *Indices of diabetic control in NIDDM patients, unsatisfactorily controlled on maximum doses of oral hypoglycaemic agents.*

	Initial profile		After 6 weeks HC diet		After 6 weeks LC diet
HbA_{1c} (%)	10.6 ± 2.1	**	8.5 ± 1.9	††	10.3 ± 2.2
Fasting blood glucose (mmol/l)	9.6 ± 4.5	**	6.8 ± 2.8	††	8.4 ± 2.8
Preprandial blood glucose[a] (mmol/l)	9.9 ± 3.9	***	7.5 ± 3.1	†††	9.5 ± 2.9
2h postprandial blood glucose[b] (mmol/l)	12.1 ± 3.8	*	10.8 ± 2.8		11.4 ± 3.5
Incremental blood glucose[c] (mmol/l)	2.2 ± 0.9		3.3 ± 1.2		1.9 ± 0.8
Mean 24-h blood glucose[d]	11.6 ± 1.5	***	9.3 ± 1.7		10.8 ± 1.3

[a] Mean values before breakfast, lunch and evening meal.
[b] Mean values 2 h after each main meal.
[c] Difference between preprandial and 2 h postprandial (mean of 3 values).
[d] Time-averaged mean value for whole 24 h.
Initial profile *vs* HC: *$P<0.05$; **$P<0.01$; ***$P<0.001$. HC *vs* LC diet: ††$P<0.01$; †††$P<0.001$.
LC = low-carbohydrate, low-fibre, high-fat diet; HC = diet high in carbohydrate and dietary fibre from various sources, especially legumes. Reprinted from Lousley et al (59) by courtesy of the Editors of *Diabetic Medicine*.

long-term Finnish experiment of guar supplementation found that the apparently lower postprandial blood glucose levels on guar were explained by a reduction in background blood glucose concentrations (54). Insulin levels on high-carbohydrate/high-fibre diets tend to be lower or not significantly higher than those observed on low-carbohydrate diets, suggesting that insulin sensitivity may be enhanced on such diets.

This alternative mechanism of action may explain the discrepancies which have been reported between the acute effects of foods on the postprandial blood glucose response and their chronic effects on overall metabolic control. This is the case, for instance, with wholemeal bread and other high-fibre cereals which are able to produce a substantial improvement in long-term glycaemic control (55) when given as part of a mixed diet, although their glycaemic index is quite unfavourable (56).

Foods with a low glycaemic index (e.g. those high in gel-forming fibre, especially various cooked dried beans, pastas and oats) seem also to have a beneficial effect in longer-term studies, and are therefore to be encouraged. However, while the glycaemic index is probably the most useful approach presently available for determining optimal carbohydrate-containing foods, not all foods with a relatively high glycaemic index are necessarily bad. The different mechanisms by which different foods might exert their beneficial effect emphasise the need for new approaches to supplement the glycaemic index.

Other aspects of appropriate nutrition for diabetic patients

Diabetic subjects, like everyone else, need to have a diet which contains adequate quantities of all essential nutrients including vitamins and minerals. Some patients may have special requirements, e.g. the elderly and those with hyperlipidaemia, but a balanced high-fibre/low-fat diet can provide all essential nutrients. Some people on high-fibre diets and various groups of diabetic patients have been shown to have a high intake of dietary sodium. Care should be taken that diabetic patients do not increase their sodium intake beyond that regarded as desirable for the general population. Recent controlled trials have shown that sodium restriction has a substantial blood-pressure-lowering effect in those with mild to moderate hypertension to the extent that such dietary advice, together with weight reduction when appropriate, should be the first line of therapy. In patients with more marked elevation of blood pressure, e.g. diastolic pressure 105-115 mmHg, the degree of blood pressure reduction is such that dietary modification should be regarded as an adjunct to conventional hypotensive therapy (57, 58).

Alcohol, diabetic foods and nutritive and non-nutritive sweeteners are all important aspects of the diabetic dietary prescription, but they have recently been reviewed elsewhere and will not be discussed again here.

Implementation of diet therapy

Most research in the field of nutrition and diabetes has, not surprisingly, been related to the scientific principles of nutrition policy and not to the practical applications. There are many issues which would be amenable to testing. Thus, in some European countries and North America diabetic patients are advised to follow a system which involves exchanging up to 10 different kinds of foods. In Britain, on the other hand, those on insulin are instructed only about carbohydrate exchanges with advice concerning regular meals of roughly equivalent energy content from day to day, the need to match times of peak insulin activity with adequate intakes of energy, and the optimal foods for people with diabetes, i.e. low in saturated fat and high in fibre-rich carbohydrate. It would be of considerable interest to compare these two approaches. In Britain patients with NIDDM are advised about total energy, the distribution of energy from various nutrients and the most appropriate carbohydrate-containing foods, but not usually about any exchange systems. Elemental diets, e.g. the Cambridge diet, are being increasingly used for overweight patients with NIDDM. Formal long-term evaluation of this diet is therefore urgently needed.

Very little attention has been given to the most appropriate means of diet teaching. The diabetic dietary prescription often involves a major change in lifestyle; physicians are rarely competent to be the sole providers of the appropriate advice and an impersonal diet sheet is probably inadequate. The diet must be tailored to individual and family requirements and new techniques of food preparation often need to be learned. It is usually assumed that the help of a dietitian or nutritionist is essential in order to give individual advice, but there are insufficient numbers of these professionals to provide this help. We need, therefore, to find ways of increasing the numbers of dietitians. As an interim measure, it is necessary to find other effective ways of providing advice concerning dietary change which, in the patient with IDDM is an essential complement to insulin therapy, and in those with NIDDM can often be more effective than oral hypoglycaemic therapy in improving glycaemic control and blood lipids.

References

1. Nutrition Sub-Committee, British Diabetic Association's Medical Advisory Committee (1982): Dietary recommendations for the 1980's - a policy statement from the British Diabetic Association. *Hum. Nutr. Appl. Nutr., 36,* 378.
2. Nutrition Sub-Committee, British Diabetic Association's Medical Advisory Committee (1987): The provision of dietetic services to diabetics in the United Kingdom. *Hum. Nutr. Appl. Nutr., 41A,* 13.
3. American Diabetes Association Committee on Food and Nutrition (1979): Principles of nutrition and dietary recommendations for individuals with diabetes mellitus: 1979. *Diabetes, 28,* 1027.

4. Special Report Committee, Canadian Diabetes Association (1981): 1980 guidelines for the nutritional management of diabetes mellitus: a special report from the Canadian Diabetes Association. *J. Can. Diet. Assoc., 42,* 110.
5. Huttunen JK, Aro A, Pelkonen R et al (1982): Dietary therapy in diabetes mellitus. *Acta Med. Scand., 211,* 469.
6. Winton R (1982): Diet and diabetes: with care, diabetics can enjoy a normal, balanced diet. *Med. J. Aust., 1,* 245.
7. Mann JI (1984): Lines to legumes. *Diabetic Med., 1,* 191.
8. Mann JI (1980): Diet and diabetes. *Diabetologia, 18,* 89.
9. Mann JI (1984): What carbohydrate foods should diabetics eat? *Br. Med. J., 288,* 1025.
10. Truswell AS, Thomas BJ, Brown AM (1975): Survey of dietary policy and management in British diabetic clinics. *Br. Med. J., 4,* 7.
11. Toeller M, Lion S (1987): Survey of the management of diet in 26 diabetes clinics in Europe. *Diabetic Med.,* in press.
12. Thompson AV, Neil HAW, Thorogood M et al (1987): Diabetes mellitus: attitudes, knowledge and glycaemic control in a cross-sectional population. *J.R. Coll. Gen. Pract.,* in press.
13. Geekie MA, Porteous J, Hockaday TDR, Mann JI (1986): Acceptability of high-fibre diets in diabetic patients. *Diabetic Med., 3,* 65.
14. Mann JI, Marmot M (1983): Epidemiology of ischaemic heart disease. In: Ledingham JJG, Warrell DA, Weatherall DJ (Eds), *Oxford Textbook of Medicine,* p. 13.151. Oxford University Press, London.
15. Colwell JA, Winocour PD, Halushka PV (1983): Do platelets have anything to do with diabetic microvascular disease? *Diabetes, 32, Suppl. 2,* 14.
16. Halushka PV, Dollery CT, MacDermott J (1983): Thromboxane and prostacyclin in disease: a review. *Q. J. Med., 208,* 461.
17. Mustard JF, Packham MA (1984): Platelets and diabetes mellitus. *N. Engl. J. Med., 311,* 665.
18. Mann JI (1986): Epidemiological and clinical studies on optimal nutrition in diabetes. *Prog. Lipid Res., 25,* 485.
19. Houtsmuller AJ, Van Hal-Ferwerda J, Zahn KJ, Henkes HE (1980): Favourable influences of linoleic acid on the progression of diabetic micro- and macro-angiopathy in adult onset diabetes mellitus. *Nutr. Metab., 24,* 105.
20. Howard-Williams J, Patel P, Jelfs R et al (1985): Polyunsaturated fatty acids and diabetic retinopathy. *Br. J. Ophthalmol., 69,*15.
21. Lopez-Espinoza I, Howard-Williams J, Mann JI et al (1984): Fatty acid composition of platelet phospholipids in non-insulin dependent diabetes randomised for dietary advice. *Br. J. Nutr., 52,* 41.
22. Chaintreuil J, Mommier L, Colette C et al (1984): Effects of dietary gamma-linolenate supplementation on serum lipids and platelet function in insulin-dependent diabetic patients. *Hum. Nutr. Clin. Nutr., 38,* 121.
23. Mikhailides DP, Kirtland SJ, Barradas MA (1986): The effect of dihomogammalenic acid on platelet aggregation and prostaglandin release, erythrocyte membrane fatty acids and serum lipids. *Diabetes Res., 3,* 7.
24. Schinke E, Hildebradt R, Bertz J (1984): Influence of cod liver oil diet in type I diabetics on fatty acid patterns and platelet aggregation. *Biomed. Biochim Acta, 43,* 8.
25. Mattson FH, Grundy SM (1985): Composition of effects of dietary saturated, monounsaturated and polyunsaturated fatty acids on plasma lipids and lipoproteins in man. *J. Lipid Res., 26,* 194.
26. Edington J, Geekie M, Carter R et al (1987): The effects of dietary cholesterol on plasma cholesterol in subjects on a reduced fat, high fibre diet. *Br. Med. J., 294,* 333.
27. Mann JI (1985): Diabetes mellitus: some aspects of aetiology and management. In: Trowell

HC, Burkitt D, Heaton K (Eds), *Refined Carbohydrate Foods, Dietary Fibre and Disease,* *2nd ed.,* p. 263. Academic Press, London.

28. Brunzell JD, Lerner RL, Hazzard WR et al (1971): Improved glucose tolerance with high carbohydrate feeding in mild diabetes. *N. Engl. J. Med., 284,* 521.

29. Coulston AM, Shislocki ALM (1985): Metabolic effects of high carbohydrate, moderate sucrose diets in patients with non-insulin dependent diabetes mellitus (NIDDM). *Diabetes, 34,* 34A.

30. Coulston AM, Liu GC, Reaven GM (1983): Plasma glucose, insulin and lipid responses to high-carbohydrate low-fat diets in normal humans. *Metabolism, 32,* 52.

31. Jellish WS, Emanuele MA, Abraira C (1984): Graded sucrose carbohydrate diets in overtly hypertriglyceridaemic diabetic patients. *Am. J. Med., 77,* 1015.

32. Chantelau EA, Gosseringger G, Sonnenberg GE, Berger M (1985): Moderate intake of sucrose does not impair metabolic control in pump treated diabetic outpatients. *Diabetologia, 28,* 204.

33. Peterson DB, Lambert J, Gerring S et al (1986): Sucrose in the diabetic diet — just another carboydrate? *Diabetic Med., 2,* 345.

34. Pelkonen R, Aro A, Nikkila EA (1972): Metabolic effects of dietary fructose in insulin dependent diabetes of adults. *Acta Med. Scand., 542, Suppl.,* 187.

35. Akerblom HK, Siltanen I, Kallio AK (1972): Does dietary fructose affect the control of diabetes in children? *Acta Med. Scand., 542, Suppl.,* 195.

36. Crapo PA, Kolterman OG (1984): The metabolic effects of 2-week fructose feeding in normal subjects. *Am. J. Clin. Nutr., 39,* 525.

37. Andersen AR, Sandahl Christiansen J, Andersen JK et al (1983): Diabetic nephropathy in type 1 (insulin dependent) diabetes: an epidemiological study. *Diabetologia, 25,* 496.

38. Viberti GC, Keen H (1984): The patterns of proteinuria in diabetes mellitus. *Diabetes, 33,* 686.

39. Mogensen CE (1971): Glomerular filtration rate and renal plasma flow in short-term and long-term juvenile diabetes mellitus. *Scand. J. Clin. Lab. Invest., 28,* 91.

40. Viberti GC, Hill RD, Jarrett RJ et al (1982): Microalbuminuria as a predictor of clinical nephropathy in insulin-dependent diabetes mellitus. *Lancet, 1,* 1430.

41. Mogensen CE, Christensen CK (1984): Predicting diabetic nephropathy in insulin dependent patients. *N. Engl. J. Med., 311,* 89.

42. Viberti GC, Bilous RW, Mackintosh D et al (1983): Long term correction of hyperglycaemic and progression of renal failure in insulin dependent diabetics. *Br. Med. J., 286,* 598.

43. Parving HH, Andersen AR, Smidt UM, Svendsen PA (1983): Early aggressive antihypertensive treatment reduce rate of decline in kidney function in diabetic nephropathy. *Lancet, 1,* 1175.

44. Attman PO, Bucht H, Larson O, Uddebom G (1983): Protein-reduced diet in diabetic renal failure. *Clin. Nephrol., 19,* 217.

45. Viberti GC, Pickup JC, Jarrett RJ, Keen H (1979): Diabetic control and renal failure. *N. Engl. J. Med., 300,* 638.

46. Wiseman MJ, Saunders AJ, Keen H, Viberti GC (1985): Effect of blood glucose control on increased glomerular filtration rate and kidney size in insulin dependent diabetes mellitus. *N. Eng. J. Med., 312,* 617.

47. Bognetti E, Wiseman MJ, Gross JL et al (1985): Renal response to protein loading and modulating effect of plasma glucose in IDDs with high and normal glomerular filtration rate. *Diabetes Res. Clin. Pract., Suppl. 1,* S556.

48. Wiseman MJ, Hunt RE, Gross JL et al (1985): Glomerular filtration rate and dietary regimens of different protein composition in healthy subjects. *Eur. J. Clin. Invest., 15,* A33.

49. McCulloch DK, Mitchell RD, Ambler J, Pattersall RB (1985): A prospective comparison of

'conventional' and high carbohydrate/high fibre/low fat diets in adults with established type 1 (insulin-dependent) diabetes. *Diabetologia, 28,* 208.

50. Hockaday TDR, Mann JI (1985): 'Conventional' and high carbohydrate/high fibre/low fat diets in adults with established type I (insulin-dependent) diabetes. *Diabetologia, 28,* 793.
51. Reckless JPD (1986): Diet and type 1 (insulin-dependent) diabetes. *Diabetologia, 29,* 205.
52. Lousley SE, Jones DB, Slaughter P et al (1984): High carbohydrate-high fibre diets in poorly controlled diabetes. *Diabetic Med., 1,* 21.
53. Simpson HCR, Simpson RW, Lousley S et al (1981): A high carbohydrate leguminous fibre diet improves all aspects of diabetic control. *Lancet, 1,* 1.
54. Aro A, Uusitupa M, Voutilainen E et al (1981): Improved diabetic control and hypocholesterolaemic effect induced by long term dietary supplementation with guar gum in type 2 (non insulin dependent) diabetes. *Diabetologia, 21,* 29.
55. Simpson RW, Mann JI, Eaton et al (1979): Improved glucose control in maturity-onset diabetes treated with high carbohydrate-modified fat diet. *Br. Med. J., 1,* 1753.
56. Jenkins DJA, Wolever TMS, Jenkins AL et al (1984): The glycaemic response to carbohydrate foods. *Lancet, 2,* 388.
57. Dodson PM, Pacy PJ, Bal P (1984): A controlled trial of a high fibre, low fat and low sodium diet for mild hypertension in type 2 (non insulin dependent) diabetic patients. *Diabetologia, 27,* 522.
58. Pacy PJ, Dodson PM, Fletcher RF (1986): Effect of high carbohydrate, low sodium and low fat diet in type 2 diabetics with moderate hypertension. *Int. J. Obesity, 10,* 43.
59. Lousley SE, Jones DB, Slaughter P et al (1984) High carbohydrate/high fibre diets in poorly controlled diabetes. *Diabetic Med., 1,* 21.
60. Peterson DB, Lambert J, Gerring S et al (1986) Sucrose in the diet of diabetic patients — just another carbohydrate? *Diabetologia, 29,* 216.

The Diabetes Annual/3
K.G.M.M. Alberti and L.P. Krall, editors
© 1987 Elsevier Science Publishers, B.V.

5 Oral hypoglycemic agents*

HAROLD E. LEBOVITZ

Introduction

The use of oral hypoglycemic agents in the management of patients with non-insulin-dependent diabetes mellitus (NIDDM) is increasing. This can be attributed to extensive investigations into the pathophysiology of hyperglycemia in NIDDM, a greater awareness of the close relationship between metabolic regulation of diabetes mellitus and its chronic complications, and increasing knowledge about the effects of oral hypoglycemic agents. Many contemporary issues concerning sulfonylurea drugs remain and answers, while elusive, are still being sought. This review tries to put these issues into focus and provides an update on our previous Chapter *(The Diabetes Annual/1)*.

Sulfonylurea treatment of patients with NIDDM

Additional insights into the mechanism by which sulfonylurea drugs ameliorate the hyperglycemia of patients with NIDDM have not been forthcoming in the last 2-3 years. Most of the clinical investigations during the last 2-3 years in this area have continued to focus on: (a) the mechanisms responsible for hyperglycemia in NIDDM; (b) the controversy over the relative importance of the extrapancreatic actions of sulfonylureas versus their insulin secretory activities in controlling hyperglycemia; (c) the relative merits of sulfonylurea therapy versus insulin treatment; and (d) the nature and significance of secondary sulfonylurea failure.

Hyperglycemia in patients with NIDDM conceptually can be separated into two distinct components: fasting and postprandial (1). These two states are quite different hormonal and metabolic entities. In the fasting state, plasma insulin levels are low, hepatic glucose production is modulated by the level of portal vein insulin, and 70% of glucose uptake is through insulin-independent mechanisms (2). The fed state, by contrast, is characterized by high plasma in-

---

*The author's own studies have been supported by grants from Pfizer Laboratories and the Division of Research Resources of the National Institutes of Health (RR00318).

sulin levels and complete or almost complete suppression of hepatic glucose production; 80-90% of glucose uptake is through insulin-dependent mechanisms (3). NIDDM is characterized by deficient glucose-mediated insulin secretion, marked resistance to the peripheral actions of physiological plasma insulin concentrations, and lesser and reversible resistance to the hepatic actions of insulin.

The consequences of the disturbance of insulin secretion and action on fasting and postprandial hyperglycemia in patients with NIDDM can be worked out from the above data. Since the bulk of glucose utilization in the fasting state is through insulin-independent mechanisms (in both normal subjects and NIDDM patients), changes in insulin action on glucose uptake can play only a minor role in increasing extracellular glucose concentrations. The main factor responsible for fasting hyperglycemia must be overproduction of glucose by the liver. Indeed, numerous studies measuring hepatic glucose production in patients with NIDDM with fasting hyperglycemia have shown a very high correlation between hepatic glucose production and fasting plasma glucose (4-6).

In the normal postprandial state, insulin action accounts for 80-90% of glucose disposal and this appears to occur predominantly in muscle. Since peripheral tissues in patients with NIDDM are resistant to insulin action, glucose disposal in response to insulin plus the deficiency in insulin secretion result in markedly reduced postprandial glucose disposal. This leads to sufficient levels of hyperglycemia to compensate for the potential intracellular fuel deficit by increasing glucose-mediated glucose uptake.

Thus the defects in patients with NIDDM (resistance to insulin action and diminished insulin secretion) differently alter the liver and peripheral tissues to cause fasting and postprandial hyperglycemia. Treatment of the hyperglycemia in patients with NIDDM must therefore be directed at correcting each of these components of hyperglycemia. It is highly likely that each may respond to therapeutic interventions differently.

The controversy as to the relative merits of increased insulin secretion versus extrapancreatic actions as the more important component in ameliorating hyperglycemia in NIDDM continues to draw considerable interest and of course is still unresolved. Several factors confound interpretation of the data in patients with NIDDM. It is now well recognized that hyperglycemia itself profoundly reduces insulin secretion (7, 8) and insulin action (9, 10). Thus, any factor which reduces hyperglycemia in patients with NIDDM will increase nutrient-mediated insulin secretion and the mere demonstration that plasma insulin or C-peptide levels increase with a treatment does not indicate causality. Many in-vivo extrapancreatic actions of sulfonylureas require either the presence of insulin or reasonably intact metabolic function to occur and the failure to demonstrate them in the absence of insulin does not mean that they do not occur in patients with NIDDM (11). Finally, the interpretation of the meaning of a change in insulin secretion as reflected in a plasma insulin level is difficult since resistance to the action of physiological levels of insulin in NIDDM is profound and changes in insulin-mediated glucose disposal impaired (12, 13).

A review by Kolterman (14) of the longitudinal effects of glyburide (glibenclamide) treatment in his patients with NIDDM essentially confirms the type of data reported in *The Diabetes Annual/1* (15). He and his colleagues studied the following parameters before and at 3 and 18 months of treatment: meal-mediated plasma glucose and insulin response; adipose tissue insulin binding and insulin-mediated glucose oxidation; peripheral glucose disposal in response to insulin infusion rates of 40, 120, 240 and 1200 $mU/m^2/min$; and basal hepatic glucose production rate. They showed that glyburide treatment increases meal-mediated insulin secretion at 3 months, but much less so at 18 months. The patients who had the best glycemic response to the treatment had the least increase in insulin secretion and there was no correlation between improved glycemic control and increased insulin secretion. Peripheral resistance to insulin action was markedly ameliorated by glyburide in patients who achieved a good glycemic response but not in those who had a poor response. The improved responsiveness to insulin was mediated predominantly by a post-receptor effect since adipose tissue insulin binding was unaltered at 3 months, even though action was markedly improved and at 18 months binding was increased in both responders and non-responders. Basal hepatic glucose output was decreased in proportion to the improvement in fasting hyperglycemia. The conclusion from the data is that the observed amelioration of glycemic control was due to extrapancreatic effects and was unrelated to any increase in insulin secretion. Ward and colleagues arrived at similar conclusions in their studies on the effect of gliclazide in obese patients with NIDDM (16), as did Canivet and Freychet in their studies with glipizide (17).

Several other investigators, however, have presented data which, they feel, support predominantly an insulin secretory effect of sulfonylureas as their major antidiabetic action (18-20). Hosker et al (18) studied patients with NIDDM before and after 3 weeks of sulfonylurea treatment with the hyperglycemic clamp technique and concluded that sulfonylurea drugs increase basal and stimulated C-peptide secretion and do not decrease insulin resistance. In a study with a very similar design, Pagano et al (21) reported results which led to the opposite conclusion.

Several studies have tried to correlate basal and stimulated serum C-peptide responses to effectiveness of sulfonylurea therapy. Grant et al (22) assessed fasting and 2-hour post-oral-glucose plasma C-peptide in 37 insulin-treated diabetic patients and then changed them to oral hypoglycemic therapy. Twenty were able to continue the oral agent for 3 months, but 17 had to re-institute insulin treatment. The group that could not be managed on oral agents had significantly lower fasting and stimulated serum C-peptide levels. Snehalatha et al

(23) measured basal and postprandial plasma C-peptide in 183 patients with NIDDM who had been treated with oral hypoglycemic drugs for more than 10 years. One hundred and forty-one (Group 1) continued to respond to the drugs, but in 42 glycemic control was not satisfactory and they had to be changed to insulin therapy (Group 2, secondary failures). Only 89 of the 183 patients had significant B-cell reserve (postprandial plasma C-peptide >0.6 pmol/ml) and 83 of them responded to oral hypoglycemic agents. Among the 94 patients with poor B-cell reserve, 58 were controlled on oral agents and 36 on insulin. Of 42 secondary failures, 36 had low plasma C-peptide levels. While the data show that good responders to oral hypoglycemic agents have better B-cell function than poor responders, there is no way of determining cause and effect and it is clear that some patients with poor B-cell reserve can respond to oral hypoglycemic agents while some with good reserve will not.

It is important to determine whether sulfonylurea drugs have a predominant effect through an extrapancreatic or insulin-secretory action. In the first instance, these drugs might be expected to have some uniqueness in their action and would achieve their actions at normal circulating insulin levels. In the latter event they would merely mimic insulin actions. Since the data are still controversial, some attention has been directed toward the practical clinical problem of whether insulin has an advantage over sulfonylureas as a first level of treatment of NIDDM after dietary management has failed to achieve euglycemia.

Newly presenting patients with NIDDM who have not achieved euglycemia (FPG <6 mmol/l) after 3 or 4 months of dietary therapy are being randomized in the U.K. Prospective Diabetes Study to continuing diet alone, diet with additional sulfonylurea, or diet with additional basal insulin supplementation. In a recent report of 195 patients studied over 1 year (24), the data show that addition of sulfonylurea drug decreased the FPG from 8.3 ± 1.9 to 6.7 ± 1.3 mmol/l (mean $\pm$ 1 SD) and HbA_{1c} from 9.1 ± 1.2 to $7.8 \pm 1.2\%$. Insulin addition resulted in a similar effect: FPG from 8.6 ± 2.2 to 6.8 ± 1.4 mmol/l and HbA_{1c} from 9.1 ± 1.9 to $8.1 \pm 1.3\%$. Both treatments were statistically more effective than diet alone (FPG 8.6 ± 1.8 to 9.3 ± 2.3 mmol/l and HbA_{1c} 8.8 ± 1.7 to $9.1 \pm 1.6\%$). This continuing study suggests that sulfonylurea therapy is as effective as insulin in management of newly presenting patients with NIDDM and that both therapies are more effective than diet alone.

A short-term cross-over study of 3 months' treatment with tolazamide or insulin in 8 patients with NIDDM examined glucose regulation, plasma C-peptide levels, hepatic glucose production and insulin-mediated glucose disposal to determine whether measurable differences in metabolic effects of sulfonylurea versus insulin treatment could be detected (25). The authors interpret their data as showing equivalent effects of either insulin or sulfonylurea treatment on metabolic regulation and improvement in insulin action.

Secondary failures to sulfonylurea treatment have remained an enigma to clinicians. Major questions which remain unanswered are: What are the causes of secondary failure? Can they be reversed? Will changing to another sulfonylurea be of benefit? Groop et al (26) examined 60 patients who were secondary drug failures. They defined secondary drug failure as a mean diurnal blood glucose >12 mmol/l after an initial good response of >2 years in patients who did not have an intercurrent illness and were not diet failures. They compared these patients with secondary failure to 60 matched sulfonylurea responders. The non-responders had basal and post-glucagon plasma C-peptide levels that were approximately 50% lower than the responders. There were extensive overlaps of individual values between the two groups, markedly limiting the value of an individual measurement. Circulating antibodies to islet cells, thyroid antigens and gastric parietal cells were noted in 12 of 53, 14 of 54 and 16 of 58 non-responders respectively in contrast to 3 of 58, 4 of 60 and 8 of 58 responders. The authors concluded that many secondary failures can be attributed to decreasing B-cell function, which in some patients may represent a form of autoimmune destruction.

By far the largest number of clinical secondary sulfonylurea failures is due to a failure of dietary compliance. A recent study by Liu et al (27) focused on the benefit of caloric restriction combined with a change in sulfonylurea on glucose regulation in obese patients thought to represent secondary sulfonylurea treatment failures. Twenty patients with FPG of 175-375 mg/100 ml (9.7-28.3 mol/l) on maximal doses of their sulfonylurea were placed on a hypocaloric diet for 4 weeks with or without glipizide, 20 mg twice a day. Patients were studied before treatment and after 2 weeks on a weight maintenance diet following the 4-week weight-loss period. Even though the weight loss and initial FPG were comparable, the group on diet plus sulfonylurea had a much greater fall in FPG and a more marked increase in glucose metabolic clearance rate than the group on diet alone. Thus, the institution of moderate weight loss seems to increase sulfonylurea action markedly in obese patients with NIDDM.

Effect of sulfonylurea on lipid metabolism in patients with NIDDM

One of the more difficult areas in managing patients with NIDDM is lipid metabolism. Numerous studies report conflicting data about the nature of the lipid abnormalities and the effect of treatment. This is particularly germaine as it pertains to sulfonylurea therapy because of the previous long-standing controversy as to whether sulfonylurea treatment has an effect on cardiovascular morbidity and mortality.

A number of investigations have been carried out to evaluate lipid metabolism and the effect of sulfonylurea therapy in Pima Indians (28-30). While this population may show unique abnormalities, it has the advantage of having comparable age-, sex- and weight-matched normal non-diabetic subjects and is uncomplicated by a heterogeneous group of genetic lipid abnormalities. NIDDM in the obese Pima Indians is associated with elevated plasma non-esterified fatty acids (NEFA) and triglycerides, increased very-low-density lipoprotein (VLDL) triglyceride, and a decreased high-density/low-density lipoprotein (HDL/LDL) cholesterol ratio. The elevated plasma NEFA seem to be due primarily to a decreased clearance from the plasma probably related to a defect in re-esterification. The increased VLDL triglyceride is the result of increased production and decreased fractional clearance. In addition, the VLDL particle is abnormal (high-triglyceride/apoprotein B ratio) since VLDL apoprotein B synthesis is not increased. The decreased VLDL triglyceride fractional clearance is due to diminished adipose tissue lipoprotein lipase activity. Treatment of these NIDDM patients with sulfonylurea drugs has a beneficial effect on many aspects of the disturbed lipid metabolism. Total serum cholesterol and triglycerides are reduced. Both VLDL and LDL cholesterol are decreased. While total HDL cholesterol is not increased to normal, HDL_2 is increased and HDL_3 is decreased. The HDL/LDL cholesterol ratio increases. Thus, sulfonylurea treatment of patients with NIDDM causes beneficial effects on lipid metabolism. The effects of sulfonylurea are probably the consequence of their action on glycemic regulation and not a unique effect of the sulfonylureas. The changes noted with sulfonylurea treatment of NIDDM in Pima Indians are similar to those reported in other patients with NIDDM. Insulin treatment of patients with NIDDM causes similar corrections to those seen with sulfonylurea treatment, although some investigators suggest that insulin increases HDL cholesterol while sulfonylureas do not (31, 32). This is a controversial issue.

Combination insulin+sulfonylurea therapy

Since sulfonylurea drugs stimulate endogenous insulin secretion and improve glucose metabolism through extrapancreatic actions, it is reasonable to ask whether the addition of sulfonylurea drugs to an insulin treatment program in a patient with diabetes mellitus has value. The patient with insulin-dependent diabetes mellitus (IDDM) usually has little or no residual insulin secretion and any improvement in glycemic regulation or reduction in the insulin dose administered would have to be attributed to extrapancreatic effects. By contrast, such changes in NIDDM patients could be due to either increased insulin secretion or improved insulin action. The potential value of combining insulin and sulfonylurea therapies in patients with diabetes mellitus would be to achieve more normal glycemia in patients who are not well regulated and/or to achieve more normal glycemia without significant peripheral hyperinsulinemia.

One would presume that it should be easy to determine whether combination insulin+sulfonylurea therapy has significant merits. Unfortunately the studies that are available are conflicting. A number of investigators have looked at the question of whether sulfonylurea drugs improve glucose metabolism in IDDM patients. Table 1 lists the results of 8 recent studies. Four studies showed no clinically significant effect of combination insulin+sulfonylurea treatment on glucose regulation (33, 34, 36, 37). Two studies clearly documented that the addition of sulfonylurea treatment to insulin therapy in IDDM patients increases insulin-mediated glucose disposal in the absence of any increase in insulin secretion. It is of note that Pernet et al (38) showed a significant increase in glucose disposal at an insulin infusion rate of 0.5 mU/kg/min with lesser and statistically insignificant effects at 1.0 and 2.0 mU/kg/min. Pontiroli et al (40) showed that sulfonylureas increased insulin-mediated glucose disposal at an insulin infusion rate of 1.67 mU/kg/min.

Clinically significant improvements in glycemic regulation have been reported by Burke et al (35) and Kabadi (39). Burke and co-workers studied combination therapy in 20 patients and measured FPG, HbA_1 and plasma C-peptide response to oral glucose. Nine of his patients had a significant plasma C-peptide response and as a group their mean FPG and HbA_1 decreased significantly on combination insulin+glibenclamide therapy. The mean change in glycemic regulation in his plasma C-peptide non-responders were not significant. The authors suggested that increased endogenous insulin was responsible for the beneficial effects of combination therapy. Careful analysis of their primary data raises significant questions about their conclusions since the correlation between changes in plasma C-peptide responses and improved glycemic control was not good and the patient with the most dramatic fall in plasma glucose (the only patient to develop hypoglycemia on combination therapy) had no significant change in plasma C-peptide response. Kabadi reported that all 12 patients who had FPG <150 mg/100 ml (8.3 mmol/l) and/or HbA_1 <9.0% could be maintained on significantly less insulin (42 ± 5 *vs* 61 ± 6 U/d) on combination insulin+tolazamide treatment and that 8 patients achieved significant improvements in FPG (126 ± 12 *vs* 253 ± 13 mg/100 ml; 7.0 *vs* 14.1 mmol/l) and HbA_1 (8.6 ± 0.3 *vs* $12.0 \pm 0.4\%$) on the same insulin dose (60 ± 10 U/d) when tolazamide was added to their treatment program.

The various investigators have sought to explain the differences in their results on the particular drug, dose of drug, or duration of treatment. Several studies which showed no effects were of short duration or did not use maximal doses of the sulfonylurea drug. The studies which did show effects used higher doses of drug and were of longer duration. The conclusions that can be drawn from the available data are that sulfonylurea drugs do seem to show extrapancreatic effects in patients with IDDM, but it is still unclear whether the addition of sulfonylurea drugs to insulin results in clinically beneficial results.

The results of investigations of combination insulin+sulfonylurea treatment

TABLE 1 *Effects of insulin+sulfonylurea treatment in IDDM*

Investigators	Number of patients	Drug	Dose (mg/d)	Duration	Parameter	Result
Grunberger et al (33)	11	chlorpropamide	250-500	3-19 d	1. FPG 2. pp PG 3. Insulin binding	no effect
Ratzmann et al (34)	7	tolbutamide	500 i.v. 2500	acutely 6 d	insulin required to maintain constant plasma glucose level	no effect
Burke et al (35)	20	glibenclamide	15	3 mth	a. daily mean blood glucose b. glycohemoglobin	9/20 significant $\downarrow$ blood glucose and HbA$_1$
Ward et al (36)	7	glibenclamide	10	4 wk	a. 24-h plasma glucose profile b. glycohemoglobin	no effect
Goldman et al (37)	14	glibenclamide	5	6 mth	a. FPG b. HbA$_{1c}$ c. insulin binding	no effect FPG $\downarrow$ HbA$_{1c}$ at 6 but not 24 wk $\downarrow$ insulin binding at 24 wk
Pernet et al (38)	8	glibenclamide	15	15 d	glucose disposal rate	$\uparrow$ at physiologic but not pharmacologic insulin concentration
Kabadi (39)	20	tolazamide	1000	12 wk	a. insulin dose b. FPG c. HbA$_{1c}$	decreased insulin dose or decreased FPG and HbA$_{1c}$ in all subjects
Pontiroli et al (40)	9	chlorpropamide glipizide	500 15	8 d 8 d	glucose disposal rate with 1.67 mU/kg/min insulin infusion	70-80% $\uparrow$ glucose disposal rate

$\uparrow$ = increase; $\downarrow$ = decrease; FPG = fasting plasma glucose; pp PG = postprandial plasma glucose.

TABLE 2 *Effects of insulin+sulfonylurea treatment in NIDDM*

Investigator	Design	No. of patients	Drug	Dose (mg/d)	Duration	Parameter	Result
Longnecker et al (41)	double-blind cross-over	11	tolazamide	500 (3) 1000 (8)	8 wk	a. HbA_{1c} b. plasma glucose c. plasma C-peptide response to meal	FPG 272±21→ 222±31 mg/100 ml; 6/11 responded 5/11 no response
Allen et al (42)	patient as own control	6	glipizide	7.5-10 (2) 40 (4)	2-10 mth	a. plasma glucose profile b. insulin tolerance test	3/6 responded well
Lardinois et al (43)	patient as own control	14	glyburide*	20	3 mth	a. plasma glucose profile b. euglycemic clamp (MCR) c. HbA_{1c}	6 ↓ FPG 30% or more; those 6 ↑ MCR glucose 18-80% 5 no signif. change FPG or MCR
Groop et al (45)	cross-over	13	glibenclamide*	10	8 wk	a. plasma glucose profile b. insulin tolerance	FPG ↓ 2&4 wk but not 8 wk urinary glucose 4 and 8 wk; HbA_{1c} 4 wk but not at 8 wk
Falko and Osei (46)	double-blind	10	glyburide*	20	16 wk	a. plasma glucose response to OGTT b. HbA_{1c} c. serum lipids	FPG + OGTT ↓ at 4 but not 16 wk HbA_{1c} at ↓ 4 and 16 wk no changes in lipid
Mauerhoff et al (47)	double blind	11	glibenclamide*	10.5	16 wk	a. insulin dose b. FPG + pp PG	insulin dose ↓ 8-10% FPG + pp PG ↓ 18%

*Glyburide and glibenclamide are different names for the same drug.
↑ = increase; ↓ = decrease; FPG = fasting plasma glucose; MCR = metabolic clearance rate; pp PG = postprandial plasma glucose.

of patients with NIDDM are equally confusing. Table 2 gives the results of 6 recent studies that are representative of the data in the literature. Several investigators have found that combination insulin+sulfonylurea treatment improves glycemic regulation (41-44), while several others have found transient improvements at 4 weeks which are not sustained at 8 weeks or longer (45-48). Neither the specific drug nor dose or duration of treatment can account for the differences (Table 2). In the studies reporting significant benefit of combination therapy, considerable heterogeneity of responses was noted. Figure 1 is a com-

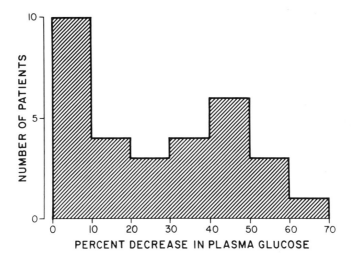

FIG. 1 *Effect of combination insulin+sulfonylurea treatment, combined data from Refs. 41-43.*

posite of the combined data from the 3 positive studies listed in Table 2 for which individual data are available. Note that 14 of 30 patients had no significant change in glycemia, while 13 of 30 had striking changes in glycemia following the institution of combined therapy.

Many investigators attribute any beneficial effects of combination therapy in patients with NIDDM to a sulfonylurea-mediated increase in insulin secretion as measured by basal and stimulated plasma C-peptide levels. However, Lardinois et al (43) and Allen et al (42) found a significant correlation between the decrease in glycemia and the improvement in insulin action (increase in glucose metabolic clearance rate or insulin-mediated glucose disposal) and not with the improvement in insulin secretion. Indeed, many individual patients in the various studies had a significant increase in basal and stimulated plasma C-peptide without a change in glycemic regulation.

We are left with the observation that some patients with NIDDM who are poorly controlled on insulin alone will have improved glycemic regulation on combination insulin+sulfonylurea therapy. It is unclear why some patients respond and others do not. It is also unclear whether the beneficial effect can be maintained beyond several months.

Pharmacokinetics of sulfonylurea drugs

Several significant pharmacokinetic studies have been published which have potential clinical relevance. Glibenclamide in the form of HB-419 has been shown to have variable and incomplete absorption (49, 50). Thus, Groop et al (49) found that comparable doses of glipizide achieved 3 times higher peak plasma levels (C_{max}) and area-under-the-curve (AUC) values than glibenclamide when administered to patients with NIDDM. The newer glibenclamide formulation (HB-420) appears to have more complete and consistent absorption. The newer formulation should result in decreased dosage and more consistent treatment.

Significant drug interactions have been reported with some sulfonylurea drugs but not with others. Tolbutamide and carbutamide enhanced and glibenclamide did not influence the incidence of digitalis intoxication in diabetic patients (51). In rabbits, glibenclamide decreased and tolbutamide and carbutamide increased strophanthidin toxicity in a dose-dependent manner. It appears that second-generation sulfonylureas may be preferable to first-generation agents in patients on digitalis therapy. Indobufen treatment inhibits glipizide metabolism in man and leads to increased plasma glipizide levels so that the dose may have to be adjusted appropriately (52). Phenylbutazone treatment of well-controlled diabetic patients treated with chlorpropamide leads to a reduction in fasting plasma glucose levels, but clinical hypoglycemia was not observed (53). Again the potential for serious side effects from this drug interaction must be appreciated.

Complications of sulfonylurea treatment

The most serious complication of sulfonylurea treatment continues to be severe and sometimes fatal hypoglycemic reactions. In *The Diabetes Annual/1*, we reviewed the Swedish experience with glibenclamide-associated hypoglycemia (15). Berger et al (54) subsequently have presented the relative incidence of severe sulfonylurea-induced hypoglycemic reactions in Switzerland in the last 25 years. In 1969 and 1984 all emergency wards in Switzerland were asked to report on the incidence of severe sulfonylurea-induced hypoglycemia in the preceding 10-year period. Period 1960-1969 was designated as 'Period A' and 1975-1984 'Period B'. There were 78 severe hypoglycemic episodes (0.22 per 1000 patient-treatment-years) in Period A. In spite of increased knowledge and different sulfonylureas, the incidence of severe hypoglycemic episodes was essentially unchanged in Period B (116 episodes which was 0.24 per 1000 patient-treatment-years). In Period A, chlorpropamide was the agent most frequently responsible, with tolbutamide and carbutamide much less so. In Period B, chlorpropamide and glibenclamide were equally responsible while tolbutamide and glibornuride were infrequently responsible. The authors concluded that chlorpropamide and glibenclamide use is associated with the greatest risk of severe hypoglycemia. Fatal hypoglycemia occurred in 6.5% of the episodes in Period A and 4.3% in Period B. Risk factors for severe sulfonylurea-induced hypoglycemia in Period B were: advanced age (77% of episodes were in patients 69 years of age or older even though they represented only 50% of sulfonylurea-treated diabetics); impaired renal function (21% of episodes) and possible drug interactions (27% of episodes). Clearly, long-acting sulfonylureas present a significant risk to NIDDM patients with advanced age or associated medical complications.

Chlorpropamide continues to be associated with rare idiosyncratic reactions such as hemolytic anemia (55, 56), cholestatic jaundice (57-59) and various skin reactions (59, 60). These events, however, are uncommon and the specific incidence is unknown. Of some importance are the observations that a second-generation sulfonylurea frequently did not give the same idiosyncratic reaction as chlorpropamide or other first-generation sulfonylureas (55, 57).

The significance and mechanism of the chlorpropamide-alcohol flush are still poorly understood. Several publications have shown that the chlorpropamide-alcohol flush is more commonly found in women than men, is highly correlated with plasma chlorpropamide levels, and is inversely correlated with body weight (61, 62). There is some suggestion that the observed sex difference is a reflection of a lower body weight in females. Recent measurements of 6-oxo-prostaglandin $F_{1\alpha}$ and thromboxane B_2 in peripheral venous plasma before and during chlorpropamide-alcohol flushing failed to show any increases and consequently a role for prostaglandins in mediating chlorpropamide-alcohol-induced flushing has been questioned (63).

Extrapancreatic effects of sulfonylureas in vitro

The demonstration of an action of sulfonylurea drugs in an in-vivo model always raises the question whether the measured effect can be explained by an action secondary to increased pancreatic insulin secretion or improved glycemic regulation rather than a direct extrapancreatic action. Perusal of the clinical literature on sulfonylurea treatment of patients with NIDDM exemplifies this phenomenon. An example of this is the effect of sulfonylurea drugs on insulin binding to the insulin receptor (15). Many studies have shown that improvement of glycemic control in NIDDM patients or animals treated with sulfonylureas is associated with an increase in insulin binding to peripheral mono-cytes, red blood cells or plasma membranes from hepatocytes or adipocytes. An almost equal number of similar investigators have shown no increase in in-sulin binding. Most studies in vitro of sulfonylurea action on insulin-sensitive cells indicate that sulfonylureas do not have a direct effect on the number or af-finity of insulin receptors, but rather that the changes observed in vivo are sec-ondary to some other effect in vivo of the drugs. A true extrapancreatic action of sulfonylurea drugs must be demonstrable in vitro as well as in vivo.

Two studies in vivo in rats have presented some interesting data about poten-tial extrapancreatic actions of sulfonylureas that may be of interest for further investigations but whose current relevance is unknown. Acute and chronic sulfonylurea but not insulin or 2-deoxy-D-glucose treatment of rats leads to rises in hypothalamic serotoninergic neuronal activity (64). Rats treated with glibenclamide for 4 months showed decreased intestinal somatostatin and en-teroglucagon content compared to control animals (65).

Considerable new information has become available about extrapancreatic actions in vitro of sulfonylureas on adipose tissue, liver and myocardium. These studies are important since they indicate that sulfonylureas can affect specific enzymes and intracellular functions. Additionally, and equally important, they show that some extrapancreatic actions of sulfonylureas are related to that molecular structure which is responsible for hypoglycemic activity, while other actions are unique to some sulfonylureas and not to others.

Adipose tissue

Isolated adipocytes have served as a valuable model for studying effects in vitro of sulfonylureas. The demonstration that insulin action on glucose transport in-volves a translocation of the glucose carrier from a microsomal storage pool to the plasma membrane was made using isolated adipocytes. Jacobs and Jung (66) have shown recently that glyburide added to adipocytes in vitro for 48 hours had no effect on basal 3-O-methyl-D-glucose flux or the glucose-sensitive cytochalasin-B-binding sites (glucose carriers) of the plasma membrane. How-ever, insulin stimulation of the glyburide-treated adipocytes increased the insu-lin-induced recruitment of the glucose carrier from the microsome to the plasma membrane by 27-31% and increased insulin stimulation of glucose transport by 31-45%. Thus, it appears that the sulfonylurea-mediated potentia-tion of insulin-stimulated glucose transport can be explained by its effect in facilitating insulin-induced translocation of the glucose carrier molecule.

This effect of sulfonylurea drugs in potentiating insulin-mediated glucose transport is not limited to insulin alone but is also seen with agents that mimic insulin action such as vitamin K_5 and H_2O_2 (67). Glyburide increases glucose-mediated uptake which is stimulated by insulin, vitamin K_5 or H_2O_2 by 30% in cultured rat adipocytes. Since the oxidants do not affect the binding portion of the insulin receptor, these data confirm that the sulfonylurea drugs do not act through changing insulin binding to its receptor but rather some post-receptor event.

Another interesting extrapancreatic effect of sulfonylureas that has been reported recently is a direct action in increasing glycogen synthase activity in cultured rat adipocytes (68). This action was demonstrated with high concentrations of glyburide, required exposure to the drug for a minimum of 10-20 hours, and was dependent on glucose concentration. Not only was basal glycogen synthase activity increased but insulin-mediated activation of glycogen synthase was also potentiated by glyburide. Altan et al (68) proposed that the sulfonylurea is probably acting to increase glucose transport, thus increasing synthase phosphatase allosterically by glucose-6-phosphate. This would increase activation of glycogen synthase by dephosphorylating it.

Hepatic metabolism

As noted earlier, hepatic glucose production is the major determinant of fasting plasma glucose and agents that reduce fasting hyperglycemia in patients with NIDDM do so by either direct or indirect effects (e.g. increased insulin secretion or decreased glucagon secretion) on hepatic glucose production. Many investigators have sought extrapancreatic actions of sulfonylurea drugs on the liver as one possible explanation for their hypoglycemic actions. The preparations in vitro used have included isolated perfused rat livers, rat hepatocytes in culture and rat liver cubes. Table 3 summarizes the results of such recent investigations.

Neither first- nor second-generation sulfonylureas increase basal rates of glycogen synthesis, but both second-generation sulfonylureas studied increased insulin-mediated glycogen synthesis independently of any changes in insulin binding to hepatic insulin receptors (69-71). These data are similar to previous data indicating that tolazamide has no effect on basal hepatic lipogenesis but increases insulin-stimulated lipogenesis (72), and are contrary to the observation that high concentrations (40 μM) of glyburide increase both basal and insulin-stimulated glycogen synthase activity in cultured adipose tissue (68).

Direct inhibition of gluconeogenesis from lactate and pyruvate and ketogenesis from long-chain fatty acids seem to be consistent effects of sulfonylurea drugs (69, 73, 74). The mechanism for the inhibition of gluconeogenesis is unknown, while the decreased long-chain fatty acid oxidation is thought to be due to an inhibition of carnitine palmitoyltransferase 1, most probably by competing with L-(−)-carnitine.

The first-generation sulfonylureas (tolbutamide and chlorpropamide) increase hepatic glycolysis (73, 75). While the same drugs are known to increase

TABLE 3   *Effects of sulfonylureas on hepatic function in vitro*

	Tolbutamide	Tolazamide	Chlorpropamide	Glyburide*	Gliquidone
Fructose 2,6-bisphosphate	↑		↑		
Glycolysis	↑		↑		
Glycogen synthesis					
Basal		○			
Insulin-stimulated				○ ←	○ ←
Gluconeogenesis					
Lactate, pyruvate	→	→	→		
Glycerol, fructose	○				
Ketogenesis					
Long-chain fatty acids	→	→		→	
Octanoate	○			○	

*Glyburide and glibenclamide are different names for the same drug.
○ = no change; ↑ = increase; ↓ = decrease.

fructose 2,6-bisphosphate (a stimulator of phosphofructokinase and an inhibitor of fructose 1,6-diphosphatase (15, 75), it is unclear whether this is the mechanism for the increased glycolysis. It would be worthwhile to know whether a drug such as gliclazide which has no effect on fructose 2,6-bisphosphate content alters glycolysis. Indeed, more information is needed on the effects of other second generation sulfonylureas on both hepatic fructose 2,6-bisphosphate content and glycolysis.

The relevance of these extrapancreatic effects demonstrated in vitro with rat liver preparations to human clinical pharmacology is unclear, but they certainly raise questions which should be explored.

Myocardial metabolism and function

The effects of sulfonylurea drugs on the heart have been studied periodically since the UGDP study suggested that tolbutamide might have detrimental effects. Studies in vitro with the isolated perfused rat heart and rabbit myocardial membranes have added considerably to our knowledge in this area (76-79). Table 4 summarizes some of the more salient features of these studies. It is noteworthy that the first-generation sulfonylurea, tolbutamide, and the second-generation sulfonylurea, glyburide, have a different spectrum of activity. Glyburide has no effect on the mechanical function of the isolated perfused rat heart (77) whereas tolbutamide has an inotropic effect and increases oxygen consumption (76, 78). This is correlated with tolbutamide inhibiting calmodulin binding to rabbit heart membranes and decreasing myocardial sarcolemmal Ca^{2+}-ATPase (79). Since tolazamide has the same effect on rabbit heart membranes, this is a property shared by other first-generation sulfonylureas and is not unique to tolbutamide.

A second point of divergence between tolbutamide and glyburide is a stimu-

TABLE 4   *Effects of sulfonylureas on myocardial metabolism and function in vitro*

	Tolbutamide	Glyburide*
Inotropic effect	+	O
Oxygen consumption	+	O
Glucose transport	+	+
Glycogenolysis	+	O
Glycolysis	+	+
Phosphofructokinase activity	+	+
Pyruvate oxidation	+	+
Membrane Ca^{2+}-ATPase	+	O

*Glyburide and glibenclamide are different names for the same drug.
O = no change; + = significant effect.

lation of myocardial glycogenolysis by tolbutamide but not by glyburide. Both, however, have direct stimulatory effects on glucose transport, glycolysis, phosphofructokinase activation and pyruvate oxidation. The data indicate that two classes of extrapancreatic actions of sulfonylurea drugs occur in the myocardium: one which accompanies the molecular components responsible for the hypoglycemic action and one which is associated with molecular components that are unrelated.

Pancreatic effects of sulfonylureas in vitro

A popular hypothesis for the mechanism of sulfonylurea action in stimulating B-cell insulin secretion which was formulated in the early 1980s (80) is as follows: (a) hypoglycemic sulfonylureas bind to a region of the plasma membrane of the B cell; (b) the binding causes a decrease in membrane potassium permeability; (c) the B-cell membrane depolarizes; (d) calcium ion influx occurs through voltage-dependent channels; (e) cytosolic calcium ion concentration increases and triggers the release of insulin; (f) the effect of the insulin-releasing signal is amplified by cyclic AMP which increases in the cell as a result of depolarization of the membrane and calcium ion influx. Several studies measuring ^{86}Rb efflux, ^{45}Ca influx or cytosolic calcium ion content in isolated islets or B cells have lent support to the depolarization theory (81-84).

Some controversy now exists as to whether sulfonylurea drugs are bound primarily to the plasma membrane or enter the cell and exert their effects intracellularly. Several groups of investigators have described specific binding sites for sulfonylureas on the plasma membranes of B-cell tumor membranes. The binding sites have high affinity and are multiple, saturable and displaced by various sulfonylureas and analogs in proportion to their hypoglycemic potency (85-87). In contrast, Carpentier et al (88) incubated [^{3}H]glibenclamide with pancreatic islet cells and found that less than 15% could be localized to the plasma membrane by autoradiographic techniques while 72-79% was localized in the cytoplasm associated with the insulin secretory granule. Thus, the cellular site of action of sulfonylurea drugs is yet to be resolved.

Several new studies have confirmed that the sulfonylurea grouping is not solely responsible for the hypoglycemic activity of these drugs (89-91). Two non-sulfonylurea analogs of sulfonylurea drugs have been shown to increase insulin release from B cells. These drugs, HB-699 (analog of glibenclamide) and UL-DF-9 (analog of gliquidone) cause decreased potassium permeability, increased membrane depolarization, increased calcium ion influx and increased cytosolic calcium ion concentration in the B cell. Thus, they seem to increase insulin release in an identical manner to sulfonylureas. It appears, therefore, that there are two active sites on the second-generation hypoglycemic sulfonylurea drugs. The implications of this second non-sulfonylurea site in the future development of drugs may be important.

Several other studies reporting potentially important effects of sulfonylureas on islet cells are worthy of note. Panten et al (92) have shown that tolbutamide lowers islet cell ATP content in the presence of 5-10 mM glucose. Sako et al (93) utilizing isolated perfused islets from normal and cysteamine-treated rats have shown that glibenclamide has a direct inhibitory effect on A-cell glucagon secretion.

References

1. Olefsky JM (1985): Pathogenesis of insulin resistance and hyperglycemia in non-insulin dependent diabetes mellitus. *Am. J. Med., 79, Suppl. 3B,* 1.
2. Baron AD, Kolterman OG, Bell J et al (1985): Rates on non-insulin mediated glucose uptake are elevated in Type II diabetic subjects. *J. Clin. Invest., 76,* 1782.
3. Ferrannini E, Reichard G, Bevilacqua S et al (1984): Oral glucose disposal in non-insulin dependent diabetes. *Diabetes, 33,* 66A.
4. Kolterman OG, Gray RS, Shapiro et al (1984): The acute and chronic effects of sulfonylurea therapy in Type II diabetic subjects. *Diabetes, 33,* 346.
5. Best JD, Judzewitsch RG, Pfeiffer MA et al (1982): The effect of chronic sulfonylurea therapy on hepatic glucose production in non insulin dependent diabetes. *Diabetes, 31,* 333.
6. De Fronzo RA, Simonson DC (1984): Oral sulfonylurea agents suppress hepatic glucose production in non-insulin dependent diabetic individuals. *Diabetes Care, 7, Suppl. 1,* 72.
7. Kosaka K, Kuzuya T, Akanuma Y et al (1980): Increase in insulin response after treatment of overt maturity-onset diabetes is independent of the mode of treatment. *Diabetologia, 18,* 23.
8. Vague P, Moulin JP (1982): The defective glucose sensitivity of the B cell in non insulin-dependent diabetes: improvement after twenty hours of normoglycemia. *Metabolism, 31,* 139.
9. Revers RR, Fink R, Griffin J et al (1984): Influence of hyperglycemia on insulin's in vivo effects in Type II diabetes. *J. Clin. Invest., 73,* 664.
10. Unger RH, Grundy S (1985): Hyperglycemia as an inducer as well as a consequence of impaired islet cell function and insulin resistance: implications for the management of diabetes. *Diabetologia, 28,* 119.
11. Lebovitz HE, Feinglos MN (1978): Sulfonylurea drugs: mechanism of action and therapeutic usefulness. *Diabetes Care, 1,* 189.
12. Olefsky JM, Ciaraldi TP, Kolterman OG (1985): Mechanisms of insulin resistance in non-insulin dependent (Type II) diabetes. *Am. J. Med., 79, Suppl. 3B,* 12.
13. Lebovitz HE, Feinglos MN (1984): Mechanism of action of the second generation sulfonylurea glipizide. *Am. J. Med., 75, Suppl. 5B,* 46.
14. Kolterman OG (1985): Longitudinal evaluation of the effects of sulfonylurea therapy in subjects with Type II diabetes mellitus. *Am. J. Med., 79, Suppl. 3B,* 23.
15. Lebovitz HE (1985): Oral hypoglycemic agents. In: Alberti KGMM, Krall LP (Eds), *The Diabetes Annual/1,* pp. 93-109. Elsevier, Amsterdam.
16. Ward G, Harrison LC, Proietto J et al (1985): Gliclazide therapy is associated with potentiation of postbinding insulin action in obese, non-insulin-dependent diabetic subjects. *Diabetes, 34,* 241.

17. Canivet B, Freychet P (1985): Le traitement par glipizide ne modifie pas les récepteurs insuliniques érythrocytaires chez le diabétique non insulino-dépendant. *Thérapie, 40,* 93.
18. Hosker JP, Burnett MA, Davies EG et al (1985): Sulphonylurea therapy doubles B-cell response to glucose in Type II diabetic patients. *Diabetologia, 28,* 809.
19. Sonksen PH, Lowy C, Perkins JR, Lim HS (1984): Noninsulin dependent diabetes: 10 year outcome in relation to initial response to diet and subsequent sulfonylurea therapy. *Diabetes Care, 7,* 59.
20. Pfeifer MA, Halter JB, Judzewitsch RG et al (1984): Acute and chronic effects of sulfonylurea drugs on pancreatic islet function in man. *Diabetes Care, 7, Suppl. 1,* 25.
21. Pagano G, Lombardi A, Pisu E et al (1984): Hyperglycaemic clamp and insulin binding to isolated monocytes before and after glibenclamide treatment of mild Type II diabetics. *Horm. Metab. Res., 16,* 215.
22. Grant PJ, Barlow E, Miles DW (1984): Plasma C-peptide levels identify insulin-treated diabetic patients suitable for oral hypoglycaemic therapy. *Diabetes Med., 1,* 284.
23. Snehalatha C, Ramachandran A, Mohan V et al (1986): Beta cell function in long term NIDDM (Type II) patients and its relation to treatment. *Horm. Metab. Res., 18,* 391.
24. U.K. Prospective Diabetes Study (1985): II. Reduction in HbA(1c) with basal insulin supplement, sulfonylurea, or biguanide therapy in maturity-onset diabetes: a multicenter study. *Diabetes, 34,* 793.
25. Firth RG, Bell PM, Rizza RA (1986): Effects of tolazamide and exogenous insulin on insulin action in patients with non-insulin-dependent diabetes mellitus. *N. Engl. J. Med., 314,* 1280.
26. Groop LC, Pelkonen R, Koskimies S et al (1986): Secondary failure to treatment with oral antidiabetic agents in non-insulin dependent diabetics. *Diabetes Care, 9,* 129.
27. Liu GC, Coulston AM, Lardinois CK et al (1985): Moderate weight loss and sulfonylurea treatment of non-insulin-dependent diabetes mellitus: combined effects. *Arch. Intern. Med., 145,* 665.
28. Howard BV, Xiaoren P, Harper I (1985): Effect of sulfonylurea therapy on plasma lipids and high-density lipoprotein composition in non-insulin-dependent diabetes mellitus. *Am. J. Med., 79, Suppl. 3B,* 78.
29. Taskinen MR, Bogardus C, Kennedy A, Howard BV (1985): Multiple disturbance of free fatty acid metabolism in non insulin-dependent diabetes: effect of oral hypoglycemic therapy. *J. Clin. Invest., 76,* 637.
30. Taskinen MR, Beltz WF, Harper I et al (1986): Effects of NIDDM on very-low density lipoprotein triglyceride and apolipoprotein B metabolism: studies before and after sul-fonylurea therapy. *Diabetes, 35,* 1268.
31. Kasim SE, LeBoeuf RC, Rockett MJ et al (1986): The effects of oral agent or insulin treat-ment on the plasma lipoproteins and the plasma lipoprotein lipase activator in diabetic pa-tients. *Horm. Metab. Res., 18,* 190.
32. Huupponen RK, Viikari JS, Saarimaa H (1984): Correlation of serum lipids with diabetes control in sulfonylurea-treated diabetic patients. *Diabetes Care, 7,* 575.
33. Grunberger G, Ryan J, Gorden P (1982): Sulfonylureas do not affect insulin binding or glycemic control in insulin-dependent diabetics. *Diabetes, 31,* 890.
34. Ratzmann K, Schulz B, Heinke P, Besch W (1984): Tolbutamide does not alter insulin requirements in Type I (insulin dependent) diabetes. *Diabetologia, 27,* 8.
35. Burke B, Hartog M, Waterfield M (1984): Improved diabetic control in insulin-dependent diabetics treated with insulin and glibenclamide. *Acta Endocrinol., 107,* 70.
36. Ward E, Ward G, Turner R (1981): Effect of sulfonylureas on insulin secretion and glucose control in insulin-treated diabetics. *Br. Med. J., 283,* 278.
37. Goldman J, Tamayo R, Whitehouse F, Kahkonen D (1984): Effect of glyburide on metabolic control and insulin binding in insulin-dependent diabetes mellitus. *Diabetes Care, 7, Suppl. 1,* 106.

38. Pernet A, Trimble ER, Kuntschen F et al (1985): Sulfonylureas in insulin-dependent (Type I) diabetes: evidence for an extrapancreatic effect in vivo. *J. Clin. Endocrinol. Metab., 61,* 247.

39. Kabadi UM (1985): Adjuvant therapy with tolazamide and insulin improves metabolic control in Type I diabetes mellitus. *Diabetes Care, 8,* 440.

40. Pontiroli AE, Alberetto M, Bertoletti A et al (1984): Sulfonylureas enhance in vivo the effectiveness of insulin in Type I (insulin dependent) diabetes mellitus. *Horm. Metab. Res., 16, Suppl. 1,* 167.

41. Longnecker MP, Elsenhans VD, Leiman SM et al (1986): Insulin and a sulfonylurea agent in non-insulin dependent diabetes mellitus. *Arch. Intern. Med., 146,* 673.

42. Allen BT, Feinglos MN, Lebovitz HE (1985): Treatment of poorly regulated non-insulin-dependent diabetes mellitus with combination insulin-sulfonylurea. *Arch. Intern. Med., 145,* 1900.

43. Lardinois CK, Liu GC, Reaven GM (1985): Glyburide in non-insulin-dependent diabetes: its therapeutic effect in patients with disease poorly controlled by insulin alone. *Arch. Intern. Med., 145,* 1028.

44. Beiser WP, Diugosch R, Rettenmeier A et al (1984): Trial of sulfonylurea in combination with insulin in the therapy of diabetes Type I and II: evidence against a primary extrapancreatic receptor effect. *Klin. Wochenschr., 62,* 631.

45. Groop L, Harno K, Nikkila EA et al (1985): Transient effect of the combination of insulin and sulfonylurea (glibenclamide) on glycemic control in non-insulin dependent diabetics poorly controlled with insulin alone. *Acta Med. Scand., 217,* 33.

46. Falko JM, Osei K (1985): Combination insulin glyburide therapy in Type II diabetes mellitus. *Am. J. Med., 79, Suppl. 3B,* 92.

47. Mauerhoff T, Ketelslegers JM, Lambert AE (1986): Effect of glibenclamide in insulin-treated diabetic patients with a residual insulin secretion. *Diabète Métab., 12,* 34.

48. Sachse G, Mriser E, Federlin K (1984): Combination therapy with insulin and sulfonylurea in secondary failure of sulfonylurea therapy. *Dtsch. Med. Wochenschr., 109,* 419.

49. Groop L, Wahlin-Boll E, Groop P-H et al (1985): Pharmacokinetics and metabolic effects of glibenclamide and glipizide in Type 2 diabetics. *Eur. J. Clin. Pharmacol., 28,* 697.

50. Ikegam H (1985): Pharmacokinetics of glibenclamide: heterogeneity in its absorption. *Med. J. Osaka Univ., 35,* 55.

51. Pogatsa G, Koltai MZ, Balkanyi I et al (1985): Effects of various hypoglycaemic sulphonylureas on the cardiotoxicity of glycosides. *Eur. J. Clin. Pharmacol., 28,* 367.

52. Elvander-Stahl E, Melander A, Wahlin-Boll E (1984): Indobufen interacts with the sulphonylurea, glipizide, but not with the beta-adrenergic receptor antagonists, propranolol and atenolol. *Br. J. Clin. Pharmacol., 18,* 773.

53. Shah SJ, Bhandarkar SD, Satoskar RS (1984): Drug interaction between chlorpropamide and non-steroidal anti-inflammatory drugs, ibuprofen and phenylbutazone. *Int. J. Clin. Pharmacol. Ther. Toxicol., 22,* 470.

54. Berger W, Caduff R, Pasquel M, Rump A (1986): Die relative Häufigkeit der schweren Sulfonylharnstoff-Hypoglykämie in den letzten 25 Jahren in der Schweiz. *Schweiz. Med. Wochenschr., 116,* 145.

55. Or R, Merin E, Stupp Y, Matzner Y (1984): Chlorpropamide-induced hemolytic anemia. *Drug. Intell. Clin. Pharm., 18,* 981.

56. Sosler Sd, Behzad O, Garratty G et al (1984): Acute hemolytic anemia associated with a chlorpropamide-induced apparent auto-anti-J. *Transfusion (Philadelphia), 24,* 206.

57. Rumboldt Z, Bota B (1984): Favorable effects of glibenclamide in a patient exhibiting idiosyncratic hepatotoxic reactions to both chlorpropamide and tolbutamide. *Acta Diabetol. Lat., 21,* 387.

58. Gupta R, Sachar DB (1985): Chlorpropamide-induced cholestatic jaundice and pseudomembranous colitis. *Am. J. Gastroenterol., 80,* 381.
59. Baciewicz AM, Dattilo R, Willis SE, Kershaw JL (1985): Jaundice and rash associated with chlorpropamide. *Diabetes Care, 8,* 200.
60. Barnett JH, Barnett SM (1984): Lichenoid drug reactions to chlorpropamide and tolazamide. *Cutis, 34,* 542.
61. Groop L, Eriksson CJP, Wahlin-Boll E, Melander A (1984): Chlorpropamide-alcohol flush: significance of body weight, sex and serum chlorpropamide level. *Eur. J. Clin. Pharmacol., 26,* 723.
62. Jerntorp P, Almer L-O (1984): On plasma chlorpropamide, body weight and sex difference in chlorpropamide alcohol flush (CPAF). *Diabetes Res., 1,* 223.
63. Johnston C, Carey F, Forder RA, Haworth D (1984): Prostacyclin and thromboxane in non-insulin dependent diabetes: the chlorpropamide alcohol flush reaction revisited. *Clin. Sci., 67,* 633.
64. Grunstein HS, Smythe GA, Bradshaw JE, Compton PJ (1986): Tolbutamide increases hypothalamic serotonin activity in the rat. *Diabetes, 35,* 475.
65. Filipponio F, Marcelli M, Gregorio R et al (1984): Reduced intestinal contents of vasoactive intestinal polypeptide, somatostatin and entero-glucagon in rats chronically treated with glibenclamide. *IRCS Med. Sci., 12,* 943.
66. Jacobs DB, Jung CY (1985): Sulfonylurea potentiates insulin-induced recruitment of glucose transport carrier in rat adipocytes. *J. Biol. Chem., 260,* 2593.
67. Maloff BL, Drake L, Riedy DK, Lockwood DH (1984): Effects of sulfonylureas on the actions of insulin and insulin-mimickers: potentiation of stimulated hexose transport in adipocytes. *Eur. J. Pharmacol., 104,* 319.
68. Altan N, Altan M, Mikolay L et al (1985): Insulin-like and insulin enhancing effects of the sulfonylurea glyburide on rat adipose glycogen synthase. *Diabetes, 34,* 281.
69. McCormick K, Williams MC, Sicoli R, Chen L (1986): Effect of tolazamide on basal ketogenesis, glycogenesis and gluconeogenesis in liver obtained from normal and diabetic rats. *Endocrinology, 119,* 1268.
70. Rinninger F, Kirsch D, Haring HU, Kemmler W (1984): Extrapancreatic action of the sulphonylurea gliquidone: post-receptor effect on insulin-stimulated glycogen synthesis in rat hepatocytes in primary culture. *Diabetologia, 26,* 462.
71. Fleig WE, Noether-Fleig G, Fussgaenger R, Ditschuneit H (1984): Modulation by a sulfonylurea of insulin-dependent glycogenesis but not of insulin binding in cultured rat hepatocytes. *Diabetes, 33,* 285.
72. Salhanick AI, Konowitz P, Amatruda JM (1983): Potentiation of insulin action by a sulfonylurea in primary cultures of hepatocytes from normal and diabetic rats. *Diabetes, 32,* 206.
73. Patel TB (1986): Effects of tolbutamide on gluconeogenesis and glycolysis in isolated perfused rat liver. *Am. J. Physiol., 250,* E82.
74. Patel TB (1986): Effect of sulfonylureas on hepatic fatty acid oxidation. *Am. J. Physiol., 251,* E241.
75. Monge L, Mojena M, Ortega JL et al (1986): Chlorpropamide raises fructose-2,6-bis-phosphate concentration and inhibits gluconeogenesis in isolated rat hepatocytes. *Diabetes, 35,* 89.
76. Lampson WG, Kramer JH, Schaffer SW (1985): Effect of tolbutamide on myocardial energy metabolism of the ischemic heart. *Biochem. Pharmacol., 34,* 803.
77. Schaffer SW, Tan BH, Mozaffari MS (1985): Effect of glyburide on myocardial metabolism and function. *Am. J. Med., 79, Suppl. 3B,* 48.

78. Tan BH, Wilson GL, Schaffer SW (1984): Effect of tolbutamide on myoca. and mechanical performance of the diabetic rat. *Diabetes, 33,* 1138.

79. Warnick PR, Davis FB, Davis PJ et al (1986): Differential effects of tolazamide and glyburide in vitro on rabbit myocardial membrane Ca^{2+} ATPase activity. *Diabetes, 35,* 1044.

80. Gylfe E, Hellman B, Sehlin J, Taljedal IB (1984): Interaction of sulfonylurea with the pancreatic B-cell. *Experientia, 40,* 1126.

81. Matthews EK, Shotton PA (1984): The control of Rb^{85}, efflux from rat isolated pancreatic islets by the sulphonylureas tolbutamide and glibenclamide. *Br. J. Pharmacol., 82,* 689.

82. Norlund L, Sehlin J (1985): Effect of tetracaine and glibenclamide on Ca^{2+} handling by isolated pancreatic islets. *Br. J. Pharmacol., 85,* 127.

83. Ferrer R, Atwater I, Omer EM et al (1984): Electrophysiological evidence for the inhibition of potassium permeability in pancreatic beta-cells by glibenclamide. *Q. J. Exp. Physiol., 69,* 831.

84. Abrahamsoon H (1985): Direct measurements of increased free cytoplasmic Ca^{2+} in mouse pancreatic B cells following stimulation by hypoglycemic sulfonylureas. *FEBS Lett., 190,* 21.

85. Geisen K, Hitzel V, Okomonopoulos R et al (1985): Inhibition of ^{3}H-glibenclamide binding to sulfonylurea receptors by oral antidiabetics. *Arzneim.-Forsch./Drug Res., 35,* 707.

86. Siconolfi L, Banerji MA, McNeil E, Lebovitz HE (1985): evidence for a specific plasma membrane sulfonylurea receptor. *Clin.Res., 33,* 574A.

87. Siconolfi-Baez L, Lebovitz HE (1985): Characteristics of a specific plasma membrane sulfonylurea receptor. *Diabetes, 34, Suppl. 1,* 228.

88. Carpentier JL, Sawano F, Ravazzola M, Malaisse WJ (1986): Internalization of ^{3}H-glibenclamide in pancreatic islet cells. *Diabetologia, 29,* 259.

89. Norlund L, Sehlin J (1984): Different effects of glibenclamide and the structural analogue HB-699 on the Ca^{2+} uptake by Ob/Ob-mouse islets. *Acta Physiol. Scand., 122,* 187.

90. Puech R, Manteghetti M, Ribes G et al (1985): Enhancement of insulin release and islet cell calcium content by an acyl-amino-alcyl benzoic acid derivative, HB 699. *Horm. Metab. Res., 17,* 1.

91. Garrino MG, Meissner HP, Henquin JC (1986): The non-sulfonylurea moiety of gliquidone mimics the effects of the parent molecule on pancreatic B-cells. *Eur. J. Pharmacol., 124,* 309.

92. Panten U, Zunkler BJ, Scheit S et al (1986): Regulation of energy metabolism in pancreatic islets by glucose and tolbutamide. *Diabetologia, 29,* 648.

93. Sako Y, Wasada T, Umeda F, Ibayashi H (1986): Effect of glibenclamide on pancreatic hormone release from isolated perifused islets of normal and cysteamine-treated rats. *Metabolism, 35,* 944.

...betes Annual/3
...M.M. Alberti and L.P. Krall, editors
©1987 Elsevier Science Publishers, B.V.

6   Insulin injection therapy

P.D. HOME

Introduction

Sixty-four years after the introduction of insulin injections in Toronto, this form of therapy remains the mainstay of treatment in the overwhelming majority of insulin-dependent diabetic patients. During this time the major advances in insulin therapy that can be identified are few, but include the introduction of the two main types of extended-action preparations, the development of highly purified insulin, and self-monitoring of blood glucose. While all these have contributed to achieving better metabolic control and/or a more flexible lifestyle for a large number of patients, the occasional personal reports of the success of many decades of intensive monitoring with multiple injection regimens (1) serve to remind us that it is still the use of injections, rather than the tools, which may determine long-term outcome.

Any analysis of developments in injection therapy must therefore still ask the questions that would have been fundamental to treatment in the 1920s, though we can now perhaps formulate them more succinctly. These major questions are:

a. Has any advance helped overcome the tyranny of giving insulin prospectively to cover a period of hours during which requirement will vary enormously and often unpredictably?
b. Are we any further forward in providing a basal supply of insulin, well matched to overnight and interprandial requirement?
c. Is insulin delivery *per se* any more acceptable to the patient as a result of recent developments?

For a small but significant number of patients a positive answer to these questions has appeared in recent years in the form of the insulin infusion pump, but cost and physical inconvenience are a barrier to the majority. Equally, islet transplantation must be a major hope for the future (see Chapter 11), but has nothing to offer today's patients.

Special problems of insulin injections

The drawing up of an insulin formulation into a syringe, precise measurement of the dose, the mixing of two preparations, and their subcutaneous delivery, all remain problems of significance in obtaining satisfactory treatment in some patients. Lester (2) continues to remind us how important these factors can be in less developed countries, where the handling of a delicate syringe by fingers accustomed to agricultural implements may itself be a daunting task. In many of these climates, deterioration of injection needles is a significant problem, as is the loss of markings on an insulin syringe worth a week's wages.

While in Ethiopia an insulin injection is generally of a single preparation for reasons of simplicity and supply, mixing of soluble and extended-acting preparations is general diabetic practice in the developed world for twice-daily injection regimens, which remain the basis of most patients' management. Mixing of preparations in a low dead-space syringe was found to lead to a mean deviation equivalent to around 1 unit of the intended insulin mixture when using 100 U/ml formulations, the variation probably not being significant in management terms (3). Interchangeable needle syringes led to much larger and more variable delivery of the two components, the range of 0.033-0.065 ml suggesting a significant dosage error which might vary between 3 and 7 units of insulin, despite good precision of the total dose delivered. Similar results have been reported by Corcoran and Yudkin (4), who noted that over 80% of patients drew up a test dose to within 5% of targets, and with a coefficient of variation of under 5% in nearly 90% of patients. These workers point out that the errors from dead-space problems are much more significant with small doses, and the variability between doses can be particularly marked if air is trapped within the dead space on occasion.

Heine and colleagues have continued to pursue the question of the importance of the mixing of soluble and zinc-complexed insulin preparations. This problem arises because it is necessary to maintain a high free zinc ion concentration in solution (approx. 50 mg/l), if the integrity of the insulin-zinc complexed crystals is to be maintained. Such free zinc can however react with added soluble insulin, precipitating it into a loose complex. The early studies in this field suggested it to be a significant effect when 40 U/ml insulin was used (5). In 100 U/ml formulations the supernatant zinc concentration is unchanged; but because the dissolved insulin concentration is 2.5 times higher, miscibility effects should be less significant. Nevertheless, it was still possible to demonstrate blunting of the rise of serum insulin concentrations in normal subjects, and plasma free insulin concentrations in diabetic patients, when human soluble insulin was mixed with human crystalline insulin-zinc suspensions in a 6:14 ratio (6). The extent of this effect was much less than that reported by Heine and colleagues for insulins from the same manufacturer at the lower concentration, though a more marked effect was seen with a zinc-insulin complex from another company.

Alternative insulin regimens

Useful comparisons of insulin regimens based on different intermediate- or long-acting insulin preparations have yet to be published. In a small but complex study Corcoran and Yudkin attempted to answer the question whether patients can be as well controlled with pre-mixed soluble (regular) and isophane (NPH) insulin as with a flexible mixture prepared in the syringe immediately before injection (7). They studied only 12 patients but crossed them also to regimens based on twice-daily lente and ultralente insulin, as well as to the isophane (NPH) insulin based regimens. None of the control parameters measured suggested any difference between the 4 regimens studied, possibly through a Type 2 statistical error in view of the small number of patients involved. When the results from the isophane (NPH) insulin regimens together were compared with the insulin-zinc suspensions, however, fasting blood glucose concentration was markedly and significantly lower on the latter. As blood glucose concentrations were again comparable after breakfast, this might suggest that while the insulin-zinc preparations give better overnight control, this advantage is lost through miscibility problems affecting the soluble (regular) insulin.

The use of isophane (NPH)/soluble (regular) premixture in multiple injection regimens is discussed below in the section on pen injectors.

Allergic reactions to insulin formulations   Reports continue to appear of allergic reactions following injections of insulin formulations, many years after the introduction of the highly purified insulins. While in many countries the move to these insulins has continued in the last 5 years, often with the additional introduction of highly purified bovine preparations, it must be remembered that recrystallized insulin is still in widespread use in many parts of the world. Nevertheless, even in these circumstances systemic allergy is rare, Granic and colleagues reporting only 4 cases in a series of 4000 other admissions of people with diabetes (8). Allergic reactions can however occur even with the most highly purified porcine and human preparations, though usually only after previous exposure to a short course of a less purified preparation. The case reported by Yap (9) appears very unusual in that the reaction apparently occurred in response to highly purified insulin on first exposure to insulin of any type. Nevertheless, injection site lipoatrophy is also an immunological phenomenon, and has been described after treatment solely with highly purified insulin preparations. Rosman (10) now describes a case in which lipoatrophy appeared during treatment with highly purified porcine insulin therapy, and continued to develop after transfer to human insulin.

An insulin formulation contains buffers and preservatives as well as insulin, however, and allergic reactions are at least theoretically possible to these. In a letter Bruni and colleagues report a patient intermittently treated with insulin who developed local cutaneous reactions to zinc-insulin complexed preparations (11). Skin testing showed an absence of any reaction to human, pork or bovine insulin, but a positive reaction to the carrier medium, and to zinc acetate.

Protamine is, after insulin, the animal protein most commonly administered to man, both for reversal of heparin anticoagulation, and as a major constituent of isophane (NPH) insulin preparations. Given that it is a foreign protein, of fish origin, and highly charged, its low antigenicity is at first sight surprising, but probably reflects its regular, smooth, 3-dimensional structure. Serious reactions to protamine do occur, however, and can be fatal. Following a fatality after sensitization during cardiac catheterization, Sharath and colleagues noted the presence of protamine-specific immunoglobulin E in the circulation of many patients treated with protamine-containing insulin preparations, but not in control patients (12). In a review of the subject these authors suggest that treatment with these insulin preparations may pose a significant if small risk of anaphylaxis during later therapeutic exposure to the protein (13).

Insulin dose adjustment

Insulin dose adjustment remains a major problem to both patients and their physicians. Many patients use ill-balanced regimens with resulting instability. Recent attention has turned towards using computers to analyse blood glucose records and to advise on dosage adjustment through defined algorithms. Patients using such devices are asked not to enter blood glucose results known to be affected by unusual patterns of exercise or eating, but the extent of the problem of under- and over-recording of blood glucose results (14) must place a limit on the success of such computer systems ('garbage in, garbage out'). Adolescence is recognised as being a period of particular difficulty in these respects, with the maturing child often not taking over responsibility for self-management as parents withdraw (15). Clinical impressions that some adolescents do take on their own management with impressive competence were however confirmed by this study of 41 patients, in whom tests of cognitive maturity correlated with both self-adjustment rates and glycosylated haemoglobin concentrations.

Schiffrin et al (16) describe their first experiences with the hand-held dosage computer developed by Albisser. This device works on a comparatively simple dose-adjustment algorithm, generally intended for patients on twice-daily insulin injection regimens mixing soluble and isophane (NPH) insulin preparations. The study was inevitably open (unblinded), but the subjects were already using self-monitoring techniques before being introduced to the computer. Nevertheless, during its use mean blood glucose concentrations fell significantly in the 7 patients, and deteriorated again after the computers were returned. Interestingly, only small changes in insulin dosage occurred (an increase in morning isophane (NPH)), giving rise to questions as to whether it was the data entry and instructions which improved control, or the algorithm itself.

The development of memory meters, and the explosion of the availability of microcomputers, has however opened another avenue of insulin dose adjustment at home, albeit less flexible than with a portable hand-held machine. Various degrees of patient interaction with the computer are possible, from machines at home, through data transmission to hospital-based computers, to data transfer and analysis only at clinic visits. Pernick and Rodbard (17) describe a flexible system based on the IBM-PC, and designed for patient use at home. This includes different means of displaying self-collected blood glucose data, making suggestions as to dose adjustment and, perhaps importantly, explanations to the patient as to the reasons for making such recommendations. It remains to be established whether such devices are capable of being adopted and used by a significant proportion of patients, even with increasing computer literacy.

Subcutaneous insulin absorption and insulin pharmacokinetics

The role and influence of circulating insulin antibodies on insulin pharmacokinetics continue to attract studies, even though few patients now have serum concentrations that on historical grounds would be considered anything but low. Thus, while a cohort of patients treated with conventional recrystallized insulin had mean concentrations of 8.2 µg/l on entry to an insulin trial in 1981, Waldhäusl and colleagues (18) were able to show only differences in the serum fractional clearance rate of insulin when studying patients with and without very high (>25 µg/l) serum insulin antibody concentrations. Gray and colleagues also noted effects of high concentrations of circulating insulin antibodies on apparent serum half-time and distribution space (19).

When patients with the antibody concentrations commonly found on treatment with highly purified insulin preparations (approx. 4 µg/l) were compared with those with moderately elevated concentrations (mean 16 µg/l), then a significant blunting of the rise in free insulin concentrations after injection of soluble human or bovine insulin was demonstrable (20). Furthermore, this was associated with exacerbation of the already abnormal rise in blood glucose concentrations after breakfast. The change in the plasma free insulin profile at this time could be explained either by the apparent prolongation in serum half-time noted by Waldhäusl and colleagues, or be an effect on insulin diffusion within the subcutaneous tissue before absorption. In this study, however, the rise to peak free insulin concentrations was slower in the patients with low antibody concentration than is generally found on subcutaneous injection of soluble insulin in normal subjects. It remains unclear whether the antibodies are significant in this respect.

Studies of the subcutaneous absorption of insulin preparations have, at last, begun to concentrate on the all-important extended-acting preparations that are so vital to effective overnight control. While this interest in itself is a reflection of the recognition of the co-called dawn phenomenon and its importance in disturbing overall diabetic control (21), the differences in the absorption characteristics of human compared with animal insulin preparations have also stimulated research. Nevertheless, many of the factors affecting absorption of the extended-acting preparations remain to be elucidated. Hildebrandt et al (22) report the disappearance rates for increasing doses of ^{125}I-porcine lente insulin, extending the original studies of Binder (23). They recorded a highly statistically significant relationship between dose and time to 50% absorption, for doses of over 12 units. Nevertheless, the extent of the change is unlikely to be clinically significant for doses of under 24 units.

Increasing interest is also being shown in the characteristics of the ultralente type of insulin preparations, in an attempt to define the extent to which they could be used to help imitate with injections the basal-bolus delivery concept introduced with infusion pumps. While the differences between human and porcine insulin preparations remain contentious, with the exception of a slightly longer duration of action for porcine zinc-complexed preparations, the differences between human and bovine insulins are much more clear-cut, even being demonstrable for the soluble (regular) insulin preparations (20). When comparing human and bovine ultralente preparations, again using the ^{125}I-label disappearance method, Hildebrandt and colleagues found large differences in absorption rates, with 50% absorption times for human ultralente of about half those found for the bovine preparation (9-15 versus 16-44 hours) (24). The authors conclude that both preparations would be suitable for basal insulin delivery as part of a multiple injection regimen, but on these figures human ultralente would have to be given in the evening or at night to achieve sufficient overnight insulinisation. It would not then provide sufficient supply through the afternoon if the midday injection was omitted. Owens et al (25) studied the absorption profiles of the different species of ultralente insulin preparations more directly, after subcutaneous injection in normal subjects, and again demonstrated large differences between the human and bovine preparations. Porcine ultralente was not shown to be different from the human preparation. In Owens' study, however, the time of peak absorption of human ultralente was 14-18 hours from injection, and the shape of the profile would suggest the possibility of its being a true 24-hour insulin.

With the bovine preparation, if short-acting insulin is omitted, then no fluctuations of plasma free insulin concentrations are demonstrable in relation to injections once steady state has been reached (26). This is not surprising given the duration of absorption of individual injections. Although theoretically it should make bovine ultralente an ideal insulin preparation for basal insulin delivery, past experience has suggested that its very long absorption time is associated with poor bioavailability (27).

Bedtime insulin injections The purpose of delaying the evening extended-action insulin injection until bedtime is to provide higher insulin concentrations at the end of the night, without having to increase insulin dosage to the extent that night-time hypoglycaemia becomes a serious problem. The demonstration of its effectiveness in adults identified as having morning hyperglycaemia as a particular problem (28) has led to its consideration as a general measure in patients on multiple injection regimens, and therefore tending to receive their pre-prandial soluble insulin injections separately. As is evident from the above absorption studies, even if human ultralente is used to provide the overnight insulin supply, the absorption characteristic of this preparation means that rising or steady plasma insulin concentrations at the end of the night can only be obtained by a late evening rather than early evening injection.

A pre-dawn rise in blood glucose concentrations is a particular problem in very young children (29), in whom insulin is often given at an early hour in the late afternoon at teatime. This early injection may be accompanied by faster absorption, partly perhaps because of the small dose needed, and partly because of the nature of subcutaneous tissue in childhood. Hinde and Johnston (30) performed a crossover trial of teatime and bedtime injections in 16 children from 3 years old upwards, but were unable to demonstrate overall improvement in blood glucose control, despite some improvement in morning hyperglycaemia. Interestingly, however, the youngest children who went to bed earlier did appear to benefit more than their older colleagues.

The dawn phenomenon is not just a problem for people with insulin-dependent diabetes, as has been known for 40 years. If, as some workers believe, the key to management of non-insulin-dependent diabetes is to restore normal basal insulin delivery, then the best timing for an insulin injection to achieve this might also be before bed. Riddle (31) suggests that use of intermediate-acting preparations alone in this fashion should give better overall control without a significant problem from hypoglycaemia.

Pen injectors

The basal-bolus concept of the pattern of insulin administration appears to have taken root after the early comparative studies of continuous subcutaneous insulin infusion with multiple injection regimens (32, 33). At that time pre-meal doses of soluble (regular) insulin had to be given by conventional syringe injection, and many patients disliked the need to ensure that they carried the necessary equipment and syringes with them for the midday meal (33). Nevertheless, with enthusiastic support even quite large numbers of patients in an unsophisticated setting can achieve very good blood glucose control when each meal-time dose is adjusted in accordance with self-monitored blood glucose levels (34).

The pen injector was introduced by Paton et al (35) as a means to carry and deliver insulin for injection in a single portable package. In its initial form the barrel of a disposable insulin syringe was utilised within a purpose-designed plastic mount and dose-regulating device, but the profusion of pen injectors now appearing on the market is generally designed around a purpose-built insulin cartridge. While pen injectors are the logical adjunct to basal insulin delivery with a long-acting insulin preparation, they can be used with a bedtime intermediate-acting insulin injection, or indeed to deliver soluble insulin in any type of regimen. It remains to be established, however, that pen injectors are themselves suitable for delivery of extended-acting insulin preparations, mainly because of the problem of even resuspension of the particles of the insulin complex.

Nevertheless, McCaughey et al (36) describe a study with the original Penject using an isophane (NPH) based pre-mixed insulin preparation, and in a difficult patient group, namely adolescents selected for having poor control (HbA$_1$ >10%). Eleven of 14 patients completed the trial in which glycosylated haemoglobin and self-monitored blood glucose levels fell over the course of 3 months. This fall was maintained in the patients randomised to continue the multiple injection regimen, but was reversed in those patients returning to conventional twice-daily syringe injections.

Formal testing of the newer cartridge-based devices has not been reported. Open evaluations of 11 'interested' adolescent patients (37) and 31 adults (38) have indicated that one such device (NovoPen) can provide control at least equivalent to that achieved on conventional injection regimens, and probably better. No special problems were encountered, and in general patients seem to have been keen to continue using the devices after completion of these evaluations. To date, claims that the pen injector allows a more flexible eating pattern have not been tested against the possibility that this can only be achieved with less good blood glucose control.

Human insulin

Comparative studies of human sequence insulin and animal insulins are now much less frequently published than 2-3 years ago, but in general cover much of the same ground. Pickup recently reviewed the first 5 years of clinical experience with human insulin preparations (39). He concluded that all new patients should be started on such insulins, although there was little indication to change over patients established on animal preparations. There is some controversy over the interpretation made of some of the research studies (40, 41), where differences between human and porcine insulin may be present. These are, however, small enough not to impede or encourage withdrawal of the animal insulin preparations by the insulin manufacturers. Furthermore, many possible differences have been studied on several occasions with differing results, a situation that is not easily amenable to resolution by further similar studies.

An example of such a controversy has been the debate about whether the counterregulatory response to hypoglycaemia induced by injection or infusion of human insulin differs from that following injection of porcine insulin. Such a question can be difficult to answer because counterregulatory responses are themselves highly variable, even when a study is repeated in the same subject. In two recent studies (42, 43) human and porcine insulins were infused or injected intravenously into 10 normal subjects. In both studies, rates of fall of blood glucose concentrations and blood glucose nadirs were similar with the two insulins, and there were no detectable differences in any of the counterregulatory hormone responses including catecholamines and ACTH. Neither study will allow the conclusion that there is no difference in this respect between human and porcine insulin, although, given the lack of physiological reason to expect such a difference, the subject is now probably closed.

There is also still some dispute as to whether human and porcine insulins differ in antigenicity when given to newly diagnosed patients. This has partly arisen because of design flaws in one of the largest and most often quoted studies, although a more recent large multicentre trial does support the hypothesis that human insulin is less antigenic in these circumstances (44). The clinical significance of this small difference remains doubtful. The authors only quote a report on the possible relationship between the development of circulating insulin antibodies and the preservation of endogenous insulin secretion in newly diagnosed patients. In a small study Olczak et al (45) randomised 39 patients between human, porcine and bovine insulin preparations, and observed no difference in antibody response or preservation of endogenous insulin secretion between human and porcine insulins. Both the antibody response and C-peptide secretion were greater in the bovine-insulin-treated patients however, an association in the opposite direction to that suggested previously.

Further metabolic studies of the responses to human insulin have, in general, been in line with previously published experience. In a small group of adolescents, transfer to human insulin was associated with a possible increase in daily insulin dosage, while blood glucose control assessed on 24-hour profiles, and glycosylated haemoglobin concentration, was unchanged (46). Nevertheless, significant differences in metabolic responses were found during 24-hour monitoring , with higher blood lactate concentrations, and lower blood glycerol and ketone body concentrations. While, with a change in insulin dose, these differences do not necessarily indicate different tissue responses to human and animal insulins, they do suggest that different pharmacokinetics may lead to a different metabolic milieu. The same workers also studied the response of blood metabolites to incremental infusions of human and porcine insulin in 6 insulin-dependent diabetic men, beginning from a state of relative insulin deprivation (47). Here, however, giving the same doses on each occasions, no differences in lactate, glycerol or ketone body responses could be found.

In an open study in which patients were simply transferred to human insulin, Marchetti and colleagues followed serum lipid and apolipoprotein concentrations for periods of 3 months (48). While minor changes in HDL-cholesterol and subfractions may have been present at the end of the first month, their overall conclusion was of no significant influence from this change of treatment.

Conclusions

1985-1986 has continued the process of improving our understanding of the pharmacokinetics of subcutaneous insulin delivery, and of developing the means for regulating insulin dosage effectively. Understanding of the pharmacokinetics of extended-acting insulin preparations is, however, still primitive, and certainly not at a stage where the information can be used intelligently by computer algorithms in advising changes to insulin regimens. These latter methods probably have enormous potential when such information is available, and provided the problems of providing a satisfactory input signal (blood glucose concentrations) can be overcome. This may have to await subcutaneous sensing devices.

Human insulin is to be welcomed for its guarantee of insulin supply, and for the explosion of interest in insulin that was associated with its introduction, but it must be doubtful whether in itself it will save any more eyes or kidneys, or make life easier for our patients. It must be regretted that the two families of extended-acting preparations date from 1936 and 1951, their limitations partly reflecting that their modern roles were never intended when originally designed. New extended-acting preparations are required.

Although the pen injector first appeared in the early 1980s, the last two years have seen a major expansion in its use, associated with the availability of ever more convenient designs. This trend must be expected to continue and, if the early promise is borne out, pens may promote a rapid expansion in the use of multiple injection regimens. However, for true flexibility in eating habits, these preprandial injections will have to be matched to more satisfactory ways of ensuring basal insulin delivery.

References

1. Eastwood JD (1986): Insulin and independence. *Br. Med. J., 293,* 1659.
2. Lester F (1985): Insulin therapy: problems in an African country. *Diabetic Med., 2,* 405.
3. Berne C, Eriksson G, Lundgren P (1986): How accurate are insulin mixtures prepared by the patient? *Diabetes Care, 9,* 23.
4. Corcoran JS, Yudkin JS (1985): How accurate is insulin mixing? Patient variability and syringe dead space effect. *Diabetic Med., 2,* 131.
5. Heine RJ, Bilo HGJ, Sikkenk AC (1985): Mixing short and intermediate acting insulins in the syringe: effect on postprandial blood glucose concentrations in type I diabetics. *Br. Med. J., 290,* 204.
6. Francis AJ, Hanning I, Alberti KGMM (1985): The effect of mixing human soluble and human crystalline zinc-suspension insulin: plasma insulin and blood glucose profiles after subcutaneous injection. *Diabetic Med., 2,* 177.
7. Corcoran JS, Yudkin JS (1986): A comparison of pre-mixed with patient mixed insulins. *Diabetic Med., 3,* 246.
8. Granic M, Pavlic Renar I, Metelko Z, Skrabalo Z (1986): Insulin allergy (Letter to Editor). *Diabetes Care, 9,* 99.
9. Yap PK (1985): Primary allergy to monocomponent porcine insulin. *Postgrad. Med. J., 61,* 629.
10. Rosman MS (1986): Fat atrophy in human insulin therapy (Letter to Editor). *Diabetes Care, 9,* 436.
11. Bruni B, Campana M, Gamba S et al (1985): A generalized allergic reaction due to zinc in insulin preparation (Letter to Editor). *Diabetes Care, 8,* 201.
12. Sharath MD, Metzger WJ, Richerson HB et al (1985): Protamine induced fatal anaphylaxis: prevalence of antiprotamine immunoglobulin E antibody. *J. Thorac. Cardiovasc. Surg., 90,* 86.
13. Weiler JM, Freiman P, Sharath MD et al (1985): Serious adverse reactions to protamine sulphate: are alternatives needed? *J. Allergy Clin. Immunol., 75,* 297.
14. Mazze R, Shamoon H, Pasmantier R et al (1984): Reliability of blood glucose monitoring by patients with diabetes mellitus. *Am. J. Med., 77,* 211.
15. Ingersoll GM, Orr DP, Herrold AJ, Golden MP (1986): Cognitive maturity and self-management among adolescents with insulin-dependent diabetes mellitus. *J. Pediatr., 108,* 620.
16. Schiffrin A, Mihic M, Leibel BS, Albisser AM (1985): Computer-assisted insulin dosage adjustment. *Diabetes Care, 8,* 545.
17. Pernick NL, Rodbard D (1986): Personal computer programs to assist with self-monitoring of blood glucose and self adjustment of insulin dosage. *Diabetes Care, 9,* 61.
18. Waldhäusl WK, Bratusch Marrain P, Kruse V et al (1985): Effect of insulin antibodies on insulin pharmacokinetics and glucose utilization in insulin-dependent diabetic patients. *Diabetes, 34,* 166.
19. Gray RS, Cowan P, Di Mario U et al (1985): Influence of insulin antibodies on pharmacokinetics and bioavailability of recombinant human and highly purified beef insulins in insulin dependent diabetics. *Br. Med. J., 290,* 1687.
20. Francis AJ, Hanning I, Alberti KGMM (1985): The influence of insulin antibody levels on the plasma profiles and action of subcutaneously injected human and bovine short acting insulins. *Diabetologia, 28,* 330.

21. Francis AJ, Home PD, Walford S et al (1985): Prevalence of morning hyperglycaemia: determinants of fasting blood glucose concentrations in insulin-treated diabetics. *Diabetic Med., 2,* 89.
22. Hildebrandt P, Birch K, Sestoft L, Volund A (1984): Human Monotard insulin: dose-dependent subcutaneous absorption. *Diabetes Res., 1,* 183.
23. Binder C (1969): The absorption of insulin. *Acta Pharmacol. Toxicol., 27, Suppl. 2,* 1.
24. Hildebrandt P, Berger A, Volund A, Kuhl C (1985): The subcutaneous absorption of human and bovine ultralente insulin formulations. *Diabetic Med., 2,* 355.
25. Owens DR, Vora JP, Heding LG et al (1986): Human, porcine, and bovine ultralente insulin: subcutaneous administration in normal man. *Diabetic Med., 3,* 326.
26. Rizza RA, O'Brien PC, Service FJ (1986): Use of beef ultralente for basal insulin delivery: plasma insulin concentrations after chronic ultralente administration in patients with IDDM. *Diabetes Care, 9,* 120.
27. Home PD, Hanning I, Capaldo B, Alberti KGMM (1983): Bioavailability of highly purified bovine ultralente insulin (Letter to Editor). *Diabetes Care, 6,* 210.
28. Francis AJ, Home PD, Hanning I et al (1983): Intermediate acting insulin given at bedtime: effect on blood glucose concentrations before and after breakfast. *Br. Med. J., 286,* 1173.
29. De Beaufort CE, Bruining GJ, Home PD et al (1986): Overnight metabolic profiles in very young insulin-dependent diabetic children. *Eur. J. Pediatr., 145,* 73.
30. Hinde FRJ, Johnston DI (1985): Bedtime insulin injections: an alternative regimen. *Arch. Dis. Child., 60,* 311.
31. Riddle MC (1985): New tactics for type 2 diabetes: regimens based on intermediate-acting insulins taken at bedtime. *Lancet, 1,* 192.
32. Reeves ML, Seigler DE, Ryan EA, Skyler JS (1982): Glycemic control in insulin-dependent diabetes mellitus: comparison of outpatient intensified conventional therapy with continuous subcutaneous insulin infusion. *Am. J. Med., 72,* 673.
33. Home PD, Capaldo B, Burrin JM et al (1982): A crossover comparison of continuous subcutaneous insulin infusion (CSII) against multiple insulin injections in insulin dependent diabetic subjects: improved control with CSII. *Diabetes Care, 5,* 466.
34. Waldhäusl W, Howorka K, Derfler K et al (1985): Failure and efficacy of insulin therapy in insulin dependent diabetic (type I) patients. *Acta Diabetol. Lat., 22,* 279.
35. Paton JS, Wilson M, Ireland JT, Reith SBM (1981): Convenient pocket insulin syringe. *Lancet, 1,* 189.
36. McCaughey ES, Betts PR, Rowe DJ (1986): Improved diabetic control in adolescents using the Penject syringe for multiple insulin injections. *Diabetic Med., 3,* 234.
37. Jefferson IG, Marteau TM, Smith MA, Baum JD (1985): A multiple injection regimen using an insulin injection pen and pre-filled cartridged soluble human insulin in adolescents with diabetes. *Diabetic Med., 2,* 493.
38. Walters DP, Smith PA, Marteau TM et al (1985): Experience with Novopen, an injection device using cartridged insulin, for diabetic patients. *Diabetic Med., 2,* 496.
39. Pickup JC (1986): Human insulin. *Br. Med. J., 292,* 155.
40. Home PD (1986): Human insulin (Letter to Editor). *Br. Med. J., 292,* 625.
41. Pickup JC (1986): Human insulin (Letter to Editor). *Br. Med. J., 292,* 626.
42. Muller-Esch G, Ball P, Bekemeyer U et al (1985): Comparative study of hormonal counter-regulation during GCIIS-guided insulin hypoglycaemic tests using human insulin (recombinant DNA) and pork insulin. *Diabetes Res., 2,* 121.
43. Perez Fernandez R, Casaneuva FF, Devesa J, Cabezas-Cerrato J (1985): Metabolic and hormonal parameters after insulin induced hypoglycemia in man: comparison between biosynthetic human insulin and purified pork insulin. *Horm. Metab. Res., 17,* 351.
44. Heding LG, Marshall MO, Persson B et al (1984): Immunogenicity of monocomponent

human and porcine insulin in newly diagnosed type 1 (insulin dependent) diabetic children. *Diabetologia, 27,* 96.

45. Olczak SA, Rainbow S, Murphy M et al (1985): Insulin antibodies do not reduce residual C-peptide secretion in newly diagnosed IDDM (Abstract). *Diabetic Med., 2,* 218A.
46. Hocking MD, Crase J, Rayner PHW, Nattrass M 81986): Metabolic rhythms in adolescents with diabetes during treatment with porcine or human insulin. *Arch. Dis. Child., 61,* 341.
47. Hale PJ, Brimble J, Crase J, Nattrass M (1986): Metabolic response to intravenous infusion of porcine and semi-synthetic human insulin in insulin-dependent diabetic men. *Diabète Mètab., 12,* 74.
48. Marchetti P, Benzi L, Cerri M et al (1986): Biosynthetic human insulin does not modify circulating lipid and apolipoprotein concentrations in type 1 diabetic patients. *Acta Diabetol. Lat., 23,* 63.

The Diabetes Annual/3
K.G.M.M. Alberti and L.P. Krall, editors
© 1987 Elsevier Science Publishers, B.V.

7   Unconventional routes of insulin administration

ALAN C. MOSES AND JEFFREY S. FLIER

Introduction

Since the early 1920s, investigators have searched for more acceptable and more physiological routes to administer insulin than subcutaneous injection (1-4). While major advances have been made in purifying animal insulins and in producing human insulin, the ability to achieve euglycemia reproducibly and safely in patients with diabetes has not kept pace with the increased awareness that such control may decrease the incidence of both the micro- and macrovascular complications in diabetes (5, 6). Intensified conventional insulin treatment regimens do improve overall glycemic control in patients with Type I and Type II diabetes (7, 8), but normalization of glycemic excursion and mean blood glucose has been difficult to achieve and the incidence of acute complications, specifically hypoglycemia, has increased in parallel (9).

This Chapter will review some of the many unconventional approaches that have been investigated to achieve a more physiologic and reproducible means of delivering insulin.

Unfortunately, absorption of insulin following subcutaneous injection is highly variable between individuals and within the same individual (10). Variability is seen with regard to the time to peak serum insulin levels, the time to peak insulin action, and the efficacy of insulin absorption as a percentage of the administered dose (10). Multiple factors contribute to this variability and include: concentration of insulin in the formulation; volume of injection; site of injection; exercises; body temperature; local insulin degradation; depth of injection; and anti-insulin antibodies. Intensive insulin treatment programs require multiple subcutaneous injections, a requirement that many patients with diabetes are reluctant to meet. Even patients willing to administer multiple injections daily, or patients on continuous subcutaneous insulin infusion, have difficulty reproducing the kinetic profile of serum insulin levels seen postprandially in non-diabetic individuals (11, 12).

Experimental approaches to insulin administration have attempted to reproduce either or both basal and bolus physiologic insulin release. No single method of insulin administration has yet achieved this goal because of the lack of a long-lived, reliable feedback control system to regulate insulin absorption and/or release to ambient blood (tissue) glucose concentration. Although not the specific subject of this Chapter, B-cell replacement either as segmental pancreatic or islet cell transplantation would appear to represent an ideal closed-loop system *if* the technology can be perfected (13) (see also Chapters 10 and 11).

Much effort has been expended in developing a reliable, implantable glucose sensor that could be coupled to an insulin delivery system to provide closed-loop insulin administration. Shichiri et al (14) have developed an implantable glucose sensor that will function up to 48 hours. This device shows promise for developing an effective closed-loop insulin delivery system, but serum insulin profiles will still be non-physiological if insulin is administered subcutaneously. Attempts to develop effective and reliable internal insulin pumps have been restricted by insulin aggregation (15), uncertainty as to the best route of administration (peripheral *vs* portal) (16, 17), the lack of an effective feedback loop system, and the impracticality of implanting large numbers of these devices in the current diabetic population.

The subsequent discussion will address methods that provide basal insulin and those that provide bolus insulin (Table 1). Some of these approaches have not been effectively tested with insulin, but have the potential to be useful in diabetes therapy.

TABLE 1. *Unconventional routes of insulin administration*

Basal insulin
   Continuous subcutaneous insulin infusion pumps
   Biodegradable insulin-polymer microspheres
   Rectal osmotic minipumps
Bolus (periprandial) insulin
   Oral (± liposomes)
   Iontophoresis
   Pulmonary inhalation
   Rectal suppository
   Nasal

Basal insulin administration

In normal man, basal insulin levels regulate hepatic glucose production, lipogenesis (and lipolysis), and amino acid release from peripheral tissues. Regulation of these processes can be achieved by administering insulin subcutaneously, intravenously or intraportally (via the peritoneum or the portal vein). Successful basal insulin administration requires rigid control of the rate of insulin administration since minor variation in rate can have major effects on fasting blood glucose concentrations.

Subcutaneously implanted insulin pellets

Insulin has been mixed with biocompatible polymers to form pellets that will release insulin at a constant fixed rate in vitro (18) and in vivo (19). The rate of insulin release depends on the physical structure of the polymer and the geometric design of the pellet. The duration of insulin release depends on the size of the pellet and the amount of insulin incorporated into it. The pellets can be packed with sufficient insulin to last for several months (19). Pellets consisting of biodegradable polymers have the advantage of not having to be physically removed when the insulin supply is expended.

This system can provide long-term, stable basal serum insulin levels (19). It is effective in producing excellent glycemic control in streptozotocin-induced diabetes in rats (19). Subcutaneous placement of the pellets would result in unphysiologically high peripheral serum insulin concentrations to achieve the desired effect. This system also suffers from the disadvantage of delivering a non-adjustable, fixed rate of insulin delivery that cannot be adjusted to changing insulin requirements. This problem may be circumvented by the development of biodegradable polymers or insulin complexes that release insulin based on ambient glucose concentrations. This approach offers some significant advantages over currently available insulin therapy, particularly among populations where daily insulin administration is not practical.

Subcutaneous liposomes

Liposome technology has been utilized in an attempt to deliver insulin perorally (21). This technology also has been utilized to prolong the absorption characteristics of insulin from the subcutaneous space (22). Insulin can be stably incorporated into liposomes of varying lipid composition and these complexes do release insulin slowly from the subcutaneous space (22). Subcutaneously administered, insulin-containing liposomes increase the duration of insulin action, but their role in diabetes therapy has not been defined.

Basal-rate insulin pumps

Several external and implantable insulin pumps have been developed that will release insulin at a constant rate. These pumps have been successfully used in both Type I and Type II diabetic subjects to supply stable basal insulin levels (23-25). Modification of the insulin solution may be necessary to prevent insulin aggregation within the pump itself (15). These pumps have delivered insulin intraportally (intraperitoneal) (16) and to the peripheral venous circulation (23-25). Current efforts are directed to coupling these pumps to computer algorithm systems in an attempt to provide meal-time boluses as well as basal insulin administration (26).

External pumps can deliver insulin into the subcutaneous space at a constant rate for prolonged periods of time. The more sophisticated of these pumps also can be programmed to deliver extra subcutaneous insulin periprandially. Convincing data exist that these pumps can effectively improve glycemic control in the majority of diabetic patients who utilize them (23). Unfortunately, these pumps have been limited in their appeal to the general diabetic population because of inconvenience, expense, infection at the site of catheter insertion (27), and an increased incidence of both hypoglycemia and diabetic ketoacidosis (28, 29). These pumps also share with conventional insulin administration the delivery of insulin into the subcutaneous space and the peripheral circulation, factors that either delay the rate of insulin absorption or produce peripheral hyperinsulinemia. The exact role that these pumps will play in diabetes therapy in the future remains undefined and will depend, in large part, on the development of effective glucose sensors to 'close' the feedback loop of insulin delivery.

Long-lasting rectal suppositories

Several investigators (see below) have demonstrated that insulin can be absorbed across the rectal mucosa in the presence of certain adjuvant molecules. While this has been viewed as a means of delivering bolus insulin at meal-times, new technology suggests that appropriate basal serum insulin levels could be achieved using long-lasting osmotic rectal minipumps (30). Such pumps can deliver drug (insulin) at a constant, predetermined rate for up to 60 hours. Rectal insulin administration has the advantage of potentially delivering insulin into the portal circulation if the drug delivery system is inserted to a level drained by the superior hemorrhoidal veins (31). This route of delivery has the disadvantages of being socially less acceptable than some other routes and of being subject to considerable variability of absorption. While some degree of variability may be of little consequence for some pharmaceuticals, normal glycemic control will not be tolerant of variability in insulin absorption in the postabsorptive state.

Iontophoresis

Iontophoresis is the technique of administering a drug across a mucosal or cutaneous surface via an electrochemical gradient. This technique has been successfully utilized to deliver therapeutically active small molecules across the epidermis. Iontophoresis of insulin can be accomplished in rabbits if the epidermis has first been abraded to decrease the thickness of the keratinized layer and to increase cutaneous blood flow (32). While this technique theoretically holds some promise for delivering insulin at a constant rate, the low bioavailability for peptides such as insulin does not favor its successful development.

Buccal insulin patch

The buccal mucosa is an advantageous surface for the absorption of pharmacologically useful drugs such as nitroglycerin and nifedipine. These drugs routinely are administered in bolus fashion across the buccal mucosa, although recent efforts have been directed toward developing sustained-release buccal patches that will provide constant serum levels of the applied pharmaceutical. Efforts have been directed toward developing a similar system for insulin administration (33). Unfortunately, the stratified squamous epithelium of the buccal cavity is not the most advantageous for absorption of large peptides and the efficiency of insulin absorption remains low (33).

Bolus insulin administration

Despite the current inadequacies of insulin administration, it is easier to achieve control of fasting blood glucose concentrations in patients with Type I diabetes mellitus than it is to achieve control of postprandial glycemic excursion. The major limitations to achieving a physiological pattern of serum insulin concentrations (and insulin biological effects) at meal-times relate to the delayed absorption of insulin from the subcutaneous space (10) and the lack of a feedback system to regulate insulin release (or absorption) by ambient glucose concentration (17).

Pressure-driven transcutaneous insulin administration

A number of mechanical devices have been developed that 'drive' insulin across the cutaneous barrier without the use of a needle. These devices offer several advantages for insulin therapy. First, they circumvent the fear of injection that dominates a small subset of patients with diabetes. Second, they promote more rapid insulin absorption than subcutaneous insulin injection (34, 35). More rapid insulin absorption presumably occurs because insulin is deposited over a wider area within the subcutaneous space. This characteristic of pressure-driven insulin administration is kinetically advantageous for improving postprandial glycemic control. In part, these advantages are negated by the expense and the bulk of the devices. Nonetheless, these devices should be considered in patients seeking better control of glucose excursions than can be achieved with conventional insulin administration.

Pen pump

The NovoPen has been developed by Novo to provide a convenient means of delivering insulin periprandially by subcutaneous injection (36). This system has been enthusiastically received by the population of patients with diabetes in Europe because of its convenience. It offers no specific advantage with regard to the kinetics of insulin absorption. Preliminary reports suggest that this device may improve overall glycemic control in Type I diabetic patients, probably by increasing patient compliance in multiple-dose regimens (36).

Transmucosal transport of insulin

The above alternative routes of insulin administration rely on improving the convenience of multiple subcutaneous injections and, in the case of the trans- cutaneous pressure-driven injection, on increasing the rate of insulin absorp- tion. Other approaches are being studied to promote insulin absorption across mucosal surfaces that normally form a barrier against such absorption (Table 2). The ultimate utility of insulin administration by one or all of these techniques will depend on the development of reproducible, efficacious and safe devices or formulations to promote absorption.

TABLE 2. *Absorption enhancers for transmucosal insulin delivery*

Saponins
Non-ionic polyoxyethylene ethers
Bile acid salts
Salicylic acid
Polyacrylic acid
Derivatives of fusidic acid

Oral insulin

Investigators have attempted to administer insulin perorally since the early 1920s (37). These efforts have been largely unsuccessful, presumably because of proteolytic degradation of insulin by digestive enzymes, either secreted by the pancreas or present on the brush border of the absorptive intestinal epithelium. Attempts to circumvent insulin degradation have involved encap- sulating insulin within liposomes (21) or instilling insulin directly into the jejunum in the presence of absorption-enhancing agents (38). In rats, direct in- stillation of insulin into the jejunum results in some absorption, but the efficiency of this absorption remains low and the approach impractical (38). Recently, Saffran et al (39) have coated insulin with divinylazobenzene cross-linked polymers and have achieved biologically effective insulin absorption across the colonic mucosa of rats following intragastric insulin administration. The slow absorption and the variability of kinetics of insulin absorption (2-8 hours) suggest that this approach will have limited application for periprandial insulin administration. It is unclear whether this approach will be useful for providing basal insulin delivery in human subjects with diabetes.

Peroral insulin administration is advantageous because of its convenience and because it allows insulin delivery into the portal circulation with a physiologically relevant first pass of insulin through the liver. Major unknowns are the kinetics of insulin absorption and the reproducibility of those kinetics. Finally, the efficiency of insulin absorption must be reproducible and must be high enough to be economically feasible.

Pulmonary inhalation

The alveoli of the lung provide a potentially important site for insulin absorption since peptides can be absorbed across this surface in the absence of adjuvant molecules. Wigley et al (40) demonstrated that sufficient nebulized insulin can be absorbed across the respiratory mucosa to produce hypoglycemia in normal volunteers. Initial experiments used very large amounts of insulin and the resulting biological effects were consistent with only a very low bioavailability. More recently, another group has demonstrated the potential utility of pulmonary absorption of insulin; however, the percent bioavailability of this system remains undefined (41). The kinetics of insulin absorption across the respiratory mucosa would favor periprandial administration; serum insulin levels peak at 15-20 min and, as assessed by blood glucose response, return to baseline by 40-60 min. The reproducibility of this system has not yet been assessed. No long-term studies have been reported in animals to assess the potential side effects of this route of insulin delivery.

Rectal administration

Many small-molecular-weight pharmaceuticals are effectively absorbed across the rectal mucosa. Polypeptides the size of insulin are not absorbed across this surface in the absence of agents that enhance this process. Several investigators have identified absorption-enhancing molecules to promote insulin absorption. These compounds differ markedly in structure and range from bile acid salts to enamines and salicylic acids (1, 42-44) (Table 2). They all produce relatively prompt absorption of insulin into the portal and/or systemic circulation depending on where the drug is placed relative to the drainage of the superior hemorrhoidal veins (portal). The mechanisms by which these agents promote insulin (peptide) absorption across the rectal mucosa remains incompletely understood.

The kinetics of insulin absorption across the rectal mucosa may differ for different adjuvant molecules and for different dissolution rates of the suppository formulations. Ideally, serum insulin levels should reach their peak at 10-30 min after rectal delivery and significant insulin absorption should not continue for more than 120 min. In dogs, serum insulin profiles with a kinetic pattern described above can be achieved. Data are limited in man (43).

Nasal administration

As early as 1923, clinicians attempted to administer insulin intranasally (45). By 1932, Collins and Goldzieher had successfully achieved sufficient insulin absorption across the nasal mucosa to produce a hypoglycemic effect in subjects with diabetes mellitus (46). Concerns about the reproducibility and efficiency of this route of insulin delivery inhibited significant progress until Hirai et al (47) began to investigate conditions that might allow insulin absorption across the nasal mucosa of animals and man. Recent investigations have demonstrated that insulin can be effectively absorbed into the systemic circulation after nasal delivery and that this route of administration can improve both fasting and post-prandial hyperglycemia in subjects with Type I and Type II diabetes mellitus (48-51). Several aspects of nasal insulin delivery suggest that it may be an advantageous means of treating diabetes mellitus (Table 3).

TABLE 3.　*Characteristics of nasal insulin*

Rapid absorption
Defined duration of action
Reproducible kinetics
High serum (hepatic) insulin levels simulating portal insulin from the normal pancreas

In recent years there has been a resurgence of interest in delivering systemic medications via the nasal route (52). Pharmaceuticals such as propranolol, progesterone and enkephalins are readily absorbed into the systemic circulation across the nasal mucosa (52). For some drugs, bioavailability and serum drug levels are higher after intranasal than after oral administration (52).

Several biologically active peptides including vasopressin (53), LHRH (54) and ACTH (55) can be absorbed across the nasal mucosa without the addition of absorption-enhancing molecules. Unfortunately, insulin by itself does not cross the nasal mucosal barrier in man (48). The factors limiting absorption are not known but have been suggested to be insulin aggregation, proteolysis, precipitation, or a mechanical barrier at the level of the lipid bilayer of the cell membrane. A number of approaches have been utilized to enhance insulin absorption across the nasal mucosa. Collins and Goldzieher demonstrated that saponins enhance insulin absorption (46). Hirai et al (56) studied a series of bile acid salts in rats and Hirata et al (48) studied glycocholate in man as potential enhancers of insulin absorption. Hirai et al (56) also demonstrated the efficacy of a group of polyoxyethylene ethers in promoting insulin absorption in rats. Interestingly, polyoxyethylene esters of the same chain length had no activity as adjuvant molecules (57). Salzman et al (51) demonstrated that a specific polyoxyethylene ether (laureth-9) potently stimulated insulin absorption across the nasal mucosa of normal and diabetic volunteers. Concentrations of laureth-9 that gave maximal serum insulin levels were not well tolerated by the human volunteers (51).

Several groups have concentrated their efforts on the ability of the glycine conjugate of cholic acid (sodium glycocholate) to enhance insulin absorption (48, 49, 51). Structure-function studies performed with a series of naturally occurring bile acid salts revealed that the ability of a bile salt to promote insulin absorption across the nasal mucosa depends on the hydrophobicity of its steroid nucleus (59). Sodium deoxycholate was the most efficacious of the unconjugated bile salts tested. Conjugation of the bile acid salts with glycine or taurine reduced the net hydrophobicity of the molecule but did not diminish its activity as an adjuvant molecule. These structure-function studies suggested that amphiphilic steroidal detergents promote insulin absorption by forming aqueous pores through the cell membrane through which insulin travels down a concentration gradient. This interpretation differs from that of Hirai et al (57) derived from experiments with nasal insulin absorption in rats. In those studies, there was a correlation between a bile salt's ability to promote insulin absorption and its ability to inhibit nasal mucosal proteases. Differences in the two model systems do not permit determination of the mechanism(s) involved in the acute transport of a peptide across the mucosal surface.

The potential local toxicity of absorption-enhancing molecules on the nasal mucosa has led to the search for efficacious and safe adjuvant molecules. Preliminary studies suggest that a derivative of the antistaphylococcal antibiotic, fusidic acid, may serve such a role (60). Fusidic acid bears structural similarities to the unconjugated bile acids. Unlike the bile acids, however, it has had extensive clinical use without significant toxicity when administered orally, intravenously and topically. Modification of this molecule to remove its antibiotic activity has not reduced its activity as a potent enhancer of insulin absorption across the nasal mucosa (60). Data in sheep and in man demonstrate that insulin can be efficaciously and reproducibly administered across the nasal mucosa and that the absorbed insulin has its expected hypoglycemic effect (60).

Whether delivered in the presence of bile acid salts, taurodihydrofusidate or laureth-9, the kinetic profile of insulin absorption resembles that following intravenous bolus injection (50, 51, 60). Serum insulin levels peak in 10-20 min and return to basal by 40-60 min and produce a serum insulin profile that is reminiscent of that seen in non-diabetic individuals following a mixed meal. With sodium taurodihydrofusidate, the kinetics are highly reproducible within a given subject and between subjects (61). This kinetic profile is particularly advantageous for periprandial insulin administration.

In normal volunteers, the bolus administration of 0.50 insulin per kg of body weight mixed with 1% sodium deoxycholate results in peak serum insulin levels of ~110 µU/ml at 10 min and a nadir of blood glucose to 45-50% of basal at 20 min (50). Hypoglycemia is followed by a rapid return of blood glucose to basal levels by 50 min. In both Type I and Type II diabetic volunteers with fasting hyperglycemia, the same dose of insulin per kg body weight produces a similar serum insulin profile but a distinctly different blood glucose response (50). In the diabetic individuals, blood glucose decreases over 60 min and achieves a new steady-state level at ~60% of basal blood glucose (62). Studies utilizing the glucose clamp technique and an infusion of ^{3}H-labelled glucose demonstrate that the prolonged lowering of fasting blood glucose following bolus insulin administration in diabetic subjects occurs secondary to prolonged suppression of hepatic glucose production compared to non-diabetic volunteers (62).

When insulin is administered intranasally at meal times to either Type I or Type II diabetic subjects, a marked blunting of postprandial glycemic excursion results (Fig. 1). This effect has been demonstrated for insulin mixed with a variety of adjuvant molecules including laureth-9 (55), glycocholate (49, 58), sodium deoxycholate (63), and derivatives of fusidic acid (60). In two separate studies, periprandial nasal insulin administration in conjunction with intermediate-acting or ultralente insulin administration provided comparable glycemic control to that of multiple daily insulin injections (51, 58).

The kinetic profile, the reproducibility, and the demonstrated efficacy in diabetic subjects suggest that intranasal insulin is a promising route for insulin administration. Many issues concerning long-term safety, efficacy, and mechanism of transport and action require investigation. Defining the mechanisms by which adjuvant molecules promote insulin transport across the nasal mucosa should lead to the development of safe and highly efficacious absorption enhancers. Understanding the mechanisms by which bolus insulin (administered by any route) alters peripheral glucose utilization and hepatic glucose production should provide a stronger rationale for this type of insulin administration. Preliminary results support a role for nasal insulin as a periprandial adjunct to some injectable form of basal insulin in Type I and in Type II diabetics (50, 51, 58, 62). The effects of bolus insulin on fasting blood glucose in subjects with Type II diabetes also suggest a role for nasal insulin alone in some patients with Type II diabetes.

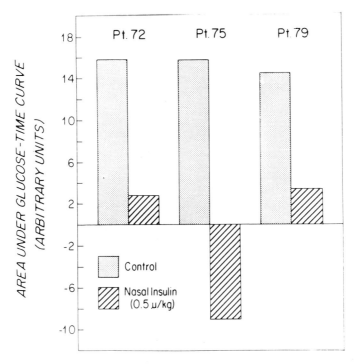

FIG. 1. *Effects of intranasal insulin in 3 subjects with Type II diabetes mellitus on postprandial glycemic excursion. The subjects received an identical 600 kcal mixed meal on each of 2 days. They received no insulin on the control day and 0.5 U/kg body weight on the study day. The area under the glucose-time curve over 3 hours is expressed in arbitrary units. Unpublished data of Silver R, Moses AC, Carey MC and Flier JS.*

Summary

Currently available insulin delivery systems do not reproduce the pattern of insulin secretion seen in non-diabetic individuals and thus do not allow patients with diabetes to maintain normal levels of blood glucose even with intensive therapy regimens. Major research efforts are underway to develop reliable, long-lasting glucose sensors to 'close the loop' for insulin infusion systems or to develop alternative routes and techniques for insulin administration. Orally active insulin remains an elusive goal, but progress has been made in developing constant-rate insulin delivery systems (subcutaneous pumps and biocompatible polymeric pellets) for basal insulin delivery. Advances also have been made in designing safe, reproducible and efficacious bolus insulin delivery systems for periprandial insulin administration.

References

1. Yamaski Y, Shichiri M, Kawamori R et al (1981): The effectiveness of rectal administration of insulin suppository in normal and diabetic subjects. *Diabetes Care, 4,* 454.
2. Fisher NF (1923): The absorption of insulin from the intestine, vagina, and scrotal sac. *Am. J. Physiol., 67,* 65.
3. Wigley FM, London OHJ, Wood SH et al (1971): Insulin across respiratory mucosa by aerosol delivery. *Diabetes, 20,* 552.
4. Collins WS, Goldzieher MA (1932): Absorption of insulin by nasal mucous membrane. *Proc. Exp. Biol. Med., 29,* 756.
5. Chiasson JL, Ducros F, Poliquin-Hamet M et al (1984): Continuous subcutaneous insulin infusion (Mill-Hill Infuser) versus multiple injections (Medi-Jector) in the treatment of insulin-dependent diabetes mellitus and the effect of metabolic control on microangiopathy. *Diabetes Care, 7,* 331.
6. White NH, Waltman SR, Krupin T et al (1983): Comparison of long-term intensive conventional therapy and pumped subcutaneous insulin on diabetic control, ocular fluorophotometry, and nerve conduction velocities. In: Brunetti P (Ed.), *Artificial Systems for Insulin Delivery,* pp. 217-225. Raven Press, New York.
7. Nathan DM, Lou P, Avruch J (1982): Intensive conventional and insulin pump therapies in adult type I diabetes. *Ann. Intern. Med., 97,* 31.
8. Tamborlane WV, Sherwin RS, Genel M, Felig P (1980): Outpatient treatment of juvenile-onset diabetes with a preprogrammed portable subcutaneous insulin infusion system. *Am. J. Med., 68,* 190.
9. DCCT Research Group, DCCT Feasibility Study (1987): *Diabetes Care, 10,* 1.
10. Galloway JA, Spradlin CT, Nelson RL et al (1981): Factors influencing the absorption, serum insulin concentration, and blood glucose responses after injections of regular insulin and various insulin mixtures. *Diabetes Care, 4,* 366.
11. Rizza R, Gerich J, Haymond M et al (1980): Control of blood sugar in insulin-dependent diabetes: comparison of an artificial pancreas, continuous subcutaneous insulin infusion and intensified conventional insulin therapy. *N. Engl. J. Med., 303,* 1313.
12. Kraegen EW, Chisholm DJ (1985): Pharmacokinetics of insulin implications for continuous subcutaneous insulin infusion therapy. *Clin., Pharmacokinet., 10,* 303.
13. Sutherland DER, Kendall D (1986): Pancreas transplantation. In: Alberti KGGM, Krall LP (Eds), *The Diabetes Annual/2,* p. 94. Elsevier, Amsterdam.
14. Shichiri M, Kawamori R, Hakui N et al (1984): Closed-loop glycemic control with a wearable artificial endocrine pancreas: variations in daily insulin requirements to glycemic response. *Diabetes, 33,* 1200.
15. Blackshear PJ, Rohde TD, Palmer JL et al (1983): Glycerol prevents insulin precipitation and interruption of flow in an implantable insulin infusion pump. *Diabetes Care, 6,* 387.
16. Eaton RP, Allen RC, Shade DS, Standefer JC (1980): 'Normal' insulin secretion: the goal of artificial insulin delivery systems? *Diabetes Care, 3,* 270.
17. Gooch BR, Abumrad NN, Robinson RP, Crofford OB (1984): Near normalization of metabolism of IDDM: comparison of continuous subcutaneous (CSII) versus intraperitoneal (CIPII) insulin delivery. *Horm. Metab. Res., 16,* 190.
18. Brown L, Siemer L, Langer R (1986): Controlled release of insulin from polymer matrices: in vitro kinetics. *Diabetes, 35,* 684.
19. Brown L, Siemer L, Munoz C et al (1986): Controlled release of insulin from polymer matrices: control of diabetes in rats. *Diabetes, 35,* 692.
20. Jeong SY, Kim SW, Holmberg DL et al (1985): Self-regulating insulin-delivery systems. III. In vivo studies. *J. Control. Release, 2,* 143.

21. Dapergolas G, Gregoriadia G (1976): Hypoglycemic effect of liposome entrapped insulin administered intragastrically into rats. *Lancet, 2,* 824.
22. Stevenson RW, Patel HM, Parsons JA et al (1982): Prolonged hypoglycemic effect in diabetic dogs due to subcutaneous administration of insulin in liposomes. *Diabetes, 31,* 506.
23. Mecklenburg RS, Benson EA, Benson Jr JW et al (1985): Long-term metabolic control with insulin pump therapy. *N. Engl. J. Med., 313,* 465.
24. Blackshear PJ, Shulman GI, Roussell AM et al (1986): Metabolic response to 3 years of continuous basal rate intravenous insulin infusion in type II diabetic patients. *J. Clin. Endocrinol. Metab., 61,* 753.
25. Pickup J, Keen H, Viberti G et al (1980): Continuous subcutaneous insulin infusion in the treatment of diabetes mellitus. *Diabetes Care, 3,* 290.
26. Irsigler K, Kritz H (1980): Long-term continuous intravenous insulin therapy with portable insulin dosage regulating apparatus. *Diabetes, 28,* 196.
27. Mecklenburg RS, Benson EA, Benson JW et al (1984): Acute complications associated with insulin pump therapy: report of experience with 161 patients. *J. Am. Med. Assoc., 252,* 3265.
28. Braaten JT, O'Leary TJ, Riedel D et al (1985): Hypoglycemia during long-term continuous subcutaneous insulin infusion (CSII) (Abstract). *Diabetes, 34,* 63A.
29. Peden NR, Braaten JT, McKendry JB (1984): Diabetic ketoacidosis during long-term treatment with continuous subcutaneous insulin infusion. *Diabetes Care, 7,* 1.
30. Fara JW (1985): Osmotic delivery systems for research. *Methods Enzymol., 112,* 470.
31. De Boer AG, Moolenar F, De Leede LGJ et al (1982): Rectal drug administration. *Clin. Pharmacokinet., 7,* 285.
32. Kari B (1986): Control of blood glucose levels in alloxan-diabetic rabbits by iontophoresis of insulin. *Diabetes, 35,* 217.
33. Nagai T (1985): Adhesive topical drug delivery system. *J. Control. Release, 2,* 121.
34. Taylor R, Home P, Alberti K (1981): Plasma free insulin profiles after administration of insulin by jet and conventional syringe injection. *Diabetes Care, 4,* 377.
35. Pehling GB, Gerich JE (1984): Comparison of plasma insulin profiles after subcutaneous administration of insulin by jet spray and conventional needle injection in patients with insulin-dependent diabetes mellitus. *Mayo Clin. Proc., 59,* 751.
36. Walters DP, Smith PA, Marteau TM et al (1985): Experience with NovoPen, an injection device using cartridged insulin for diabetic patients. *Diabetic Med., 2,* 496.
37. Harrison GA (1923): Insulin in alcoholic solution by mouth. *Br. Med. J., 2,* 1204.
38. Nishihata T, Rytting JH, Kamada A et al (1981): Enhanced intestinal absorption of insulin in rats in the presence of sodium 5-methoxysalicylate. *Diabetes, 30,* 1065.
39. Saffran M, Kumar GS, Savariar C et al (1986): A new approach to the oral administration of insulin and other peptide drugs. *Science, 233,* 1081.
40. Wigley FM, Londono JH, Wood SH et al (1971): Insulin across respiratory mucosae by aerosol delivery. *Diabetes, 20,* 552.
41. Kohler D, Enzmann F, Kerp L (1984): Pulmonary administration of human insulin in volunteers and type I diabetics. *Diabetics, 33, Suppl. 1,* Abstract 298.
42. Ichikawa K, Ohata I, Mitomi et al (1980): Rectal absorption of insulin suppositories in rabbits. *J. Pharm. Pharmacol., 32,* 314.
43. Yamasaki Y, Shichiri M, Kawamori R et al (1981): The effectiveness of rectal administration of insulin suppository on normal and diabetic subjects. *Diabetes Care, 4,* 454.
44. Kim S, Nishihata T, Kawabe S et al (1984): Effect of gelatin in the formulation of rectal insulin absorption in the presence of enamine in normal rats and depancreatized dogs. *Int. J. Pharm., 21,* 179.
45. Woodyatt RT (1922): The clinical use of insulin. *J. Metab. Res., 2,* 793.

46. Collins WS, Goldzieher MA (1932): Absorption of insulin by nasal mucous membrane. *Proc. Soc. Exp. Biol. Med., 29,* 756.
47. Hirai S, Ikenaga T, Matsuzawa T (1978): Nasal absorption of insulin in dogs. *Diabetes, 27,* 296.
48. Hirata Y, Yokosuka T, Kasahara T (1978): Nasal administration of insulin in patients with diabetes. In: Baba S, Kaneko T, Yanaihara N (Eds), *Proceedings, Symposium on Pro-insulin. Insulin and C-Peptide,* p. 319. ICS No. 468, Excerpta Medica, Amsterdam.
49. Pontirolli AE, Alberetto M, Secchi et al (1982): Insulin given intranasally induces hypoglycemia in normal and diabetic subjects. *Br. Med. J., 284,* 303.
50. Moses AC, Gordon GS, Carey MC et al (1983): Insulin administered intranasally as an insulin-bile salt aerosol: effectiveness and reproducibility in normal and diabetic subjects. *Diabetes, 32,* 1040.
51. Salzman R, Manson JE, Griffing GT et al (1985): Intranasal aerosolized insulin: mixed-meal studies and long-term use in type I diabetes. *N. Engl. J. Med., 312,* 1078.
52. Chang SF, Chien YW (1984): Intranasal drug administration for systemic medication. *Pharm. Int., 5,* 287.
53. Dashe AM, Kleeman CR, Czarzkes CR et al (1964): Synthetic vasopressin nasal spray in the treatment of diabetes insipidus. *J. Am. Med. Assoc., 190,* 113.
54. Solbach HG, Wiegelmann W (1973): Intranasal application of luteinizing-hormone releasing hormone. *Lancet, 1,* 1259.
55. Baumann G, Walser A, Desaulles PA et al (1975): Corticotropic action of an intranasally applied synthetic ACTH derivative. *J. Clin. Endocrinol. Metab., 42,* 60.
56. Hirai S, Yashiki T, Mima H (1981): Effect of surfactants on the nasal absorption of insulin in rats. *Int. J. Pharm., 9,* 165.
57. Hirai S, Yashiki T, Mima H (1981): Mechanisms for the enhancement of the nasal absorption of insulin by surfactants. *Int. J. Pharm., 9,* 173.
58. Frauman AG, Cooper ME, Seeman E (1985): Long-term use of aerosolized intranasal insulin. *Proc. Endocr. Soc. Aust., 28,* Abstract No. 123.
59. Gordon GS, Moses AC, Silver RD et al (1985): Nasal absorption of insulin: enhancement by hydrophobic bile salts. *Proc. Natl Acad. Sci. USA, 82,* 7419.
60. Silver R, Moses AC, Carey MC et al (1985): Derivatives of fusidic acid: novel adjuvants for transnasal peptide absorption. *Clin. Res., 33,* 288A.
61. Nolte MS, Taboga C, Salamon E (1987): Euglycemic clamping to determine the bioavailability of intranasally administered insulin in normal subjects. *Clin. Res., 35,* 156A.
62. Chaiken RL, Moses AC, Silver RD et al (1985): The prolonged hypoglycemic effect of an insulin-adjuvant nasal spray in diabetes is secondary to prolonged suppression of hepatic glucose output. *Clin. Res., 33,* 426A.
63. Silver RD, Moses AC, Carey MC (1984): Insulin-bile salt nasal aerosol markedly reduces postprandial glycemic excursion in diabetics. *Diabetes, 33, Suppl. 1,* 300.

The Diabetes Annual/3
K.G.M.M. Alberti and L.P. Krall, editors
© 1987 Elsevier Science Publishers, B.V.

8   Brittle diabetes — current approaches to diagnosis and treatment

DAVID S. SCHADE AND GEORGES M. ARGOUD

Introduction

There have been many reviews of 'brittle diabetes' within the past 10 years detailing the various causes and treatments of this complication of diabetes. In the same period, new approaches to the diagnosis and therapy of brittle diabetes have been developed. This Chapter will focus on these new approaches which have recently become available.

Definition

The term 'brittle diabetes' is frequently credited to Woodyatt based on his book chapter on diabetes mellitus published in 1938 (1). The exact location of this term in his work is however not clear. The term has been commonly used since the 1950s to refer to a subset of diabetic patients who appear to have greater fluctuations in blood glucose concentration than are observed in the majority of diabetic subjects (2). Furthermore, the term is usually applied to insulin-dependent diabetic patients, but since all diabetic patients have glucose fluctuations, this criterion may not always be applicable.

Is it important to define the term 'brittle diabetes'? Prior to 1970, the answer to this question was probably negative. However, since 1975, precise definition of 'brittle diabetes' has become of greater importance for several reasons. First, an increasing number of studies have been published on brittle diabetes. Comparisons between the results of these published studies is extremely difficult when the study groups may be markedly different. Second, improved clinical methods for detecting the etiology of brittle diabetes involve a multistep diagnostic evaluation which may be expensive and invasive. A clear definition of brittle diabetes would assist the physician in deciding when such a diagnostic evaluation is indicated. Third, and most important, new, invasive treatments

121

are being utilized (e.g. implanted insulin pumps, Hickman catheters, Portocaths) and inappropriate use of these devices in a diabetic patient will lead to unnecessary patient morbidity.

For the above reasons, the physician must make a decision as to which diabetic patient is 'brittle'. Attempts at formulating an unambiguous definition of 'brittle diabetes' have been made. Most successful was the effort in 1977 by Tattersall who restricted 'brittle diabetes' to *'the patient whose life is constantly being disrupted by episodes of hypo- or hyperglycemia, whatever their cause'* (3). This definition was later expanded by Pickup and colleagues who separated brittle diabetic patients into two categories — those that are predominantly characterized by hyperglycemia and those principally characterized by hypoglycemia (4). This was an improvement on the definition by Tattersall, but classification problems and diagnostic confusion still exist. In addition, changes in treatment strategies and techniques during the last 5 years require a revision in the definition.

An inherent limitation in the definition of 'brittle diabetes' is that it is a clinical definition: i.e., the diagnosis is not made based on the result of an impartial laboratory test. However, the low sensitivity and specificity involved in labeling a patient as a brittle diabetic based on the above definition can be resolved partially by establishing careful clinical criteria which the patient must meet before applying this diagnosis. This approach has been adopted for the separation of Type I and Type II diabetes mellitus by the American Diabetes Association (5). Even so, these clinical criteria are not absolute and a few patients cannot be definitely classified as having Type I or Type II diabetes mellitus. Hopefully, as better diagnostic methods for brittle diabetes become available, clinical criteria will be replaced by or supplemented with objective laboratory testing.

The definition of brittle diabetes published by Tattersall in 1977 is no longer adequate to define a specific population. Thus, the 10 brittle diabetic patients described by Pickup and associates in 1983 (4) are markedly different from the 50 brittle diabetic patients described by Lev-Ran 5 years earlier (2). The results observed by Pickup and associates cannot be compared with the previous results of Lev-Ran. A working classification of brittle diabetes is proposed which extends the definitions of Tattersall and Pickup (Table 1). Specifically, a brittle diabetic patient is defined as one who is either incapacitated (Type A) or whose life is disrupted more than 3 times per week (Type B) by repeated episodes of hyperglycemia *after the patient has been trained in the techniques of intensive insulin therapy.*

Using this definition, the patients of Pickup et al (4) would fall into Class A, those of Lev-Ran (2) into Class B. The key to this definition is the word 'incapacitated' which means that the patient is unable to maintain gainful employment, raise a family, remain out of the hospital, attend school, or perform duties necessary to maintain self-sufficiency. In contrast, Type B brittle diabe-

TABLE 1   *Definition of brittle diabetes**

Type A - Incapacitated** by glucose excursions
       1. Primarily hyperglycemic
       2. Primarily hypoglycemia
       3. Mixed

Type B - Not incapacitated by glucose excursions but lifestyle interrupted by decompensation of
       glucose control more than 3 times per week
       1. Primarily hyperglycemic
       2. Primarily hypoglycemia
       3. Mixed

Type C - Unclassified

*Only applies after the patient has been seen by a diabetic specialist and received diabetic education from skilled personnel.

**Unable to maintain gainful employment, attend school, raise a family, perform duties to maintain self-sufficiency, or prevent admission to hospital at least once per month.

tic patients are not incapacitated but do have their usual lifestyle disrupted more than 3 times per week. The latter criteria separates the Type B patient from patients undergoing intensive insulin therapy who may have occasional hypoglycemia. Class C brittle diabetic subjects are patients who do not fit readily into category A or B. These may be patients who have intermittent brittle diabetes induced by the occurrence of a periodic stress or intermittent insulin resistance.

Before classification as 'brittle' patients should have been evaluated and treated by a physician specializing in the treatment of diabetes. Many diabetic patients diagnosed as having 'brittle diabetes' may become 'non-brittle' by modern methods of diabetes care such as home blood glucose monitoring and multiple insulin injections (6, 7). Thus, a diabetic patient on an inappropriate insulin regimen (e.g. 1 injection per day) will frequently show wide swings in plasma glucose concentration (8). Such a patient should not be classified as brittle.

Does brittle diabetes exist?

It is conceivable that brittle diabetes as a primary diagnosis would not exist if all the known secondary 'causes' could be identified and corrected. This is a fundamental question which has been examined previously (2), but not adequately answered.

The experiment to resolve this issue must meet several criteria. First, any known mechanism of brittle diabetes must be corrected. Second, brittle diabetic subjects must be placed in a standardized metabolic state prior to study with normal hydration and adequate insulinization to achieve normal glycemia. Third, the administration of the insulin infusion must be unbiased, e.g. a computer-controlled insulin infusion system. Fourth, the control group must be matched identically with the brittle diabetic subjects. Several studies which have now been published directly or indirectly attempt to resolve whether brittle diabetic patients are quantitatively different from other diabetic subjects.

Service investigated 5 'brittle' diabetic patients under hospitalized conditions and treated them with either subcutaneous (intermediate- and short-acting insulin) or intravenous insulin with pulses before each meal (9). Predictably, all patients improved on intravenous insulin (as their insulin profiles were normalized) compared to subcutaneous insulin. A non-brittle control group was not studied, so the specific relationship of this improvement to brittle diabetes is not clear. A similar approach was utilized in one patient by Conner and colleagues who placed a brittle diabetic patient on the Biostator with excellent results (10). This approach was expanded by Deckert and Lorup who demonstrated that 11 brittle diabetic patients could be well controlled with intravenous insulin delivery (11). These data suggest that brittle diabetic patients can be controlled with programmed intravenous insulin delivery (in the short term), but they do not prove that non-brittle diabetic patients cannot also achieve a significant improvement with subcutaneous insulin.

Attempts to find pathophysiological differences between brittle diabetic subjects and non-brittle subjects have been published. Williams et al (12) studied blood flow in the skin of brittle diabetic subjects and suggested that abnormalities in subcutaneous blood flow at the insulin injection site existed (although no direct measurements of insulin absorption were performed). Subsequent studies by these authors demonstrated no abnormalities in insulin absorption (13), a finding consistent with our own data (14). Taylor et al (15) measured subcutaneous adipose tissue insulin binding, and also sensitivity to stimulation of lipogenesis in adipose tissue biopsies from brittle diabetic subjects. These authors demonstrated lower maximum adipocyte insulin binding and also resistance to insulin stimulation of lipogenesis in the brittle diabetic patients compared to non-brittle diabetic patients. They suggested that the abnormalities of insulin sensitivity in adipose tissue could exacerbate the brittle diabetic syndrome in some patients. This is an interesting observation which suggests a difference between stable and diabetic subjects. Recently, Husband et al (16) demonstrated that during insulin withdrawal in brittle diabetic subjects, their rate of rise in plasma glucose concentration was slightly greater than in stable diabetic subjects, although the change in other metabolic variables (including ketone bodies) was not different. Since the difference in the rate of glucose elevation was small, this difference is probably not sufficient to explain why some patients are 'brittle'.

To summarize, most diabetologists believe (from clinical observation and experience) that brittle diabetic patients are a separate population from stable diabetic patients. There are a few studies which have been performed suggesting that brittle diabetes may be characterized by specific metabolic abnormalities. However, exactly what abnormality separates the brittle diabetic patient from the non-brittle diabetic patient is not known and additional studies are eagerly awaited.

Mechanisms of brittle diabetes

The most common approach to brittle diabetes is to assume that abnormalities in insulin action are leading to wide swings in plasma glucose concentration. Indeed, this may be true, but in our experience it is an unusual mechanism (<10%). It is not surprising, therefore, that long-term solutions to brittle diabetes involving alterations in insulin injection regimens are usually unsuccessful. If, however, insulin resistance is causing the brittle diabetes, then several locations of this abnormality may exist.

The most controversial cause of insulin resistance-induced brittle diabetes is the syndrome of subcutaneous insulin resistance. This syndrome, first reported in detail by Paulsen et al in 1977 (17), has as its basis an abnormality of subcutaneous insulin absorption which leads to unpredictable (often unmeasurably low) levels of free insulin in the blood. The resulting insulin deficiency leads to diabetic ketoacidosis. In some studies the cause has been linked to an increase in a subcutaneous insulin protease which hydrolyzes the insulin prior to absorption into the circulation. Positive associations have been shown between the presence of metabolic decompensation and the level of insulin protease in subcutaneous tissue biopsies (17-19). Only one study has demonstrated abnormalities in insulin absorption patterns in these patients (20). In contrast, we have not been able to confirm the presence of this syndrome in 16 brittle diabetic patients, specifically referred to us with this diagnosis (14). Other investigators have also not been able to measure increased levels of insulin-degrading activity in this type of patient (13). Proving that this syndrome exists is not easy because it requires evidence that all other causes of subcutaneous insulin non-responsiveness have been excluded (such as factitious disease), documentation that the subcutaneously injected insulin is not absorbed systemically, and proof that systemic insulin responsiveness is normal. To date, these 3 criteria have not yet been unequivocally documented for any patient reported to have this syndrome.

If the patient has a subnormal glycemic response to subcutaneously injected insulin but the subcutaneous absorption of insulin is normal, then systemic insulin resistance must exist. This may be caused by one of several mechanisms.

First, high titers of circulating insulin antibodies may bind the insulin, preventing it from interacting with the cellular insulin receptor (21). This mechanism has become a rare cause of brittle diabetes with the advent of purified insulin. Second, resistance to the action of insulin at the receptor or post-receptor level can also cause brittle diabetes by decreasing the responsiveness to injected insulin (22). Receptor-mediated insulin resistance has been reported in patients with antibodies to the insulin receptor which results in severe insulin resistance (23). We have observed one brittle diabetic subject with antibodies to the insulin receptor and concomitant systemic lupus erythematosus. This patient failed to display a hypoglycemic response to massive doses of injected insulin (24).

If normal responsiveness to subcutaneously injected insulin is documented under rigidly controlled conditions, then other causes of brittle diabetes must be pursued. The majority of cases of brittle diabetes are the result of underlying abnormalities other than insulin resistance. Foremost among these other causes is the presence of psychological abnormalities.

Much has been written about the psychological causes of brittle diabetes and the reader is referred to previously published reviews (25-30). Two points deserve emphasis. First, insulin-dependent diabetes mellitus (IDDM) is a disease in which the patient must actively participate in management. Anything that impairs the ability of the diabetic patient to follow accurately the instructions of the physician and to make appropriate therapeutic judgments may result in metabolic decompensation and brittle diabetes. Thus, psychological abnormalities which interfere with mental functioning are a leading cause of brittle diabetes. Second, it has not been proven that the psychopathology always antedates the onset of the brittle diabetes. In some patients, the stress of having brittle diabetes may exacerbate psychological problems. For this reason, even if a brittle diabetic patient has identifiable psychological abnormalities, other causes of brittle diabetes must always be excluded. In our experience, patients with incapacitating brittle diabetes usually have more than one contributing factor to their metabolic instability (31).

In this Chapter, the term 'psychological abnormalities' is used in the broadest sense, i.e. any abnormality in mental functioning. For brittle diabetes, these abnormalities usually segregate into one of three categories: (a) factitious disease, (b) manipulative behavior, and (c) communication disorders, although other categories such as personality disorders may coexist.

Factitious disease is probably a rare cause of brittle diabetes in general but common in a referral population of brittle diabetic patients. We were able to identify 5 brittle diabetic patients with factitious disease as the etiology of their metabolic instability (32). The important difference between factitious disease and manipulative behavior as a cause of brittle diabetes is that, in the former, no reason can be identified to explain why the patient performs the self-destructive behavior (33). Obviously, if the diabetic patient intentionally omits his/her insulin injection, metabolic decompensation will result. Usually, the factitious acts are more dramatic than simply not following the prescribed therapeutic regimen: thus, patients may dilute the insulin with water or septic material (32, 34).

In contrast to factitious disease, manipulative behavior (malingering) is performed by the brittle diabetic patient to achieve a specific goal such as being absent from school, gaining increased parental attention, or avoiding difficult social situations. Since the insulin-dependent diabetic patient can easily induce ketoacidosis and be hospitalized, short-term removal from society's pressures is often attractive. Because manipulative behavior is prevalent in teenagers, it is not uncommon to observe this behavior in the majority of teenage diabetic patients (35). This mechanism of brittle diabetes should always be suspected in any psychologically immature diabetic patient.

The third psychological mechanism capable of inducing brittle diabetes is a communication disorder. This is a very broad term encompassing all aspects of patient interactions (see also Refs. 36-38). In our series of diabetic patients, the presence of a communication disorder was very common (31). Communication and social interaction require many sequential steps as illustrated in Figure 1. Relative to diabetic therapy, the patient must first properly receive the diabetic instructions from the physician (e.g. by hearing or observing them). The patient must then process the information through a complicated series of events which

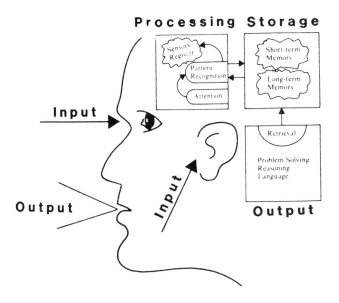

FIG. 1 *Schematic diagram of the complicated mental processes which occur in a patient receiving instructions in diabetic management. Abnormalities at any level can cause a communication disability and result in metabolic instability and brittle diabetes. Adapted from Ellis and Hunt (72).*

are incompletely understood. Finally, the patient must choose the correct instructions at the right time and apply the information to manage his diabetes appropriately. This complicated series of events is not often considered when giving instructions to a patient. A simple example of a daily task which may be problematic for a diabetic patient with a communication disorder is the process of injecting insulin. If a patient has difficulty with following these steps, then inappropriate insulin injections will result (38). All patients with brittle diabetes should be tested for a possible underlying communication disorder.

In addition to insulin resistance and psychological abnormalities, there are several other mechanisms which may result in brittle diabetes. Identification and treatment of these may result in resolution of the metabolic instability in brittle diabetic patients. A short summary of these follows below.

Gastroparesis is a cause of brittle diabetes which is often overlooked (31). The success of intensive insulin therapy regimens is based on the physiological approach of matching the absorption of food (i.e. the rise in plasma glucose concentration) to the absorption of injected insulin (8). A mismatch between these two factors will result in recurrent swings in blood glucose between hyperglycemia and hypoglycemia (i.e. brittle diabetes). An example of such a mismatch is the injection of insulin 30 min prior to the meal in a patient with delayed gastric emptying. The injected insulin will reach maximal blood concentrations 1-2 hours post-injection whereas the peak in meal-induced hyperglycemia may be delayed for hours. We have been referred two brittle diabetic patients who had undergone numerous invasive procedures (multiple Hickman catheters) for subcutaneous insulin resistance when in fact they had gastroparesis as the mechanism of their brittle diabetes (31).

Surreptitious drug ingestion can lead to brittle diabetes by inducing metabolic instability (31). The actual pathophysiological mechanisms may be multiple, and may well be related to the signs and symptoms of drug withdrawal. A cycle of drug dependence → withdrawal → stress → ketoacidosis → more drug is not uncommon. Since many brittle diabetic patients have a background of medical training (e.g. nurses and paramedical personnel), there is facilitated access to addictive drugs. Most frequent, however, is the intermittent use of narcotics prescribed by the physician for painful diabetic neuropathy.

The dawn phenomenon has not itself been reported as a mechanism of brittle diabetes *per se,* but many brittle diabetic patients have a dramatic increase in early morning hyperglycemia (39). This may be related to falling levels of circulating insulin and/or a rise in growth hormone during the night (40). This potential mechanism needs further study as a cause of hyperglycemia in brittle diabetic patients.

The Somogyi phenomenon is a controversial mechanism of brittle diabetes (41, 42). This phenomenon is initiated by the insulin dose taken being excessive for the caloric intake or activity pattern, thereby inducing hypoglycemia. The physiological response to hypoglycemia is the secretion of counterregulatory hormones which in turn induce hyperglycemia (43). Rosenbloom and Clarke (44) have suggested that this mechanism is a common cause of recurrent hyperglycemia in brittle diabetic patients although they did not document the occurrence of preceding hypoglycemia in their patients. Others have doubted the importance and frequency of the Somogyi phenomenon (41, 42). Recent data, however, suggest that the Somogyi phenomenon does exist, although this cause of diabetic instability should be readily correctable with changes in the insulin regimen (40).

Excesses or deficiencies of counterregulatory hormones have profound effects on blood glucose concentration and should always be considered as etiological mechanisms of brittle diabetes. Such mechanisms include endocrine tumors producing excessive amounts of counterregulatory hormones or endocrine gland failure resulting in hormonal deficiency. Since catecholamines have a marked stimulatory effect on both lipid and carbohydrate metabolism, pheochromocytoma should be considered in the differential diagnosis of brittle diabetes, although it has not yet been described (45). Recently, a deficiency of epinephrine secretion together with a deficiency of glucagon secretion during hypoglycemia has been described in many diabetic patients having diabetes for more than 7 years (46). This combination may cause severe recurrent hypoglycemia in patients treated with intensive insulin therapy. We have been referred one stable diabetic patient who became brittle when placed on multiple doses of regular insulin to achieve euglycemia. Thyroid hormone excess can also cause hyperglycemia and mobilization of non-esterified fatty acids (47). The only single counter-regulatory hormone deficiency (in adult diabetic patients) to cause serious metabolic instability is adrenal insufficiency. Lack of glucocorticoids alone frequently results in hypoglycemia (48). Lack of both glucocorticoids and mineralocorticoids can result in severe volume depletion and dehydration, leading to metabolic instability including severe hypoglycemia (48). Clinical signs and symptoms should alert the physician to these underlying causes of brittle diabetes.

Differential diagnosis

The first step in evaluation is the exclusion of an inappropriate treatment regimen. The evaluation must also include direct interview and clinical examination. Delineation of eating habits, insulin injection schedules, exercise routines, and current life stresses are all important in assessing the adequacy of the patient's current insulin treatment schedule (49). At a minimum the diabetic patient should perform home blood glucose monitoring, be on two injections of insulin per day (short-acting plus intermediate action) and follow a consistent meal and exercise schedule. If the diabetic patient is not adhering to these minimal therapeutic guidelines, then applying the diagnosis of brittle diabetes is inappropriate.

If the therapeutic regimen is appropriate, but the patient still meets the definition of brittle diabetes, hospitalization is the next logical step (34, 50). This approach is the only way to ensure that the cause of the brittle diabetes is not an error (intentional or non-intentional) in diabetic management. A formal diagnostic algorithm is then useful (Fig. 2). Changes in this may be necessary depending upon resources (50).

The first step following hospitalization is a complete history, physical examination and routine blood screening tests to rule out chronic infection and underlying diseases. Although in the past chronic infection was a major cause of brittle diabetes, improved methods of screening and diagnosis have permitted this to be detected and treated early in the course of unstable diabetes. In our series of 30 brittle diabetic patients, not one had a chronic infection (31). Similar results were observed by Gill et al (34).

The sensitivity of the patient to injected insulin under rigidly controlled conditions is next determined (Fig. 3). The details of this test have been published (14, 50). Several points should be emphasized while testing insulin sensitivity in brittle diabetic patients. First, assume that factitious disease is present. Second, the physician (not the nurse or patient) should inject all test doses of insulin taken from a bottle to which the patient has not had access. Third, to exclude manipulative acts, at no time during the test should the patient be left alone. Fourth, both the change in plasma free insulin and in the blood glucose concentration should be measured as an assessment of insulin absorption and action. Fifth, the brittle diabetic patient must be in good metabolic control prior to testing to exclude the effects of dehydration, hyperglycemia, and counterregulatory hormone excess on insulin absorption and action.

If the patient has an abnormal response to injected insulin, then the site of the abnormality is next determined (skin, plasma or peripheral tissues). By contrast, if the patient demonstrates a normal response to subcutaneously injected insulin (in our experience, approx. 90% of referred brittle diabetic patients have normal responses), then it should be assumed that the cause of the brittle diabetes is not directly related to insulin resistance.

The next step in the patient with normal insulin responsiveness is psychological assessment. Such an evaluation may take many forms, but the least productive is an interview with a psychiatrist unless the latter has a specific interest in brittle diabetes. The patient should rather be interviewed and tested by a trained psychologist or speech/language pathologist. Many objective psychological tests exist which provide important information about the patient's psychological status when administered and interpreted by a trained professional (51). At least 50% of brittle diabetic patients in our series had psychological abnormalities (31).

During hospitalization, the patient should be placed on an appropriate inten-

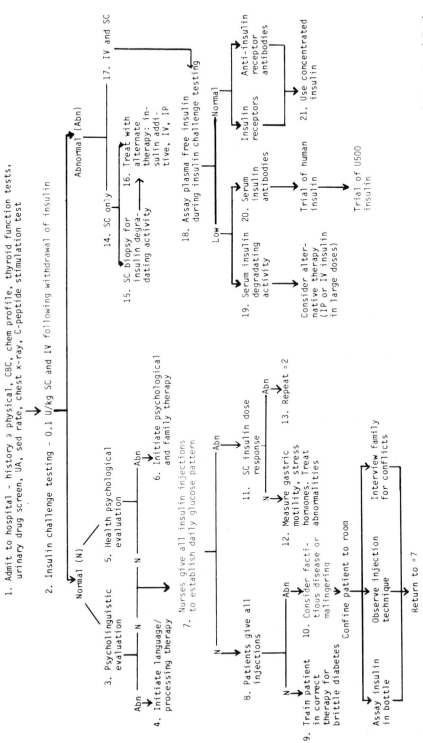

FIG. 2   *A diagnostic algorithm which can be utilized to identify the etiology of brittle diabetes. This algorithm should only be initiated (in the hospital) after the patient has not responded to diabetic education (50).*

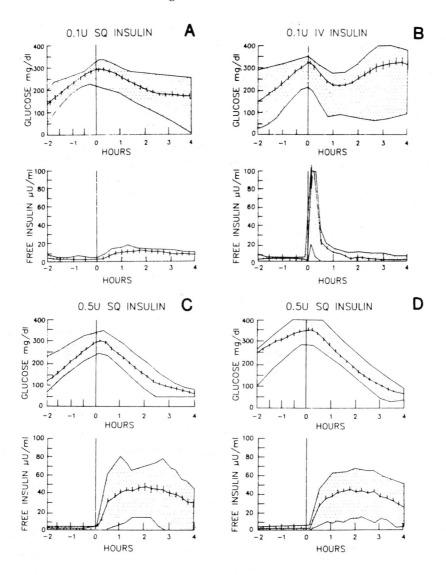

FIG. 3   *Plasma glucose and free insulin concentration in 16 brittle diabetic subjects with normal responsiveness to exogenous insulin. The patients are withdrawn from overnight maintenance intravenous insulin until their plasma glucose exceeds 250 mg/100 ml (13.8 mmol/l). At time 0 they are challenged with either subcutaneous or intravenous insulin at the dose indicated. The response in 11 diabetic controls is shown as ±2 SD. Panel A shows the response in brittle and non-brittle diabetic patients to 0.1 U of regular insulin given subcutaneously; Panel B to 0.1 U of regular insulin given intravenously; Panel C to 0.5 U of regular insulin given subcutaneously; and Panel D to 0.5 U of regular insulin given subcutaneously after the patient's blood glucose concentration was permitted to rise to approx. 250 mg/100 ml (13.8 mmol/l). Reprinted from Schade and Duckworth (14) by courtesy of the Editors of New England Journal of Medicine.*

sive therapeutic regimen (49) under close supervision. Even so, it may be extremely difficult to identify the patient with manipulative behavior or factitious disease who may not perform self-destructive acts when under scrutiny.

If, during the week of intensive monitoring, the patient's blood glucose concentrations do not demonstrate unexpected glycemic excursions, the physician can tentatively conclude that some aspect of the patient's management is causing the brittle diabetes. In this case, the patient is kept in hospital for an additional 2 weeks and placed in charge of their diabetic management. The patient is encouraged to leave the hospital during the day but to return for meals and sleep. During this period, close interaction between the patient and the diabetic teaching nurse will often expose the etiology of the brittle diabetes.

If the patient cannot be well controlled on subcutaneous insulin injections during the week when diabetic management has been assumed by the nurses, then there are several mechanisms for brittle diabetes which must be considered. These etiologies are not uncommon but constitute a heterogeneous group. They include gastroparesis (31), surreptitious drug addiction (31), an exaggerated dawn phenomenon (39), recurrent Somogyi phenomenon (43), and counterregulatory hormone insufficiency (48).

Gastroparesis, a manifestation of diabetic autonomic neuropathy, is identifiable with a technetium-99 colloid meal (52). This diagnosis should be suspected in any brittle diabetic patient with diabetes of greater than 5 years' duration who gives a history of fullness and nausea after meals.

Surreptitious drug administration should be suspected in all brittle diabetic subjects. The patients are usually unaware of a connection between their drug intake and brittle diabetes (see above). Urinary drug screening for narcotics and amphetamines is recommended in all brittle diabetic subjects undergoing etiological testing for brittle diabetes (50).

The dawn phenomenon is intermittent, which makes diagnosis often difficult. Frequent monitoring of blood glucose between 0600 and 0800 will indicate the magnitude of the dawn phenomenon in a brittle diabetic patient.

A recently identified cause of metabolic instability (primarily hypoglycemia) is the lack of catecholamine response to hypoglycemia (46). Since most Type I diabetic patients have an inadequate glucagon response to hypoglycemia, the presence of insufficient epinephrine secretion in response to low blood glucose impairs the patient's recovery from severe hypoglycemia. Defective counterregulation to hypoglycemia is usually observed in diabetic patients placed on an intensive insulin therapy regimen aimed at achieving normoglycemia. This deficiency can be diagnosed utilizing either an intravenous (53) or subcutaneous (54) insulin challenge test.

Adrenal insufficiency is more common in diabetic individuals than in the general population. The lack of glucocorticoids may result in severe hypoglycemia and/or dehydration. Replacement therapy with cortisol in adrenal insufficiency has precipitated diabetic ketoacidosis (55). An 0800 hour serum cortisol should be measured in brittle diabetic patients who manifest signs or symptoms of adrenal insufficiency (56). If low values suggest adrenal insufficiency, additional hormonal stimulation studies are warranted.

If no cause of the brittle diabetes is identified during the initial hospitalization, then prolonged close medical follow-up is required. In our own series, we were able to identify a cause in all but 1 of 30 brittle diabetic patients using the above approach. The 1 patient in whom no cause could be identified had a 'spontaneous remission' immediately prior to a planned hospitalization for repeat testing. Factitious disease was strongly suspected.

Treatment

There are two general approaches to the treatment of brittle diabetic patients: (a) empirical therapy and (b) etiological therapy. The former is indicated when a specific cause cannot be established. In this situation, treatment should be as non-invasive as possible. Appropriate changes in the subcutaneous insulin dose and food intake schedules can control almost all compliant brittle diabetic patients. Frequent monitoring of the patient is necessary both to assess the effect of therapy and to continue to seek the underlying cause. In contrast to empirical therapy, etiological therapy is based on correcting the specific cause(s) of the brittle diabetes. This may be simple or complex and require substantial physician effort.

Empirical therapy has often resulted in short-term success. Based on the assumption that the brittle diabetic patient would be controllable if his exact insulin needs were known, patients have been connected to a glucose-controlled insulin delivery device (Biostator) for 24 hours (57). From the insulin profile, the total daily dose of insulin calculated and the 24-hour pattern of exogenous insulin administration determined. Since no long-term controlled studies are available to assess the effectiveness of this approach, it is not known whether it is superior to using a standard (and less expensive) intensive insulin therapy regimen. Several points should be considered. First, this approach assumes that the abnormality in a brittle diabetic patient is related to insulin delivery, which may be true in only a small minority. Second, despite the drastically different environment of the hospital compared with that of the home, it is assumed that insulin requirements determined in the hospital will be applicable to the home and work environment of the patient. Third, it is assumed that the intravenous insulin dose will approximate the subcutaneous insulin dose in spite of the known differences in insulin responsiveness and availability by these different routes (58).

Another empirical approach which also provides an insulin profile uniquely tailored to the patient is the multiple fixed basal dose concept. Only a few patients have been reported, using this method of insulin delivery successfully (59). The rationale behind this approach is that the patient is insulinized continuously and thus avoids the variable rise and fall of plasma insulin which inevitably occurs with multiple insulin injections. Since no long-term controlled studies are available, the success rate is not known. Several potential hazards should be recognized. First, a fixed infusion of basal insulin lacks the flexibility required by most patients: e.g., a patient who exercises may experience severe hypoglycemia because of increased muscle glucose utilization combined with the insulin-induced decreased hepatic glucose output. Second, long-term metabolic effects of continuous hyperinsulinemia are unknown, but may be detrimental (60). Third, this approach also assumes that a major cause of brittle diabetes is related to insulin delivery abnormalities, which is probably not true.

A third empirical approach is to administer insulin at a concentration of 500 U/ml. Reports of the successful use of this concentration of insulin are scarce (61, 62), and there are no long-term reports of efficacy.

The second general approach is causal therapy, which is initiated by an attempt to diagnose underlying abnormalities which may lead to brittle diabetes. Frequently, multiple abnormalities are present (31) and each one has to be dealt with. This approach is intellectually more satisfying and leads to long-term patient improvement in 50% of brittle diabetic patients (31). The drawbacks are that studies evaluating the etiology of brittle diabetes are difficult to perform and that the expertise necessary to perform these tests correctly may not be available. Because of these pitfalls, all incapacitated brittle diabetic subjects should be referred to a medical center experienced in the assessment and treatment of brittle diabetes.

The diagnostic evaluation will depend upon the expertise available to the center, the demographic characteristics of the patient, and the tests that have previously been performed. We prefer an algorithmic approach based on the patient's sensitivity to exogenous insulin as outlined in Figure 2 (50). Whatever the approach, testing and close observation must be continued until an abnormality is discovered. Even factitious disease, perhaps the most difficult diagnosis to establish, usually becomes evident with prolonged observation (32).

It must be emphasized that appropriate clinical trials of various treatments for brittle diabetes are not available, so that much of the published data on therapeutic interventions is based on clinical experience. Since the spontaneous cure rate for brittle diabetes is not known, a successful outcome may not always be secondary to a specific treatment. Nonetheless, because brittle diabetes is disruptive to the patient's lifestyle and often incapacitating, available therapeutic options should be attempted as long as the least invasive approach is used.

A successful outcome is not always achieved. The reasons for failure are often multiple and unavoidable, even if the correct etiology is established. The

most difficult to treat is factitious disease because, by definition, the patient induces metabolic instability for no apparent reason. Similarly, factitious disease
unrelated to diabetes is also often unresponsive to therapy (63). A second cause
of brittle diabetes — manipulative behavior — may also be resistant to treatment (26-30). Such patients, usually young females, are poorly responsive to
psychotherapy and often use the hospital as a haven from the outside world. A
third cause of treatment failure of brittle diabetes is rarely acknowledged, i.e.
the failure of the patient and/or the referring physician to accept the cause and
follow the treatment regimen. It is suggested that the brittle diabetic patient stay
in close communication with and receive therapeutic guidelines from the diabetes center which made the etiological diagnosis.

The following have been used:

Insulin resistance Approximately 10% of brittle diabetic patients have resistance to insulin as assessed by either overnight basal insulin requirements or a
subnormal response to injected insulin. The very existence of the syndrome of
subcutaneous insulin resistance is debatable (14). Patients who were reported
to have this syndrome were not adequately tested for systemic insulin resistance
and/or psychological abnormalities. Systemic and subcutaneous insulin resistance can have a similar presentation and can only be differentiated when the
appropriate tests are performed under controlled conditions.

Systemic insulin resistance is not an uncommon cause of brittle diabetes requiring therapeutic intervention. Such resistance to insulin may be induced by
obesity or by one of the many causes of decreased insulin action. These causes
are usually categorized as being at the level of circulating factors (i.e. insulin
antibodies), insulin receptor abnormalities, and post-receptor abnormalities.
Treatment usually involves increasing the concentration of insulin at the target
cell, either by giving the insulin intravenously or intraperitoneally or by injecting
large doses of short-acting insulin subcutaneously. The latter approach is less invasive and causes less patient morbidity. This does, however, require compliance on the part of the patient to match the timing of the insulin dose with the
ingestion of the meal.

Factitious disease There is no proven therapy for factitious disease. Both our
group (31) and Alberti's group (34) have identified a small subset of young adult
female brittle diabetic patients who induced brittle diabetes without any identifiable rational cause. Many other factitious diseases have been reported with no
proven therapy (63). The usual approach involves both direct confrontation by
the physician and referral to a psychiatrist, but neither has been shown to be
completely successful. None of the 5 brittle diabetic patients that we identified
to have factitious disease would consent to long-term psychiatric counseling.
The best approach is for all physicians involved in the patient's care to stay in

communication so that invasive procedures are avoided. This is not always possible as the patient frequently finds new physicians who are unaware of the factitious behavior.

Manipulative behavior   This is a common cause of brittle diabetes. It is usually observed in teenagers or immature adults. There should be a high level of suspicion of this as a cause in any brittle diabetic teenager. Manipulative behavior is the performance of acts to attain a desired goal. This is common behavior in all teenage diabetic patients (35) but is carried to the extreme in patients whose behavior induces brittle diabetes (31). Treatment is difficult because the physician cannot remove the 'crutch', i.e. the diabetes. The patient can therefore always avoid life stresses by omitting his or her insulin and finding a refuge in the hospital. Several strategies have been developed to handle manipulative behavior in teenagers: e.g., contracts between the child and the parents can be established. Professional intervention (e.g. by a child psychologist) is required for effective implementation of such contracts. Parents are almost always incapable of correcting the problem without professional help, and indeed, the parents usually deny that the child is manipulating the diabetes. Such patients often improve, either because they have responded to psychological therapy or because they have matured. Invasive procedures should not be used to treat this form of brittle diabetes.

Communication disorders   Until recently, communication disorders were overlooked as a cause of brittle diabetes (38). The lack of detection of these disorders is unfortunate because they responded to corrective therapy. Diagnosis and treatment of communication disorders require professional intervention. Patients must be taught coping skills to compensate for their specific decifit. The physician can help by providing all instructions in writing and encouraging the patient to write down all diabetic treatments in a carefully kept ledger (38). Close examination of these ledgers will often reveal the type of communication problem affecting the patient. In our series of brittle diabetic patients, results of the treatment of communication deficits have been encouraging — more than 75% of patients improve with appropriate follow-up therapy.

Somogyi phenomenon   This is a rare cause of brittle diabetes. Since the initiating cause of the Somogyi phenomenon is overinsulination, a reduction in insulin dosage is needed. A change in the type of insulin given at night or a change in the timing of the insulin injection may be tried. Alternatively, ingestion of additional carbohydrates may be appropriate. This cause of brittle diabetes should always be correctable with appropriate changes in the therapeutic regimen.

The dawn phenomenon   The dawn phenomenon is present in all individuals, both diabetic and non-diabetic (40). However, because the C-peptide-negative patient cannot secrete endogenous insulin to counteract it, this individual may have the greatest rise in early morning hyperglycemia. Several approaches to therapy of the dawn phenomenon exist. Pickup and colleagues give a relatively high overnight subcutaneous insulin infusion to their patients to eradicate the dawn phenomenon (64). Alternatively, a late night injection of intermediate-acting insulin can be given so that its hypoglycemic effect occurs after 0400 hours. However, because the magnitude of the dawn phenomenon appears to be related to the degree of growth hormone secretion during sleep, both of these approaches can cause hypoglycemia if growth hormone secretion is minimal. We prefer to check the blood glucose concentration upon awakening and to take short-acting insulin at that time to suppress the hyperglycemia. In addition, breakfast is delayed until the blood glucose is below 200 mg/100 ml (11.1 mmol/l).

Counterregulatory hormone insufficiency   Counterregulatory hormone insufficiency (i.e. glucagon and epinephrine) is not amenable to currently available treatment. Therefore, patients with this complication of long-standing diabetes should not be treated with intensive insulin therapy with the goal of achieving euglycemia. These patients are prone to severe episodes of recurrent hypoglycemia if aggressively treated with multiple injections of insulin (53, 54).

Drug addiction   This may be treated by standard medical methods. Drug addiction was the cause of brittle diabetes in 2 patients referred to us with the diagnosis of subcutaneous insulin resistance.

Invasive procedures   Several invasive procedures have become popular for treating brittle diabetic subjects. These range from the insertion and reinsertion of Hickman catheters for intravenous insulin delivery (65) to plasmaphoresis to remove an unknown 'inducing substance' (66). Such procedures are frequently misused and result in unacceptable patient morbidity. These procedures are usually employed in patients in whom a cause for the brittle diabetes has not been identified (usually because of inadequate clinical testing).

Several points should be considered before resorting to an invasive procedure. First, diabetic patients are more prone to infection than non-diabetic patients, in part secondary to hyperglycemic inhibition of leukocyte function (67). Second, brittle diabetic patients may also be leukopenic, for reasons that are unknown (unpublished observations). Third, clinical experience with many invasive procedures in brittle diabetic patients indicates a high rate of failure and sepsis (65, 68). Fourth, it has been demonstrated that long-term therapy with chronic intravenous insulin via a central venous line does not correct the brittle diabetes (68). Experience with intraperitoneal access devices is similar, i.e. a high rate of failure and infection was observed (69). Because there are many hazards associated with invasive procedures in brittle diabetes patients, they should only be done by medical centers experienced in brittle diabetes treatment.

One invasive procedure which may be appropriate in a small subset of brittle diabetic patients is the use of the implanted Infusaid insulin pump (70, 71). This constant intravenous (or intraperitoneal) insulin infusion pump prevents the brittle diabetic subject from becoming totally insulin-deficient. Since it is implanted, the risk of infection may be reduced. However, 5 brittle diabetic subjects who were referred to us have had their Infusaid pump removed due to infection of the pump pocket. Whether this infection was secondary to direct patient subterfuge or was related to infection introduced at the time of surgery was not clear. This therapeutic modality will require further study, but its use should be restricted to the few centers with experience in implanting this type of insulin pump.

References

1. Woodyatt RT (1938): Diabetes mellitus. In: Cecil R (Ed.), *A Textbook of Medicine, 4th ed.*, p. 620. Saunders, Philadelphia.
2. Lev-Ran A (1978): Clinical observation on brittle diabetes. *Arch. Intern. Med., 138*, 372.
3. Tattersall R (1977): Brittle diabetes. *Clin. Endocrinol. Metab., 6*, 403.
4. Pickup J, Williams G, Johns P, Keen H (1983): Clinical features of brittle diabetic patients unresponsive to optimized subcutaneous insulin therapy (continuous subcutaneous insulin infusion). *Diabetes Care, 6*, 279.
5. National Diabetes Data Group (1979): Classification and diagnosis of diabetes mellitus and other categories of glucose intolerance. *Diabetes, 28*, 1039.
6. Gill GV, Alberti KGMM (1986): The ups and downs of brittle diabetes. *Diabetes Forecast, 39*, 45.
7. Rizza R, Zimmerman B, Service J (1985): Brittle diabetes. *Diabetes Care, 8*, 93.
8. Eaton RP, Spencer W, Schade DS et al (1978): Diabetic glucose control: matching plasma insulin concentration to dietary and stress hypoglycemia. *Diabetes Care, 1*, 40.
9. Service JF (1978): Normalization of plasma glucose of unstable diabetes: studies under ambulatory, fed conditions with pumped intravenous insulin. *J. Lab. Clin. Med., 91*, 480.
10. Connor H, Atkin G, Attwood E (1982): Short-term control of brittle diabetes using a Biostator. *Br. Med. J., 285*, 1316.
11. Deckert T, Lorup B (1976): Regulation of brittle diabetics by a pre-planned insulin infusion programme. *Diabetologia, 12*, 573.
12. Williams G, Pickup J, Clarck A et al (1983): Changes in blood flow close to subcutaneous insulin injection sites in stable and brittle diabetics. *Diabetes, 32*, 466.
13. Williams G, Pickup JC (1985): Subcutaneous insulin degradation. In: Pickup JC (Ed.), *Brittle Diabetes*, p. 154. Blackwell, Oxford.
14. Schade DS, Duckworth WC (1986): In search of the subcutaneous-insulin-resistance syndrome. *N. Engl. J. Med., 315*, 147.
15. Taylor R, Husband DJ, Marshall SM et al (1984): Adipocyte insulin binding and insulin sensitivity in 'brittle' diabetes. *Diabetologia, 27*, 441.

16. Husband DJ, Pernet A, Gill GV et al (1986): The metabolic response to insulin deprivation in idiopathic brittle diabetes. *Diabetes Res., 3,* 193.
17. Paulsen EP, Courtney III JW, Duckworth WC (1979): Insulin resistance caused by massive degradation of subcutaneous insulin. *Diabetes, 28,* 640.
18. Maberley GF, Wait GA, Kilpatrick JA et al (1982): Evidence for insulin degradation by muscle and fat tissue in an insulin resistant diabetic patient. *Diabetologia, 23,* 333.
19. Blazar BR, Whitley CB, Kitabchi AE et al (1984): In vivo chloroquine-induced inhibition of insulin degradation in a diabetic patient with severe insulin resistance. *Diabetes, 33,* 1133.
20. Home PD, Massi-Benedetti M, Gill GV et al (1982): Impaired subcutaneous absorption of insulin in 'brittle' diabetics. *Acta Endocrinol., 101,* 414.
21. Rennie A, Hamilton RG, Adkinson NF, Rendell MS (1981): Hyperlabile diabetes accompanied by insulin resistance. *Clin. Chem., 27,* 1463.
22. Kahn CR, Rosenthal AS (1979): Immunologic reactions to insulin-insulin allergy, insulin resistance and the autoimmune insulin resistance syndrome. *Diabetes Care, 2,* 283.
23. Flier JS, Kahn CR, Roth J, Bar R (1975): Antibodies that impair insulin receptor binding in an unusual diabetic syndrome with insulin resistance. *Science, 190,* 63.
24. Eaton RP, Friedman N, Allen RC, Schade DS (1984): Insulin removal in man: in vivo evidence for a receptor-mediated process. *J. Clin. Endocrinol. Metab., 58,* 555.
25. White K, Kolman M, Wexler P et al (1984) Unstable diabetes and unstable families: a psychological evaluation of diabetic children with recurrent ketoacidosis. *Pediatrics, 73,* 749.
26. Bradley C (1982): Psychophysiological aspects of the management of diabetes mellitus. *Int. J. Ment. Health, 11,* 117.
27. Bradley C (1985): Psychological aspects of diabetes. In: Alberti KGMM, Krall LP (Eds), *The Diabetes Annual/1,* p. 374. Amsterdam, Elsevier.
28. Fisher EB, Delamater AM, Bertelson AD, Kirkely BG (1982): Psychological factors in diabetes and its treatment. *J. Consult. Clin. Psychol., 50,* 993.
29. Tattersall R, Walford S (1984): Brittle diabetes, a spectrum of illness in response to life stress: the place of 'cheating and manipulation'. In: Pickup JC (Ed.), *Brittle Diabetes,* p. 76. Blackwell, Oxford.
30. Wilkinson G (1986): Psychological factors in brittle diabetes: diagnosis and treatment. *Pract. Cardiol., 12 (9),* 93.
31. Schade DS, Drumm DA, Duckworth WC, Eaton RP (1985): The etiology of incapacitating, brittle diabetes. *Diabetes Care, 8,* 12.
32. Schade DS, Drumm DA, Eaton RP, Sterling WA (1985): Factitious brittle diabetes mellitus. *Am. J. Med., 78,* 777.
33. Committee on Nomenclature and Statistics (1980): *Diagnostic and Statistical Manual of Mental Disorders,* p. 286. American Psychiatric Association, Washington.
34. Gill GV, Walford S, Alberti KGMM (1985): Brittle diabetes — present concepts. *Diabetologia, 28,* 579.
35. Stearns S (1959): Self-destructive behavior in young patients with diabetes mellitus. *Diabetes, 8,* 379.
36. Hamburg BA, Lipsett LF, Inoff GE, Drash AL (Eds) (1979): *Behavioral and Psychosocial Issues in Diabetes.* NIH Publication No. 80-1993, National Institute of Arthritis, Metabolism, and Digestive Diseases, National Diabetes Information Clearinghouse, Madison, WS.
37. Crystal D (1982): *Profiling Linguistic Disability,* p. 1. London.
38. Drumm DA, Schade DS (1986): How communication disorders destabilize diabetes. *Clin. Diabetes, 4,* 16.
39. Schmidt MI, Hadji-Georgopoulos A, Rendell M et al (1981): The dawn phenomenon, an early morning glucose rise: implications for diabetic intraday blood glucose variation. *Diabetes Care, 4,* 579.

40. Campbell PJ, Bolli GB, Cryer PE, Gerich JE (1985): Pathogenesis of the dawn phenomenon in patients with insulin-dependent diabetes mellitus. *N. Engl. J. Med.*, *312*, 1473.
41. Gale EAM, Kurtz AB, Tattersall RB (1980): In search of the Somogyi effect. *Lancet*, *2*, 279.
42. Raskin P (1984): The Somogyi phenomenon: sacred cow or bull? *Arch. Intern. Med.*, *144*, 781.
43. Bloom ME, Mintz DH, Field JB (1969): Insulin-induced posthypoglycaemic hyperglycaemia as a cause of 'brittle' diabetes. *Am. J. Med.*, *47*, 891.
44. Rosenbloom AL, Clarke DW (1985): Excessive insulin treatment and the Somogyi effect. In: Pickup JC (Ed.), *Brittle Diabetes*, p. 103. Blackwell, Oxford.
45. Christensen NJ (1974): Norephinephrine and epinephrine in untreated diabetics during fasting and after insulin administration. *Diabetes*, *23*, 1.
46. Bolli GB, Dimitriadis GD, Pehling GB et al (1984): Abnormal glucose counterregulation after subcutaneous insulin in insulin-dependent diabetes mellitus. *N. Engl. J. Med.*, *310*, 1706.
47. Lakin AM, Bradley RF, Bell GO (1961): Acute hyperthyroidism in severe diabetic ketoacidosis. *Am. J. Med. Sci.*, *241*, 443.
48. Luft R, Olivecrona H, Sjogren B (1955): Hypophysectomy in man: experience in severe diabetes mellitus. *J. Clin. Endocrinol.*, *15*, 391.
49. Schade DS, Santiago JV, Skyler JS, Rizza RA (Eds) (1983): *Intensive Insulin Therapy*. Excerpta Medica, Princeton, NJ.
50. Schade DS, Eaton RP, Drumm DA, Duckworth WC (1985): A clinical algorithm to determine the etiology of brittle diabetes. *Diabetes Care*, *8*, 5.
51. Thorum AR (1981): *Language Assessment Instruments Infancy Through Adulthood*, p. 3. Charles C Thomas, Springfield, IL.
52. Malmud LS, Fisher RS, Knight LC, Rock E (1982): Scintigraphic evaluation of gastric emptying. *Sem. Nucl. Med.*, *12*, 116.
53. White NH, Skor D, Cryer PE et al (1983): Identification of type I diabetic patients at increased risk for hypoglycemia during intensive therapy. *N. Engl. J. Med.*, *308*, 485.
54. Bolli G, DeFeo P, DeCosmo S et al (1984): A reliable and reproducible test for adequate glucose counterregulation in type I (insulin-dependent) diabetes mellitus. *Diabetes*, *33*, 732.
55. Baird I, Munro DS (1954): Addison's disease with diabetes mellitus: a case treated with cortisone. *Lancet*, *1*, 962.
56. Cryer PE (Ed.) (1979): *Diagnostic Endocrinology, 2nd ed.*, p. 77. Oxford University Press, New York.
57. Lambert AE, Buysschaert M, Marchand E et al (1978): Determination of insulin requirements in brittle diabetic patients by the artificial pancreas. *Diabetes*, *27*, 825.
58. Stevenson RW, Tsakok TI, Parsons JA (1980): Matched glucose responses to insulin administered subcutaneously and intravenously. *Diabetologia*, *18*, 423.
59. Nathan DM (1982): Successful treatment of extremely brittle, insulin-dependent diabetes with a novel subcutaneous insulin pump regimen. *Diabetes Care*, *5*, 105.
60. Stout RW (1979): Diabetes and atherosclerosis — the role of insulin. *Diabetologia*, *16*, 141.
61. Baumann G, Drobny (1984): Enhanced efficacy of U-500 insulin in the treatment of insulin resistance caused by target tissue insensitivity. *Am. J. Med.*, *76*, 529.
62. Nathan DM, Axelrod L, Flier J, Carr DB (1981): U-500 insulin in the treatment of antibody-mediated insulin resistance. *Ann. Intern. Med.*, *94*, 653.
63. Reich P, Gottfried LA (1983): Factitious disorders in a teaching hospital. *Ann. Intern. Med.*, *99*, 240.
64. Bending JJ, Pickup JC, Collins ACG, Keen H (1985): Rarity of a marked 'dawn phenomenon' in diabetic subjects treated by continuous subcutaneous insulin infusion. *Diabetes Care*, *8*, 28.

65. Freidenberg GR, White N, Cataland S et al (1981): Diabetes responsive to intravenous but not subcutaneous insulin: effectiveness of aprotinin. *N. Engl. J. Med., 305,* 363.
66. Antony G, Berdoukas VA, Charlton B et al (1983): Plasmapheresis in intractable insulin-resistant diabetes. *Lancet, 2,* 1148.
67. Bagdade JD, Root RK, Bulger RJ (1974): Impaired leukocyte function in patients with poorly controlled diabetes. *Diabetes, 23,* 9.
68. Williams G, Pickup JC, Keen H (1985): Continuous intravenous insulin infusion in the management of brittle diabetes: etiologic and therapeutic implications. *Diabetes Care, 8,* 21.
69. Schade DS, Eaton RP (1985): Intraperitoneal insulin administration in brittle diabetes. In: Pickup JC (Ed.), *Brittle Diabetes,* p. 275. Blackwell, Oxford.
70. Gill GV, Husband DJ, Wright PD et al (1986): The management of severe brittle diabetes with 'Infusaid' implantable pumps. *Diabetes Res., 3,* 135.
71. Buckwald H, Chute EP, Goldenberg FJ et al (1985): Implantable insulin pump management of insulin treatment diabetes mellitus. *Ann. Surg., 202,* 278.
72. Ellis HC, Hunt RR (1983): *Fundamentals of Human Memory and Cognition, 3rd ed.* Brown, Dubuque.

The Diabetes Annual/3
K.G.M.M. Alberti and L.P. Krall, editors
© 1987 Elsevier Science Publishers, B.V.

9   Assessment of diabetic control

ROBERT TATTERSALL AND IAN PEACOCK

Self-monitoring of blood glucose (SMBG)

New equipment

The recent comparison of 5 blood glucose meters by Gifford-Jorgensen et al (1) concluded: 'the future of SMBG appears to hold smaller and better meters striving competitively for the diabetes market, requiring consistent updating for the health care provider caring for diabetic patients' (presumably this latter phrase means doctors and nurses!). Consistent updating is undoubtedly necessary since the pace of change in the market is so fast that by the time an evaluation of a strip or meter has been published, the product has often been superseded by 'the new improved' version. The article by Gifford-Jorgensen is a case in point: they concluded that the Glucoscan II meter was less accurate than four others but had to add as a postscript that it was being replaced by the Glucoscan Plus.

The major obstacle to more widespread use of SMBG has always been the cost of strips: each test costs nearly 10 times as much as a urine test. Cutting strips in half lengthwise is one economy which many units have been forced to make and there are meters specially adapted to read half-strips. However, many have hoped that the cost of SMBG would be reduced by an increased volume of sales and the introduction of genuine competition. Whether this hope will be realised may now be put to the test: we know of at least 4 new strips marketed in the past year. It is to be expected that evaluations of them will be published in 1987.

New meters or updated versions of old ones are continually appearing and gradually approaching the ideal: 'small, slim, light, compact, mains-independent with long battery life, and containing the minimum of mobile parts or buttons... A built-in memory with up to one hundred automatic recordings would also be useful. With modern technology these requirements should be easily attainable at a low cost' (2). The main developments in meter technology over the past year have been a reduction in size, memories and, in some, automatic internal calibration. A memory is certainly useful, but should be 'patient proof': values must be recorded automatically; the need to press a button to enter blood glucose in the memory allows censorship (see below).

Most strip and meter manufacturers provide aqueous control solutions to allow accuracy to be checked. Unfortunately, results with these control solutions frequently lie at or beyond the 'acceptable' limits, possibly because their physical properties differ from those of whole blood. The use of calibration solutions is regarded by most patients as a nuisance and automatic calibration by a bar code on the strip is to be welcomed. It is worth noting, however, that in one study meter reliability did not seem to be affected by the use of the 'incorrect' calibration strip (1).

Does SMBG improve glycaemic control?

The Diabetes Annual/1 concluded there was little evidence that SMBG *per se* improved glycaemic control; in most studies which purported to show such an improvement the crucial factor was almost certainly increased input and interest from patients, nurses and doctors. Up to 1984 SMBG had only once been tested in a prospective trial as an independent variable (3). There is now more evidence bearing on this issue, though much of it is at first sight contradictory. Three studies (one short-term and prospective but randomised, and the other two longer-term but retrospective) suggest that the introduction of SMBG in children does not improve mean HbA_1 concentrations. In Pittsburgh (4) 16 children took part in a 26-week double-cross-over study with and without SMBG added to their usual treatment. No significant differences in control between the two groups were detected at any stage. In a retrospective study of 282 children in the same clinic (5) there was no difference in control between those who monitored urine as opposed to blood glucose, or between those who performed SMBG often as opposed to rarely. Similarly, in Linköping Sweden, SMBG was preferred by most of the 160 children, but over 3 years did not 'automatically lead to an improvement in metabolic balance in comparison to the situation with conventional glucosuria testing' (6).

By contrast SMBG may improve control in adults, at least in small selected groups. In a randomised trial of 24 patients with insulin-dependent-diabetes mellitus (IDDM) (only 3 less than 25 years old) Peterson and colleagues found a significant fall in HbA_1 when patients measured blood glucose and 'had the ability to adjust insulin, food and activity based on the values obtained' (7). A similar improvement was not seen with urine testing. In a trial which included virtually all adults with IDDM in a Swedish community (only 37 patients, but unselected) Terent and co-workers found that SMBG produced a significant decrease in HbA_1 compared to formal education which was equally time-consuming but ineffective (8). To underscore the difference between adults and children, it should be remembered that a previous randomised study in poorly controlled adolescents showed that neither education nor SMBG caused any change in HbA_1 levels over 18 months (9).

A simplistic summary of the literature on SMBG and blood glucose control would be that it works in adults but not in adolescents or children, in small groups (less than 20) but not in large ones (more than 100), and in prospective but not in retrospective studies. There are a number of possible explanations for these findings:

Patient selection   In retrospective studies the possibility cannot usually be ruled out that the worst-controlled patients were preferentially selected for SMBG in the hope of improving control. In the study of Wing et al (5) this seemed un-likely, however, because those who were taught SMBG but never used it had similar control to those who actually used it. Every physician could probably name at least one patient in his clinic who would wreck a trial of SMBG or any-thing else. In prospective studies of small groups, these 'wreckers' never seem to have appointments when the consecutive series is chosen.

Attempts have been made to identify those who cannot or will not benefit from SMBG. For example, Gardner et al (10) found that high HbA_1 levels cor-related with more severe psychological abnormalities, but not with intelligence. They also confirmed, what many have suspected, that patients with 'anxiety neurosis' achieved the best glycaemic control, presumably because of their ob-sessional and meticulous attention to detail.

Non-compliance   Most children and adults with IDDM claim to prefer SMBG to urine testing, but in practice find monitoring repetitive and boring. One explanation for the failure of SMBG to improve control may be that patients simply do not test their blood sugar as frequently as they claim. Self-reported es-timates of long-term compliance vary widely. Wing and co-workers found that 26% of their children tested 3 or more times a day and 37% once or twice (5). This is better than in St. Louis where after 6 months only 8% of children were monitoring twice or more each day (11). In adults compliance (or the gullibility of investigators in accepting self-reported rates) seems better. According to Scobie and colleagues, 'even in the long term, 80% of 55 adults tested once or more a day while 62% managed twice or more' (12). These reports should, like self-reports of alcohol consumption, be treated with an appropriate degree of scepticism. In *The Diabetes Annual/2* we mentioned how meters surreptitiously modified with memory chips showed that three-quarters of patients reported fictitiously low values at least once, 10% omitted meter readings from their log book, and 40% added imaginary values (13). A similar study in London (14) showed discrepancy rates of 1 in 5 in nearly half the 21 subjects. The patterns of unreliable reporting were mixed, with some patients under- and others over-re-porting; it was reassuring that, in general, clinic staff had recognised the unreli-able patients, only two inaccurate reporters being unsuspected. A high HbA_1 was associated with misreporting. Half the children given memory meters by

Wilson and Endres fabricated test results (15).

Mazze and colleagues have carried their 1984 study (13) a stage further by telling patients that their performance would be checked by a memory chip in the meter (16). The result was greatly improved recording, with an error rate of only 1/100 log book entries. However, the authors noted: 'despite these substantial findings and important changes in behaviour, we did not observe a significant change in metabolic control either during the six week period with the memory meter or in comparison with our earlier blind study'. This conclusion was vigorously challenged in the correspondence columns since the patients were apparently not given any instructions on insulin adjustment, which led Davidson to comment on the futility of SMBG without algorithms for adjusting insulin doses (17).

Failure to act on the results Even if performed religiously, SMBG will not improve control unless the results are assessed and acted upon. Hermansson et al (6) point out that: 'many factors have an impact on the degree of metabolic control including... a more flexible and individual approach to the insulin regimen and possibly a less authoritative attitude among doctors and other members of the diabetic team.' The latter is important but has never been tested; it needs to be established how many doctors who claim to want their patients to be independent, actually give them a different message non-verbally. Patients who perform SMBG month after month without getting any feedback from doctors or nurses will become frustrated and discontinue monitoring.

The failure of SMBG to improve control could be because 'tools are lacking to assist the physician and guide the patient in exploiting these valuable data most advantageously' (18). Optimum teaching of the skills and tools required to establish relatively physiological blood glucose levels may require as much as 40 hours of professional input (19). Even if this estimate is correct, it is doubtful whether the ordinary patient can retain the principles for more than a month or two. One obvious solution is to supplement teaching with algorithms (step-by-step instructions for problem-solving). In practice, printed algorithms, like those of Skyler et al (20), are self-defeating, either because they are too simple and exclude important variables, or because they do take everything into account but then become so complex that no ordinary person can use them.

Computers for adjusting insulin dose

Computers may be the answer because, at least in theory, programs for insulin dose adjustment can be customised to 'know their owners' — gender, weight and body composition, metabolic status, activity pattern, insulin, diet — and what the physician expects.

Several programs have been published for home computers or pocket-sized programmable calculators. Pernick and Rodbard (21) have devised micro-computer programs in BASIC for the IBM-PC or compatible personal computers which 'provide a convenient means of data collection, display and analysis; suggestions about insulin dose based on an individually customised algorithm, and explanations of the logic used in adjusting insulin dose.' The physician can choose the targets and strategy and 'select from several standard prescriptions to provide a nearly continuous gradation of levels of tightness of control and aggressiveness of therapy'. This system has not been tested in a formal trial and one worry is that the program is too complicated, tends to be intimidating and requires too much time for input of data.

Others have put their algorithms into hand-held personal computers (17, 22). These are relatively cheap and portable, but their memory is too small to take account of anything except routine life. In the sequential study of Schiffrin et al (18) there were significant reductions in mean capillary blood glucose, HbA_1 and variability of blood glucose before meals in 7 subjects who used the device for 8 weeks. However, it should be noted that during computer use, all subjects increased (? had to) the frequency of SMBG. In the 8 weeks following the trial blood glucose and HbA_1 reverted to baseline, suggesting that the algorithms had not been assimilated by the subjects, presumably because they were too complicated. Computer systems for insulin adjustment will undoubtedly be a growth area over the next few years; a first international symposium has already been held (23).

Accuracy

In *The Diabetes Annual/1* we concluded: 'paramedical personnel and patients can measure blood glucose accurately under test conditions with either visually read strips or a meter. However, there is a nagging suspicion that 'free range' patients obtain less accurate results, or, if the results are accurate, that they are not used appropriately.' Further evidence continues to accumulate to support this proposition.

Evaluations of accuracy often have shortcomings that interfere with their extrapolation to routine patient use (24). These include: (a) using medical staff instead of patients; (b) reporting only overall accuracy over the entire blood glucose range; and (c) evaluating statistical rather than clinical significance.

Error grid analysis is a useful way of assessing the significance of errors. Both Clarson et al (25) and Cox et al (26) found that between 25% and 33% of SMBG measurements deviated by more than 20% from reference readings. However, by error grid analysis only 1.9% were sufficiently wrong to have clinical consequences. The most common error was not detecting hypoglycaemia which, when the test is done by a hypoglycaemic patient, may be more a matter of brain dysfunction than machine malfunction (26). Undoubtedly the hypoglycaemic patient may make mistakes, but several studies have shown that strips overestimate blood glucose in the hypoglycaemic range. Thus, both Southgate and Marks (27) and Rayman et al (28) found that Reflocheck, a machine intended for hospital use, overestimated 'blood' glucose by an unpredictable amount in the range below 3 mmol/l.

There is concern about the possibility of gross errors when SMBG techniques are used (inappropriately, as we suggested in *The Diabetes Annual/2*) in hospital for diagnostic purposes. Last year we cited the report of 4 cases when Chemstrip estimations by 'trained' emergency department nurses were dangerously misleading (29). Cohen et al (30) underlined the difficulties of quality control when blood glucose measurements become decentralised from the central clinical chemistry laboratory to the wards; one of their patients, an elderly man being treated with hyperalimentation, became comatose and would certainly have been inappropriately treated had the ward measured blood glucose of 266 mg/100 ml (14.8 mmol/l) been acted on, when the simultaneously measured laboratory plasma glucose was 1392 mg/100 ml (77.3 mmol/l). The American Diabetes Association have published a position statement on bedside blood glucose monitoring in hospitals (31) in which they suggest that safeguards should include: (a) a training programme for those doing the testing; (b) a well-defined procedures manual; (c) quality control; and (d) a fixed maintenance schedule for the equipment. They caution that bedside blood glucose monitoring should only be used for patient-management decisions and not to establish the diagnosis of diabetes. We would add that these techniques should not be used to diagnose anything else either, e.g. the cause of unconsciousness.

There is little to suggest that gross errors are due to anything other than poor technique. Thus, even the extremes of blood urea and haematocrit which occur during dialysis do not interfere with the accuracy of either Dextrostix or Chemstrip (32). Wickham et al (33) did find a major discrepancy between capillary blood glucose measured by a stick and simultaneous venous values in a patient with peripheral cyanosis, which they attributed to continued glucose utilization by peripheral tissues in face of vascular stasis. It has been stressed many times that nurses and patients will only obtain accurate results with SMBG if they are carefully and systematically taught; there are many examples of how intensive and repetitive this teaching must be to ensure continuing accuracy. It seems self-evident, but has been shown by a randomised controlled trial, that patients who learned SMBG merely by reading the package insert had a 22-37% error rate, compared to 9% in those taught by a diabetes educator (34). We remain sceptical about the feasibility of assuring quality control on all wards in a hospital. It is easy to assume that because nurses are highly skilled in other roles, they are also competent in SMBG. That this is not so is shown by the study of Laus et al (35), where specialist nurses operating a Biostator but only 'casually trained' in SMBG obtained inaccurate (over 15% deviation from the reference method) results in 63% of cases.

We are apprehensive about suggestions that the inaccuracy of meters at the upper or lower end of the range can be overcome by diluting blood samples or shortening the incubation time (36).

The present status of SMBG

SMBG is not a panacea for bad glycaemic control. Nevertheless, it does have considerable advantages over urine testing, especially in the following cases:
a. Patients receiving intensive insulin therapy whose blood glucose is usually within the normal range. Here it is the only method of monitoring which can measure, as opposed to infer, low blood glucose concentrations (with the provisos listed earlier).
b. Women who are pregnant or planning pregnancy.
c. Patients with insulin-dependent diabetes who have lost their 'warning' of hypoglycaemia.
d. Those with an unusually high or low renal threshold for glucose.
e. Those who dislike urine testing but are prepared to do regular monitoring.

Guidelines for the use of SMBG have recently been published by the American Diabetes Association (31). We would add two further points:
a. Urine testing for ketones is still essential where blood glucose concentrations are persistently elevated or where the patient has an intercurrent illness: one disadvantage of SMBG is that it may blind patient and doctor to normoglycaemic ketoacidosis.
b. SMBG can be used either for monitoring or problem-solving. Monitoring is a continuous, potentially monotonous, process in which diabetes control is checked day by day to provide continuous feedback to the patient. Problem-solving is an intensive short-term exercise, for specific purposes.

Glycated proteins

As discussed by Peterson and Formby in *The Diabetes Annual/2*, many, if not all, proteins with suitably reactive amino groups can be modified by hyperglycaemia. The term 'glycation' is now preferred to glycosylation, or glucosylation, as it describes the chemistry more correctly (37). Protein glycation may be a cause of complications, but is useful in assessing chronic glycaemic control, since the level of glycation of any protein is proportional to the average glucose concentration during its lifespan in the circulation or tissues.

Methods for measuring glycated haemoglobin are well established, but have many drawbacks, and newer techniques for measuring other glycated proteins, which are assuming greater importance, will be discussed in this section. Glycation of nail (38), skin from the sole of the foot (39) and maternal hair during pregnancy (40) have been reported as useful measures of control, but glycated plasma proteins currently offer the most promise.

Glycated haemoglobin

Glycated haemoglobin (HbA_1) has been used to assess control for almost 10 years, since the introduction of practicable and commercially available methods. For routine purposes, most laboratories now use mini-column ion-exchange chromatography, phenylboronate affinity chromatography, agar gel electroendosmosis or the thiobarbiturate colorimetric technique. These have been reviewed several times in the past year (41-44). No method has clear superiority over the others; the cost (of equipment and labour) must be balanced against reliability. The cheaper assays are difficult to standardise and control. High-pressure liquid chromatography offers greater precision, at higher cost, for research purposes.

Problems with assay precision and reproducibility have led to doubts about the clinical value of glycated haemoglobin measurement. Column methods, in particular, are unreliable unless assay conditions are carefully controlled. Their temperature dependence has been well described (45) though Bisse and colleagues have described a new, less temperature-sensitive microchromatographic method using a non-cyanide buffer system (46).

A major problem has been finding suitable and stable standards for assay control and comparison of results from clinic to clinic. Mosca et al (47) found no significant change in glycated haemoglobin level in ethylene-glycol-stabilized haemolysates during 10 months storage at $-20°C$. Little et al (48) also used erythrocyte haemolysates as standards, but noted the impossibility of preparing a common standard for all the various HbA_1 assays, some of which measure different glycated haemoglobin species.

Another problem is to avoid being misled by the concentration of labile aldimine intermediate, which is usually less than one-twentieth of that of stable HbA_{1c}, but can increase rapidly by up to 4-fold when blood glucose rises unusually high (49). This labile fraction should be removed by dialysis, saline incubation (the simplest technique) or one of the several available chemical methods (50). The suggestion that stable HbA_{1c} can be calculated from total HbA_{1c} and co-incident serum glucose (51) seems to overlook the variable time course of glycaemic excursions.

Other distortions have been reported. Burden (52) cautioned that direct glycation by fructose can cause spuriously raised glycated haemoglobin levels in patients who include fructose in their diet. Eberentz-Lhomme (53) has again drawn attention to the influence of haemoglobinopathies, which may be the cause of unexpected HbA_1 results, as can transfused blood stored in dextrose (54).

Glycated haemoglobin is an index of control not directly available to patients, though samples posted on filter paper (55) or in special collector bottles (56) can be assayed. Results can either be posted back by the laboratory, or be available for the next clinic visit.

Glycated plasma protein

Glycation of plasma proteins was first described in 1979 (57, 58), and may be more valuable than glycated haemoglobin as an index of diabetic control. Plasma proteins are a complex mixture with variable half-life (mean 30 days). Albumin has a half-life of 15-20 days, and therefore serves as a short rather than a medium-term index of diabetic control (59).

Available methods include colorimetry (based on the thiobarbituric reaction first described by Fluckiger (60), furosine/HPLC (61), and affinity chromatography on aminophenylboronic acid agarose columns (62, 63). Rendell (64) has suggested that results with crude plasma are essentially the same as those after extensive purification of albumin. Hence the affinity procedure can quantitate percent glycated albumin without prior purification of albumin (64). Unfortunately, since these assays are labour-intensive and time-consuming, and cannot be automated, they are unsuitable for large numbers of samples. Only the methods of Moore et al (65) (a semi-automated colorimetric technique), and Hayashi et al (66) (a fluorimetric assay which does not require prior separation of albumin) are feasible for routine use. Little and colleagues have measured glycated protein in filter-paper spots (67).

Fructosamine

The term 'fructosamine' (a name for the ketoamine products of protein glycation formed when glucose bound to protein by aldimine linkage undergoes the Amadori rearrangement) was brought into widespread use by Baker and colleagues. They exploited the reducing properties of fructosamines in alkaline solution to pioneer a novel colorimetric technique (68), the first assay of glycated serum proteins to have widespread potential as a routine test. It depends on the colour developed by reduction of nitroblue tetrazolium, in carbonate buffer at pH 10.8 (optimal reaction conditions are still debated, more recent publications suggesting a slightly lower pH) (69). Kinetic analysis (measurement of the rate of colour development) after initial preincubation of sample and reagents eliminates the contribution of most non-specific reductants in plasma (71). The assay is quickly becoming popular with laboratories as a simpler, cheaper and more reliable test than HbA$_1$. It can be performed on autoanalysers (69, 71-73), with obvious savings of time and money. Within-batch variation of around 1%, and 3% between batches, can be expected (74), better figures than those for most generally available HbA$_1$ assays.

A solution of 1-deoxy-1-morphilinofructose (DMF; a synthetic fructosamine which can be prepared in pure crystalline form) in albumin shows similar reducing activity and can be used as a primary standard (69). Most commercial kits now provide secondary standards prepared using glycated bovine serum albumin, which are less sensitive to changes in reaction conditions. Despite the availability of these apparently robust standards, there is alarming disparity between the 'normal' ranges (in non-diabetics) published by different laboratories. Thus, while Zeyen and colleagues quote a reference range of 1.93-2.54 mmol/l (74) and Baker and colleagues 1.87-2.87 (69), Hindle and colleagues found a mean of 0.69 in adults, and a lower figure (0.59) in children (75). It is to be hoped that the reasons for these differences can be identified, and international agreement on methodology and standards reached.

Zeyen and colleagues have reported that haemolysis (≤ 0.4 mmol/l), hyperbilirubinaemia (342 μmol/l), hyperglycaemia (≤ 50 mmol/l) and α-ketoglutaric acid (≤ 10 mmol/l) do not affect the assay, though lipaemia (triglycerides > 3.5 mmol/l) causes interference (74). However Baker and colleagues did find interference in icteric samples (bilirubin > 60 μmol/l), but no other problems from 28 potentially interfering substances, including common drugs (69). It is generally agreed that fructosamine measured in heparinised or EDTA plasma is 7-15% lower than in serum (69, 74), but fluoride oxalate has no effect on the result.

Technically the assay seems satisfactory, but few clinical studies have been published, and much work remains to be done. The kinetics of protein glycation are not established: Are all plasma proteins glycated at the same rate? Is the relation of blood glucose to fructosamine direct and linear? Is there a threshold? Can the mechanism become saturated, as has been suggested for haemoglobin? Periods of hypoglycaemia during the night will not 'undo' glycation, but may lead to misleadingly low results and a false impression that all is well.

Both glycated albumins *and* globulins are measured as fructosamines. Although albumin molecules predominate in plasma, the longer half-life of globulins increases their contribution to total fructosamine. Lloyd et al (76) confirmed that colorimetric assay of serum fructosamine corresponds equally to serum glycated albumin and glycated total protein (determined by affinity chromatography). The effect of abnormal plasma protein concentration on fructosamine results has not been settled. No significant effect was seen in studies of sick hypoalbuminaemic patients (73), and women on oestrogens, or pregnant (71), and other patients with albumin < 30 g/l (74). However, McCance et al (77) have recently described an effect of hypoalbuminaemia, and

have proposed that results should be reported as an index: (fructosamine ×
100)/albumin. This index has the incidental merit that results are expressed in
whole numbers.

So far the only clinical studies of fructosamine are simple cross-sectional surveys at a single point in time; longitudinal studies with well-documented
changes in glycaemic control are not yet available. Ross et al (78) found the
fructosamine assay discriminated between 3 groups of patients (defined by clinical criteria as well, moderately or poorly controlled) better than colorimetric
HbA_1 or glycated plasma protein assays. HbA_1 and fructosamine reflect blood
glucose over different time periods, so it is to be expected that results will not
always correlate closely.

At first sight, the fructosamine assay seems of particular value during diabetic
pregnancy. Six to 8 weeks of improved glycaemic control must pass before the
concentration of glycated haemoglobin will fall significantly. Reduced glycation
of albumin gives earlier confirmation of improved diabetic control. Five studies
have looked at glycated plasma proteins in pregnancy (79-83). Given the known
fall of plasma albumin levels, especially during the latter stages of pregnancy, it
is surprising that fructosamine levels have been reported not to decline. Perhaps
the explanation is the simultaneous increase in globulin levels, indicating the
need for a more complex protein 'correction' of fructosamine results than an
index based on albumin alone.

Conclusions

Even experienced physicians frequently misjudge how well patients are controlled. Such mistakes can have serious consequences, at worst unwarranted
advice to take more insulin. The appeal of a simple, reliable, objective estimate
of chronic glucose control from a single blood sample is obvious, both in routine
practice, and especially in research.

Still the question must be asked: Has the measurement of HbA_1 and other
glycated proteins been of any value in the control of diabetes? As with SMBG,
the information is but a starting point — a recipe for action.

Doctors must be experienced in the limitations of available monitoring
techniques and interpretation of the results. Maximal benefit to the patient
cannot be obtained unless all the physiological and technical factors which influence the results are properly considered. Use of these tests should be limited to
the most appropriate clinical situations (40); laboratories must ensure that the
results are reliable.

The attraction of a single-sample test has encouraged the use of glycated
proteins in diagnosis of diabetes (84-88), but Albutt et al (84) conclude that the
glucose tolerance test (although time-consuming and poorly reproducible) still
remains the test of choice. At present, the lack of a commonly agreed method

and of reference materials preclude standard application of the new tests, which are neither sufficiently sensitive nor specific. However, HbA_1 uniquely offers the possibility of retrospective diagnosis — it is stable post-mortem! (89).

References

1. Gifford-Jorgensen RA, Borchert J, Hassanein R et al (1986): Comparison of five glucose meters for self-monitoring of blood glucose by diabetic patients. *Diabetes Care, 9*, 70.
2. Petranyi G, Kyne DA, Alberti KGMM (1986): Evaluation of four modern home blood glucose meters including two memory meters. *Diabetic Med., 3*, 187.
3. Worth R, Home PD, Johnston DG et al (1982): Intensive attention improves glycaemic control in insulin-dependent diabetics without further advantage from home blood glucose monitoring: a controlled trial. *Br. Med. J., 285*, 1233.
4. Daneman D, Siminerio L, Transue D (1985): The role of self-monitoring of blood glucose in the routine management of children with insulin-dependent diabetes mellitus. *Diabetes Care, 8*, 1.
5. Wing RR, Lamparski DM, Zaslow S et al (1985): Frequency and accuracy of self-monitoring of blood glucose in children: relationship to glycaemic control. *Diabetes Care, 8*, 214.
6. Hermansson G, Ludvigsson J, Larsson Y (1986): Home blood glucose monitoring in diabetic children and adolescents: a 3 year feasibility study. *Acta Peadiatr. Scand., 75*, 98.
7. Peterson CM, Jones RL, Drexler AJ et al (1984): A randomised comparative crossover evaluation of glucose monitoring technologies. *Diabetes Res., 1*, 195.
8. Terent A, Hagfall O, Cederholm V (1985): The effect of education and self-monitoring of blood glucose on glycosylated haemoglobin in type I diabetes: a controlled 18 month trial in a representative population. *Acta Med. Scand., 217*, 47.
9. Mann N, Noronha J, Johnston DI (1984): A prospective study to evaluate the benefits of long-term self-monitoring of blood glucose in diabetic children. *Diabetes Care, 7*, 322.
10. Gardner DF, Eastman BG, Mehl TD (1985): Effect of psychosocial factors on success in a program of self-glucose monitoring. *Diabetes Res., 2*, 89.
11. Carney RM, Schecter R, Homa M et al (1983): The effects of blood glucose testing versus urine sugar testing on the metabolic control of insulin-dependent diabetic children. *Diabetes Care, 6*, 378.
12. Scobie IN, Bowden UK, Lowy C et al (1985): A consumer-orientated survey of long-term home blood glucose monitoring. *Pract. Diabetes, 2*, 33.
13. Mazze RS, Shamoon H, Pasmantier R et al (1984): Reliability of home blood glucose monitoring by patients with diabetes mellitus. *Am. J. Med., 77*, 211.
14. Williams CD, Scobie IN, Till S et al (1986): Use of memory meters to measure compliance with home blood glucose monitoring. Submitted for publication.
15. Wilson DP, Endres RK (1986): Compliance with blood glucose monitoring in children with type 1 diabetes mellitus. *J. Pediatr., 108*, 1022.
16. Mazze RS, Pasmantier R, Murphy JA et al (1985): Self-monitoring of capillary blood glucose: changing the performance of individuals with diabetes. *Diabetes Care, 8*, 207.
17. Davidson MB (1986): Futility of self-monitoring of blood glucose without algorithms for adjusting insulin doses. *Diabetes Care, 9*, 320.
18. Schiffrin A, Mihic M, Liebel BS et al (1985): Computer assisted insulin dosage adjustment. *Diabetes Care, 8*, 545.
19. Jovanovic L, Peterson CM (1984): Comparison of educational programs to normalise the glycosylated haemoglobin levels in insulin-dependent diabetic patients. *Diabetes Educ., 10*, 40.

20. Skyler J, Skyler DS, Seigler D et al (1981): Algorithms for adjustment of insulin dosage by patients who monitor blood glucose. *Diabetes Care, 4,* 311.
21. Pernick NL, Rodbard D (1986): Personal computer programs to assist with self-monitoring of blood glucose and self-adjustment of insulin dosage. *Diabetes Care, 9,* 61.
22. Chanoch LH, Jovanovic L, Peterson CM (1985): The evaluation of a pocket computer as an aid to insulin dose determination by patients. *Diabetes Care, 8,* 172.
23. Albisser AM, Beyer J (1986): Meeting report: First International Symposium on Computer Systems for Insulin Adjustment in Diabetes Mellitus. *Diabetes Care, 9,* 208.
24. Pohl SL, Gonder-Frederick L, Cox DJ et al (1985): Self-measurement of blood glucose: clinical significance of patient generated measurements. *Diabetes Care, 8,* 617.
25. Clarson C, Daneman D, Frank M et al (1985): Self-monitoring of blood glucose: how accurate are children with diabetes at reading Chemstrip bG? *Diabetes Care, 8,* 354.
26. Cox DJ, Clarke WL, Gonder-Frederick L et al (1985): Accuracy of perceiving blood glucose in IDDM. *Diabetes Care, 8,* 529.
27. Southgate HJ, Marks V (1986): Measurement of hypoglycaemia by Reflocheck. *Pract. Diabetes, 3,* 206.
28. Rayman G, Spencer PD, Tillyer CR et al (1984): Evaluation of a self-calibrating blood glucose monitoring. *Diabetes Care, 7,* 378.
29. Coppack SW, Mitchell D, McIntosh CS (1985): Accuracy of BM Test Glycemie 20-800 strips. *Diabetic Med., 2.* 146.
30. Cohen FE, Sater B, Feingold KR (1986): Potential danger of extending SMBG techniques to hospital wards. *Diabetes Care, 9,* 320.
31. American Diabetes Association (1986): Position statement: bedside blood glucose monitoring in hospitals. *Diabetes Care, 9,* 89.
32. Wason CJ, Green J, Miller C (1985): Reagent strip glucose monitoring methods in chronic hemodialysis. *Diabetes Care, 8,* 603.
33. Wickham NWR, Achar KN, Cove DH (1986): Unreliability of capillary blood glucose in peripheral vascular disease. *Pract. Diabetes, 3,* 100.
34. Ward KW, Haas LB, Beard JC (1985): A randomised controlled comparison of instruction by a diabetes educator versus self-instruction in self-monitoring of blood glucose. *Diabetes Care, 8,* 284.
35. Laus VG, Dietz MA, Levy RP (1984): Potential pitfalls in the use of Glucoscan and Glucoscan II meters for self-monitoring of blood glucose. *Diabetes Care, 7,* 590.
36. Umpierrez GE, Reed JC, Tacker SV (1986): Preliminary studies of diabetic decompensation assessed with bedside glucose-monitoring techniques. *Diabetes Care, 9,* 77.
37. Roth M (1983): 'Glycated hemoglobin', not 'glycosylated' or 'glucosylated'. *Clin. Chem., 29,* 1991.
38. Bakan E, Bakan N (1985): Glycosylation of nail in diabetics: possible marker of long-term hyperglycaemia. *Clin. Chim. Acta, 147,* 1.
39. Delbridge L, Ellis CS, Robertson K et al (1985): Non-enzymatic glycosylation of keratin from the stratum corneum of the diabetic foot. *Br. J. Dermatol., 112,* 547.
40. Paisey RB, Lewin IG, Hopton M et al (1985): Glycosylation of maternal hair and cord skin during pregnancy in diabetic and non-diabetic women. *Diabetic Med., 2,* 367.
41. Ashby JP, Deacon AC, Frier BM (1985): Glycosylated haemoglobin. I. Measurement and clinical interpretation. *Diabetic Med., 2,* 83.
42. Kortland W, Van Rijn HJM, Hoeke JOO et al (1985): Comparison of three different assay procedures for the determination of HbA_1 with special attention to the influence of pre-HbA_{1c}, temperature and haemoglobin concentration. *Ann. Clin. Biochem., 22,* 261.
43. Meskar A, LeBras R, L'Emeillat M et al (1985): Glycated haemoglobin: comparison between methods based upon 5-hydroxymethylfurfural determination (colorimetric or

HPLC) and ion exchange chromatography (HbA₁). *J. Clin. Chem. Clin. Biochem., 23*, 197.

44. National Diabetes Data Group (1984): Report of the expert committee on glucosylated hemoglobin. *Diabetes Care, 7,* 602.
45. Fluckiger R, Woodtli T (1985): Effect of temperature on quantifying glycated (glycosylated) hemoglobin by cation-exchange chromatography. *Clin. Chem., 31,* 114.
46. Bisse E, Abraham EC (1985): New less temperature-sensitive microchromatographic method for the separation and quantitation of glycosylated hemoglobins using a non-cyanide buffer system. *J. Chromatogr., 344,* 81.
47. Mosca A, Carpinelli A, Paleari R et al (1985): Preparation and control of ethylene glycol-stabilised haemolysates for glycated haemoglobin assay. *J. Clin. Chem. Clin. Biochem., 23,* 361.
48. Little RR, England JD, Wiedmeyer H-M et al (1986): Interlaboratory standardisation of glycated hemoglobin determinations. *Clin. Chem., 32,* 358.
49. Kennedy L (1985): Labile glycosylated haemoglobin — is it clinically important? *Diabetic Med., 2,* 86.
50. Bannon P, Joly J-G, Lessard F et al (1985): Comparison of three methods for the elimination of the labile fraction of HbA₁. *Clin. Biochem., 18,* 114.
51. Kawahara R, Amemiya T, Komori T et al (1985): The effect of blood glucose concentration on labile A₁c in diabetic patients. *Diabetes Care, 8,* 375.
52. Burden AC (1984): Fructose and misleading glycosylation data. *Lancet, 2,* 986.
53. Eberentz-Lhomme C, Ducrocq R, Intrator S et al (1984): Haemoglobinopathies: a pitfall in the assessment of glycosylated haemoglobin by ion-exchange chromatography. *Diabetologia, 27,* 596.
54. Weinblatt MK, Kochen JA, Scimeca PG (1986): Chronically transfused patients with increased hemoglobin A₁c secondary to donor blood. *Ann. Clin. Lab. Sci., 16,* 34.
55. Little RR, McKenzie EM, Wiedmeyer H-M et al (1986): Collection of blood on filter paper for measurement of glycated hemoglobin by affinity chromatography. *Clin. Chem., 32,* 869.
56. Moore JC, Bown E, Outlaw MC et al (1986): Glycosylated haemoglobin: comparison of five different methods, including measurement on capillary blood samples. *Ann. Clin. Biochem., 23,* 85.
57. Kennedy AL, Kandell TW, Merimee TJ (1979): Serum protein-bound hexose in diabetes: the effect of glycemic control. *Diabetes, 28,* 1006.
58. McFarland KF, Cataland EW, Day JF et al (1979): Nonenzymatic glucosylation of serum proteins in diabetes mellitus. *Diabetes, 28,* 1011.
59. Kennedy L, Mehl TD, Riley WJ et al (1981): Non-enzymatically glycosylated serum protein in diabetes mellitus: an index of short-term glycaemia. *Diabetologia, 21,* 94.
60. Fluckiger R, Winterhalter KH (1976): In vitro synthesis of hemoglobin A₁c. *FEBS Lett., 71,* 356.
61. Schleicher ED, Gerbitz KD, Dolhofer R et al (1984): Clinical utility of nonenzymatically glycosylated blood proteins as an index of glucose control. *Diabetes Care, 7,* 548.
62. John WG, Jones AE (1985): Affinity chromatography: a precise method for glycosylated albumin estimation. *Ann. Clin. Biochem., 22,* 79.
63. Rendell M, Kao G, Mecherikunnel P et al (1985): Aminophenylboronic acid affinity chromatography and thiobarbituric acid colorimetry compared for measuring glycated albumin. *Clin. Chem., 31,* 229.
64. Rendell M, Kao G, Mecherikunnel P et al (1985): Use of aminophenylboronic acid affinity chromatography to measure glycosylated albumin levels. *J. Lab. Clin. Med., 105,* 63.
65. Moore JC, Outlaw MC, Barnes AJ et al (1986) Glycosylated plasma protein measurement by a semi-automated method. *Ann. Clin. Biochem., 23,* 198.
66. Hayashi Y, Makino M (1985): Fluorometric measurement of glycosylated albumin in human serum. *Clin. Chim. Acta, 149,* 13.

67. Little RR, Wiedmeyer H-M, England JD et al (1985): Measurement of glycosylated whole-blood protein for assessing glucose control in diabetes: collection and storage of capillary blood on filter paper. *Clin. Chem., 30*, 213.

68. Johnson RN, Metcalf PA, Baker JR (1982): Fructosamine: a new approach to the estimation of serum glycosylprotein: an index of diabetic control. *Clin. Chim. Acta, 127*, 87.

69. Baker JR, Metcalf PA, Johnson RN et al (1985): Use of protein-based standards in automated colorimetric determinations of fructosamine in serum. *Clin. Chem., 31*, 1550.

70. Seng LY, Staley MJ (1986): A 10-min pre-incubation is required for measurement of fructosamine in plasma. *Clin. Chem., 32*, 403.

71. Hindle EJ, Rostron GM, Gatt JA (1985): The estimation of serum fructosamine: an alternative measurement to glycated haemoglobin. *Ann. Clin. Biochem., 22*, 84.

72. San-Gil F, Schier GM, Moses RG et al (1985): Improvement estimation of fructosamine, as a measure of glycated serum protein, with the Technicon RA-1000 analyser. *Clin. Chem., 31*, 2005.

73. Lim YS, Staley MJ (1985): Measurement of plasma fructosamine evaluated for monitoring diabetes. *Clin. Chem., 31*, 731.

74. Zeyen LJJM, Vermes I, Van der Veen EA (1986): Serum fructosamine, een nieuwe parameter voor diabetescontrole. *Tijdschr. Ned. Ver. Klin. Chem., 11*, 8.

75. Hindle EJ, Rostron GM, Clark SA et al (1986): Serum fructosamine and glycated haemoglobin measurements in diabetic control. *Arch. Dis. Child., 61*, 113.

76. Lloyd DR, Nott M, Marples J (1985): Comparison of serum fructosamine with glycosylated serum protein (determined by affinity chromatography) for the assessment of diabetic control. *Diabetic Med., 2*, 474.

77. McCance DR, Coulter D, Smye M et al (1986): Effect of minor fluctuations in serum albumin levels on serum fructosamine. *Diabetic Med., 3*, 576A.

78. Ross IR, Mitchell AF, Stroud RE (1986): Glycated haemoglobin and glycated plasma protein: a comparative study. *Clin. Chim. Acta, 156*, 329.

79. John WG, Webb AMC, Jones AE (1985): Glycosylated haemoglobin and glycosylated albumin in non-diabetic and diabetic mothers, and their babies. *Diabetic Med., 2*, 103.

80. Leiper JM, Talwar D, Robb DA et al (1985): Glycosylated albumin and glycosylated proteins: rapidly changing indices of glycaemia in diabetic pregnancy. *Q. J. Med., 218*, 225.

81. Morris MA, Grandis AS, Litton J (1985): The correlations of glycosylated serum protein and glycosylated hemoglobin concentrations with blood glucose in diabetic pregnancy *Am. J. Obstet. Gynecol., 153*, 257.

82. Morris MA, Grandis AS, Litton JC (1986): Longitudinal assessment of glycosylated blood protein concentrations in normal pregnancy and gestational diabetes. *Diabetes Care, 9*, 107.

83. Nelson DM, Barrows HJ, Clapp DH et al (1985): Glycosylated serum protein levels in diabetic and nondiabetic pregnant patients: an indicator of short-term glycemic control in the diabetic patient. *Am. J. Obstet. Gynecol., 151*, 1042.

84. Albutt EC, Natrass M, Northam BE (1985): Glucose tolerance test and glycosylated haemoglobin measurement for diagnosis of diabetes mellitus — an assessment of the criteria of the WHO Expert Committee on Diabetes Mellitus 1980. *Ann. Clin. Biochem., 22*, 67.

85. Hall PM, Cook JGH, Sheldon J et al (1984): Glycosylated hemoglobins and glycosylated plasma proteins in the diagnosis of diabetes mellitus and impaired glucose tolerance. *Diabetes Care, 7*, 147.

86. John WG, Richardson RW (1986): Glycosylated haemoglobin levels in patients referred for oral glucose tolerance tests. *Diabetic Med., 3*, 46.

87. Lester E, Frazer AD, Shepherd CA et al (1985): Glycosylated haemoglobin as an alternative to the glucose tolerance test for the diagnosis of diabetes mellitus. *Ann. Clin. Biochem., 22*, 74.

88. Simon D, Coignet MC, Thibult N et al (1985): Comparison of glycosylated hemoglobin and fasting plasma glucose with two-hour post-load plasma glucose in the detection of diabetes mellitus. *Am. J. Epidemiol., 122,* 589.
89. Hindle EJ, Rostron GM, Gatt JA (1985): The diagnostic value of glycated hemoglobin levels in post-mortem blood. *Ann. Clin. Biochem., 22,* 144.

The Diabetes Annual/3
K.G.M.M. Alberti and L.P. Krall, editors
© 1987 Elsevier Science Publishers, B.V.

10 Pancreas transplantation: an update

DAVID E.R. SUTHERLAND

Introduction

The frequency by which pancreas transplants are being performed has continued to increase (1). In *The Diabetes Annual/2* the results of 561 pancreas transplants performed from 1966 through 1984 were summarized (2). As of October 17, 1986, 1001 pancreas transplants had been reported to the International Pancreas Transplants Registry, including 218 for all of 1985 and 220 during less than 10 months in 1986 (3).

Refinements in surgical techniques and immunosuppression have led to a gradual improvement in results, and observations on the effect of pancreas transplantation on the complications of diabetes are beginning to emerge. In addition, animal experiments have led to advances in organ preservation, have shown differences in the effects of various techniques on function and physiological response to the graft, and have provided methods for early detection and treatment of pancreas graft rejection that are of immediate clinical relevance.

In the following sections an updated report of the Pancreas Transplant Registry is given, the results of clinical pancreas transplantation as reported in the literature by various institutions are summarized, the relevant animal experiments are cited, and advances in knowledge in selected areas of importance for pancreas transplantation are discussed.

Pancreas Transplant Registry Report

From December 17, 1966, to October 17, 1986, 1001 pancreas transplants in 932 diabetic patients were reported to the International Pancreas Transplant Registry (3). One year actuarial graft function (insulin-independent) and recipient survival rates for all cases were 35 and 75%, respectively. Of the 329 grafts that were functioning at the time of the analysis, 169 were less than 1 year after transplantation, while 160 were more than 1 year, including 16 that were more than 4 years, the longest being 8.2 years.

159

In an analysis by era of 1966-1977 (n = 64), 1978-1982 (n = 201), 1983-1984 (n = 298) and 1985-1986 (n = 438), cases, 1-year actuarial graft function rates were 3, 21, 39 and 44% and recipient survival rates were 42, 72, 76 and 83%, respectively ($P \leq 0.05$ for all comparisons except patient survival for 1983-1984 versus 1985-1986).

In a separate analysis of 1983-1986 cases (n = 736), overall 1-year graft function and patient survival rates were 42 and 79%, respectively. The results according to multiple variables during this period are given in Table 1 and in the following paragraphs.

Graft functional survival rates were similar whether a whole or a segment of the pancreas was transplanted (Table 1). The technical failure rate was also similar ($P > 0.3$) for whole versus segmental grafts (24% vs 27%). There also were no significant differences in the incidence of thromboses (11.8% vs 12.2%) or infections (5.1% vs 8.3%) for whole versus segmental grafts.

With regard to management of the pancreatic duct and graft exocrine secretions, functional survival rates were similar for the most common techniques, namely duct injection, intestinal drainage and bladder drainage (Table 1). Within each of these categories there were no significant differences in functional survival rates for whole versus segmental grafts. The technical failure rates were 20% for polymer injection, 31% for intestinal drainage, 38% for stomach drainage, 23% for bladder drainage, and 22% for ureter drainage. The differences in technical failure rates were significant ($P < 0.05$) for duct injection versus stomach and intestinal drainage, but not for the other comparisons. The thrombosis rates for polymer injection, intestinal drainage, stomach drainage, bladder drainage and ureter were 11, 14, 16, 12 and 0%, respectively (all nonsignificant).

Functional survival rates according to duration of preservation were significantly higher for grafts stored less than 6 hours than those stored more than 6 hours (Table 1). The functional survival rates were not significantly different for grafts stored 6-12 hours and those stored for more than 12 hours. It is apparent that storage for more than 12 hours is compatible with normal function, but the success rate is reduced with increasing duration of preservation.

With regard to immunosuppression, graft functional survival rates were significantly higher in recipients who were treated with cyclosporine than in those who were not (Table 1). Cyclosporine was used in different ways, either as the sole immunosuppressant, initially in combination with prednisone, initially in combination with azathioprine alone or in combination with both azathioprine and prednisone; or as a late addition to an initial course of azathioprine and prednisone in the early post-transplant period. Functional survival rates for technically successful grafts were significantly higher in recipients treated with cyclosporine than in those not so treated. In recipients treated with cyclosporine and prednisone the graft survival rates were significantly higher for those who

TABLE 1   *Pancreas graft actuarial functional (insulin-independent) survival rates at 1 year for transplants reported to the Registry between January 1, 1983, and October 17, 1986*

Category (n)	Percent functioning at 1 year	P-values <0.05
A. All cases (736)	42	
B. Method		
1. Whole (280)	41	none
2. Segmental (456)	42	
C. Duct management		
1. Polymer injection (254)	43	1 *vs* 3b
2. Enteric drainage (254)	42	2 *vs* 3b
		2a *vs* 3b
a. Intestinal drainage (228)	43	2a *vs* 3b
b. Stomach drainage (26)	37	
3. Urinary drainage (214)	39	
a. Bladder drainage (196)	47	
b. Ureter drainage (18)	16	
D. Preservation time		
1. < 6 hours (460)	46	1 *vs* 2
2. 6-12 hours (146)	39	
3. > 12 hours (52)	30	
E. Recipient immunosuppression (all cases)		
1. All cyclosporine (CsA) (670)	43	
		1b *vs* 1c
a. CsA alone (30)	49	1b *vs* 1c
b. CsA + pred (232)	37	
c. CsA + Aza + pred (338)	46	
d. CsA + Aza (7)	71	
e. Aza + Pred + CsA (delayed) (63)	45	
2. No CsA (Aza + Pred) (56)	34	
F. Recipient immunosuppression (technically successful cases only)		
1. All cyclosporine (495)	59	1 *vs* 2
		1a *vs* 2
a. CsA alone (21)	70	1b *vs* 1c
b. CsA + Pred (165)	51	1b *vs* 1e
c. CsA + Aza + Pred (263)	60	1c *vs* 2
d. CsA + Aza (4)	100	1e *vs* 2
e. Aza + Pred + CsA (delayed) (41)	70	
2. No cyclosporine (Aza + Pred) (44)	41	
G. Presence or absence of ESDN		
1. No ESDN (127)	31	none
2. ESDN (609)	44	
a. Px simultaneously with Kx (465)	46	
b. Px after Kx (141)	39	

Aza = azathioprine; ESDN = end-stage diabetic nephropathy; Kx = kidney transplant; Pred = prednisone; Px = pancreas transplant.

also received azathioprine than for those who did not, whether analyzed for all or for technically successful cases. The initial triple-therapy groups (cyclosporine + azathioprine + prednisone combination) also had significantly higher graft survival rates than the groups not treated with cyclosporine. The combination of cyclosporine and azathioprine does not have a detrimental effect on patient survival; for all cases the 1-year survival rate for recipients treated with both cyclosporine and azathioprine was 85%, versus 76% for those treated with cyclosporine without azathioprine and 60% for those treated with azathioprine without cyclosporine ($P<0.05$).

There were no significant differences in functional survival rates for pancreas grafts placed in recipients with end-stage diabetic nephropathy (ESDN) versus those without. There were also no significant differences in functional survival rates for pancreas grafts transplanted simultaneously with kidneys versus those transplanted after kidney grafts (Table 1). However, patient survival rates were significantly ($P<0.05$) higher in recipients without than in those with ESDN (87% *vs* 77% at 1 year). Patient survival rates were also significantly ($P<0.05$) higher in recipients of pancreas transplants alone or of pancreas transplants after a kidney than in those who received pancreas and kidney transplants simultaneously (87, 87 and 75% at 1 year, respectively).

The kidney graft survival rate in recipients of simultaneous pancreas transplants (n = 465) was 63% at 1 year. This outcome is similar to that reported by the UCLA Kidney Transplant Registry for kidneys transplanted alone to uremic diabetic recipients (4).

The Registry documents a progressive improvement in pancreas transplant results. Since 1983, overall graft functional survival rates have been greater than 40%. Results have been similar for the 3 most common duct-management techniques. Preservation times below 6 hours have been associated with higher graft survival rates than preservation times above 6 hours, but the difference is small. Combination immunotherapy with cyclosporine, azathioprine and prednisone is associated with higher graft survival rates than the immunosuppressive regimens of cyclosporine and prednisone without azathioprine or azathioprine and prednisone without cyclosporine. Combination immunotherapy does not have a detrimental effect on patient survival rates. Pancreas graft survival rates are no longer significantly different between patients who do and do not receive kidney transplants, but patient survival rates are higher in recipients with pancreas transplants alone than in those with ESDN who receive a kidney simultaneously with a pancreas. The overall improvement in pancreas graft survival rates is encouraging, but the success rate is still less than that of other solid organs.

Clinical pancreas transplant results reported in the literature by individual institutions with the largest experience

The general trend of improvement in pancreas transplant results as documented in the Registry statistics is also reflected in reports from individual institutions on their most recent cases. A summary of the results at the institutions (3 American, 4 European) with more than 30 pancreas transplant cases during 1983-1986 is given below.

The *University of Minnesota* performs pancreas transplants in both kidney transplant recipients and in non-uremic, non-kidney-transplant diabetic recipients (5). This transplant group has used a variety of techniques, but since 1984 has gradually converted to using the bladder drainage method (6). This group also began using a triple or quadruple drug regimen of cyclosporine, azathioprine and prednisone with or without antilymphocyte globulin for immunosuppression in 1983 (7). These changes in protocol have been associated with improvements in graft survival rates. For all cases from January 1, 1983, through the first 9 months of 1986 (99 pancreas transplants), the overall 1-year patient survival rate was 88% and the graft functional survival rate was 40% (5). When the results were analysed according to surgical technique, the 1-year graft survival rates were 42% for 63 enteric-drainage grafts and 63% for 23 bladder-drained grafts. The differences in functional survival rates for grafts transplanted by the two techniques did not relate solely to differences in complication rates. For 32 enteric-drained and 17 bladder-drained grafts that were technically successful, the 1-year actuarial functional survival rates were 64 and 100%, respectively. This difference suggests that there is an advantage for monitoring for rejection with the bladder-drained grafts.

The University of Minnesota transplant group is the only one in which the majority of the patients are non-uremic non-kidney-transplant diabetic recipients (8). Of 62 transplants in this category during 1983-1986, the 1-year patient survival rate was 92% and the 1-year graft survival rate was 46%. According to surgical technique, the 1-year graft survival rate for 48 enteric-drained and 14 bladder-drained grafts was 38 and 80%, respectively. This reflects primarily differences in the ability to monitor for rejection. In the absence of the transplanted kidney, the only parameter to monitor for rejection with enteric-drained grafts is hyperglycemia, while in the bladder-drained grafts urinary amylase can be monitored. For technically successful cases only, the 1-year graft survival rate for 32 enteric-drained and 13 bladder-drained grafts was 57 and 100%, respectively. Again, these results suggest that the ability to monitor rejection is enhanced with the bladder drainage technique (9). The results have continued to improve. For 1985-1986, 39 of the pancreas transplants were in non-uremic, non-kidney-transplant recipients of the pancreas alone (5). The 1-year patient survival rate was 95% and the 1-year graft survival rate was 52%.

Again, a striking advantage for bladder drainage was seen in this subset of patients; 1-year graft survival rate for 26 enteric-drained and 13 bladder-drained grafts was 36 and 100%, respectively.

The *University of Wisconsin* has the second largest series of pancreas transplants in the United States (10). Most transplants have been performed in patients who have had previously received a kidney transplant, but recently pancreas grafts have been performed simultaneously with kidney transplants as well. There has been a progressive improvement in results. The University of Wisconsin has used exclusively the bladder drainage technique, with a gradual shift from segmental to whole pancreas transplants and evolution of a quadruple immunosuppressive regimen consisting of cyclosporine, azathioprine, prednisone and a temporary course of antilymphocyte globulin (11). In the most recent report from the University of Wisconsin, a total of 57 pancreas transplants have been performed, of which 11 were segmental, 9 were pancreaticosplenic and 37 were whole pancreas without the spleen (11). In the overall series for 1983-1986, the 1-year graft survival rate was 62% and the 1-year patient survival rate was 91% (1). The best results were in the latest series in 28 patients, of whom 18 received a pancreas transplant after a kidney and 10 had a simultaneous kidney and pancreas transplant (11). For the combined groups, the 1-year patient survival rate was 96% and the 1-year graft survival rate was 74%. For pancreas transplants after a kidney transplant, the 1-year pancreas graft survival rate was 72%, while for those performed simultaneously with a kidney the actuarial graft survival rate at 10 months was 80%. Of the 7 grafts that failed from the latest series, 3 were due to rejection and 4 were for technical reasons. Again, rejection losses are infrequent and this outcome may reflect the ability to monitor for rejection episodes by urine amylase measurements.

The *University of Iowa* has the third largest series of pancreas transplants in the United States (12), including 40 cases for 1983-1986, with an overall 1-year pancreas graft survival rate of 46% and patient survival rate of 76% (1). The whole pancreaticoduodenal transplant method has been used (12), with enteric drainage technique in most of the cases. Recently there has been a shift to the bladder drainage technique (13). For 1983-1986 cases, the graft survival rate at 1 year was 48% for 31 enteric-drained and 42% for 15 bladder-drained transplants (1). In 33 pancreases transplanted simultaneously with the kidney, the 1-year pancreas graft function was 53%, while it was 30% for 11 pancreas transplants after a kidney. In the most recent publications from Iowa, the results of 29 pancreas transplants simultaneously with a kidney from March, 1984, to May, 1986, were reported, with a 1-year pancreas transplant survival rate of 57%, kidney graft survival rate of 86% and patient survival rate of 78% (14). Pancreas graft losses were from rejection in 4 cases and from death (myocardial infarct with a functioning graft) in 4 cases; the other losses were technical. Corry et al (14) stressed the importance of careful screening for cardiac disease prior to assessing uremic diabetic patients for pancreas transplantation.

There are several relatively large series of pancreas transplants in Europe. Unlike the United States, where almost all groups are now using the bladder drainage technique for cadaver pancreas transplants, the duct injection or enteric drainage techniques have continued to be used by the centers in Europe with the most experience. Some of the newer centers, however, are using urinary drainage (1).

Huddinge Hospital in Stockholm, one of the pioneers in the field of pancreas transplantation, uses the segmental method with enteric drainage, usually to a Roux-en-Y limb of intestine (15), although a few grafts have been drained into the stomach (16). For 52 pancreas transplants during 1983-1986, the overall 1-year graft and patient survival rates were 41 and 83%, respectively (1). The best results were in the subgroup of 37 patients who received segmental grafts drained into a Roux-en-Y loop of intestine simultaneously with a kidney transplant, with a 1-year pancreas graft function rate of 52%. Tyden et al (17) have recently reported that the results have been improved by reduction in non-immunological graft failures. In 28 consecutive combined renal and pancreas transplants with enteric exocrine drainage performed between June, 1984, and May, 1986, the 1-year actuarial survival rates were 69% for the pancreas grafts, 67% for the kidney grafts and 90% for the patients. Only 2 of the losses were attributable to non-immunological causes. Of the 9 losses, 2 were from patient deaths, 4 due to rejection, 1 from an abscess secondary to cytomegalovirus infection, 1 primary abscess and 1 from bleeding. The 19 grafts that were functioning at the time of the report included 9 for more than 1 year and 10 for less than 1 year.

The *University of Munich* has a large experience with prolamine duct-injected segmental grafts, almost all of them placed simultaneously with the kidney in uremic recipients (18). In a report on the results of 44 pancreas transplants since 1981, the 1-year pancreas graft survival rate was 45%, kidney graft survival rate 64%, and patient survival rate 84% (18). In a recent analysis of 1983-1986 cases, 1-year pancreas graft function rates for all cases (n = 53) was 56%, and for 49 pancreases transplanted simultaneously with a kidney was 59% (1).

Herriot Hospital in Lyon is also one of the pioneer institutes in pancreas transplantation (19). Until recently this institution used exclusively the segmental technique with duct injection. Currently, this group is conducting a prospective trial of segmental neoprene duct-injected grafts versus whole pancreas enteric-drained grafts (20). In recent years, almost all of the pancreas grafts have been placed simultaneously with the kidney in uremic diabetic recipients. For 1983-1986, the overall 1-year graft and patient survival rates for 42 cases were 55 and 73%, respectively; of 29 duct-injected grafts placed simultaneously with a kidney, the 1-year function rate was 51% (1). In one of the most recent reports from the Lyon series (19), several changes in immunosuppressive protocols were described that have contributed to the progressive improvement in results. The pancreas graft survival rate at 1 year was 51% for 27 patients treated initially with azathioprine followed by conversion to cyclosporine, and for 6 patients treated with cyclosporine and azathioprine from the onset the 1-year graft survival rate was 60%. Again, the Lyon group is following the trend to use multiple-drug combination immunotherapy for prevention of allograft rejection.

The next largest series of pancreas transplants in Europe is at the *University of Oslo* (21), and includes 39 cases for 1983-1986 with an overall 1-year graft and patient survival rate of 55% and 91% (1). The Oslo group has used exclusively the segmental technique with duct injection with neoprene, and almost all pancreas grafts have been placed simultaneously with a kidney in uremic recipients. In the subgroup of 34 pancreas transplants placed simultaneously with the kidney during 1983-1986, the 1-year pancreas graft survival rate was 61% (1). Their most recent publication describes 25 double transplanted cases, with 1-year pancreas, kidney and recipient survival rates of 60, 79 and 96%, respectively; however, 4 of the 17 patients counted as functioning pancreas grafts were receiving some insulin (21).

Several other institutions have active pancreas transplant programs, but have performed fewer than 30 cases during 1983-1986. The experiences with either duct injection (22, 23), enteric drainage (24), or urinary drainage (25-27), are of interest. Thus, the University of Cambridge team has used the stomach for drainage of the graft exocrine secretions, and the portal system for drainage of the graft venous effluent (24). The University of Zurich (22) and the University of Innsbruck groups (23) have used the duct injection technique, but have delayed injecting the duct until several weeks after the transplant, draining the excretions externally via a catheter in the interim. The University of Cincinnati workers have used both the ureter and bladder drainage techniques (26), and is the only group to have described a detrimental effect of activation of the pancreatic enzymes on the urine excretory system (28). The University of Maastricht team is the only group currently transplanting the spleen *en bloc* with the pancreas graft; the spleen is irradiated ex vivo prior to implantation (27) and so far graft-versus-host disease has not occurred. The small number of cases at these institutions does not lend itself to accurate calculation of graft survival rates; in general, they are similar to those described for the institutions with relatively large numbers of cases. More follow-up is needed, however, to determine whether or not the innovations that these groups have introduced will lead to further improvements in pancreas graft functional survival rates.

Results of pancreas transplant experiments in animals relevant to the clinical situation

Numerous papers have been published on pancreas transplantation in experimental animal models. The impact of pancreas transplant techniques on methods of duct management and functional outcome has been studied, advances in graft preservation have been made, the perturbations associated with pancreas graft rejection have been defined, methods for detection and early treatment of rejection developed, and the effects of pancreas transplantation on metabolism and secondary complications have been further delineated.

Experimental studies in relation to pancreas transplant technique

Dogs, rats and baboons have been used for recent pancreas transplant experiments. The duct and exocrine secretions have been managed by either free drainage into the peritoneal cavity, duct injection with synthetic polymers, enteric drainage or bladder drainage.

Leaving the duct open to drain freely into the peritoneal cavity of dogs has been a standard technique for years. Exocrine secretions are absorbed, and the duct eventually closes, followed by fibrosis. The consequences of this process may be minimal. In a long-term study by Cutfield et al (29) of canine recipients of segmental pancreas autografts, all dogs were euglycemic 4 years after transplantation and intravenous glucose tolerance test results were no different from those in age-matched controls. The pancreas transplant recipients had slightly increased insulin levels, although C-peptide levels were lower than in the controls. Graft biopsies showed atrophy of exocrine pancreas, mild fibrosis and coalescence of islets containing all of the relevant endocrine cell types. The fact that deterioration of endocrine function did not occur over time is encouraging for clinical application of pancreas transplantation, and consistent with clinical observations.

These observations are in contrast to those of Van Goor et al (30) in which deterioration of canine heterotopic function pancreas autografts was seen in 40% of the recipients after 1 year. It is difficult to reconcile these conflicting observations, but similar discrepancies are encountered in the islet transplant literature. Thus, Alejandro et al (31) found that in some euglycemic canine recipients of intraportal islet autografts, there was gradual deterioration of function and eventual recurrence of hyperglycemia. On the other hand, Alderson et al (32) found that the function of islet autotransplants in dogs improved with time. Thus, it appears that both pancreas and islet autografts can function long-term with maintenance of the recipient in the normoglycemic state, but that deterioration of function may occur in some cases for reasons that are not related to rejection.

Gooszen et al (33) studied the effect of duct obliteration with neoprene on the histological appearance and endocrine function of canine pancreas autografts. Although the recipients had some abnormal test results, progressive deterioration did not occur, and normoglycemia was maintained over the 12-month period of study. Serial histological observations showed a rapid and total replacement of the exocrine pancreas by fibrosis with a progressive increase in the proportion of the pancreas comprised of endocrine tissue (from 2 to 16% by 1 year). The proportions of the various endocrine cells related to one another remained constant. A similar study was conducted by Squifflet et al (34) in isologous rats using two different substances for duct injection, namely prolamine and silastic. Even though the histological changes induced in the pancreas were severe, there were no differences between the two agents and all of the recipients were normoglycemic 3 months after transplantation, with insulin levels and intravenous glucose tolerance test K-values within the normal range. These studies do not support the concept that fibrosis induced by duct injection leads to a progressive deterioration in function, even though the histological changes produced are severe.

Pancreas transplantation methods that maintain duct patency remain conceptually appealing, and the most physiological technique is enteric drainage. Diliz-Perez et al (35) in dogs, and Lee et al (36) and Orloff et al (37) in rats, had a high success rate with pancreaticoduodenal grafts, as did Liu et al (38) and Senninger et al (39) with segmental grafts in dogs. Orloff et al (37) documented life-long reversal of the metabolic abnormalities of streptozotocin-induced diabetes by whole pancreaticoduodenal transplantation in rats. Lindsey et al (40) reported a relatively high incidence of infections in cyclosporine-treated rat recipients of enteric-drained pancreas grafts. Senninger et al (39) in dogs used the novel method of intestinalization of the pancreatic segment, inserting the entire graft into a Roux-en-Y limb of intestine with the vessels exiting through the bowel wall. Whether this technique reduces the complications relative to other methods of enteric drainage was not clear, since a comparative study was not done.

The bladder drainage technique is rapidly becoming the most frequently used clinical technique for pancreas transplantation, and the soundness of this approach is supported by studies in dogs. With segmental grafts a mucosa-to-mucosa anastomosis ensures that the pancreatic duct will remain patent (38), a physiological response of the exocrine pancreas to hormonal stimuli can be demonstrated by an increase of pancreatic enzyme activity in the urine following administration of cholecystokinin (41), the incidence of infections is low (42), and long-term normoglycemia can be maintained (43). Nghiem et al (44) drained whole pancreaticoduodenal grafts into the bladder, and showed normal healing at the site of the duodenocystostomy with maintenance of a normal bladder mucosa. In general, urine amylase activity remains high as long as the graft is viable.

A number of investigators have compared the various pancreas transplant techniques in either the dog (38, 45), or rat (34, 46-48) models. Overall, the authors concluded that methods establishing duct drainage are better than those that do not. Such statements were, however, usually based on the fact that the histological appearance of the duct-injected pancreas was much less esthetic than that of the duct-drained pancreas, since differences in graft function as determined by plasma glucose levels or glucose tolerance test results were minimal (46-48) or non-existent (34, 38, 45).

The question whether or not the thrombosis rate in segmental pancreas grafts could be lowered by creation of an arteriovenous fistula between the graft splenic artery and splenic vein has finally been subjected to controlled studies (49, 50). Neither experiment showed a beneficial effect.

Another area of controversy is whether islet grafts and pancreas grafts can provide equivalent metabolic effects in diabetic recipients. There are 3 reports where such a comparison was made in the same laboratory: two in rats (51, 52) and one in dogs (53). Florack et al (53) found that heterotopic segmental transplants with systemic drainage produced a metabolic state closer to that of normal dogs than did intrasplenic islet transplants, even though the latter resulted in portal delivery of insulin. Squifflet et al (51) found no differences in the metabolic effect of intraportal islet grafts and standard segmental pancreas transplants in rats followed $\geq$ 3 months in terms of plasma glucose levels or intravenous glucose tolerance test K-values. On the other hand, Orloff et al (52) found that whole pancreas transplants reversed all the metabolic abnormalities in diabetic rats, while intraportal islet transplants were associated with abnormal glucose tolerance test results and elevation of basal glucose levels beginning 4 months after transplantation.

The results of the above experiments indicate that all of the standard pancreas transplant techniques can establish a permanent normoglycemic state in diabetic recipients, that deterioration of function is exceptional, and that differences in functional outcome are minor. The choice of technique for clinical application cannot be based solely on the results of animal experiments. However, the fact that urinary drainage is safe and provides a parameter other than plasma glucose concentrations or insulin levels for monitoring of graft function supports the increase in clinical application of this technique.

Experimental studies of pancreas graft preservation

The limits of organ preservation are the main logistical restriction on clinical application of pancreas transplantation. Presumably methods that extend the preservation limits of animal pancreas grafts will also extend those of human pancreas grafts. Florack et al (54) originally showed that canine pancreas grafts could be reliably preserved for up to 48 hours in a hyperosmolar, silica-gel-filtered plasma solution (SGF). That pancreas grafts can be preserved at least this long in a hyperosmolar colloid solution has been confirmed (55).

Intracellular electrolyte solutions (Collins or their equivalent) have been used successfully for preservation for no more (56) or somewhat less (57) than 24 hours, although there is one report that storage for 72 hours was successful in dogs (58). Pancreas preservation by machine perfusion has not been extended beyond 24 hours (59). Otherwise, consistently successful storage of pancreas grafts for 72 hours has been reported only by Wahlberg et al (60). This group used hydroxethyl starches as the colloid and raffinose as the osmotic agent in the preservation solution. A comparative study between the colloid solution of Wahlberg et al (60) and the plasma-based solution of Florack et al (54) has not been made. The latter solution, however, has been tested under a variety of adverse conditions, including subjection of the canine pancreas to warm ischemia prior to preservation (61). Normal function was observed in the canine pancreas grafts subjected to ½ hour of warm ischemia followed by 24 hours of cold storage in SGF; 1 hour of warm ischemia followed by 24 hours of cold storage was also successful, but graft function was not normal until 1 week following transplantation. Pancreas grafts have exhibited a surprising tolerance to warm ischemia, and appear to be less sensitive than the kidney to such insult (62).

Experimental pancreas allotransplantation, immunosuppression and rejection

Experimental studies are conflicting on whether the pancreas is or is not more susceptible to rejection than other organs. In the rat, pancreas grafts appear to be more readily rejected than the heart, liver or kidney. Klempnauer et al (63) found that in non-immunosuppressed rat recipients of pancreas or heart allografts from donors differing with the recipient at the major histocompatibility complex (MHC) both organs were rejected, the heart slightly sooner than the pancreas; however, in donor-recipient strain combinations that had only non-MHC differences, heart grafts were not rejected while pancreas grafts were. This group also found a differential effect of donor-recipient differences at the RT1.C region in heart and pancreas rejection in rats (64). Timmerman et al (65), using a protocol that was uniformly successful at permanently preventing rejection of heart, liver and kidney allografts found that a limited course of cyclosporine delayed, but did not prevent, rejection of pancreas allografts in rats across both major or minor barriers. These experiments confirmed the early observations of Rynasiewicz and his group (66), but he had also shown that a temporary course of cyclosporine did not permanently prevent rejection of heart allografts in certain donor-recipient strain combinations (67). Cyclosporine can, however, prevent rejection of pancreas grafts in rats if administered indefinitely (68). Again this effect may also depend upon the strengths of the histocompatibility barrier breeched (67). Perhaps the pancreas is more susceptible to rejection than other immediately vascularized grafts, but even so the pancreas appears to be less susceptible to rejection than islets as free grafts in the absence of manipulations to reduce graft immunogenicity or recipient responsiveness (69).

In large animals, comparative studies of rejection have been done only between the pancreas and the kidney, and the physiological manifestations of rejection appear earlier in the kidney than in the pancreas (70). Interestingly, in combined kidney-pancreas transplants, Florack et al (71) found that the duration of pancreas graft function was longer than when the pancreas was transplanted alone. Nakayama et al (72) confirmed the observations of Florack and colleagues in non-immunosuppressed animals, but in immunosuppressed dogs an advantage of combined pancreas and kidney transplant compared to pancreas transplant alone could not be shown.

The histological features of pancreas graft rejection have now been studied in detail (73-79). Schulak and Drevyanko (74) correlated the histological features of rejection with the physiological manifestations in the rat pancreas allograft model. Perivascular infiltration was seen by day 3, lymphocytic infiltration in the exocrine pancreas by day 6, and islets were infiltrated by day 9. Anti-rejection treatment begun when the glucose levels rose did not reverse the process, while anti-rejection treatment begun on day 3, at the onset of histological rejection, prolonged graft functional survival.

The histological features of rejection have also been studied in relationship to whether exocrine function has or has not been preserved (75). Although duct ligation results in a non-specific inflammatory process, the features of allograft rejection can be distinguished and are similar no matter what method of pancreas transplant is used. Perivascular, interstitial and finally islet lymphocytic infiltration occurs sequentially. Another group found, however, that the physiological manifestations of rejection, i.e. hyperglycemia, occurred earlier in order in rats with duct-ligated-segmental versus duct-ligated-whole versus enteric-drained-whole pancreaticoduodenal grafts (76, 77). Interestingly, in whole pancreaticoduodenal grafts, the sequence of vasculitis, exocrine infiltration, and islet infiltration preceded duodenal destruction, and the myth that the duodenum is particularly susceptible to rejection no longer seems tenable (78).

The most sophisticated study on the histology of pancreas rejection is that of Steiniger et al (79), who used modern immunocytochemical techniques not only to identify the various cell types that infiltrate the islets, but also to determine the distribution of Class I and II major histocompatibility antigens during acute pancreas allograft rejection in rats. Exocrine acinar cells, normally being Class I antigen negative, strongly express these antigens during rejection. Class II antigens, which are normally not found in pancreatic endothelial or parenchymal cells, appear in duct epithelium, acinar cells and endothelial vessels, an early phenomenon characteristic of a continuing immune response. The increase in donor Class I and Class II antigen positive interstitial cells may amplify the rejection process.

Whether this histological information could be used in the clinical situation is uncertain because of the difficulties in obtaining biopsies (80). Steiner et al (81) had attempted fine needle aspiration of pancreas allografts in dogs, but had only a 10% technical success rate and the investigators were not able to evaluate the condition of the graft or to correlate the inflammatory cells with the outcome.

Early diagnosis of rejection is, of course, important, and Schulak and Drevyanko (74) showed the importance of early treatment. The urinary drainage method of pancreas transplantation provides the opportunity to monitor exocrine function as a marker of rejection other than hyperglycemia (82). Gotoh et al (83) and Prieto et al (43) have shown the value of urinary amylase monitoring, with a decrease in urinary amylase preceding an increase in plasma glucose levels and with the interval being greatest in immunosuppressed animals (43). Initiation of anti-rejection treatment at the time that the urinary amylase level decreases will prolong pancreas allograft survival in dogs (84).

Prophylactic measures to prevent rejection include recipient immunosuppression or graft pretreatment to reduce immunogenicity. Generalized immunosuppression with cyclosporine can prolong pancreatic allograft survival in animals (43, 65-68, 70-72, 76, 77, 84). The effect of cyclosporine by itself is variable, and additional maneuvers have also been used such as total lymphoid irradiation in dogs (85) or baboons (86). Cyclosporine may also be more effective at preventing rejection when administered at certain times and in certain doses determined chronobiologically (87, 88). Other adjunctive measures, such as splenectomy, did not help in the rat pancreas allograft model (89).

Inclusion of the spleen with pancreas allografts has been associated with prolonged pancreas functional survival in some (90) but not in other (91) donor-recipient strain combinations. In the one experiment where such a maneuver has been tested in a large animal allograft model, it was not effective; indeed inclusion of the spleen shortened pancreas allograft survival times in pigs (92). There is also the risk of graft-versus-host disease with spleen allotransplantation, although this occurrence can be prevented by ex vivo irradiation of the spleen in rats (93), a maneuver also used clinically by Koostra et al (27). With regard to graft-versus-host disease, it might be expected that inclusion of the duodenum could result in such an occurrence, but such does not appear to be the case (94).

Methods to reduce immunogenicity of the pancreas have been attempted. Asano et al (59) added anti-Ia antibodies to the solution used for machine perfusion-preservation of canine pancreas allografts, but the rejection time following transplantation was not altered. These results are not surprising in light of the recent demonstration by Gores et al (95) that anti-Ia treatment of isolated mouse islets with elimination of Ia-positive cells does not abrogate their ability to incite a rejection response and does not prolong their survival in the renal subcapsular position. Ex vivo irradiation of rat pancreas allografts has also not been effective on prolonging their functional survival (96).

The pancreas allotransplant experiments in animals have provided information on the rejection process. Maneuvers to prevent rejection complement protocols being employed clinically. The increased tendency to use urinary drainage for pancreas allografts clinically is also supported by the observations in animals that rejection can be diagnosed earlier and treated more effectively, by continuous monitoring of the exocrine function of pancreas allografts.

Metabolic effects of pancreas transplants in animals

Although it has been well documented that pancreas transplants can establish an euglycemic, insulin-independent state in diabetic recipients, the degree to which metabolism is normalized continues to be the subject of experimental studies. Albisser et al (97) compared the glycemic control that a heterotopic segmental pancreas autotransplant could provide with that achievable by administration of exogenous insulin in totally pancreatectomized dogs. The glucose values in both the transplant recipients and the insulin-treated animals were slightly but significantly higher than those in normal dogs. The mean values were no different between the pancreas transplant recipients and the insulin-treated animals, but the glycemic excursions were much narrower in the transplanted animals. In contrast, Orloff et al (37) found that rat recipients of systemically drained whole pancreas transplants had glucose levels that were entirely normal. The differences in these results may reflect the difference in B-cell mass for whole versus segmental transplants, but a control group of partially pancreatectomized dogs was not included in the studies of Albisser et al (97) to determine whether or not this hypothesis is correct. This issue has been addressed by earlier studies in which glucose levels in partially pancreatectomized dogs and in totally pancreatectomized dogs with heterotopic segmental autotransplants were identical (98).

The same considerations also pertain to measurement of serum insulin levels. Thus, Orloff et al (37) found that insulin values were higher in rat recipients of whole pancreas grafts, while Gooszen et al (99) found that the levels were similar. On the other hand, Florack et al (98) found that the levels were lower in canine recipients of systemically drained segmental transplants compared to normal dogs but not in relationship to partially pancreatectomized dogs, again emphasizing the need to consider both B-cell mass and the site of venous drainage when interpreting the results of pancreas transplant experiments.

Calhoun et al (100) performed intravenous glucose tolerance tests (IVGTTs) in totally pancreatectomized canine recipients of segmental pancreas auto-transplants with systemic drainage and found that the area under the glucose and insulin curves was normal, but K-values were less negative than in normal dogs. Falholt et al (101) found just the opposite: K-values were normal, but the total areas under the insulin and glucose curves were increased. These investigators did not make comparisons with partially pancreatectomized dogs. Gooszen et al (99) and Florack et al (98) did make such a comparison and found no differences in the quantitative and qualitative response to intravenous glucose, again emphasizing the effect of B-cell mass on the results of metabolic tests. Calhoun et al (100) also found that the shape of oral glucose tolerance test curves in the transplant recipients were different from those of normal dogs, but the glucose values were not significantly different at any time point.

The effects of pancreas transplantation on intermediary metabolism have also been studied. Albisser et al (102) measured the concentrations of 10 metabolites in totally pancreatectomized dogs with segmental pancreas transplants or insulin and found that 8 of the 10 values were normal in transplanted dogs while only 5 of 10 were normal in the insulin-treated dogs. Calhoun et al (100) measured other islet hormones in canine recipients of segmental pancreas transplants, and found no alterations from normal. Falholt (101) found elevated triglyceride levels in canine recipients of pancreas autotransplants, results in contrast with those of Kruszynska et al (103) in which islet transplants normalized lipid metabolism in rats.

The question of the relative advantage of portal versus systemic drainage of pancreas graft venous effluent continues to be examined, but no recent experiments have directly compared recipients in which intact pancreas grafts were transplanted with drainage to either of these two sites. Experiments that indirectly studied this question have been reported. Albisser et al (104) compared the glucose levels in transplanted dogs with systemic drainage to pancreatectomized dogs treated with insulin by either the systemic or portal route. The mean glucose levels were lowest in dogs receiving insulin via the portal route. However, the transplanted dogs had narrower glycemic excursions than dogs treated with either mode of insulin delivery, and intermediary metabolism was more nearly normalized in the transplanted dogs than in either of the two insulin-treated groups. With fetal pancreas transplants in rats to sites providing either portal or systemic drainage, there were no metabolic differences (103). Gooszen et al (105) provided data indicating that systemic drainage of segmental pancreas transplants compensated for changes in insulin and intravenous glucose tolerance K-values induced by reduction in B-cell mass. Conversely, Van Goor et al (30) presented data indicating that autotransplanted segments with drainage underwent progressive deterioration that was not seen when the left limb of the canine pancreas was left *in situ* with portal drainage. Florack et al (53) compared systemically drained pancreas grafts with portally drained islet grafts and found no significant differences, but the B-cell mass of the islet graft may have been less. Squifflet et al (51) examined this problem in rats with quantitation of B-cell mass by measurement of tissue insulin content following completion of the studies, and found that portal drainage was better if the B-cell mass was marginal; however, with a larger B-cell mass there were no differences in IVGTT K-values or other parameters for systemic versus portally drained grafts. Although the data, interpretations and conclusions of the various studies on portal versus systemic drainage are in conflict, the differences are minor and suggest that choosing one route over another will not have practical consequences, and that the differences are of physiological interest only.

The last metabolic problem to be investigated relates to the effect that immunosuppression may have on metabolism. Several investigators have reported an effect of cyclosporine on insulin secretion or on peripheral metabolism, particularly in rats where cyclosporine administration can result in impaired glucose tolerance and decreased insulin content of the pancreas (106, 107). Histological changes are also induced in the pancreas by cyclosporine, although the lesions are reversible (108). Van Schilfgaarde et al (109) found no effect of azathioprine and prednisone on the function of segmental pancreas transplants in dogs, but did find an effect of cyclosporine (110). In contrast, Hesse et al (111) found no effect of cyclosporine on the metabolic function of autotransplants in dogs. Again, the results of the various studies are in conflict and further investigations will be needed to determine whether or not cyclosporine has a significant effect on the function or the metabolic effect of pancreas transplants. Although it has been suggested that cyclosporine influences IVGTTs in human pancreas transplant recipients (112), the possible perturbations in metabolism induced by cyclosporine do not outweigh its advantage in preventing rejection.

Effect of experimental pancreas transplantation on the complications of diabetes in animal models

A plethora of papers extending back to the early 1970s have shown that normalization of metabolism by either islet or pancreas transplantation can prevent the occurrence or induce the regression of early lesions affecting the eye, nerves and kidneys in diabetic rats (2). Confirmation and extension of these observations have recently been provided by Orloff et al (113) in which reversal of glomerular mesangial enlargement in rats with long-standing diabetes was achieved by whole pancreas transplantation. Indeed, the salutary effect was seen at a later stage than has been possible with islet transplants, which Orloff et al (113) attributed to a superior normalization of metabolism by pancreas transplants (52).

With regard to vascular complications, Falholt et al (101) studied canine recipients of pancreas autotransplants. The animals were hyperinsulinemic and in addition had increased triglycerides in the arterial smooth muscle 4 years after the transplant. These results contrast with those of Kruszynska et al (104) in which lipid metabolism was normalized.

In an unique study of a complication previously ignored, Limmer et al (114) found that pancreas transplants could reverse the exocrine dysfunction associated with streptozotocin-induced diabetes in rats, suggesting that the abnormality in exocrine function of the pancreas in diabetic animals is not a result of loss of a paracrine effect from B-cell-deficient islets, but is secondary to the metabolic disturbance.

Clinical progress on selected issues of importance in pancreas transplantation

The issues discussed in *The Diabetes Annual/2* (2) continue to be investigated in the clinical arena. Progress or changes are being made in patient selection, surgical methods, graft preservation, diagnosis of rejection, and management of immunosuppression; new information on metabolism and the effect of pancreas transplantation on diabetic complications is slowly being gathered.

Recipient and donor selection

The majority of pancreas transplant recipients continue to be those with end-stage diabetic nephropathy (3, 115), but the Minnesota group has accumulated a relatively large experience with pancreas transplantation in non-uremic diabetic patients who have not received kidney transplants (8). The patients have largely been those with proteinuria or preproliferative retinopathy; whether the complications can be influenced by pancreas transplantation at this stage remains the subject of studies. Selection of uremic patients who should receive simultaneous pancreas and kidney transplants as opposed to kidney transplants alone continues to be debated (116), but the only contraindication at this time appears to be uncorrected coronary artery disease (14).

Generally any non-diabetic donor suitable for heart, kidney and liver donation is suitable as a pancreas donor (117). Amylase levels are often high in brain of cadavers and glucose levels may also be high from administration of steroids or fluids containing dextrose. However, the function of grafts obtained from such donors has been satisfactory (117).

Surgical techniques and complications

No new surgical techniques have been introduced since the last review on pancreas transplantation (2), but the bladder drainage technique has become the most popular (10). The relatively high infection rate with enteric drainage (118) prompted some groups to adapt the bladder drainage technique, lessening the risk of bacterial contamination from the transplant procedure (13, 26, 27). Although the Registry data do not show a difference in the rate of complications for enteric- versus urinary-drained grafts, individual groups adapting this technique have experienced a decrease in complications (119). Nevertheless, the enteric drainage technique continues to be used with good results (120), as does the duct injection technique (18).

The main advantage of the bladder drainage technique has been the ability to monitor for rejection using urinary amylase as a marker (6). Exocrine function can also be monitored temporarily with enteric drainage and the duct injection technique if a catheter in the duct is temporarily brought externally, but ultimately the catheter must be removed (17, 22, 23). With bladder drainage the graft exocrine function can be monitored indefinitely (9).

When complications related to the pancreas graft do occur, computerized tomography has been an aid in diagnosis and management (121). Abdominal fluid collections can be localized and drained if necessary.

Koostra et al (27) have continued to include the spleen with pancreas grafts, irradiating the spleen in order to avoid graft-versus-host disease. The latter has been described by other groups when the spleen was transplanted with the pancreas (122, 123). Even if classic graft-versus-host disease does not develop, if the spleen from a blood type O donor is transplanted to a blood type A recipient, immune hemolysis can occur (124, 125). With appropriate donor and recipient matching and irradiation of the spleen these problems may be avoided, but whether there is an advantage or not to transplanting the donor spleen *en bloc* with the pancreas remains to be shown.

Preservation of the pancreas

Most groups have continued to preserve pancreas grafts by cold storage in an intracellular electrolyte solution and to limit preservation time to less than 6 hours. The logistical constraints are justified by the Registry data showing higher failure rates with increasing length of preservation. However, the situation may be changing as groups adopt the solutions developed by Florack et al (54) and Wahlberg et al (60). Hyperosmolar colloid solutions are clearly superior to the intracellular electrolyte solutions developed for kidney preservation. The modified hyperosmolar silica-gel-filtered plasma solution developed by Florack et al (54) has been used for cold storage of human pancreas grafts at the University of Minnesota in their most recent cases, with adequate function of grafts stored for 12-24 hours (126). Nineteen of 20 grafts stored for 6-12 hours functioned as did 18 of 19 stored for 12-24 hours, a primary non-function rate of only 5%. Glucose tolerance and metabolic profile results were indistinguishable from those obtained in recipients with grafts preserved for shorter periods.

Observations of rejection and changes in immunosuppression for pancreas transplant recipients

It is still not clear whether the pancreas is more or less susceptible to rejection than other organs. With combined kidney and pancreas transplants, the kidney has been rejected while the pancreas from the same donor has continued to function (18). The physiological manifestations of rejection may appear earlier with the kidney than the pancreas, leading to earlier treatment of pancreas rejection in the situation when both organs were transplanted simultaneously from the same donor (127). In non-uremic, non-kidney transplant patients, pancreas grafts have been rejected very vigorously (8). The diagnosis of rejection of solitary pancreas grafts is facilitated with urinary drainage of the exocrine secretions (9). Prior to the use of this technique, clinical diagnosis of rejection was usually not made until hyperglycemia recurred (80, 128). The University of Minnesota team adopted the policy of performing graft biopsies in order to confirm the diagnosis of rejection, and the clinical features and correlations with the pathological process and response to treatment have been described (80). The histological features of recurrence of disease and islet inflammation in non-immunosuppressed or minimally immunosuppressed diabetic recipients of segmental pancreas grafts from identical-twin and HLA-identical-sibling donors have also been described (129). Recurrence of disease has not been seen in pancreas graft recipients of living related donors treated with an adequate immunosuppressive regimen (cyclosporine, azathioprine and prednisone in combination) (130).

Several groups have now adopted triple-drug or quadruple-drug immunotherapy for pancreas transplant recipients (7, 11, 17, 29). Such an approach is associated with less toxicity than single or double drug therapy because the doses of the individual drugs can be lower. Quadruple drug therapy consists of a temporary course of antilymphocyte globulin with maintenance immunosuppression by cyclosporine, azathioprine and prednisone. The reported graft and patient survival rates have been highest with this regimen (3).

Metabolic studies in pancreas transplant recipients

Formal studies such as those performed by Albisser et al (97, 102, 104) in diabetic dogs comparing glycemic control and the effects on intermediary metabolism of treatment by exogenous insulin versus pancreas transplantation have been carried out in humans by Pozza et al (131). Although glucose values could be maintained within a nearly normal range over the short term with exogenous insulin, the constant normalization or near-normalization possible with pancreas transplantation could not be sustained on a week-to-week or month-to-month basis. Circadian hormonal and metabolic patterns in pancreas transplant recipients showed mildly elevated plasma glucose levels, hyperinsulinemia between meals and at night, with delayed postprandial insulin peaks compared with normal individuals, but lactate and glucagon levels were normal. The minor differences compared with normal individuals could be due to a decrease in islet mass, denervation, peripheral hormone delivery, immunosuppression or, in the patients of Pozza et al (132), mild renal insufficiency.

An effect of cyclosporine on metabolism similar to that described by Gunnerson et al (112) was not seen in the studies by Pozza et al (113). The results of metabolic studies were similar in azathioprine- or cyclosporine-treated patients except for slightly increased insulin values in the cyclosporine group, a finding opposite to that described in animals (106, 107). The influence of cyclosporine on metabolism in pancreas transplant patients may be complex. Thus, Ost et al (134) found that cyclosporine enhanced the effect of prednisone in transplant patients, and interactions between the various drugs administered has to be taken into consideration when interpreting the results of metabolic studies.

More observations on the differences in results of metabolic studies in recipients of pancreas transplants with the graft venous effluent draining into the systemic versus the portal circulation have been made. Brons et al (135) compared the results of glucose tolerance tests performed in patients with paratopic segmental pancreas transplants drained into the recipient splenic vein with the results in non-transplant patients who had undergone a Whipple procedure; the glucose curves for these two groups were superimposed, but the results were different from those in normal individuals, confirming an effect on metabolism from reduction of B-cell mass. Patients with segmental grafts drained systemically had glucose tolerance curves that deviated even more from the normal than those with paratopic grafts. By contrast, Sutherland et al (136) studied 4 patients with segmental grafts drained via the inferior mesenteric vein to patients with systemically drained segmental pancreas grafts. Although glucose values tended to be lower in the portally drained group and a higher proportion had normal glucose tolerance test results, the differences were not statistically significant. Thus, efforts to establish portal drainage should not be based on a need to influence the results of metabolic tests, but rather on other considerations. It has been well established that segmental grafts with systemic drainage can result in fasting and postprandial glucose levels within the normal range, that glycosylated hemoglobulin levels are normal in pancreas transplant recipients with functioning grafts, and that glucose tolerance test results will be normal in at least half of the recipients (137).

Observations on the effect of pancreas transplantation on the complications of diabetes

It still is not clear what effect normalization of plasma glucose levels by pancreas transplantation has on the course of pre-existing secondary complications in diabetic recipients. Bohman et al (138) showed that kidneys transplanted to diabetic patients with end-stage renal disease did not develop lesions of diabetic nephropathy if the recipients also underwent simultaneous pancreas stimulation. Thus, development of new lesions may be prevented.

Most of the studies of complications in diabetes and pancreas transplant recipients have been in patients who also underwent kidney transplants. Thus, not only must the effect of immunosuppression be taken into account, but also the effect of correction of uremia, a correction that by itself has been shown to influence the course of diabetic retinopathy (139) and neuropathy (140). Nevertheless, it is apparent that diabetic recipients of pancreas and kidney transplants have an improvement in neuropathy (141-145). Kampik et al (146) found that visual acuity improved in more than half of the recipients of combined transplants, and proliferative retinopathy stabilized in the vast majority. In non-uremic recipients of pancreas transplants alone, however, Ramsay et al (147) found no differences in the incidence of stabilization or progression of retinopathy over the first year of follow-up in patients with functioning versus those with failed grafts. Long-term follow-up in larger numbers of patients will be necessary in order to discern the beneficial effects, if any, on progression of diabetic complications following successful pancreas transplantation.

Miscellaneous observations in pancreas transplant recipients

Although the objective of pancreas transplantation is to provide a permanent euglycemic state that will favorably influence the complications of diabetes affecting the eye, nerves and kidneys, the change in life style made possible by obviating the need for balancing insulin injections with meals and activities should not be dismissed as trivial (115). Elimination of the need for exogenous insulin comes at the expense of a requirement for life-long immunosuppression, but in many such patients, a normal life style is possible. Indeed, pregnancy with delivery of a normal child has been accomplished by a cyclosporine-treated recipient of a pancreas transplant (148).

Summary

The incidence of pancreas transplants and the success rate have continued to increase. The majority of pancreas transplants continue to be placed in diabetic recipients of kidney transplants with end-stage renal disease, but interest in application to non-uremic, non-kidney-transplant recipients is slowly mounting. Drainage of the graft duct into the bladder, allowing direct assessment of exocrine function, leads to earlier diagnosis and treatment of rejection episodes and has been associated with an improvement in graft survival rates, as has been the use of combination immunotherapy with cyclosporine and other immunosuppressants. Data on the effect of successful pancreas grafts on the specific complications of diabetes is just beginning to emerge, but preliminary evidence suggests that a salutary effect is achieved if the transplant is performed sufficiently early in the course of the disease.

References

1. Sutherland DER (1987): Pancreas transplantation. *Curr. Probl. Surg.*, in press.
2. Sutherland DER, Kendall DM (1986): Pancreas transplantation: clinical aspects. In: Alberti KGGM, Krall LP (Eds), *The Diabetes Annual/2*, pp 94-119. Elsevier, Amsterdam.
3. Sutherland DER, Moudry KC (1987): Pancreas Transplant Registry Report — 1986. *Clin. Transplant., 1*, 3.
4. Cats S, Gallon J (1985): Effect of original disease on kidney transplant outcome. In: Terasaki PI (Ed.), *Clinical Kidney Transplantation — 1985*, p. 35. University of California at Los Angeles Press.
5. Sutherland DER, Goetz FC, Najarian JS (1987): Pancreas transplant donor and recipient selection, management and outcome. *Transplant. Proc.*, in press.
6. Prieto M, Sutherland DER, Fernandez-Cruz L et al (1987): Experimental and clinical experience with urinary amylase monitoring for earlier diagnosis of rejection in pancreas transplantation. *Transplantation, 43*, 71.
7. Sutherland DER, Goetz FC, Najarian JS (1986): Improved pancreas graft survival rates by use of multiple drug combination immunotherapy. *Transplant. Proc., 18*, 1770.
8. Sutherland DER (1986): Transplantation in nonuremic diabetic patients. *Transplant. Proc., 18*, 1747.
9. Prieto M, Sutherland DER, Fernandez-Cruz L et al (1987): Diagnosis of rejection in pancreas transplantation. *Transplant. Proc., 19*, 2348.
10. Sollinger H, Kalayoglu M, Hoffman RM (1986): Experience with whole pancreas transplantation and pancreaticoduodenocystostomy. *Transplant. Proc., 18*, 1759.
11. Sollinger HW, Kalayogly M, Hoffman RM (1987): Quadruple immunosuppressive therapy in whole pancreas transplantation. *Transplant. Proc., 19*, 2297.
12. Corry RJ, Nghiem DD, Schulak JA et al (1986): Surgical treatment of diabetic nephropathy with simultaneous pancreatic duodenal and renal transplantation. *Surg. Gynec. Obstet., 162*, 547.
13. Nghiem DD, Beutel WD, Corry RJ (1986): Duodenocystostomy for exocrine pancreatic drainage and experimental and clinical pancreatico-duodenal transplantation. *Transplant. Proc., 18*, 1762.
14. Corry RJ, Nghiem DD, Schanbacher B (1987): Critical analysis of mortality and graft loss following simultaneous renal-pancreaticoduodenal transplantation. *Transplant. Proc., 19*, 2305.
15. Groth C, Lundgren G, Wilczek H et al (1984): Segmental pancreas transplantation with duct ligation or enteric diversion: technical aspects. *Transplant. Proc., 16*, 724.

16. Tyden G, Wilczek H, Lundgren G et al (1985): Experience with 21 intraperitoneal segmental pancreatic transplants with enteric or gastric exocrine diversion in humans. *Transplant. Proc., 17,* 331.
17. Tyden G, Brattstorm C, Lundgren G et al (1987): Improved results in pancreatic transplantation by avoiding non-immunological graft failures *Transplantation,* in press.
18. Landgraff R, Landgraff-Leurz MML, Burg D et al (1986): Long-term followup of segmental pancreas transplantation in Type I Diabetes. *Transplant. Proc., 18,* 1118.
19. Dubernard JM, Monti LD, Faure JL et al (1986): Report on 63 pancreas and kidney transplants in uremic diabetic patients. *Transplant. Proc., 18,* 1111.
20. Dubernard JM, Faure JL, Gelet A et al (1987): Simultaneous pancreas and kidney transplantation: long-term results and technical discussion. *Transplant. Proc., 19,* 2285.
21. Brekke IR, Dyrbekk D, Jakobsen A (1986): Combined pancreas and kidney transplantation for diabetic nephropathy. *Transplant. Proc., 18,* 1125.
22. Baumgartner D, Bruhlmann W, Largarider F (1986): Technique and timing of pancreatic duct occlusion with prolamine in recipients of simultaneous renal and intraoperative segmental pancreas alloimplants. *Transplant. Proc., 18,* 1134.
23. Steiner E, Klima J, Niederwieser D et al (1987): Monitoring of the pancreatic allograft by analysis of exocrine secretion. *Transplant. Proc., 19,* 2336.
24. Brons LGM, Calne RY, Rolles K et al (1986): Paratopic segmental pancreas transplantation with segmental kidney transplantation in diabetic recipients. *Transplant. Proc., 18,* 1757.
25. Gil-Vernet JM, Fernandez-Cruz L, Andreu D et al (1986): Urinary tract diversion clinical pancreas transplantation. *Transplant. Proc., 18,* 1132.
26. Munda R, First MR, Weiss MA et al (1987): Synchronous pancreatic and renal allografts with urinary tract drainage of the pancreas. *Transplant. Proc. 19,* 2343.
27. Koostra G, Von Hooff JP, Jorning PJG et al (1987): A new variant for whole pancreas grafting. *Transplant. Proc., 19,* in press.
28. Munda R, Tom WW, First MR et al (1987): Pancreatic allograft exocrine urinary tract diversion: pathophysiology. *Transplantation, 43,* 95.
29. Cutfield RG, Polonsky K, Olson L et al (1985): Long-term followup of canine segmental pancreatic autografts. *Diabetes, 34,* 174.
30. Van Goor HM, Floof MGH, Wijfels RPM et al (1986): Beta cell response and insulin sensitivity after segmental pancreas autotransplantation with systemic drainage. *Transplant. Proc., 18,* 1790.
31. Alejandro R, Cutfield RG, Shenvold FL (1986): Natural history of intrahepatic canine islet cell autografts. *J. Clin. Invest., 87,* 1339.
32. Alderson D, Farndon JR, Alberti KGMM et al (1984): Islet auto-transplantation in the pancreatectomized dog: effect of time on graft function. *World J. Surg., 8,* 590.
33. Gooszen HG, Bosman FT, Van Schilfgaarde R (1984): The effect of duct obliteration on histology and endocrine function of the canine pancreas. *Transplantation, 38,* 13.
34. Squifflet JP, Sutherland DER, Florack G (1986): Pancreas transplantation in the rat: long-term followup studies following different methods of management of exocrine drainage. *Transplant. Proc., 18,* 1143.
35. Diliz-Perez HS, Han HQ, De Santibanes E et al (1984): Total pancreatectomy duodenal homotransplantation in dogs immunosuppressed with cyclosporine and steriods. *Am. J. Surg., 147,* 677.
36. Lee S, Scott M, DeMacedo AR (1986): Pancreaticoduodenal transplantation in the rat: a technical update. *Transplantation, 42,* 327.
37. Orloff MJ, Greenleaf GE, Urban P et al (1986): Lifelong reversal of the metabolic abnormalities of diabetes in rats by whole pancreaticoduodenal transplantation. *Transplantation, 41,* 556.

38. Liu T, Sutherland DER, Heil J et al (1985): Beneficial effects of establishing pancreatic duct drainage into a hollow organ (bladder, jejunum, or stomach) compared to free intraperitoneal drainage or duct injection. *Transplant. Proc., 17,* 366.
39. Senninger N, Moody FG, Van Buren DH et al (1986): Intestinalization of pancreas fragments in dogs. *Surg. Gynecol. Obstet., 162,* 355.
40. Lindsey NJ, Ingram MS, Nolan PF et at (1984) Infection as a complication of Roux-en-Y loop jejunal draining rat pancreas grafts, including the effect of cyclosporine. *Transplant. Proc., 16,* 797.
41. MacAulay MA, Frasier RB, Morais A et al (1985): Acinar structure and function in canine pancreatic autografts with duct drainage into the urinary bladder. *Transplantation, 39,* 490.
42. MacDonald AS, MacAulay MA, Mackinnon SC et al (1984): Duct to bladder anastomosis pancreatic transplants: the effect of enzymuria and bacteruria. *Transplant. Proc., 16,* 1130.
43. Prieto M, Sutherland DER, Fernandez-Cruz L et al (1986): Urinary amylase monitoring for early diagnosis of pancreas allograft rejection in dogs. *J. Surg. Res., 40,* 597.
44. Nghiem DD, Beutel WD (1986): Duodenocystostomy for exocrine drainage in total pancreas transplantation in dogs. *Transplant. Prog., 18,* 1874.
45. Nghiem DD, Pitzen RH, Corry RJ (1985): Evaluation of techniques of controlling exocrine drainage after segmental pancreatectomy in dogs: implications for pancreatic transplantation. *Arch. Surg., 8120,* 1132.
46. Ingram MP, Nolan MS, Lindsey MJ et al (1984): Advantage of exocrine drainage on long-term endocrine function in the transplanted rat pancreas. *Transplant. Proc., 16,* 747.
47. Klempnauer J, Steingeer B, Lund R (1986): Importance of different surgical techniques on graft function, morphology and endocrine function following pancreas transplantation in rats. *Transplant. Proc., 18,* 1149.
48. Schang T, Timmerman W, Thiede A (1985): Models and perspectives on pancreas transplantation in rats: comparison of different transplantation models in the syngeneic system. *Langenbecks Arch. Chir., 363,* 227.
49. Garvin PJ, Castenada NA, Niehoff ML (1985): An in situ evaluation of distal splenic arterial venous fistula on pancreas function in an isolated pancreas segment. *Arch. Surg., 120,* 1148.
50. Steiner HE (1986): Pancreas transplantation: an experimental study of clinical problems. *Fortschr. Med., 104,* 40.
51. Squifflet JP, Sutherland DER, Florack G et al (1985): Physiologic comparison of segmental pancreas and islet transplants in rats. *Transplant. Proc., 17,* 378.
52. Orloff MJ, Maceda A, Greenleaf G et al (1987): Comparison of metabolic control of diabetes achieved by whole pancreas transplantation and pancreatic islet transplantation in rats. *Ann. Surg.,* in press.
53. Florack G, Sutherland DER, Hesse U et al (1986): Metabolic studies after heterotopic segmental pancreas and intrasplenic islet cell transplantation: a comparison. *Transplant. Proc., 18,* 1164.
54. Florack G, Sutherland DER, Heil J et al (1982): Long term preservation of segmental pancreas autografts. *Surgery, 92,* 260.
55. Toledo-Pereyra LH, Bach G, Schneider A (1985): Pancreas preservation with TP-4: a hyperosmolar colloid solution. *Cryobiology, 22,* 40.
56. Van Schilfgaarde R, Gooszen HG, Bosman FT et al (1984): Effect of 24 hour cold storage on the histology and long-term endocrine function of autografted canine left pancreatic segments. *Transplant. Proc., 16,* 809.
57. Nolan MS, Lindsay MJ, Ingrim MD et al (1984): Hypothermic preservation of rat pancreas with a view to maintaining endocrine function using either cold storage of pulsatile perfusion. *Transplant. Proc., 16,* 807.

58. Kanai Manden M, Gotoh M (1986): Successful 72 hour preservation of canine pancreas by simply hypothermia. *Transplant. Proc., 17,* 536.
59. Asano T, Watanabe K, Ohtsuka M (1985): Preservation of the segmental pancreas by non-pulsatile machine perfusion and anti-Ia monoclonal antibody treatment during the perfusion period. *Transplant. Proc., 17,* 1491.
60. Wahlberg JA, Love R, Landegaard L (1987): 72 hour preservation of the canine pancreas. *Transplantation, 43,* 5.
61. Florack G, Sutherland DER, Dunning M et al (1984): Function of segmental pancreas grafts subjected to warm ischemia prior to hypothermic preservation. *Transplant. Proc., 16,* 111.
62. Florack G, Sutherland DER, Ascherl R (1986): Definition of normothermic ischemia limits for kidney and pancreas grafts. *J. Surg. Res., 40,* 550.
63. Klempnauer J, Hoins L, Steiniger B et al (1984): Evidence for a differential importance of MHC and non-MHC alloantigens in pancreas and heart transplantation in the rat. *Transplant. Proc., 16,* 778.
64. Klempnauer J, Wonigeit K, Steiniger B (1985): Transplantation of effects of the RTI.C region in rat heart and pancreas grafting. *Transplant. Proc., 17,* 1893.
65. Timmerman W, Schang T, Thiede A (1984): The course of pancreatic allografts with physiologic secretion drainage in rats temporarily treated with cyclosporin A. *Transplant. Proc., 16,* 794.
66. Kawahara K, Sutherland DER, Rynasiewicz JJ, Najarian JS (1980): Prolongation of heterotopic cardiac allografts in rat by cyclosporin A. *Surgery, 88,* 594.
67. Rynasiewicz JJ, Sutherland DER, Ferguson RM et al (1982) Cyclosporine for immuno-suppression: observations in rat heart, pancreas and islet allograft models and in human renal and pancreas transplantation. *Diabetes, 31, Suppl. 4,* 92.
68. Domerque J, Douhaddioui N, Barneon GA (1984): Indefinite survival of pancreatic allografts under the cover of cyclosporin A in the rat. *J. Chir., 121,* 195.
69. Squifflet JP, Sutherland DER, Morrow CE et al (1983): Comparison of rejection of intra-portal islet versus immediately vascularized segmental pancreatic allografts in rats in relation to beta cell mass engrafted. *Transplant. Proc., 15,* 1344.
70. Severyn W, Olson L, Miller J et al (1982): Monitoring the kidneys for early diagnosis of pancreas rejection in canine recipients of combined pancreas and kidney transplants. *Transplantation, 33,* 606.
71. Florack G, Sutherland DER, Sibley RK et al (1985): Combined kidney and segmental pancreas allotransplantation in dogs. *Transplant. Proc., 17,* 374.
72. Nakayama Y, Uchida H, Yokopa K et al (1986): Combined pancreas and kidney transplantation with or without cyclosporine. *Transplant. Proc., 18,* 1798.
73. Steiniger B, Klempnauer J (1986): Distinct histological patterns of acute, prolonged and chronic rejection and vascularized rat pancreatic allografts. *Am. J. Pathol., 124,* 253.
74. Schulak JA, Drevyanko TF (1985): Experimental pancreas allograft rejection: correlation between histologic and functional rejection and the efficacy of antirejection treatment. *Surgery, 98,* 330.
75. Steiniger B, Klempnauer J, Brusch U et al (1984): Histology of rejection in rat pancreas allografts with suppressed or preserved exocrine function. *Transplant. Proc., 16,* 783.
76. Schang T, Timmerman W, Thiede A (1986): Influence of the technique for pancreatic transplantation on long-term function and the course of rejection. *Transplant. Proc., 18,* 1147.
77. Timmerman W, Schang T, Thiede A (1986): The influence of transplantation technique and the duration of endocrine function of pancreas allograft in the rat model. *Transplantation, 41,* 650.

78. Timmerman W, Schang T, Thiede A (1985): Models and perspectives of pancreas transplantation in rats to the course of the rejection of pancreaticoduodenal grafts to varying degrees of histoincompatibility and the influence of temporary treatment with cyclosporine. *Langenbeks Arch. Chir., 363*, 235.
79. Steiniger B, Klempnauer J, Wonigeit K (1985): Altered distribution of Class I and Class II MHC antigens during acute pancreas allograft rejection in the rat. *Transplantation, 40*, 234.
80. Sutherland DER, Casanova D, Sibly RK (1987): Role of pancreas graft biopsies and the diagnosis of treatment of rejection after pancreas transplantation. *Transplant. Proc., 19*, 2329.
81. Steiner E, Hammer C, Land W et al (1984): Fine needle biopsy of canine pancreas graft: an attempt at cytologic diagnosis in graft rejection. *Transplant. Proc., 16*, 789.
82. Cook K, Sollinger HW, Warner T et al (1983): Pancreaticocystostomy: an alternative method for exocrine drainage of segmental pancreatic allografts. *Transplantation, 35*, 634.
83. Gotoh M, Monden N, Motoki Y et al (1984): Early detection of rejection in the allografted pancreas. *Transplant. Proc., 16*, 781.
84. Prieto M, Fernandez-Cruz L, Sutherland DER et al (1986): Early diagnosis and treatment of rejection in pancreas transplantation. *Transplant. Proc., 18*, 1805.
85. Steward GJ, Williamson P, Garvey JFW (1985): Total lymphoid irradiation in canine pancreatic allograft recipients. *Transplant. Proc., 17*, 1731.
86. Du Toit DF, Heydenrych JJ, Schmidt B et al (1985): Segmental pancreatic allograft survival in baboons treated with combined irradiation and cyclosporine. *Surgery, 97*, 447.
87. Lui T, Cavallini M, Halberg F et al (1986): More on the need for circadian, circaseptan, and circannual optimization of cyclosporine therapy, *Experientia, 42*, 20.
88. Cavallini M, Halberg F, Cornelissen G et al (1986): Organ transplantation and broader chronotherapy with implantable pump and computer program for marker rhythm assessment. *J. Controlled Release, 3*, 3.
89. Schulak JA, Engelstad KM (1985): Splenectomy in experimental pancreas transplantation. *Transplantation, 40*, 564.
90. Bitter-Suermann H, Brynger J, Wikstrom I et al (1979): A new technique of orthotopic en bloc transplantation of the porcine liver and duct ligated pancreas. *J. Surg. Res., 27*, 105.
91. Squifflet JP, Sutherland DER, Florack G et al (1985): Physiologic comparison of segmental pancreas and islet transplants in rats. *Transplant. Proc., 17*, 378.
92. DaFoe DC, Campbell DA, Marks WH et al (1985): Association of inclusion of the donor spleen and pancreaticoduodenal transplantation with rejection. *Transplantation, 40*, 579.
93. Schulak JA, Sharp WJ (1986): Graft irradiation abrogates graft versus host disease in combined pancreas-spleen transplantation. *J. Surg. Res., 40*, 326.
94. Timmerman EG, Schubert T, Schang T et al (1986): Incidence of graft versus host reactions after pancreaticoduodenal transplantation in the rat. *Transplant. Proc., 18*, 1177.
95. Gores PF, Sutherland DER, Platt JL Bach FH (1986): Depletion of donor Ia+ cells before transplantation does not prolong islet allograft survival. *J. Immunol., 137*, 1482.
96. Cavallini M, Sutherland DER (1985): Ex vivo irradiation of the pancreas and treatment with cyclosporine: effects on graft rejection in an experimental model of allografts in rats. *Policlin. Sez. Chir., 92*, 21.
97. Albisser AM, Nomura M, McPhedran NT (1985): Glycemic control in diabetic dogs treated with pancreatic autotransplants and insulin pumps. *Diabetes Res., 2*, 145.
98. Florack G, Sutherland DER, Squifflet JP et al (1982): Effect of graft denervation, systemic venous drainage, and reduction of beta cell mass on insulin levels after heterotopic pancreas transplantation in dogs. *Surg. Forum., 33*, 351.
99. Gooszen HG, Van Schilfgaarde R, Frolich M et al (1985): The effects of duct obliteration and of autotransplantation on the endocrine function of canine pancreatic segments. *Diabetes, 34*, 1008.

100. Calhoun P, Brown KS, Crusch DA et al (1986): Evaluation of insulin secretion by pancreas autotransplants by oral or intravenous glucose challenge. *Ann. Surg., 204*, 585.
101. Falholt K, Cutfield R, Alejandro R et al (1985): The effects of hyperinsulinemia on arterial wall and peripheral muscle metabolism in dogs. *Metab. Clin. Exp., 34*, 1146.
102. Albisser AM, Nomura M, McPhedran NT (1986): Intermediary metabolism in diabetic dogs treated with pancreatic autotransplants and insulin pumps. *Metab. Clin. Exp., 35*, 378.
103. Kruszynska YT, Home PD, Alberti KGMM (1985): Comparison of portal and peripheral insulin delivery on lipid metabolism in streptozotocin diabetic rats. *Diabetes, 34*, 611.
104. Albisser AM, Nomura M, Greenberg GR et al (1986): Metabolic control on diabetic dogs treated with pancreatic autotransplants and insulin pumps. *Diabetes, 35*, 97.
105. Gooszen HG, Van Schilfgaarde R, Vanderburg MPM et al (1986): Does normal glucose tolerance after transplantation of the duct-obliterated pancreas reflect normal beta cell function? *Transplant. Proc., 18*, 1155.
106. Hahn HJ, Laube F, Lucke S et al (1986): Toxic effect of cyclosporine on the endocrine pancreas of Wistar rats. *Transplantation, 41*, 44.
107. Yale JF, Roy RD, Grose M et al (1985): Effects of cyclosporine on glucose tolerance in the rat. *Diabetes, 34*, 1309.
108. Mirkovitch V, Augstburger M, Telmer E et al (1986): Influence of cyclosporine on the function and morphology of the rat pancreas. *Transplant. Proc., 18*, 1171.
109. Van Schilfgaarde R, Gooszen HG, Frolich M et al (1984): The effect of prednisone and azathioprine on endocrine function of the canine segmental pancreatic autografts. *Transplant. Proc., 16*, 802.
110. Van Schilfgaarde R, Van der Burg MPM, Van Suylichem PTR et al (1986): Does cyclosporine influence beta cell function? *Transplant. Proc., 18*, 1175.
111. Hesse UJ, Stock P, Sutherland DER et al (1986): Cyclosporine and glucose metabolism. *Transplant. Proc., 18*, 1154.
112. Gunnerson R, Klintmalm G, Lundgren G et al (1984): Deterioration of glucose metabolism in pancreas transplant recipients after conversion from azathioprine to cyclosporine. *Transplant. Proc., 16*, 709.
113. Orloff MJ, Yamanaka N, Greenleaf G et al (1986): Reversal of mesangial enlargement in rats with long-standing diabetes by whole pancreas transplantation. *Diabetes, 35*, 347.
114. Limmer J, Beischer W, Buchler M et al (1985): Heterotopic pancreas transplantation in the rat. *Transplant. Proc., 17*, 400.
115. Landgraff R (1986): General considerations in pancreatic transplantation. *Transplant. Proc., 18, Suppl. 3*, 50.
116. Pozza G, Secchi A, Bonisolli L (1986): Prognostically poor signs in Type I diabetes mellitus and how to identify high risk patients. *Transplant. Proc., 18, Suppl. 3*, 52.
117. Hesse UJ, Najarian JS, Sutherland DER (1985): Amylase activity and pancreas transplantation. *Lancet, 2*, 726.
118. Hesse UJ, Sutherland DER, Simmons RL, Najarian JS (1986): Intra-abdominal infections in pancreas transplant recipients. *Ann. Surg., 203*, 153.
119. Hesse UJ, Sutherland DER, Simmons RL et al (1986): Graft infection in pancreas transplant recipients. *Transplant. Proc., 18*, 1755.
120. Groth CG, Lundgren G, Wilczek H (1984): Segmental pancreatic transplantation with duct ligature or impaired diversion: technical aspects. *Transplant. Proc., 16*, 724.
121. Maile CW, Crass CR, Frick MP (1985): Computerized tomography of pancreas transplantation. *Invest. Radiol., 20*, 609.
122. DaFoe DC, Campbell DA, Marks WH et al (1985): Karyotypic chimerism and rejection in a pancreaticoduodenal splenic transplant. *Transplantation, 40*, 572.
123. Deierhoi MH, Sollinger HW, Bozdec MJ et al (1986): Lethal graft versus host diaease in a recipient of a pancreas-spleen transplant. *Transplantation, 41*, 544.

124. Starzl TE, Iwatsuki S, Shaw BW (1984): Pancreaticoduodenal transplantation in humans. *Surg. Gynecol. Obstet., 159,* 265.
125. Salamon DJ, Ramsay G, Nusbacher J et al (1985): Anti-A production by a Group O transplanted to a Group A recipient. *Vox Sang., 48,* 309.
126. Abouna GM, Sutherland DER, Florack G et al (1987): Function of transplanted human pancreatic allografts after preservation in cold storage for 6-26 hours. *Transplantation,* in press.
127. Traeger J, Dubernard JM, Piatti PM et al (1984): Clinical aspects of pancreatic rejection and pancreaticorenal allotransplants. *Transplant. Proc., 16,* 718.
128. Tyden G, Lundgren G, Gunnarson R (1984): Laboratory findings during rejection of segmental pancreatic allografts. *Transplant. Proc., 16,* 715.
129. Sibley RK, Sutherland DER, Goetz FC, Michael AF (1985): Recurrent diabetes mellitus in the pancreas iso- and allograft: A light and electron microscopic and immunohistochemical analysis of four cases. *Lab. Invest., 53,* 132.
130. Sutherland DER, Kendall DM, Najarian JS (1985): One institution's experience with pancreas transplantation. *West. J. Med., 143,* 838.
131. Pozza G, Secchi, Bosi E et al (1985): Artificial insulin delivery systems versus pancreas transplantation: effect on metabolic control. *Transplant. Proc., 17,* 358.
132. Pozza G, Bosi E, Secchi A et al (1985): Metabolic control of Type I diabetes after pancreas transplantation. *Br. Med. J., 291,* 510.
133. Pozza G, Bosi E, Secchi A et al (1985) Metabolic control of Type I diabetes after pancreas transplantation. *Br. Med. J., 291,* 510.
134. Ost L, Klintmalm G, Ringden O (1985): Mutual interactions between prednisolone and cyclosporine in renal transplant patients. *Transplant. Proc., 17,* 1252.
135. Brons IGM, Calne RY, Rolles K et al (1986): Paratopic segmental pancreas with simultaneous kidney transplantation in diabetics. *Transplant. Proc., 18,* 757.
136. Sutherland DER, Goetz FC, Mandry KC et al (1987): Use of recipient mesenteric vessels for revascularization of segments of pancreas grafts: technical and metabolic considerations. *Transplant. Proc., 19,* 2300.
137. Tyden G (1986): What can be achieved by pancreatic transplantation? *Transplant. Proc., 18, Suppl. 3,* 55.
138. Bohman SO, Wilczeck H, Tyden G et al (1987): Recurrent diabetic nephropathy in renal transplants placed in diabetic patients and the protective effect of simultaneous pancreatic transplantation. *Transplant. Proc., 19,* 2290.
139. Ramsay RC, Cantrill HC, Knobloch WH et al (1983): Visual parameters in diabetic patients following renal transplantation. *Diabetic Nephropathy, 2,* 26.
140. Barbosa J, Burke B, Buselmeier TJ et al (1974): Neuropathy, retinopathy and biopsy findings in transplanted kidney and diabetic patients. *Kidney Int., 6, Suppl. 1* S32.
141. Tyden G, Lundgren G, Oste L et al (1986): Progress in segmental pancreas transplantation. *World J. Surg., 10,* 404.
142. Traeger J, Monti LD, Dubernard JM et al (1986): Metabolic studies in followup of degenerative complications in patients with a long-term functioning pancreatic graft (more than one year). *Transplant. Proc., 18,* 1139.
143. Tzakis AG, Carrol PB, Makowaka L et al (1987): Effect of pancreatic transplantation on diabetic complications in adults. *J. Surg. Res.,* in press.
144. Schafferhan SK, Heidbreder E, Land W et al (1986): Diabetic automatic neuropathy after simultaneous kidney and pancreas transplantation. *Transplant. Proc., 18,* 1136.
145. Kennedy WR, Fries TJ, Sutherland DER et al (1986): Thermosensitivity in patients with diabetes mellitus. *Transplant. Proc., 18,* 775.
146. Kampik A, Ulberg M (1986): Is proliferative diabetic retinopathy an indication for pancreatic transplantation? *Transplant. Proc., 18,* 62.

147. Ramsay RC, Rice SW, Sutherland DER et al (1986): Visual status following pancreas transplantation for Type I diabetes mellitus. *Transplant. Proc., 18,* 1774.
148. Castro LA, Baltzer U, Hillebrand G et al (1986). Pregnancy in juvenile diabetes mellitus under cyclosporine treatment after combined kidney and pancreas transplantation. *Transplant. Proc., 18,* 1780.

The Diabetes Annual/3
K.G.M.M. Alberti and L.P. Krall, editors
© 1987 Elsevier Science Publishers, B.V.

11 Islet transplantation

PAUL E. LACY

Introduction

Since transplantation *per se* has not been reviewed previously in *The Diabetes Annual*, a brief overview of the past accomplishments as well as more recent developments will be presented. Several detailed reviews on islet transplantation have been published recently (1-3). In approximately one decade, it has been shown that transplants of islets will reverse experimental diabetes to normal and will prevent or reverse early complications of diabetes as they occur in animals; methods have been developed for the prevention of rejection of islet allografts in animals without using immunosuppressive drugs; isolation techniques have been developed for the mass isolation of human islets; and human clinical trials are being initiated using either adult islets or human fetal pancreas for transplantation. This is a remarkably rapid rate of development in a scientific field. Each of these areas of accomplishment will be reviewed in the following sections.

Adult islet transplants

Effect of islet isografts on complications of diabetes in animals After the development of the collagenase technique for the isolation of rat islets (4, 5), many laboratories demonstrated that transplants of normal islets in inbred strains of rats would reverse experimentally induced diabetes to normal and maintain normoglycemia indefinitely in the recipients (6-9). The sites that have been used effectively for isografts of islets are the liver (by injecting the islets into the portal vein), spleen, intraperitoneal cavity, and the subcapsular space of the kidney. Methods have been developed for the mass isolation of canine islets, and autotransplants of islets in dogs following total pancreatectomy have maintained normoglycemia in the recipients (10-14).

Isografts of islet in rats have not only produced normoglycemia in the recipients, but they have also prevented or reversed early complications of diabetes in these animals involving the eye, kidney, autonomic nervous system, and the articular cartilage (15-20). These findings raised the hope that islet transplantation could be used as a therapeutic approach to human diabetes. Before this could be attempted, several problems had to be resolved. One was to attempt to prevent rejection of islet transplants in animals without the use of immunosuppressive drugs. This was a particularly key problem, since it would not be appropriate to maintain diabetic patients on immunosuppressive therapy for decades with the hope that the islet transplants would prevent complications but with the knowledge that serious toxic side effects could occur from long-term immunosuppression. Thus, procedures were sought which might prevent rejection of islets without the use of immunosuppressive drugs.

Prevention of rejection of islet allografts   In 1957, Snell (21) suggested that passenger leukocytes carried along with transplanted organs might be responsible for initiation of immune rejection, whereas the parenchymal cells of the organ would not initiate rejection. This suggestion lay fallow for many years until 1974 when Jacobs (22) reported that culture in vitro of the ovary for several days would prolong the survival of ovarian grafts transplanted across major histocompatibility barriers in mice. A year later, Lafferty et al (23) found that incubation of donor thyroid in the presence of 95% oxygen for 3 weeks prior to transplantation would prevent rejection of thyroid allografts in mice. Subsequently, our laboratory demonstrated that rejection of islet allografts in rats transplanted across a major histocompatibility barrier could be prevented by culturing the donor tissue at 24°C for 7 days and giving 1 injection of antilymphocyte serum to the recipients at the time of transplantation (24, 25). These in vitro culture procedures were apparently altering or destroying passenger leukocytes within the grafts.

In the ensuing years several procedures have been developed for the destruction or alteration of passenger leukocytes in the islets and have been shown to be effective in preventing rejection of islets in mice and rats (Table 1). These methods include: culture of aggregates of islets in the presence of 95% oxygen (26); treatment of the donor islets with specific Ia antiserum and complement (27) or anti-dendritic-cell antibody and complement (28); ultraviolet irradiation of the donor islets (29); separation in vitro of purified populations of donor B cells (30); and transplantation of the donor islets into partially immunologically privileged sites, such as the testes (31) and brain (32).

Studies on the immunologic status of animals receiving transplants of endocrine grafts devoid of passenger, Ia$^+$ lymphoid cells have shown that a state of specific immune unresponsiveness or tolerance has been induced in the recipients (33-36). The development of tolerance in the recipient animals bearing established endocrine allografts is apparently due to induction of suppressor T cells; however, these suppressor cells have not been specifically demonstrated in this transplant model. The finding that transplants of islets devoid of Ia$^+$ cells induced specific tolerance in the recipient raised the possibility that preimmuni-

TABLE 1   *Methods for prevention of rejection of islet allografts in rodents*

Animals	Pretreatment recipients	Pretreatment donor islets	Treatment recipients post-transplant	Site of islet implantation
Rats	none	culture 24°C, 7 days	one injection ALS	liver via PV (24)
Mice	none	culture islet aggregates 95% O_2, 7 days	none	kidney capsule (26)
Mice	none	Ia antibody + C′	none	liver via PV (27)
Mice	none	antidendritic cell antibody + C′	none	liver via PV (28)
Rats	none	UV irradiation	cyclosporin A, 30 mg/kg, 3 days	liver via PV (29)
Rats	none	separation of pure islet cells	none	liver via PV (30)
Mice	none	none	L3T4 antibody, 4 days	liver via PV (61)
Mice	Ia-depleted donor blood	none	none	liver via PV (37)
Rats	UV-irradiated donor blood	none	none	liver via PV (38)
Rats	none	none	3 injections ALS	testes, intra-abdominal (31)
Rats	none	none	none	brain (32)

PV = portal vein

zation with Ia⁻ cells might be used as a means of inducing tolerance in the recipients and thus being able to transplant untreated donor islets. Preimmunization of recipient mice with donor blood depleted of Ia^+ lymphoid cells by treatment with Ia antibody and complement prevented rejection of transplants of untreated donor islets (37). Irradiation of donor rat blood with ultraviolet light to inactivate the antigen-presenting cells has also been shown to prevent rejection of untreated donor rat islets (38).

It is easier to prevent rejection of islet allografts between different strains of mice than of rats. In the mouse it is possible to prevent rejection of islet allografts by direct treatment of the donor islets with procedures that will alter or destroy the passenger leukocytes. In contrast, in the rat it is necessary not only to destroy or alter passenger leukocytes in the islets, but to provide temporary immunosuppression of the recipient rats with either antilymphocyte serum or cyclosporin to prevent rejection when the recipient strain is a strong immune responder (24, 25, 39). This finding is of importance with respect to human islet transplantation, since undoubtedly both alteration and destruction of passenger leukocytes in donor human islets will be required in addition to immunosuppressive therapy of the recipient patient for a period of time.

Prevention of rejection of islet xenografts   The passenger leukocyte concept also applies to the prevention of rejection of islet xenografts transplanted between closely related species. Culture in vitro of rat islets at 24°C in conjunction with either a single injection of antilymphocyte serum or a short course of cyclosporin A therapy will prevent rejection of the rat islets transplanted into diabetic mice (40, 41). Culture in vitro of aggregates of rat islets in the presence of 95% oxygen for 7 days will also prolong survival of rat islet xenografts in mice (42). Nakajima et al (43) have reported prolongation of hamster islet xenografts in rats with cyclosporin A therapy. Recent studies in our laboratory have shown that low-temperature culture of donor hamster islets transplanted beneath the renal capsule of diabetic mice produces a marked prolongation of islet xenograft survival. Eloy et al (44) reported that intrahepatic transplants of 15-day-old chick embryo pancreases into diabetic rats improved the diabetic state of the recipients for as long as 18 months. In contrast, intrahepatic transplants of 18-day-old chick embryo pancreases were rapidly rejected. To my knowledge, these intriguing observations have never been confirmed in other laboratories.

Lymphokines in islet rejection   Normal human, rat, mouse, dog and pig islets do not express Class II antigens (Ia antigens) (45-47). Scattered Ia$^+$ expressing B cells have been described in the pancreas following the onset of Type I diabetes, and it has been suggested that the induction of Ia expression on the islet cells may have a role to play in autoimmunity with resultant destruction of the islet cells (48, 49). Thus, the key questions are whether Ia expression can be induced in vitro on islet cells and, if this is possible, whether these Ia$^+$ islet cells are capable of antigen presentation.

Several lymphokines are involved in an immune reaction leading to the production of cytotoxic T lymphocytes. One of these lymphokines is interferon-γ (IFN-γ). IFN-γ has been shown to induce Ia antigens on cells that do not normally express Class II antigens (such as mast cells, endothelial cells, fibroblasts, and melanoma cells) (50-53). Our laboratory has shown recently that Ia expression can be induced on mouse islet cells from B10.BR and Balb/c mice by culture in vitro of isolated islets in the presence of IFN-γ for 5-6 days (54). Studies are now needed to determine whether islet cells with induced Ia expression are capable of antigen presentation.

Another lymphokine that is released during an immune reaction is inter-leukin-1 (IL-1). Culture in vitro of rat islets in the presence of IL-1 for 6 days causes disintegration of the islets and impairment of insulin secretion (55-57). Culture in vitro of islets with IL-1 for 30 minutes causes an enhancement of glucose-induced insulin release, whereas exposure of the islets to IL-1 for 15 hours causes a significant inhibition of glucose-induced insulin release (58). These findings suggest that IL-1 released during an inflammatory reaction in the islets may affect the structure and function of islet cells.

Interleukin-2 (IL-2) is another lymphokine involved in immune reactions. IL-2 induces IL-2 receptors on activated lymphocytes, which provides a specific marker for these lymphocytes. Kirkman et al (59) obtained a marked prolonga-tion of cardiac allograft survival in mice following the administration of an anti-IL-2 receptor antibody. Another activation marker on lymphocytes is L3T4, which is shown to be present on helper T lymphocytes (60). Shizuru et al (61) have prevented rejection of islet allografts in mice by repeated injections of a monoclonal antibody to L3T4 in the recipient animals. The availability of monoclonal antibodies to the different lymphokines and to the activation markers on lymphocytes provides another approach to the prevention of rejec-tion of islet allografts by specific reagents.

Human islet isolation　The collagenase technique for isolation of islets from the rodent pancreas is not effective for the mass isolation of islets from the pancreases of large animals or from the human pancreas. Modifications of this procedure have been developed recently for the mass isolation of islets from the dog, beef and pork pancreas (11, 62-64). Further modifications of the techniques for isolating islets from large animals have led to the development of several procedures for the mass isolation of islets from the human pancreas (65-68). The development of these methods for human islet isolation has made it possible to initiate studies on human islet transplantation.

Human islet transplants　Soon after the development of the collagenase technique for isolation of rodent islets and the demonstration that transplants of the islets would reverse diabetes in animals, attempts were made to use this procedure for isolating human islets and transplanting them into diabetic patients. None of these premature attempts was successful, since the rodent islet isolation procedure is not effective when applied to the human pancreas. The development of methods in the last few years for the mass isolation of human islets has now made it possible to attempt more definitive studies on human islet transplants.

Our laboratory developed a method for human islet isolation which yielded 100,000-150,000 islets per human pancreas; however, the preparation was impure and contained only 20% islet tissue and 80% acinar tissue (66). The islets isolated by this procedure were functional in vitro; thus, initial studies on transplanting islets into diabetic patients who had a kidney transplant and were already receiving immunosuppressive drugs was initiated. Because of the impurity of the preparation, it was necessary to implant the islets directly into the parenchyma of the spleen in these individuals. Six human transplants were accomplished and 3 of the recipients had islet function as indicated by plasma C-peptide levels in the lower limits of normal and diminished insulin requirements for 1-2 months after transplantation.

Mintz and his associates used a different method for human islet isolation and were able to transplant islets into the liver via the portal vein in similar types of diabetic patients. Initial reports from these studies indicated that temporary function lasting one to several months occured following transplantation of the human islets (69).

Procedures have now been developed in our laboratory for the purification of the human islet preparation so that it contains 60-90% islets; this preparation can be maintained in culture with determination of islet function prior to transplantation. In addition, we have found that the purified human islets will survive and function after 7 days of culture at 24°C similar to what had been demonstrated with rat islets. These new developments will make it possible to initiate the second phase of human clinical trials in which the islets are cultured at low temperature to attempt to destroy alter passenger leukocytes and to transplant these via the portal vein into the liver in patients who will receive immunosuppression for a limited period of time.

A key question in this second phase of human islet transplantation will be whether the presumed autoimmune state in Type I diabetes will cause destruction of the islet transplants when immunosuppression is stopped. Sibley et al (70) reported that segmental pancreas transplants between non-diabetic and diabetic identical twins without the use of immunosuppressive drugs resulted in destruction of the B cells in the grafts and a return to a diabetic state. If the destruction of pancreatic B cells in autoimmunity is cell-mediated, then recognition of the B cells by activated lymphocytes would be linked to a close similarity of the histocompatibility antigens expressed on both the donor B cells and the recipient lymphocytes. It is possible that this cell-mediated reaction might be avoided if the donor islets expressed histocompatibility antigens different from the recipient.

Histologic studies in BB rats have shown that transplants of rat islets from a different strain would be infiltrated with lymphocytes and destroyed when transplanted into diabetic BB rats (71, 72). In contrast, Woehrle et al (73) found that allografts of Lewis islets transplanted into BB rats of the Wistar-Furth strain were not rejected when the islets were incubated at low temperature culture for 1 week and a single injection of antilymphocyte serum was given to the recipient. This pretreatment procedure did not prevent the rejection of transplants of Wistar-Furth islets which have the same histocompatibility antigens as the BB rat. The differences in these two findings may well be due to the methods that were used to prevent rejection of rat islet allografts. The histologic studies utilized high oxygen culture of aggregates of rat islets which is not effective in preventing rejection of rat islet allografts; however, low-temperature culture and a single injection of ALS is an established effective method for prevention of rat islet allograft rejection.

Selawry et al (31) utilized the testis as a semi-immunologically privileged site and found that transplants of islet allografts into the testis of diabetic BB rats in conjunction with a short course of immunosuppressive therapy prevented rejection of the transplants. If the BB rat model has similarities to Type I diabetes in man, then the findings on mismatching the donor and recipient tissue in conjunction with low-temperature culture and temporary immunosuppression provide hope that such an approach might be helpful in preventing destruction of human islet transplants via an autoimmune process following cessation of immunotherapy.

Fetal pancreas transplants

Prevention of rejection of fetal pancreas allografts   An advantage of the fetal pancreas for transplantation is that the fetal islets are capable of replication and comprise a high proportion of the pancreas as compared to the adult. Isografts of fetal pancreas in rodents have been used successfully in reversing diabetic states to normal within inbred strains of rodents (74). Prevention of rejection of allografts of the fetal pancreas by culture in vitro has not been as successful as that with allografts of isolated adult islets (75). Culture in vitro of donor fetal pancreas in the presence of 95% oxygen for 3 weeks produced only a slight to moderate reduction in immunogenicity of the fetal allografts and low-temperature culture caused damage to the endocrine portion of the fetal pancreas (76). Simeonovic et al (77) have developed a method for the isolation of pro-islets from the fetal mouse pancreas. Pro-islets are composed of undifferentiated tissue elements that will subsequently differentiate into islets following transplantation as isografts. Culture in vitro of fetal pro-islets in the presence of 95% oxygen has produced a 50% survival of pro-islet allografts at 4 weeks after transplantation (78). Further procedures that have been found to be effective in preventing rejection of adult islet allografts need to be applied to the fetal pancreas.

Human fetal pancreas transplants   Several years ago, Groth et al (79) obtained evidence of urinary C-peptide secretion following transplants of micro-fragments of cultured human fetal pancreases injected into the vascular system of the liver of a diabetic patient. The measurable levels of urinary C-peptide occurred at 1 month after transplantation and persisted for 3 months with a slight decrease in insulin requirements. Tuch et al (80) transplanted cultured explants of two human fetal pancreases into the forearm of a diabetic patient and biopsy of the transplant site at 13 months demonstrated A and D cells at the transplant site with an absence of B cells. No change occurred in insulin requirements and plasma C-peptide levels did not increase following transplantation.

Yuan-feng et al (81) have transplanted cultured fetal human pancreatic tissue into twenty-four diabetic recipients. Ten fetal pancreases were used for each transplant and the tissue was implanted either intramuscularly or intraperitoneally. A marked reduction in insulin requirements was reported for these patients. It will be of importance to learn of the change in plasma C-peptide levels in these studies. Farkas and Karacsonyi (82) have reported a reduction in insulin requirements in two diabetic patients at 8 months after transplantation of cultured fetal pancreas in the liver.

The problems that are being addressed in several centers concerning fetal pancreas transplants are: the effect of immunosuppressive agents on the differentiation of the fetal pancreas; the optimum site for implantation of the pancreas; histologic studies on the differentiation of fetal pancreas transplants; the number of fetal pancreases that should be utilized for transplantation; and the development of effective means of preventing rejection of fetal pancreas transplants without the use of immunosuppressive drugs. These are important issues and more definitive information on the use of human fetal pancreas transplants should be available in the future.

References

1. Progress Symposium (1984): Transplantation of pancreatic islet cells. *World J. Surg., 8,* 135.
2. Lacy PE, Davie JM (1984): Transplantation of pancreatic islets. *Ann. Rev. Immunol., 2,* 183.
3 Lafferty KJ, Prowse SJ, Simeonovic CJ et al (1983): Immunobiology of tissue transplantation: a return to the passenger leucocyte concept. *Annu. Rev. Immunol., 1,* 143.
4. Lacy PE, Kostianovsky M (1967): A method for the isolation of intact islets of Langerhans from the rat pancreas. *Diabetes, 16,* 35.
5. Lacy PE, Walker MM, Fink CJ (1972): Perifusion of isolated rat islets in vitro: the participation of the microtubular system in the biphasic release of insulin. *Diabetes, 21,* 987.
6. Ballinger WF, Lacy PE (1972): Transplantation of intact pancreatic islets in rats. *Surgery, 72,* 175.
7. Kemp CB, Knight MJ, Scharp DW et al (1973): Transplantation of isolated pancreatic islets into the portal vein of diabetic rats. *Nature (London), 244,* 447.
8. Reckard CR, Barker CF (1973): Transplantation of isolated pancreatic islets across strong and weak histocompatibility barriers. *Transplant. Proc., 5,* 761.
9. Leonard RJ, Lazarow A, Hegre OD (1973): Pancreatic islet transplantation in the rat. *Diabetes, 22,* 413.

10. Mirkrovitch V, Campiche M (1977): Intrasplenic autotransplantation of canine pancreatic tissues. *Eur. Surg. Res., 9,* 173.
11. Horaguchi A, Merrel RC (1981): Preparation of viable islet cells from dogs by a new method. *Diabetes, 30,* 455.
12. Alderson D, Farndon JR, Alberti KGMM et al (1984): Islet autotransplantation in the pancreatectomized dog: effect of time on graft function. *World J. Surg., 8,* 590.
13. Merrel RC, Marincola F, Maeda M et al (1985): The metabolic response of intrasplenic islet autografts. *Surg. Gynecol. Obstet., 160,* 552.
14. Merrell RC, Maeda M, Basadonna G et al (1985): Suppression, stress and accommodation of transplanted islets of Langerhans. *Diabetes, 34,* 667.
15. Mauer SM, Sutherland DER, Steffes MW et al (1974): Pancreatic islet transplantation: effects on the glomerular lesions of experimental diabetes in the rat. *Diabetes, 23,* 748.
16. Steffes MW, Brown DM, Basgen JM et al (1980): Amelioration of mesangial volume and surface alterations following islet transplantation in diabetic rats. *Diabetes, 29,* 509.
17. Federlin KF, Bretzel RG (1984): The effect of islet transplantation on complications in experimental diabetes of the rat. *World J. Surg., 8,* 169.
18. Krupin T, Waltman SR, Scharp DW et al (1979): Ocular fluorophotometry in streptozotocin diabetes mellitus in the rat: the effect of pancreatic islet isografts. *Invest. Ophthalmol. Visual. Sci., 18,* 1185.
19. Silberberg R, Hirchberg GE, Lesker P (1977): Enzyme studies in the articular cartilage of diabetic rats and of rats bearing transplanted pancreatic islets. *Diabetes, 26,* 732.
20. Schmidt RE, Plurad SB, Olack BJ et al (1983): The effect of pancreatic islet transplantation and insulin therapy on experimental diabetic autonomic neuropathy. *Diabetes, 32,* 532.
21. Snell GD (1957): The homograft reaction. *Annu. Rev. Microbiol., 2,* 439.
22. Jacobs BB (1974): Ovarian allograft survival: prolongation after passage in vitro. *Transplantation, 18,* 454.
23. Lafferty KJ, Cooley MA, Woolnough J et al (1975): Thyroid allograft immunogenicity is reduced after a period in organ culture. *Science, 188,* 259.
24. Lacy PE, Davie JM, Finke EH (1979): Prolongation of islet allograft survival following in vitro culture (24°C) and a single injection of ALS. *Science, 204,* 312.
25. Lacy PE, Davie JM, Finke EH (1979): Induction of rejection of successful allografts of rat islets by donor peritoneal exudate cells. *Transplantation, 28,* 415.
26. Bowen KM, Lafferty KJ (1980): Reversal of diabetes by allogeneic islet transplantation without immunosuppression. *Aust. J. Exp. Biol. Med. Sci., 58,* 441.
27. Faustman D, Hauptfeld V, Lacy PE et al (1981): Prolongation of murine islet allograft survival by pretreatment of islets with antibody directed to Ia determinants. *Proc. Natl Acad. Sci. USA, 78,* 5156.
28. Faustman DL, Steinman RM, Gebel HM et al (1984): Prevention of rejection of murine islet allografts by pretreatment with anti-dendritic cell antibody. *Proc. Natl Acad. Sci. USA, 81,* 3864.
29. Lau H, Reemtsma K, Hardy MA (1984): Prolongation of rat islet allograft survival by direct ultraviolet irradiation of the graft. *Science, 223,* 607.
30. Pipeleers D, Pipeleers-Marichal M, Gepts W et al (1986): Purified islet cell grafts are tolerated without immunosuppressive treatment in allotransplanted diabetic rats. In: *Abstracts. Second Assisi International Symposium on Advanced Models for the Therapy of Insulin-Dependent Diabetes, Assisi, Italy, 1986.*
31. Selawry H, Fajaco R, Whittington K (1985): Intratesticular islet allografts in the spontaneously diabetic BB/W rat. *Diabetes, 34,* 1019.
32. Tze WJ, Tai J (1983): Successful intracerebral allotransplantation of purified pancreatic endocrine cells in diabetic rat. *Diabetes, 32,* 1185.

33. Donohoe JA, Andrus L, Bowen KM et al (1983): Cultured thyroid allografts induce a state of partial tolerance in adult recipient mice. *Transplantation, 35*, 62.
34. Zitron IM, Ono J, Lacy PE et al (1981): Active suppression in the maintenance of pancreatic islet allografts. *Transplantation, 32*, 156.
35. Talmage DW, Dart G, Radovich J et al (1976): Activation of transplant immunity: effect of donor leukocytes on thyroid allograft rejection. *Science, 191*, 385.
36. Faustman D, Hauptfeld V, Lacy PE et al (1982): Demonstration of active tolerance in maintenance of established islet of Langerhans allografts. *Proc. Natl Acad. Sci. USA, 79*, 4153.
37. Faustman D, Lacy PE, Davie JM, Hauptfeld V (1982): Prevention of allograft rejection by immunization with donor blood depleted of Ia-bearing cells. *Science, 217*, 157.
38. Lau H, Reemtsma K, Hardy MA (1983): Pancreatic islet allograft prolongation by donor-specific blood transfusions treated with ultraviolet irradiation. *Science, 221*, 754.
39. Terasaka R, Lacy PE, Hauptfeld V et al (1986): The effect of cyclosporine-A, low temperature culture and anti-Ia antibodies on prevention of rejection of rat islet allografts. *Diabetes, 35*, 83.
40. Lacy PE, Davie JM, Finke EH (1980): Prolongation of islet xenograft survival without continuous immunosuppression. *Science, 209*, 283.
41. Terasaka R, Lacy PE, Bucy RP et al (1986): Effect of cyclosporine A and low temperature culture on prevention of rejection of islet xenografts (rat to mouse). *Transplantation, 41*, 661.
42. Lacy PE, Finke EH, Janney CG et al (1982): Prolongation of islet xenograft survival by in vitro culture of rat megaislets in 95% O_2. *Transplantation, 33*, 588.
43. Nakajima Y, Kessler M, Nakano H et al (1985): Restoration of T cell responsiveness to interleukin-2 in recipients of pancreatic islet xenografts treated with cyclosporine. *Transplantation, 40*, 73.
44. Eloy R, Haffen K, Kedinger M et al (1979): Chick embryo pancreatic transplants reverse experimental diabetes of rats. *J. Clin. Invest., 64*, 361.
45. Faustman D, Hauptfeld V, Davie JM et al (1980): Murine pancreatic β-cells express H-2K and H-2D but not Ia antigens. *J. Exp. Med., 151*, 1563.
46. Baekkeskov S, Kanatsuna T, Klareskog L et al (1981): Expression of major histocompatibility antigens on pancreatic islet cells. *Proc. Natl Acad. Sci. USA, 78*, 6456.
47. Shienvold FL, Alejandro R, Mintz DH (1986): Indentification of Ia-bearing cells in rat, dog, pig and human islets of Langerhans. *Transplantation, 41*, 364.
48. Bottazzo GF, Pujol-Borrell R, Hanafusa T et al (1983): Role of aberrant HLA-DR expression and antigen presentation in induction of endocrine autoimmunity. *Lancet, 2*, 1115.
49. Bottazzo GF, Dean BM, McNally JM et al (1985): In situ characterization of autoimmune phenomena and expression of HLA molecules in the pancreas in diabetic insulitis. *N. Engl. J. Med., 313*, 353.
50. Wong GHW, Clark-Lewis I, McKimm-Breschkin JL et al (1982): Interferon-γ-like molecule induces Ia antigens on cultured mast cell progenitors. *Proc. Natl Acad. Sci. USA, 79*, 6989.
51. Prober JS, Gimbrone Jr MA, Cotran RS et al (1983): Ia expression by vascular endothelium is inducible by activated T cells and by human γ interferon. *J. Exp. Med., 157*, 1339.
52. Collins T, Korman AJ, Wake CT et al (1984): Immune interferon activates multiple class II major histocompatibility complex genes and the associated invariant chain gene in human endothelial cells and dermal fibroblasts. *Proc. Natl Acad. Sci. USA, 81*, 4917.
53. Fossati G, Taramelli D, Balsari A et al (1984): Primary but not metastatic human melanomas expressing DR antigens stimulate autologous lymphocytes. *Int. J. Cancer, 33*, 591.

54. Wright JR, Lacy PE, Unanue ER, Muszynski C, Hauptfeld V (1986): Induction of Ia antigens on isolated murine islet cells with interferon-γ. Paper presented at: Annual Meeting of the American Diabetes Association, Anaheim, June, 1986.
55. Mandrup-Poulsen T, Bendtzen K, Nielson JH et al (1985): Cytokines cause functional and structural damage to isolated islets of Langerhans. *Allergy, 40,* 424.
56. Mandrup-Poulsen T, Bendtzen K, Nerup J et al (1986): Affinity-purified human interleukin-I is cytotoxic to isolated islets of Langerhans. *Diabetologia, 29,* 63.
57. Bendten K, Mandrup-Poulsen T, Nerup J et al (1986): Cytotoxicity of human pI 7 interleukin-I for pancreatic islets of Langerhans. *Science, 232,* 1545.
58. Comens PG, Wolf BA, Sullivan FP et al (1986): Effects of interleukin-I on insulin secretion. Paper presented at: Annual Meeting of the American Diabetes Association, Anaheim, June, 1986.
59. Kirkman RL, Barrett LV, Gaulton N et al (1985): Administration of an anti-interleukin-2 receptor monoclonal antibody prolongs cardiac allograft survival in mice. *J. Exp. Med., 162,* 358.
60. Dialynas DP, Quan ZS, Wall KA et al (1983): Characterization of the murine T cell surface molecule, designated L3T4, identified by monoclonal antibody GK 1.5: similarity of L3T4 to the human Leu-3/T4 molecule. *J. Immunol., 131,* 2445.
61. Shizuru JA, Gregory AK, Chao CT et al (1986): Anti-L3T, mediated tolerance induction for allogeneic islet transplantation. *Diabetes, 35,* 350.
62. Alejandro R, Cutfield R, Shienvold FL et al (1985): Successful long-term survival of pancreatic islet allografts in spontaneous or pancreatectomy-induced diabetes in dogs: cyclosporine-induced immune unresponsiveness. *Diabetes, 34,* 825.
63. Lacy PE, Lacy ET, Finke EH et al (1982): An improved method for the isolation of islets from the beef pancreas. *Diabetes, 31,* 109.
64. Ricordi C, Finke E, Lacy PE (1986): A method for the mass isolation of islets from the adult pig pancreas. *Diabetes, 35,* 649.
65. Harrison DE, Christie MR, Gray DWR (1985): Properties of isolated human islets of Langerhans: insulin secretion, glucose oxidation and protein phosphorylation. *Diabetologia, 28,* 99.
66. Scharp DW, Lacy PE (1985): Human islet isolation and transplantation. Paper presented at: Annual Meeting of the American Diabetes Association, Baltimore, June, 1985.
67. Kuhn F, Schulz HJ, Lorenz D et al (1985): Morphological investigations in human islets of Langerhans isolated by the Velcro technic. *Biomed. Biochim. Acta, 44,* 149.
68. Campbell IL, Colman PG, Harrison LC (1985): Adult human pancreatic islet cells in tissue culture: function and immunoreactivity. *J. Clin. Endocrinol. Metab., 61,* 681.
69. *Current Status — Future Directions. Proceedings, JDFI First World Conference on Diabetes Research, Monaco, November, 1985.* 125 pp.
70. Sibley RK, Sutherland DER, Goetz F et al (1985): Recurrent diabetes mellitus in the pancreas iso- and allograft: a light and electron microscopic immunohistochemical analysis of four cases. *Lab. Invest., 53,* 132.
71. Weringer EJ, Like AA (1985): Immune attack on pancreatic islet transplants in the spontaneously diabetic BioBreeding/Worcester (BB/W) rat is not MHC restricted. *J. Immunol., 134,* 2383.
72. Prowse SJ, Bellgrau D, Lafferty KJ (1986): Islet allografts are destroyed by disease occurrence in the spontaneously diabetic BB rat. *Diabetes, 35,* 110.
73. Woehrle M, Markmann JF, Silvers WK et al (1986): Transplantation of cultured pancreatic islets to BB rats. *Surgery, 100,* 334.
74. Brown J, Molnar IG, Clark W et al (1974): Control of experimental diabetes mellitus in rats by transplantation of fetal pancreases. *Science, 184,* 1377.

75. Simeonovic CJ, Bowen KM, Kotlarski I et al (1980): Modulation of tissue immunogenicity by organ culture. *Transplantation, 30,* 174.
76. Mandel TE, Koulmanda M (1985): Effect of culture conditions on fetal mouse pancreas in vitro and after transplantation in syngeneic and allogeneic recipients. *Diabetes, 34,* 1082.
77. Simeonovic CJ, Lafferty KJ (1982): The isolation and transplantation of foetal mouse proislets. *Aust. J. Exp. Biol. Med. Sci., 60,* 383.
78. Simeonovic CJ, Lafferty JH (1982): Immunogenicity of isolated foetal mouse proislets. *Aust. J. Exp. Biol. Med. Sci., 60,* 391.
79. Groth CG, Andersson A, Bjorken C et al (1980): Attempts at transplantation of fetal pancreas to diabetic patients. *Transplant. Proc., 12,* 208.
80. Tuch BE, Sheil AGR, Ng ABP et al (1986): Long-term survival of human fetal pancreatic tissue transplanted into an insulin dependent diabetic patient. *Diabetic Med., 3,* 24.
81. Yuan-feng H, Hong Z, Hong-de Z et al (1985): Culture of human fetal pancreas and islet transplantation in 24 patients with Type 1 diabetes mellitus. *Chin. Med. J., 98,* 236.
82. Farkas GY, Karacsonyi S (1985): Clinical transplantation of fetal human pancreatic islets. *Biomed. Biochim. Acta, 44,* 155.

The Diabetes Annual/3
K.G.M.M. Alberti and L.P. Krall, editors
© 1987 Elsevier Science Publishers, B.V.

12   Diabetes in children

ARLAN L. ROSENBLOOM

Introduction

Pediatric diabetology has evolved over the past 15 years from an apologetic encumbrance on pediatric endocrinology to a major emphasis. The need for programs and teams to deal with the complex problems of children with diabetes and their families and the evolution of exciting clinical and basic research related to Type I, insulin-dependent diabetes mellitus (IDDM) have moved this field to the forefront of pediatric endocrinology. Developments in childhood diabetes since the previous review in *The Diabetes Annual/1* have been in the understanding of etiology and pathogenesis, in immunotherapy, in the appreciation of the heterogeneity of diabetes in the young, in the recognition of increasing incidence of IDDM, in understanding of the apparent universality of preclinical cerebral edema in ketoacidosis, in appreciating the psychosocial aspects of IDDM in families, in recognizing the limitations and possibilities of self-monitoring of blood glucose, and in appreciating the early manifestations of complications as they appear in childhood and adolescence.

Etiology and pathogenesis *(see also Chapter 2)*

Etiologic and racial heterogeneity

Insulitis — inflammatory infiltration of the islets of Langerhans — has been considered the hallmark of IDDM since Gepts' classic study. Reported numbers have been too small to estimate the incidence of this lesion, however. Recently Foulis et al (1) reviewed over 100 pancreatic specimens from IDDM deaths under 20 years of age in the United Kingdom, finding that 78% of those with recent onset had insulitis. The lesion was only present in those islets which were still producing insulin, supporting the concept that insulitis is an immunologically mediated destruction of insulin-secreting B cells. The frequency of insulitis is similar to that reported for islet cell antibody (ICA) positivity in the first few months of diabetes in most series. It is also noteworthy that 4 patients appeared to have a different disease from classical IDDM with no evidence of insulitis despite all islets containing insulin. All of these patients had diabetes onset at 18 months of age or less.

It has long been recognized that a substantial minority of diabetes in childhood will not be typical autoimmune disease by the presence of diabetes as part of various syndromes, often with clinical characteristics different from typical IDDM, such as the diabetes that occurs in cystic fibrosis. Najjar et al (2) described 7 patients with the rare syndrome of diabetes insipidus, diabetes mellitus, optic atrophy, neurosensory deafness, atony of the urinary tract, and other abnormalities. Diabetes mellitus and optic atrophy were constant features with diabetes insipidus absent in only one. Severity of diabetes varied and all required insulin. None had haplotypes associated with IDDM. The syndrome of acanthosis nigricans, obesity, insulin resistance, and hyperandrogenemia is also being increasingly recognized in children and was described in 22 patients by Richards et al (3). Seventeen girls and 5 boys were affected. All had obesity as their initial feature, beginning at an average age of 7.3 years. Fasting insulin concentration was 5.25 μU/ml in lean controls, 19.6 μU/ml in obese controls and 49.8μ U/ml in study patients.

Not only is IDDM less frequent in the black population than among Caucasians (4), but the frequency of ICA at onset of diabetes in black children is half that of Whites (5). A substantial number of black youngsters have a non-HLA-associated diabetes which presents in a manner indistinguishable from IDDM but subsequently is not as insulin-dependent. This 'Type 1.5' diabetes is strongly familial, but differs from the Mason-type diabetes of youth in mode of onset, occurrence of complications, insulinopenia, and racial distribution (6).

Autoimmunity against B cells, insulin, and other tissues

A cross-sectional study of islet cell antibodies in Japanese IDDM gave a prevalence of 32%, with most ICA-positive subjects having short duration, similar to Western populations (7).

A recent addition to the spectrum of autoimmunity with IDDM has been the binding of autoantibodies to insulin (IAA) preceding the administration of insulin. Wilken et al (8) described IAA in 38% of 40 newly diagnosed IDDM. Unusual and inexplicable was the finding of IAA in 27 of 58 unaffected twins. Since many of these were long-standing discordant twins, who are not likely to develop IDDM, the IAA was thought to reflect inherited autoimmune tendencies. Among 124 newly diagnosed IDD children, Arslanian et al (9) found that those with the higher titers had the most symptomatic diabetes. In contrast to the studies of Wilken et al (8) only 2 of 446 siblings had elevated insulin binding, one of whom developed IDDM within a few weeks. Overall, about one-third had binding greater than 2 standard deviations above the control mean.

To determine whether the IAA reflect B cell damage, Karjalainen et al (10) studied 60 newly diagnosed IDDM with a mean age of 9.5 years. Insulin binding exceeded the upper range of age-matched controls in 28% and these subjects were younger, had lower C-peptide concentrations, were more frequently HLA-DR4 and had lower glycosylated hemoglobin levels than the other children. There was no association between IAA and ICA, either conventional or complement fixing. Thus, these authors considered the IAA to be an indicator of clinical and genetic heterogeneity within IDDM, rather than a marker of B cell destruction. Similar conclusions were reached by McEvoy et al (11). They found a highly significant negative correlation between age at onset of diabetes and insulin binding before insulin treatment. They concluded that the insulin binding was a late event in the pathogenesis of IDDM, occurring soon before the symptoms developed, as determined in 4 siblings who experienced a significant increase in serum insulin binding preceding metabolic decompensation. They also found a negative association with HLA-DR3. In their long-standing patients, the development of antibodies to exogenous insulin was negatively associated with homozygosity for DR3.

In sum, the recent finding of spontaneous anti-insulin antibodies preceding treatment for IDDM is another manifestation of the autoimmune nature of the disorder, and appears to be a function of the varying HLA associations that characterize autoimmune IDDM. Other associated autoimmunities are now well recognized, particularly involving thyroid, gastric parietal cells, and adrenal cortex. Maclaren and Riley (12) have reviewed their findings among 1456 caucasian IDDM and 240 black patients, 1467 relatives, and 1519 controls. Thyrogastric antibodies were more common in female subjects in all the groups and in the control group with advancing age, affecting one-third of caucasian women after age 60. The age-augmented increase was prematurely expressed in patients with IDDM and their relatives. In most cases, among patients with IDDM, the antibodies appeared at the time of onset and were more common among those with later age of onset. Thyroid microsomal (TMA) were present in 30% of female caucasian patients and 16% of males, while only 11% of black females and 8% of males were positive. In contrast, parietal cell antibodies (PCA) were present in 13% of white females, 8% of white males, and in precisely the same percentages of Blacks. Adrenal autoimmunity was present in only 2% of both races, still a substantial increase over the control population. At least one-third of young patients with TMA will have overt or chemical hypothyroidism and one-half of those with PCA will demonstrate achlorhydria and appear to be at risk for late development of pernicious anemia. The inheritance of thyrogastric autoimmunity was unrelated to HLA haplotype sharing with the diabetic sibling, indicating that the inherited predisposition to thyroid and gastric autoimmunity was not HLA-related.

In a group of 77 children from Italy, approximately 12% were TMA-positive and 15% PCA-positive (13). In a cross-sectional study of 130 adolescent children in the Federal Republic of Germany, 15.4% were TMA-positive, among whom 70% had thyroid enlargement (14).

The clinical importance of these and earlier reports is to emphasize the need for testing all IDDM patients for TMA and PCA. Adrenal cortical auto-immunity can be ascertained in those who are positive for one or the other of these antibodies. Since a substantial percentage of PCA-positive individuals will have achlorhydria, serum ferritin levels need to be checked periodically in those who are positive and, of course, thyroid function needs to be followed in those who are TMA-positive. Riley's studies indicate that these antibodies are present at the start of the diabetes and need not be repeatedly checked for, unless specific indications arise such as thyroid enlargement (15).

HLA genetics

It is now well recognized that heterozygocity for the high-risk HLA-DR types (3/4) confers a much greater risk (1 in 40) than the presence of either of these genes alone or in the homozygous state (1 in 400) (6). This observation had led to the concept that there may be 2 genes in the DR region which confer diabetes susceptibility. In other populations, it would not be surprising to find linkages to different genes. Among 147 Chinese IDDM patients, Chan et al (16) found only a weak association with DR4, while Lee et al (17) found a nearly 4-fold increase in the frequency of DR3 among 23 Chinese children with IDDM compared to controls. They also found no increase in DR4. It was suggested that these differences might explain the lower frequency of IDDM in Chinese children.

Eberhardt et al (18) reviewed 172 patients who had HLA-DR typing and found that DR3 was more frequent among males and DR4 among females, and that DR4-positive IDDM presented with a more severe clinical picture, more likely to be acidotic, and to be associated with a recent viral infection, substantiated by a greater frequency of antibodies to Coxsackie-B viruses. These findings again suggest heterogeneity on the basis of HLA-DR type.

Numerous investigators are attempting to identify restriction fragment length polymorphisms within the HLA-D region, either to find more precise markers for susceptibility to IDDM or to identify the gene or genes responsible for diabetes susceptibility. Thus far, evidence is only that these polymorphisms can serve as markers in particular families because of their closer linkage to predisposing genes (19).

Environmental factors

There is substantial clinical and experimental evidence that diabetes can be caused by environmental agents, including viruses (congenital rubella), toxins (Vacor), and malnutrition (J-type diabetes). However, the autoimmune basis of most IDDM and the recognition that there is usually a long latency between the beginning of autoimmune destruction and clinical onset, makes identification of specific environmental etiologies difficult. Those events surrounding the clinical onset of diabetes are likely to be simply the last in a series of hits, or the stressors that results in decompensation.

Frisk et al (20) reported a high frequency of Coxsackie-B virus (CBV) specific IgM in 24 consecutive children developing IDDM. Thirteen of them had symptoms of acute infection within two months before diagnosis. Controls were age-matched non-diabetic children scheduled for elective procedures during the same period, none of whom showed antibody rises (21). These studies were carried out during a time of high IDDM incidence among children and the CBV was thought to play an induction role. It is noteworthy that only 3 of the 16 IgM-positive patients had a significant rise in neutralizing antibody titre against the CBV type, suggesting defective immune response as part of the picture of IDDM onset.

Prediction and prevention

The evidence that most IDDM is of autoimmune pathogenesis and the success of immune suppressive therapy in such conditions and in spontaneous autoimmune rodent diabetes have led to attempts to induce remission before complete B cell destruction, using immune suppressive therapy. The only justification for preclinical detection, which now appears feasible by screening for ICA, and testing for failure of first-phase insulin response to intravenous glucose (22) would be for early intervention to prevent the progression of diabetes. Before such attempts can be undertaken, however, it will be necessary to demonstrate that there is a substantial benefit and low risk for treating newly diagnosed patients.

The drug that has been most extensively used for this purpose is cyclosporin A. In the initial uncontrolled pilot study, over half became insulin-independent during treatment and 80% achieved and maintained C-peptide levels above 0.6 pmol/ml (23). Patients in this pilot study had a more rapid decrease in ICA titers than did those treated with insulin alone, and cessation of cyclosporin A resulted in reappearance of ICA in titers higher than were present at the onset. Because of lack of correlation between the disappearance of ICA and the C-peptide response, it was not felt that the ICA were directly involved in the pathogenic process and that their reappearance may or may not signal clinical relapse (24). The Cyclosporin/Diabetes French Study Group has issued its first report of a double-blind study of 122 patients (25). An unimpressive difference of 25% and 19% not requiring insulin at 6 months differentiated the cyclosporin A group from the placebo group, although at 9 months 24% of the cyclosporin

A group but only 6% of the placebo group remained off insulin. A serious concern was the observation of a significant rise in creatinine and a significant fall in hemoglobin after 9 months of treatment with cyclosporin A. Renal tubular and glomerular damage from cyclosporin A therapy for only 2 years has been reported and such nephrotoxicity would be particularly unacceptable in diabetes (26).

Epidemiology

The increasing incidence of IDDM has been documented in Sweden (27) and Finland (28). Not only do Finland, Norway and Sweden have the highest incidence and prevalence of IDDM in the under-15-year-old group, but there are regional variations within these countries which remain unexplained. Neither is the cause of the increasing incidence known. Laporte et al (29) have summarized the wide range of childhood diabetes incidence, noting that children in Finland have 35 times the risk of developing IDDM as children in Japan. They stress the importance of population-based registries with consistent criteria for documentation of diabetes. Lorenzi et al (30) have confirmed and expanded earlier studies indicating a lower risk for Blacks than Whites in the United States (4). They found a lower incidence among Mexicans, Blacks, and Orientals than among Caucasians in Southern California (30).

There is accumulating evidence that male sex is a risk factor for the development of diabetes, as well as for its transmission. Among children developing diabetes under the age of 5 years, the sex ratio of males to females is 1.5. Furthermore, although 16% had a first-degree relative with diabetes, none of such affected relatives was a mother (31). This is consistent with the original report by Warram et al (32) that women with IDDM had less than a quarter the chance of transmitting diabetes to their offspring than did men with IDDM. A similar observation was made among Swedish children, 13% of whom had a first-degree relative affected, who was twice as likely to be a father as a mother (27).

Management

Ketoacidosis

Low-dose insulin infusion, improved bedside monitoring of treatment, limited indications for the infusion of bicarbonate, and intensive care environments have not prevented the continued rare, but devastating, occurrence of cerebral edema. Subclinical brain swelling has been demonstrated in 6 unselected children treated for ketoacidosis (33). An initial CT scan was done when the blood glucose had fallen to below 14 mmol/l or pH had gone above 7.3, with repeat after resolution of the acute episode and just before discharge from hospital. All 6 patients showed substantial narrowing without, however, obliteration of the ventricles. These findings are consistent with earlier reports showing increased cerebral spinal fluid pressure (34) and echoencephalographic decreases in the lateral ventricle width (35) during treatment. What is not known from these studies, however, is if these changes are present before correction.

If it can be assumed that these findings of subclinical cerebral edema are the early stages of what rarely develops as the clinical syndrome, a tool is available for evaluating modifications of the treatment program to prevent cerebral edema. Because of the rarity of clinically apparent cerebral edema, it has not been possible to test methods for preventing this condition in practice. Exactly what those modifications should be remains unknown (see also Chapter 27).

First stage of treatment

The assumption that all newly diagnosed patients with diabetes need to be hospitalized was initially challenged on the grounds of efficacy. It was felt that hospital settings increased anxiety and decreased receptiveness to education, and that they created an image of illness and dependency that could be deleterious to successful long-term management (36). Hospital settings may provide multiple sources of confusing information, orders for insulin may be late, the food may be unattractive or culturally unacceptable, physical activity is reduced, and the youngster is missing school with increasing anxiety. All of these factors contribute to making dose adjustments which will be inappropriate for home and school life. Regional programs for children and youth with diabetes adopted an outpatient approach to management of newly diagnosed patients as beneficial in cost terms, as well as more effective (37). Duncan and Malone (38) have described their experience with 47 children managed as outpatients in their regional diabetes program. They emphasized the need for a staff specially trained in diabetes home management, including administration of insulin, monitoring, recognition of hypoglycemia, meal planning, and sick day management. They do their teaching in a 5-day program coordinated by a medical social worker who provides continuing support and counseling. Fifteen hours of individualized training are provided over the 5-day period.

Drawing on data from the Colorado IDDM registry, Hamman et al (39) compared 37 children who had not been hospitalized at the time of diagnosis to 268 who had, between the years 1978-1982. The non-hospitalized youngsters had subsequent hospitalization and ketoacidosis rates 2-3.7 times lower than those of children who received any inpatient care in the first 2 weeks after diagnosis. Regardless of care setting, children classified as 'severe' at onset, or with parents of lower education and income, or who were age 10-14 years at diagnosis, had 2-4 times higher subsequent acute complication rates after onset than did children without these characteristics. The authors suggested that a 42% reduction in total nights hospitalized could occur if the non-severe patients were treated principally as outpatients.

As pointed out by Etzwiler in *The Diabetes Annual/1* the cost-containment trend may dictate outpatient management for newly diagnosed diabetes without ketoacidosis.

Monitoring (see also Chapter 9)

In *The Diabetes Annual/2*, Scott and Tattersall suggested that there remains a role for urine testing for glucose and proposed that '... algorithms [be] prepared so that the patient knows what to do in response to any given test result.' There are, unfortunately, no suggestions of how to develop such algorithms from the typically confusing results (40).

Hermansson et al (41) are also unwilling to relegate urine testing to the scrapheap of medical technology. They offered 160 children and adolescents the opportunity to participate in a feasibility study of home blood glucose testing. Seventeen girls and 15 boys aged 4-21 years accepted and did 20-22 diurnal blood glucose profiles, each consisting of 7 blood samples, during a 3-month period. Subsequently they were encouraged to continue blood glucose measurement and their performances were evaluated 3 years later. The patients liked blood testing because it provided immediate answers to problems, but their overall metabolic control, measured by HbA_1, was not altered. Surprisingly, only 6.4% of the patients preferred blood testing to urinalysis for long-term use and the main problem appeared to be pain from daily use. The failure to demonstrate substantial improvement in control is similar to other studies summarized in *The Diabetes Annual/2* by Tattersall (p. 132). However, preference for self-monitoring of blood glucose (SBGM) has been shown by a substantial majority in previous investigations, e.g. 69% in a Canadian study (42).

The acceptance of SBGM by young patients has been impressive in our own experience, confirming the long-recognized esthetic, as well as intellectual, antipathy to urine testing. One suspects that there is certainly no less compliance with SBGM than with urine testing in the past.

The memory reflectance meter has the ability to record and store blood glucose measurements done at home for up to 3 months. This information can be transferred to a desktop computer for rapid and detailed analysis and the information can be stored for long-term study of the relationship between control and complications (43). Another use for the recording meter is to monitor compliance. Wilson and Endres (44) studied 18 children using a memory-equipped meter with and without the child's knowledge. Poor compliance was demonstrated by fabricated test results in 40% and failure to record test results in 18%. In addition to the compliance issue, the accuracy of measurement by children is an important question. Clarson et al (45) found that 62 youngsters with a mean age of 14 ± 3 years had 68% of their readings (each subject did 20) within 20% of the correct figure, by visual examination. This was felt to be reasonable accuracy. One of the problems with analysis of accuracy of SBGM methods is the definition of accuracy. The purpose of these tests is to provide sufficiently reliable data for decision-making. Thus, analyses should be done which determine how many times a reading is considered low when it should be normal or *vice versa*, or high when it should be normal or *vice versa*.

An interesting use of SBGM was a study carried out by Freund et al (46) with 25 adolescent campers to determine their ability to estimate their blood glucose levels and the subjective symptoms they were using to do so. They completed a rating checklist and estimated their glycemia immediately before finger-prick testing 4 times daily for 11 days. As a group, no consistent relationships were detected between blood glucose levels and symptoms. However, with analysis of each camper's data separately, 23 of them had at least one significant glycemia-symptom correlation. Only one of these symptoms was significantly related to blood glucose for more than half of the youngsters studied, the symptom hunger. Otherwise each camper seemed to have a unique glucose-symptom pattern and virtually all of these were for low rather than high blood glucose. It was also noteworthy that few campers could accurately identify which symptoms are reliably associated with low or high blood glucose, despite the frequent emphasis on these symptoms in diabetes education and the wide availability of the classic lists. Better-controlled patients were more aware of the influence of the timing of their insulin injection, the quantity and timing of their food intake, and the duration and type of exercise, and were using these clues, rather than internal symptoms, to estimate blood glucose more accurately than did poorly controlled campers. This and previous studies have cast doubt on the reliability of the widely distributed list of symptoms for hyper- and hypo-glycemia. Headache, for example, can occur with either. One of the lessons that emerges from this study is the value of SBGM for determination of individual responses, to hypoglycemia in particular. Distinguishing these symptoms from simple anxiety is not always easy and the symptoms may vary in the same individual depending on the speed with which hypoglycemia has developed.

Psychosocial aspects

Pediatric investigators have for many years recognized the pre-eminent influence of psychosocial factors on diabetes control, expressed as non-compliance (e.g. omitting insulin) or as destabilization due to presumed counter-regulatory responses to emotional upset. Over recent years, increasing numbers of investigators in behavior have become interested in diabetes and the challenge it poses to the child and the family.

Fashions come and go to explain 'brittle' diabetes, including insulin anti-bodies and, more recently, subcutaneous insulin resistance (47). These expla-nations are always more attractive than nebulous psychosocial factors and com-plex manipulative techniques. The work of Baker and Minuchin emphasized the uniform reversibility of 'brittleness' upon removal of the youngster from the stressful environment of an intact but non-communicating family (48). Such has also been the experience of the residential homes for young people with dia-betes in Europe (49) and the United States (50), dealing with a wide variety of non-coping home situations (see also Chapter 13).

One of the important lessons to emerge from the involvement of psychologi-cal investigators is that compliance and control are not synonymous terms (51), and that compliance in one realm may be sufficient to obtain good control (giving insulin regularly), whereas total non-compliance in another area (blood glucose monitoring) may have no deleterious effect in an individual who has generally good health behaviour. The obverse is also frequently seen, particu-larly where the parents are inducing anxiety by frequent blood testing and ad-justment of insulin according to algorithms that may not be appropriate for a child.

One of the effects of systematic psychosocial investigations has been the ex-purgation of long-held myths, such as the 'diabetic personality'. The not surpris-ing fact is that emotional and coping responses to diabetes are as individual as the youngsters and families who must deal with it.

Kovacs et al (52) have systematically evaluated coping behavior in 74 newly diagnosed IDDM for several weeks following stabilization of their diabetes and over the subsequent year, on 3 or 4 occasions, and then at 8-monthly intervals. Life stress and prevalence of psychiatric disorders preceding IDDM were within the normal range and there was no characteristic pre-existing 'diabetic personality'. Two modes of copyng were seen initially, the predominant reac-tion in 64% of the children including mild sadness, anxiety, sense of friendless-ness, and social withdrawel. The other 36% had reactions that were consistent with a psychiatric disorder with depressive syndrome being the most common. Recovery from both the mild and more severe reactions occurred over the first 7-9 months. Parents' responses did not relate to how the children themselves coped. However, the more severe reactions were more likely in the lower socioeconomic group and in those families where there was marital distress. These investigators also examined parents' adjustment to the illness in a lon-gitudinal study. Over the first year of IDDM, they found no blatantly neurotic or pathologic behavior resorted to for coping. Instead, the initial strain of living with diabetes elicited mild depression, anxiety and distress. The principal care-giver, the mother, was more affected than the father; mothers had more symptoms, including a mild grief reaction in at least one quarter. The initial emotional upheaval resolved in approximately 6 months and the authors felt optimistic about the resilience of families during the first year of IDDM (53). The clinician will recognize that the 'subclinical' depression of children and their parents is persistent and ebbs and flows throughout the life of a person with diabetes. It needs to be recognized not just by pediatricians, but by the family physicians and internists that take care of the patients as adults.

An interesting manifestation of the despair and guilt surrounding diabetes in the child was pointed out by Kirk and Savage (54) in noting that 6 of 8 children who had a parent with IDDM had serious management problems. The experienced clinician will again recognize his/her own experience with children of parents with IDDM, whose habits may be the furthest from those one wishes to have emulated.

Although one might quibble with the psychosocial research as being simple confirmation of the obvious, such is also true of much physiologic research. A scientific basis for clinical impressions is necessary to develop appropriate tools for measuring coping behaviors, knowledge, skills, compliance and control in order to quantify these variables in relation to each other and to risk factors such as socioeconomic level, source of medical care, race and age.

Pediatrics is becoming increasingly devoted to dealing with children with chronic disease and the stresses placed on their development as independent individuals and on their families. One of the expressions of this stress in children with chronic disease is the increased incidence of child abuse and neglect, reported to be 15-20% of abused youngsters having chronic diseases such as diabetes or multiple sclerosis. Horan et al (55) raised the provocative question: 'Insulin-dependent diabetes mellitus and child abuse: is there a relationship?' They tabulated family psychosocial variables which have been cited in both the child abuse and the IDDM literature, including family organization, cohesion among family members, marital discord, number of positive child contacts, degree of stress, parental ability to cope with stress, parental feelings of inadequacy, flexibility and appropriateness of parental expectations for child behavior, tolerance for child deviations from parental control, and inadequacy of disciplinary procedures.

Another insight is becoming current among pediatric diabetologists and others who work with children with chronic disease is the concept of health locus of control. Perrin and Shapiro (56) have looked at the locus of control beliefs at different ages and in relation to different illness experiences, finding consistent variation according to these variables. Younger children, as expected, see the control of their health to be by chance and by powerful others, compared to the view of older children. Particularly noteworthy was that children with diabetes, similar to those with asthma, did not demonstrate any differences from healthy children in their health locus of control beliefs (powerful others *versus* chance *versus* internal). This was in marked contrast to those with seizures and orthopedic conditions who saw themselves much more under the influence of powerful others and chance. This is an encouraging note for diabetologists, because it suggests that the efforts to place patients and families in control of the diabetes has largely positive effects on self concept. It is of interest that the health locus of control scales for the mothers were not at all correlated with those of the youngsters and that the mothers of children with diabetes had significantly higher scores for significant others and chance than did the mothers of children without chronic disease.

Education program

The importance of the personal meaning of diabetes to the individual and how this influences his or her dealing with the condition is emphasized by Anderson (57). He deplores the transfer of the schoolroom approach to the diabetes education setting and suggests that patient education should be learner-centered rather than educator-centered. Such an approach promotes a tolerant classroom environment with such productive activities as self-exploration and self-expression, personal sharing, role playing, and values clarification exercises. The philosophical approach of patient educators is more important in the outcome of the education process than the actual educational method used. Anderson's plea that valid and reliable measures of personal meaning of diabetes must be employed in research echoes the call of investigators who have developed tools for measuring parent and child attitude toward the diabetes (51).

Golden et al (58), focusing on reduction of recurrent diabetic ketoacidosis (DKA), instituted educational programs specifically to promote adherence to insulin therapy which they found to be the most common problem precipitating admission for DKA. They obtained a major decrease in the rate of recurrence of DKA in 44 patients who had a history of this problem and also noted a decrease in mean HbA_1 as a result of intervention. These results are similar to those previously reported for reduction in hospital days attendant on the introduction of a nurse-specialist coordinated regional diabetes program (37).

These kinds of reports are extremely important in emphasizing the need for program support for specialized teams dealing with youngsters with diabetes as a cost-beneficial investment. One can well ask whether the effect of these efforts is in the education imparted or in the effects of more frequent visits to the clinic and availability by telephone to deal with problems as they arise. Everyone who systematically measures knowledge among patients validates what they have been impressed with on an individual basis, that the information transmitted is not held onto for very long.

Confirming this experience and emphasizing Anderson's concern, Lucey and

Wing (59) found that their 8- to 14-year-old patients who attended clinic regularly had poor theoretical and practical skills, regardless of the duration of diabetes. They organized two 6-hour educational sessions which included a novel participatory component, self-made videos, as well as peer-group participation, and assessed their effort by questionnaires. Even with this interactive approach, the information imparted was only remembered over the short term. They found the problem-solving approach to be more easily tackled in participative teaching. Those children who had previously attended British Diabetic Association camps had a better general knowledge of their diabetes than did non-attenders, but they had no better performances on problem-solving day-to-day practical difficulties. The lesson would appear to be that skill and knowledge need to be periodically assessed. As originally emphasized by Travis, it is important that the cognitive developmental level be recognized as an important factor (60).

Diet

A study from Newcastle, U.K. (61) and one from Uppsala, Sweden (62) have looked at the dietary intake of children with diabetes. The 168 English children consumed expected amounts of energy but more fat and fiber than is considered usual for non-diabetic children, and consequently less sugars and carbohydrates. Noteworthy was that they consumed more carbohydrate than had been prescribed, but this was less than current recommendations. There was a correlation between diabetic control and the amount of fiber consumed as well as with compliance with the prescribed diet, but not to the proportion of energy taken as carbohydrate. It would appear that the concept of carbohydrate as poison to the child with diabetes remains a resistent myth. The Swedish investigators, in a much smaller population of only 14 children with diabetes, found that they were getting 40% of their energy from fat compared to 36% in controls. They were also consuming more protein, accounting for 18% of their energy intake compared to 14% in controls. Thus, these children were also consuming less carbohydrate than their peers and less than is currently recommended.

A method for more actively involving children in improving their diets was studied by Maryniuk et al (63) at a camp for children with diabetes. Campers prepared plain yogurt as part of their lesson in trying new foods, while another group had a traditional lecture/discussion on trying new foods, with a focus on yogurt, and a control group attended general nutrition class. When these campers were given a choice of a fruited yogurt pudding or peanut butter and crackers for snack, children in the active group were more likely to select the yogurt than were the children in the other groups. These investigators suggest that diabetes educators consider ways of incorporating hands-on nutrition learning to encourage improved eating behaviors.

Insulin resistance and intensive management

Resistance to the effects of insulin in persons with IDDM has been clinically suspected because of the need for larger doses of insulin than endogenous production would dictate. However, this impression is confounded by the non-physiologic presentation of exogenous insulin. In the non-diabetic state, 20-80% of B cell secretion is taken up by the liver directly from the portal drainage of the pancreas, whereas exogenous insulin therapy would have to produce peripheral hyperinsulinemia to achieve comparable hepatic insulinization. Newer methods of studying the effects of insulin on peripheral tissues make it possible to evaluate such possibilities more precisely. The euglycemic insulin clamp technique involves infusing insulin at a constant rate and determining the amount of glucose needed to maintain constant levels of blood glucose during such exogenous hyperinsulinemia. Using this technique, Finnish investigators (64) did a longitudinal study over the first year of IDDM with approximately 20 patients and at various intervals greater than 1 year duration for 53 others. Two weeks after diagnosis, glucose uptake was 32% lower in patients with diabetes than in controls, but it rose to normal during the subsequent 3 months, by which time 43% of the patients were in clinical remission and did not require insulin therapy. In the remitting group, insulin action was 40% greater than in those who continued to require insulin treatment. Despite the remission, fasting plasma C-peptide levels were only slightly, but not significantly, higher in those in remission than in the other patients. In patients with diabetes for 1 year or more, insulin action was also reduced by a mean 40%, although there was con-siderable variation between patients and this resistance was inversely related to glycemic control and relative body weight. Thus, patients with newly diagnosed IDDM may experience transient normalization of insulin action after initial re-duction, along with partial recovery of endogenous insulin secretion, which may contribute to the clinical remission period. A majority of those with long duration of diabetes have varying degrees of peripheral insulin resistance which appears to be related to the degree of metabolic control.

The etiology of this insulin resistance is unclear. Certainly body weight is a factor. In the Finnish study, both control and IDDM subjects demonstrated an inverse correlation between insulin action and relative body weight. Of greatest interest is the relationship to diabetic control. Might a substantial portion of this resistance be the result of the higher levels of counterregulatory hormones seen in poorly controlled patients? Amiel et al (65) looked at a typically difficult group of patients with unstable diabetes, namely pubertal children. They compared the results of euglycemic insulin clamp studies between adults and prepubertal and pubertal children, with and without IDDM. They found that non-diabetic pubertal children had sharply decreased insulin-stimulated glu-cose metabolism compared with prepubertal children and adults, despite comparable elevated levels of insulin (80-90 µU/ml). A similar difference was found in those with IDDM, a 25-30% lower response to insulin in the pubertal group compared to the prepubertal children and adults. At each stage of pubertal development, the stimulating effect of insulin on glucose metabolism was decreased by 33-42% in those with diabetes. These data indicate that insulin resistance occurs during puberty in both normal children and children with diabetes. The pubertal IDDM had higher glycosylated Hb levels than the prepubertal subjects, despite higher insulin dosages. However, the authors did not report correlation with control measures as in the previous paper. They were unable to explain this insulin resistance, citing other studies indicating no effect of sex steroids, and their finding of basal levels of catecholamines and cortisol being similar, tending to rule out a stress difference. Elevated growth hormone levels would explain the relationship of insulin resistance to both puberty and metabolic control, since growth hormone elevation is related to degree of control and growth hormone levels are higher in those with IDDM than in non-diabetic controls at each stage of development. Furthermore, growth hormone elevation will suppress insulin-stimulated glucose metabolism in both normal subjects and those with diabetes.

The clinical significance of this well-documented insulin resistance in overall diabetes control is questionable. Exercise training of adolescents for 12 weeks produced significant improvement in fitness and insulin sensitivity without altering HbA_1 (66).

In addition to overall insulin resistance, there appears to be a diurnal variaton in insulin sensitivity with an increase in the amount of insulin required to maintain normal blood glucose level between 02.00 and 07.00 hours, the so-called 'dawn phenomenon'. Blood glucose rises during this time of the day can be due to posthypoglycemic hyperglycemia (the Somogyi phenomenon), or the waning of available insulin from the subcutaneous sites. However, the dawn phenomenon appears to be a distinct physiologic event which will appear during constant insulin infusion and without preceding falls in blood glucose. Campbell et al (67) have attributed this to nocturnal surges in growth hormone (GH) secretion, based on studies of GH secretion and sympathoadrenal activity during the night in 7 adults with IDDM. Nocturnal surges of GH secretion were prevented by infusing somatostatin plus replacement glucagon. Surges of GH were stimulated by hourly injections of GH during this infusion. In the control experiments, with the infusion of insulin alone, plasma glucose levels increased from 5.4 ± 0.3 mmol/l to 12.9 ± 1.8 mmol/l between 02.30 and 08.00 hours and glucose production increased by 65%. When the nocturnal surges in GH were suppressed, neither plasma glucose levels nor glucose production increased significantly. When GH surges were simulated, plasma glucose levels and glucose production increased again. These studies suggest that a portion of insulin resistance that occurs in IDDM can be attributable to GH, and that better control of the diabetes could ameliorate this problem.

In very young patients with IDDM, however, waning insulin levels in the early morning are associated with a striking dawn phenomenon. Nine children had overnight metabolic profiles measured and demonstrated a steep rise in glucose level from 04.30 hours (6.2 ± 1.3 mmol/l) to 09.30 hours (17.8 ± 2.4 mmol/l). There was an associated change in β-hydroxybutyrate and glycerol. Analysis of the time relationship suggested a delay of 2-6 hours between free insulin levels and their effects (68).

Well documented in this and many other studies of older patients was the remarkable difference between the 05.00 hour and pre-breakfast blood glucose levels; the respective means were approximately 6 and 10 mmol/l. Few would argue with the goal of decreasing such a fasting morning level to a more normal range. However, the risk of hypoglycemia beween 01.00 and 05.00 hours is readily apparent and dictates a far more sophisticated approach than simply increasing the evening insulin dose.

Intensive therapy using insulin pumps would appear to be the sophisticated approach needed. However, their use in pediatric patients has been greatly limited by the discipline required for intensive therapy in general and pump use in particular. Brink and Stewart (69) reported on their experience with 24 children and young adults, aged 8-26 years, with continuous subcutaneous insulin infusion (CSII). The use of CSII was dictated by persistently high glycohemoglobin values or wide swings in blood glucose values despite serious efforts to improve glycemia. CSII was discontinued by 30%. Significant improvement was noted by 3 months for glycohemoglobin and blood glucose values, but there was no further improvement thereafter. Only 3 of the patients attained a normal value for glycohemoglobin. There was no greater frequency of diabetic ketoacidosis with CSII. Half of the young people had electromechanical problems with the devices, erred in their use, or had local skin problems, although none of these problems resulted in ketoacidosis or severe hypoglycemia. Dietary non-compliance and decreased intensive home monitoring were important factors in the lack of success in most cases. The authors felt that better ways were needed to predict success or failure if normalization is a goal in young patients.

Investigators in Sheffield had a similar experience with a group of adolescent patients (70). Of these, 45 were offered CSII, only 13 of them chose the treatment, 11 actually started, and only 4 continued CSII for 1 year. In contrast, 30% of adults chose CSII and they had half the discontinuation rate of the adolescents. No improvement in glycemic control was demonstrable and the teenage pump users had diabetic ketoacidosis, serious hypoglycemia, and skin infections at higher rates than conventionally treated teenagers and adults using CSII. CSII remains a mode of therapy rarely applicable to the child or adolescent.

Growth

It has been accepted wisdom for half a century that children who develop diabetes are taller than average. Songer et al (71) have examined the height at the time of diagnosis in 200 children, 187 of their non-diabetic siblings, and 169 parents. They found that those 5-9 years of age at the time of diagnosis were consistently taller than the national average, but non-diabetic siblings of the same age were also tall. In contrast, those aged 14 or over at the time of diagnosis of IDDM were short while their siblings and parents were of normal height. Non-diabetic siblings at increased risk for diabetes because of HLA association with the proband were closer in height to these diabetic children than were lower-risk, non-diabetic siblings. It is possible that there are stature-determining genes linked to HLA, as well.

The relationship of growth and pubertal development to diabetes control has been of great concern to pediatricians. As with the other complications of diabetes, delayed maturation and short stature have not appeared to be directly related to the degree of metabolic control. Clarson et al (72) have looked at growth and pubertal development in 122 children with a mean age of 13 ± 3 (SD) years who had had diabetes for 6 ± 4 years. The means and distributions of height and height-velocity percentiles were normal for both sexes. Similarly, timing of onset of Tanner II development in boys and girls was normal, as was the age of menarche. This group appeared to be typical of pubertal IDDM with a mean HbA_1 of $11.1 \pm 2\%$ (normal $< 7.5\%$). There was no correlation of mean HbA_1 levels, calculated from 4 or more measurements for each child, with height velocity or weight velocity percentiles or with mean height or weight percentiles. Thus, diabetic control did not appear to be a major determinant of growth in this group of children with IDDM who, as a group, displayed a normal growth pattern and pubertal development, despite a wide range of control reflected in their HbA_1 levels. The normal distribution of this population is unusual. Our own review of a large clinic population revealed marked skewing of the heights to the lower percentiles (73).

Malone et al (74) have considered the role of hypercalciuria and hyperphosphaturia in the growth retardation of children with IDDM (n = 157) whose mean height was less than that of 37 non-diabetic siblings of similar age. Sixty-one percent were at or below the 50th percentile and 11% were shorter than would be anticipated by a normal distribution. Duration of diabetes had the greatest influence upon the children's height and this effect appeared by the 4th year of diabetes, becoming statistically significant after 7 years of diabetes. The degree of hypercalciuria and hyperphosphaturia was more closely associated with reduced height in children with diabetes than was the degree of hyperglycemia, even though the loss of calcium and phosphorus in the urine was related to glucosuria. In contrast to the study among exclusively pubertal

children from Canada (72), these authors found a statistical correlation between growth failure and glycosylated Hb levels. They also found a correlation
with duration of diabetes which could be confounding the correlation with
glycosylated Hb, since duration correlated with HbA_1 levels.

The precise explanation for short stature in IDDM remains uncertain. The
elevated growth hormone levels with unstable diabetes are not associated with
elevated somatomedin-C levels, but levels are typically low-normal. Nonetheless, improved glycemic control increases somatomedin-C levels and growth
velocity. It is likely that the complex process of growth is affected via more than
one mechanism in diabetes.

Complications

Risk factors

It has long been recognized that development of diabetes in childhood is associated with markedly reduced longevity. One of the most striking analyses
has been that of Deckert et al (75), which demonstrated that only 20% of those
developing diabetes under the age of 10 are alive at a point when 90% of the
non-diabetics of the same age population have survived. Dorman et al (76) have
found a 7-fold increased risk of dying compared to non-diabetic individuals of
the same age and have sought risk factors using a case control method. Shorter
relative height at onset, frequent diabetes-related readmissions to hospital,
presence of complications, a family history of diabetes, premature familial mortality, non-participation in school sports, and lower educational level were related to subsequent mortality among males. However, among females, only a
shorter duration of diabetes clinic attendance and the presence of complications
were significant associations with mortality.

There are numerous hypothetical bases for the relationship of diabetes control to complications and none would argue that the achievement of true
metabolic control from the outset would not abolish complications, or that
those atrociously controlled patients with difficult social situations are not at
markedly increased risk for complications. What is arguable is whether the
quality of control achievable under the best of circumstances with current
methodologies, in most cases, carries any greater risk than tight control measures, which are rarely achievable in young patients.

In all children, hyperlipidemia and elevated blood pressure are considered
risk factors for later problems and these would be especially pertinent in the
much higher risk group, children with diabetes. Strobl et al (77) found that the
atherogenic serum lipids were significantly higher in 30 youngsters with IDDM
than in controls and that these correlated with degree of metabolic control as

measured by HbA_{1c} and glycosylated serum protein. Correlation with glycosylated serum protein suggested that some of these changes might be due to glycosylation of low-density lipoprotein. Among 163 IDDM subjects aged 4-32 years, compared to 232 of their non-diabetic siblings and 292 of their natural parents, systolic pressures were not significantly increased. However, Phase IV diastolic pressure was slightly, but significantly, higher in the diabetic males than in the sibling group overall, a difference also shown individually within the 16-20 year age band. No effect was seen of duration of diabetes on blood pressure in either sex, but 20% of male IDDM subjects had mean blood pressures above the 90th percentile for age compared with only 9% of their siblings. These small differences were not thought to be major contributors to the incidence of diabetic vascular disease, but rather to reflect altered vascular regulation in IDDM (78).

Kobbah et al (79) studied vascular reactivity during the first year of diabetes in 24 children by looking at postocclusive reactive hyperemia using a transcutaneous CO_2 method. There was impairment before insulin treatment, but this improved to the point where there was no significant difference between diabetic and control children at 30 and 180 days. These changes do not appear to be related to degree of metabolic control and are of doubtful significance in the evolution of vascular complications. These same investigators studied ADP-stimulated platelet aggregation, a phenomenon noted to be increased in diabetes and hypothesized to be a pathogenic factor in both microvascular and macrovascular disease. Twenty-four children with IDDM were studied over the first year after diagnosis and compared to 20 healthy children of similar age and sex. There was no difference from controls in this measure. However, aggregation by low-dose collagen increased significantly in IDDM during the first year from seemingly normal to clearly supernormal, indicating that hypothesized risk factors for vascular disease are already present during the first year of diabetes. It also appears that collagen stimulation operates by a different mechanism to induce platelet aggregation from that stimulated by ADP (80).

Neuropsychological and neuropathic complications

Pediatric investigators have been concerned with the psychological performance of children with early-onset diabetes for more than 25 years (81). Consistent with previous studies, Holmes and Richman (82) found lower WISC-R performance IQ for children with onset of under 7 years of age and duration greater than 5 years, although IQ scores were in the average range. Performance subtest was uniformly lower for this group. Children with early-onset/long-duration also had higher rates of reading and memory impairment. There is electrophysiologic evidence of reduced central conduction velocity as a manifestation of diabetic neuropathy to explain these findings (83). More recently,

Oda et al (84) found prolonged peak latencies for auditory brainstem responses in 68 IDDM subjects aged 5-20 years.

Peroneal motor nerve conduction velocity has been studied in 61 IDDM children and adolescents with onset before 14 years of age. Approximately one-third had values greater than 2 standard deviations below the mean for normal subjects, with a highly significant negative correlation demonstrated between velocity and glycosylated Hb levels, either concomitant with the measurement or the mean annual value preceding measurement. The authors make a plea for clinical use of peroneal motor nerve conduction velocity measurement as a simple and sensitive tool to monitor young patients and motivate both physician and patient (85).

Autonomic neuropathy has been studied by Mitchell et al (86) in 38 children with IDDM aged 12 ± 3 (SD) years. The IDDM group had a faster heart rate at rest, reduced heart rate variation during quiet respiration, a smaller change in heart rate following a single deep breath, a lower Valsalva ratio, and a lower maximum/minimum R-R ratio in response to standing. These reflexes become increasingly important with aging and require careful consideration when exercise programs are undertaken.

Retinopathy

Malone and associates were the first to look at a large population of children using fluorescein injection, describing definite changes of retinopathy in 18% of youngsters with less than 5 years duration of diabetes, increasing to 70% between 11 and 16 years duration. The ophthalmologic complications of IDDM in children and adolescents have recently been reviewed by Malone (87) who notes that adolescent females are at particular risk, as are those with limited joint mobility. Burger et al (88) reported on the prevalence and development of retinopathy in 231 children with IDDM aged 18 ± 4 years with a diabetes duration of 9 ± 5 years at the end of the study. Prevalence and development of retinopathy were studied over a period of 5 years with ophthalmologic examination and fluorescein angiography. By the end of the study, 47% had developed retinal changes, half of which were classified as minimal, i.e. fewer than 5 microaneurysms. Ten of the patients had proliferative retinopathy. Lesions were rare under 15 years of age and with diabetes for less than 5 years. Median individual risk was calculated by life table analysis to be 9.1 years duration.

In a companion paper, the same investigators analyzed risk factors and found overall glycemic control from the onset of diabetes to affect the time of onset significantly, with minimal lesions developing by 8 years duration with poor control, 10.5 years with fair control and 12.5 years with good control. Only 4 of 14 variables were found to exert significant independent influences in the development of retinopathy: diabetes duration, long-term glycemic control, serum triglyceride and age. Duration was far and away the most influential factor (89).

Although Malone described female gender as a risk factor for the development of retinopathy in young patients, the Kleins and Moss (90) in a prevalence study among 1200 insulin-using patients diagnosed under 30 years of age found equal sex prevalence. Retinopathy was found in 72% of women and 69% of men with 12% of the men and 7% of the women having severe proliferative disease. Longer duration of diabetes, higher glycosylated Hb levels, older age at examination, higher diastolic blood pressure, male gender, and presence of proteinuria were all significant contributors to the severity of retinopathy.

Nephropathy

Diabetic nephropathy is a principal cause of increased morbidity and mortality in IDDM. Identification of the earliest functional changes that signal later progession can provide important information on risk factors and the effects of metabolic control or other interventions. IDDM is associated with increased glomerular filtration rate (GFR) and renal size, particularly in the early years. This increased GFR can be normalized by lowering of the blood glucose level. The relationship of this increased GFR to subsequent proteinuria and progressive nephropathy is unknown. Brouhard et al (91) have demonstrated normal GFR response to a short-term protein load (increase) in 9 patients 13-25 years old with diabetes for at least 10 years compared to 5 non-diabetic controls. These were not particularly well-controlled patients, with HbA_{1c} levels of 7.8-13.9% (controls 4.2-5.4). This study would suggest that the increased GFR, in and of itself, is not a pathologic factor.

The development of persistent proteinuria is unmistakably abnormal and of pathologic significance. Microalbuminuria, excretion of quantities below the level detected by routine methods, strongly predicts the development of nephropathy. Thus, there is great interest in reliable measurement in children. An enzyme immunoassay has been reported, which defined a marked difference between 10 healthy children and 24 with diabetes in both the supine and the standing position, in microalbuminuria excretion. Fifteen of the 24 patients had negative albuminuria by routine assays, but ELISA levels for microalbuminuria greater than the mean + 2 SD for controls. Six of 11 children with diabetes of more than 5 years had high urinary albumin excretion (92). This brief paper, which provides no data on the ages or duration of diabetes in these youngsters, suggests that 21 of 24 patients had either gross albuminuria or microalbuminuria by ELISA; this is a nearly 90% prevalence of 'nephropathy'. The clinical value of such a determination is dubious. It is certainly true that by 15 or 20 years of diabetes some degree of proteinuria and retinopathy is present in such proportion, but obviously only a subset of such individuals have progressive disease. On the other hand, if such early abnormalities are reversible by appropriate intervention, these highly sensitive methods would be of considerable value.

The proximal tubule lysosomal enzyme, N-acetyl-β-D-glucosaminidase (NAG), has also been used as an indicator of subtle renal injury. Brouhard et al (93) have studied 28 children 5-16 years of age with IDDM and 27 age-matched controls under a variety of exercise conditions. They found no significant differences in albumin excretion between IDDM and controls after exercise and urinary albumin excretion did not increase significantly in either group. NAG excretion did increase in the IDDM group compared to controls; indeed, there was a consistent mild decrease in controls and a substantial increase in excretion in those with diabetes. Thus, in contrast to studies that have been carried out in older patients, urinary albumin excretion with excercise does not detect subtle changes, but enzymuria during exercise does. The predictive value of such enzymuria remains to be determined.

Other investigators have looked at total albumin excretion during day-time and night-time. As has been well documented by others, GFR was increased, and correlated with duration of disease, but not with albumin excretion or blood pressure. Day-time albumin excretion also correlated with duration of disease, but also with glycosylated Hb, but not with age, GFR or blood presure. Night-time albumin excretion was significantly raised and correlated with duration of disease, glycosylated Hb, mean blood glucose concentration, and M value, but not with age, GFR or blood pressure. Although diastolic blood pressure was significantly elevated, it did not correlate with any other measured variable (94).

The suggestion that overnight albumin excretion is a sensitive measure of early nephropathy offers a method that is readily available in most clinical laboratories. Patients (n = 102) attending two diabetes clinics collected overnight timed urine samples for albumin analysis by radioimmunoassay, with 95% compliance. The results were compared to those of 36 healthy children matched for age and sex. Of the patients 20% had microalbuminuria defined as overnight albumin excretion rates above the upper normal level of 14 μg/min in two separate collections. Such excretion was only demonstrated in patients aged more than 5 years, among whom the prevalence was 37%. Arterial blood pressure was elevated in this group compared to the age-matched normoalbuminuric IDDM subjects. There was no difference in the prevalence of background retinopathy between those with and those without microalbuminuria. Glycosylated Hb was only slightly higher in the microalbuminuric patients and this was not significant (95). This methodology appears to identify the risk group, using a level of excretion that has previously been determined to identify those at high risk for progression to renal failure. Focusing intensive efforts on such patients, including treatment of mild elevations in blood pressure and improved diabetic control will provide more valuable information than such efforts directed more broadly.

The report by Luetscher et al (96) of plasma inactive renin being increased in IDDM includes a substantial number of young patients among the 235 tested and compared to 90 non-diabetic controls. There was an impressive increase with both age and duration of diabetes and a close correlation with the presence of complications involving the eye or kidney. Conventional treatment was associated with a steady increase in levels over 1-3 years while intensive treatment resulted in a rise in only 7% and a fall in 43% so managed. This study emphasizes the value of these discrete quantitative measures for monitoring the effects of improved control.

Limited joint mobility

Limited joint mobility (LJM), a recently recognized complication of diabetes in young patients, originally described among American IDDM patients (for review see Ref. 97), has subsequently been reported to be a frequent finding among IDDM patients in Japan, Ireland, England, Italy and, recently, Ethiopia (98). Further, as with other complications, LJM has been recognized to be prevalent among NIDDM patients as well. This condition is distinguished from other problems affecting the joints seen with diabetes which are rarely, if ever, seen in young patients, such as Dupuytren contracture, flexor tenosynovitis, carpal tunnel syndrome, the stiff hand syndrome, and reflex sympathetic dystrophy. It is noteworthy that only the stiff hand syndrome and LJM are peculiar to diabetes, and only LJM and Dupuytren contracture are unassociated with pain. The clinical findings of the other conditions are obviously different from LJM: Dupuytren contracture is characterized by thickened palmar fascia; flexor tenosynovitis involves the first, third, and fourth fingers with tendon thickening and locking while LJM involves principally the fifth finger and extends radially and also may involve large joints; carpal tunnel syndrome (also called the diabetic hand syndrome) affects all fingers equally; the stiff hand syndrome is associated with muscle atrophy and calcification of the small arteries of the hand; and the stiff hand syndrome, the diabetic hand, and reflex sympathetic dystrophy are associated with disabling pain, muscle atrophy, and neuropathies (97).

The importance of LJM lies in its correlation with microvascular complications; the presence of LJM appears to characterize a high-risk group for the early development of microvascular disease (99-101). In addition to associations with retinopathy and proteinuria, LJM has been associated with decreased pulmonary function (102). The original description of this manifestation included thick, tight, waxy skin (scleroderma-like) (97), and this has been repeatedly verified as a common association (103). A direct correlation of LJM to changes on renal biopsy has also been noted (104).

This generalized involvement of connective tissue and its correlation with microvascular disease suggests that a generalized abnormality in collagen, with functional alteration, underlies these complications (see chapters on glycosylated proteins in previous volumes). Biopsy studies have shown thickening of the dermis and epidermis with accumulation of collagen. Glycosylated skin collagen has been found to correlate with HbA_1 level but not with LJM (105, 106). However, fluorescence of skin collagen, an indirect measure of advanced glycosylation end products, has been found to increase linearly with age and to be abnormally increased for age in 95% of IDDM, reflecting increased cross-linkage. This fluorescence correlated with retinopathy, nephropathy, and LJM (106). Thus, the significance of these skin and joint changes lies in the insight provided about mechanisms of development of microvascular complications and the potential to thwart the process by direct intervention in the biochemical process.

References

1. Foulis AK, Liddle CN, Farquharson MA et al (1986): The histopathology of the pancreas in Type I (insulin-dependent) diabetes mellitus: a 25-year review of deaths in patients under 20 years of age in the United Kingdom. *Diabetologia, 29,* 267.
2. Najjar SS, Saikaly MG, Zaytoun GM et al (1985): Association of diabetes insipidus, diabetes mellitus, optic atrophy, and deafness: the Wolfram or DIDMOAD syndrome. *Arch. Dis. Child., 60,* 823.
3. Richards GE, Cavallo A, Meyer WJ et al (1985): Obesity, acanthosis nigricans, insulin resistance, and hyperandrogenemia: pediatric perspective and natural history. *J. Pediatr., 107,* 893.
4. LaPorte RE, Fishbein HA, Drash AL et al (1981): The Pittsburgh insulin-dependent diabetes mellitus (IDDM) registry: the incidence of insulin-dependent diabetes in Allegheny County, Pennsylvania (1965-1976). *Diabetes, 30,* 279.
5. Neufeld M, Maclaren NK, Rily WJ et al (1980): Islet cell and other organ-specific antibodies in U.S. Caucasians and Blacks with insulin-dependent diabetes mellitus. *Diabetes, 29,* 589.
6. Winter WE, Maclaren NK (1985): Type I insulin dependent diabetes: an autoimmune disease that can be arrested or prevented with immunotherapy? In: Barness L (Ed.), *Advances in Pediatrics,* p. 159. Year Book Medical Publishers, Chicago.
7. Notsu K, Oka N, Note S et al (1985): Islet cell antibodies in the Japanese population and subjects with Type I (insulin-dependent) diabetes. *Diabetologia, 28,* 660.
8. Wilken T, Armitage M, Casey C et al (1985): Value of insulin autoantibodies as serum markers for insulin-dependent diabetes mellitus. *Lancet, 1,* 480.
9. Arslanian SA, Becker DJ, Rabin B et al (1985): Correlates of insulin antibodies in newly diagnosed children with insulin-dependent diabetes before insulin therapy. *Diabetes, 34,* 926.
10. Karjalainen J, Knip M, Mustonen A et al (1986): Relation between insulin antibody and complement-fixing islet cell antibody at clinical diagnosis of IDDM. *Diabetes, 35,* 620.

11. McEvoy, Witt ME, Ginsberg-Fellner F et al (1986): Anti-insulin antibodies in children with Type I diabetes mellitus: genetic regulation of production and presence at diagnosis before insulin replacement. *Diabetes, 35,* 634.

12. Maclaren NK, Riley WJ (1985): Thyroid, gastric, and adrenal autoimmunities associated with insulin-dependent diabetes mellitus. *Diabetes Care, 8, Suppl. 1,*34.

13. DeLuca F, Vanelli M, Magazzu G et al (1985): Thyrogastric autoimmunity in a peadiatric group of Type I diabetics. *Minerva Pediatr., 37,* 391.

14. Kehr S, Gastauer R, Winkler G (1985): Type I diabetes, thyroid autoimmunity, thyroid function and HLA state. *Monatsschr. Kinderheilkd., 133,* 738.

15. Riley WJ, Winer A, Goldstein D (1983): Coincident presence of thyro-gastric autoimmunity at onset of Type I (insulin-dependent) diabetes. *Diabetologia, 24,* 418.

16. Chan SH, Lui KF et al (1985): HLA and Chinese patients with juvenile onset diabetes mellitus. *Ann. Acad. Med. Singapore, 14,* 209.

17. Lee BW, Tan SH, Wong HB et al (1985): HLA-DR antigens in Chinese children with insulin-dependent diabetes mellitus. *Ann. Acad. Med. Singapore, 14,* 219.

18. Eberhardt MS, Wagener DK, Orchard TJ et al (1985): HLA heterogeneity of insulin-dependent diabetes mellitus at diagnosis: the Pittsburgh IDDM study. *Diabetes, 34,* 1247.

19. Henson V, Maclaren N, Winter W et al (1986): Molecular genetics of insulin-dependent diabetes mellitus. *Mol. Biol. Med., 3,* 129.

20. Frisk G, Fohlman J, Kobbah M et al (1985): High frequency of Coxsackie-B virus-specific IgM in children developing Type I diabetes during a period of high diabetes morbidity. *J. Med. Virol., 17,* 219.

21. Friman G, Fohlman J, Frisk G et al (1985): An incidence peak of juvenile diabetes: relation to Coxsackie-B virus immune response. *Acta Paediatr. Scand., 74, Suppl. 320,* 14.

22. Orchard TJ, Rosenbloom AL (1985): The development of insulin-dependent diabetes mellitus among relatives. *Diabetes Care, 8, Suppl. 1,* 45.

23. Stiller CR, Dupre J, Gent M et al (1984) Effects of cyclosporin immunosuppression in insulin-dependent diabetes mellitus of recent onset. *Science, 223,* 1362.

24. Mandrup-Poulsen T, Stiller CR, Bille G et al (1985): Disappearance and reappearance of islet cell cytoplasmic antibodies in cyclosporin-treated insulin-dependent diabetics. *Lancet, 1,* 599.

25. Feutren G, Assan R, Karsenty G et al (1986): Cyclosporin increases the rate and length of remissions in insulin-dependent diabetes of recent onset. *Lancet, 1,* 119.

26. Palestine AG, Austin HA, Barlow JE et al (1986): Renal histopathologic alteration in patients treated with cyclosporin for uveitis. *N. Engl. J. Med., 314,* 1293.

27. Dahlquist G, Blom L, Holmgren G et al (1985): The epidemiology of diabetes in Swedish children 0-14 years — a six-year prospective study. *Diabetologia, 28,* 802.

28. Akerblom HK, Reunanen A (1985): The epidemiology of insulin-dependent diabetes mellitus (IDDM) in Finland and in Northern Europe. *Diabetes Care, 8, Suppl. 1,* 10.

29. LaPorte RE, Tajima N, Akerblom HK et al (1985): Geographic differences in the risk of insulin-dependent diabetes mellitus: the importance of registries. *Diabetes Care, 8, Suppl. 1,* 101.

30. Lorenzi M, Cagliero E, Schmidt NJ (1985): Racial differences in incidence of juvenile-onset Type I diabetes: epidemiologic studies in southern California. *Diabetologia, 28,* 734.

31. Jefferson IG, Smith MA, Baum JD et al (1985): Insulin dependent diabetes in under 5 year olds. *Arch. Dis. Child., 60,* 1144.

32. Warram JH, Krolewski AS, Gottlieb MS et al (1984): Differences in risk of insulin-dependent diabetes in offspring of diabetic mothers and diabetic fathers. *N. Engl. J. Med., 311,* 149.

226 *A.L. Rosenbloom*

33. Krane EJ, Rockoff MA, Wallman JK et al (1985): Subclinical brain swelling in children during treatment of diabetic ketoacidosis. *N. Engl. J. Med., 312*, 1147.
34. Clements Jr RS, Blumenthal SA, Morrison AD et al (1971): Increased cerebrospinal fluid pressure during treatment of diabetic ketoacidosis. *Lancet, 2*, 671.
35. Fein IA, Rackow EC, Sprung CL et al (1982): Relation of colloid osmotic pressure to arterial hypoxemia and cerebral edema during crystalloid volume loading of patients with diabetic ketoacidosis. *Ann. Intern. Med., 96*, 570.
36. Rosenbloom AL (1977): Diabetes mellitus in childhood and adolescence. In: Conn HF (Ed.), *Current Therapy*, p. 438. Saunders, Philadelphia.
37. Giordano B, Rosenbloom AL, Heller D et al (1977): Regional services for children and youth with diabetes. *Pediatrics, 60*, 492.
38. Duncan JA, Malone JI (1986): An out-of-hospital approach to the newly diagnosed diabetic. *Contemp. Pediatr., 3*, 79.
39. Hamman RF, Cook M, Keefer S et al (1985): Medical care patterns at the onset of insulin-dependent diabetes mellitus: association with severity and subsequent complications. *Diabetes Care, 8, Suppl. 1*, 94.
40. Tattersall R, Walford S, Peacock I et al (1980): A critical evaluation of methods of monitoring diabetic control. *Diabetes Care, 3*, 150.
41. Hermansson G, Ludvigsson J, Larsson Y (1986): Home blood glucose monitoring in diabetic children and adolescents: a 3-year feasibility study. *Acta Paediatr. Scand., 75*, 98.
42. Daneman D, Sinrinerio L, Transue D et al (1985): The role of self-monitoring of blood glucose in the routine management of children with insulin dependent diabetes mellitus. *Diabetes Care, 8*, 1.
43. Smith MA, Greene SA, Kuykendall VG et al (1985): Memory blood glucose reflectance meter and computer: a preliminary report of its use in recording and analysing blood glucose data measured at home by diabetic children. *Diabetic Med., 2*, 265.
44. Wilson DP, Endres RK (1986): Compliance with blood glucose monitoring in children with Type I diabetes mellitus. *J. Pediatr., 108*,1022.
45. Clarson C, Daneman D, Frank M et al (1985): Self-monitoring of blood glucose: how accurate are children with diabetes at reading Chemstrip bG? *Diabetes Care, 8*, 354.
46. Freund A, Johnson SB, Rosenbloom A et al (1986): Subjective symptoms, blood glucose estimation, and blood glucose concentrations in adolescents with diabetes. *Diabetes Care, 9*, 236
47. Schade DS, Duckworth WC (1986): In search of the subcutaneous-insulin resistance syndrome. *N. Engl. J. Med., 315*, 147.
48. Minuchin S, Baker L, Rosman BL et al (1975): A conceptual model of psychosomatic illness in children: family organization and family therapy. *Arch. Gen. Psychiatry, 32*, 1031.
49. Rosenbloom AL (1983): Residential treatment centers in Europe for children and youth with diabetes mellitus. *Clin. Pediatr., 22*, 760.
50. Johnson SB, Davidson N, Spillar R et al (1982): What determines success in a residential treatment center? *Diabetes, 31, Suppl. 1*, 17A.
51. Johnson SB (1984): Knowledge, attitudes, and behavior: correlates of health in childhood diabetes. *Clin. Psychol. Rev., 4*, 503.
52. Kovacs M, Feinberg TL, Paulauskas S et al (1985): Initial coping responses and psychosocial characteristics of children with insulin-dependent diabetes mellitus. *J. Pediatr., 106*, 827.
53. Kovacs M, Finkelstein R, Feinberg TL et al (1985): Initial psychologic responses of parents to the diagnosis of insulin-dependent diabetes mellitus in their children. *Diabetes Care, 8*, 568.
54. Kirk CR, Savage DCL (1985): The diabetic with a diabetic parent. *Arch. Dis. Child., 60*, 572.

55. Horan PF, Gwynn C, Renzi D (1986) Insulin-dependent diabetes mellitus and child abuse: is there a relationship? *Diabetes Care, 9,* 302.

56. Perrin EC, Shapiro E (1985): Health locus of control beliefs of healthy children, children with a chronic physical illness, and their mothers. *J. Pediatr., 107,* 627.

57. Anderson RM (1986): The personal meaning of having diabetes: implications for patient behaviour and education or kicking the bucket theory. *Diabetic Med., 3,* 85.

58. Golden MP, Herrold AJ, Orr DP (1985): An approach to prevention of recurrent diabetic ketoacidosis in the pediatric population. *J. Pediatr., 107.* 195.

59. Lucey D, Wing E (1985): A clinic based educational programme for children with diabetes. *Diabetic Med., 2,* 292.

60. Johnson SB, Pollak RT, Silverstein JH et al (1982): Cognitive and behavioral knowledge about insulin-dependent diabetes among children and parents. *Pediatrics, 69,* 708.

61. Hackett AF, Court S, McCowen C et al (1986): Dietary survey of diabetics. *Arch. Dis. Child., 61,* 67.

62. Kylberg E, Ewald U, Tuvemo T et al (1985): Dietary intake in Swedish diabetic children. *Acta Paediatr. Scand., 74, Suppl. 320,* 32.

63. Maryniuk MD, Kauwell GPA, Thomas RG (1986): A test of instructional approaches designed to influence food selection. *Diabetes Educator, 12,* 34.

64. Yki-Jarvinen H, Koivisto VA (1986): Natural course of insulin resistance in Type I diabetes. *N. Engl. J. Med., 315,* 224.

65. Amiel SA, Sherwin RS, Simonson DC et al (1986): Impaired insulin action in puberty: a contributing factor to poor glycemic control in adolescents with diabetes. *N. Engl. J. Med., 315,* 215.

66. Loudt KW, Campaigne BN, James FW et al (1985): Effects of exercise training on insulin sensitivity in adolescents with type I diabetes. *Diabetes Care, 8,* 461.

67. Campbell PJ, Bolli GB, Gryer PE et al (1985): Pathogenesis of the dawn phenomenon in patients with insulin-dependent diabetes mellitus: accelerated glucose production and impaired glucose utilization due to nocturnal surges in growth hormone secretion. *N. Engl. J. Med., 312,* 1473.

68. De Beaufort CE, Bruining GJ, Home PD et al (1986): Overnight metabolic profiles in very young insulin-dependent diabetic children. *Eur. J. Pediatr., 145,* 73.

69. Brink SJ, Stewart C (1986): Insulin pump treatment in insulin-dependent diabetes mellitus: children, adolescents, and young adults. *J. Am. Med. Assoc., 255,* 617.

70. Knight G, Boulton AJM, Ward JD (1986): Experience of continuous subcutaneous insulin infusion in the outpatient management of diabetic teenagers. *Diabetic Med., 3,* 82.

71. Songer TJ, LaPorte RE, Tajima N et al (1986): Height at diagnosis of insulin dependent diabetes in patients and their non-diabetic family members. *Br. Med. J., 292,* 1419.

72. Clarson C, Daneman D, Ehrlich RM (1985): The relationship of metabolic control to growth and pubertal development in children with insulin-dependent diabetes. *Diabetes Res., 2,* 237.

73. Rosenbloom AL, Silverstein JH, Lezotte DC (1982): Limited joint mobility in diabetes mellitus of childhood: natural history and relationship to growth impairment. *J. Pediatr., 101,* 847.

74. Malone JI, Lowitt S, Duncan JA et al (1986): Hypercalciuria, hyperphosphaturia, and growth retardation in children with diabetes mellitus. *Pediatrics, 78,* 298.

75. Deckert T, Poulsen JE, Larsen M (1979): The prognosis of insulin-dependent diabetes mellitus and the importance of supervision. *Acta Med. Scand., 624,* 48.

76. Dorman JS, Tajima N, LaPorte RE et al (1985): The Pittsburgh insulin-dependent diabetes mellitus (IDDM) morbidity and mortality study: case control analyses of risk factors for mortality. *Diabetes Care, 8, Suppl. 1,* 54.

77. Strobl W, Widhalm K, Schober E et al (1985): Apolipoproteins and lipoproteins in children with Type I diabetes: relation to glycosylated serum protein and HbA1. *Acta Paediatr. Scand.*, *74*, 966.
78. Tarn AC, Drury PL (1986): Blood pressure in children, adolescents and young adults with Type I (insulin-dependent) diabetes. *Diabetologia*, *29*, 275.
79. Kobbah M, Ewald U, Tuvemo T (1985): Vascular reactivity during the first year of diabetes in children. *Acta Peadiatr. Scand.*, *74, Suppl. 320*, 56.
80. Kobbah M, Ewald U, Tuvemo T (1985): Platelet aggregation during the first year of diabetes in childhood. *Acta Paediatr. Scand.*, *74, Suppl. 320*, 50.
81. Ack M, Miller M, Weil M (1961): Intelligence of children with diabetes mellitus. *Pediatrics*, *28*, 764.
82. Holmes CS, Richman LC (1985): Cognitive profiles of children with insulin-dependent diabetes. *Dev. Behav. Pediatr.*, *6*, 323.
83. Donald MW, Erdahl DLW, Surridge DHC et al (1984): Functional correlates of reduced central conduction velocity in diabetic subjects. *Diabetes*, *33*, 627.
84. Oda K, Murata R, Isshiki G et al (1986): Clinical and experimental studies of auditory brainstem responses in insulin-dependent diabetes mellitus. *No To Hattatsu*, *18*,29.
85. Dorchy H, Noel P, Kruger M et al (1985): Peroneal motor nerve conduction velocity in diabetic children and adolescents. *Eur. J. Pediatr.*, *144*, 310.
86. Mitchell EA, Wealthall SR, Elliott RB (1985): Tests for autonomic neuropathy in diabetic children. *Aust. Paediatr. J.*, *21*, 105.
87. Malone JI (1985): Ophthalmologic complications of insulin-dependent diabetes mellitus in children and adolescents. *Pediatrician. 12*, 194.
88. Burger W, Hovener G, Dusterhus R et al (1986): Prevalence and development of retinopathy in children and adolescents with Type I (insulin-dependent) diabetes mellitus: a longitudinal study. *Diabetologia*, *29*, 17.
89. Weber B, Burger W, Hartmann R et al (1986): Risk factors for the development of retinopathy in children and adolescents with Type I (insulin-dependent) diabetes mellitus. *Diabetologia*, *29*, 23.
90. Klein R, Klein BEK, Moss SE (1985): A population-based study of diabetic retinopathy in insulin-using patients diagnosed before 30 years of age. *Diabetes Care, 8, Suppl. 1*, 71.
91. Brouhard BH, LaGrone LF, Richards GE et al (1986): Short-term protein loading in diabetics with a ten-year duration of disease. *Amer. J. Dis. Child.*, *140*, 473.
92. Coppo R, Gerutti F, Amore A et al (1985): An enzyme immunoassay to detect microalbuminuria in diabetic patients. *Diabetes Care, 8*, 525.
93. Brouhard BH, Allen K, Sapire D et al (1985) Effect of exercise on urinary N-acetyl-beta-D-glucosaminidase activity and albumin excretion in children. *Diabetes Care, 8*, 466.
94. Davies AG, Price DA, Postlethwaite RJ et al (1985): Renal function in diabetic mellitus. *Arch. Dis. Child.*, *60*, 299.
95. Mathiesen ER, Saurbrey N, Hommel E et al (1986): Prevalence of microalbuminuria in children with Type I (insulin-dependent) diabetes mellitus. *Diabetologia*, *29*, 640.
96. Luetscher JA, Kraemer FB, Wilson DM et al (1985): Increased plasma inactive renin in diabetes mellitus: a marker for microvascular complications. *N. Engl. J, Med.*, *312*, 1412.
97. Rosenbloom AL (1984): Skeletal and joint manifestation of childhood diabetes. *Pediatr. Clin. North Am.*, *31*, 569.
98. Mengistu M, Abdulkadir J (1985): Limited finger joint mobility in insulin-dependent and non-insulin-dependent Ethiopian diabetics. *Diabetic Med.*, *2*, 387.
99. Rosenbloom AL, Silverstein JH, Lezotte DC et al (1981): Limited joint mobility in childhood diabetes mellitus indicates increased risk for microvascular disease. *N. Engl. J. Med.*, *305*, 191.

100. Kennedy L, Archer DB, Campbell SR et al (1982): Limited joint mobility in type I diabetes mellitus. *Postgrad. Med. J., 48,* 481.
101. Rosenbloom AL, Malone JI, Yucha J et al (1984): Limited joint mobility and diabetic retinopathy demonstrated by fluorescein angiography. *Eur. J. Pediatr., 141,* 163.
102. Schapf BM, Bank RA, Silverstein JH et al (1984): Pulmonary function in insulin-dependent diabetes mellitus with limited joint mobility. *Am. Rev. Respir. Dis., 130,* 930.
103. Buckingham B, Perejda AJ, Sandborg C et al (1986): Skin, joint, and pulmonary changes in type I diabetes mellitus. *Am. J. Dis. Child., 140,* 420.
104. Silverstein JH, Fennell R, Donnely W et al (1985): Correlates of biopsy-studied nephropathy in young patients with insulin-dependent diabetes mellitus. *J. Pediatr., 106,* 196.
105. Lyons TJ, Kennedy L (1985): Non-enzymatic glycosylation of skin collagen in patients with type I (insulin-dependent) diabetes mellitus and limited joint mobility. *Diabetologia, 28,* 2.
106. Monnier VM, Vishwanath V, Frank KE et al (1984): Relation between complications of type I diabetes mellitus and collagen-linked fluorescence. *N. Engl. J. Med., 314,* 403.

The Diabetes Annual/3
K.G.M.M. Alberti and L.P. Krall, editors
© 1987 Elsevier Science Publishers, B.V.

13 Education*

STEWART M. DUNN AND JOHN R. TURTLE

Education alone is ineffective

In previous editions of *The Diabetes Annual,* several authors have commented on the need for integration of the biomedical, psychosocial and educational aspects of diabetes care (1, 2). Responsibility for this lack of integration was assigned to all levels of the medical care system, from the doctor's office to the physicians organizing national and international meetings on diabetes. No mention was made of the tacit belief amongst many diabetologists that patient education was 'unscientific' and therefore irrelevant to the clinical management of diabetes.

In the 3 years from 1984 to 1986, rapid developments aimed at restoring this imbalance have occurred from within the ranks of diabetes education itself. In Europe, the influential activities of the Diabetes Education Study Group of the European Association for the Study of Diabetes (EASD), and its subsidiary organizations, have resulted in a proliferation of professional workshops generating an active quality assurance programme and the publication of specific journals, whose effect has been to improve the scientific quality of educational research (3). In the United States, the momentum established by the publication of National Standards in Diabetes Care, and recommendations for the treatment and prevention of major complications (4), led to the development and implementation of National Standards for Patient Diabetes Education Programs (5), and, in some states, to third-party reimbursement for the costs of education. In some countries, professional criteria for the training and accreditation of diabetes educators have accompanied the establishment of professional educators' associations, together with the publication of specific 'Diabetes Educator' journals. Formative evaluation is seen increasingly as an integral component in the development of patient education programmes. At the policy level diabetes education is active and productive; this review will address the more fundamental issue of the effectiveness of diabetes education as demonstrated by critical, scientific research.

Research in diabetes education has suffered from 3 related problems: (a) the

*Preparation of this chapter was supported by grants from the National Health & Medical Research Council of Australia, and the Rebecca L. Cooper Medical Research Foundation.

absence of experimental controls and objective outcomes, (b) inadequate cost-benefit evaluation, and (c) the lack of a research model which integrates education within the total scheme of patient care.

Developing a scientific approach to diabetes education

The value of experimental controls A recent report in the general health literature illustrates the misleading conclusions which may result from uncontrolled studies (6). The authors evaluated a 16-hour outpatient education programme by assessing knowledge, attitude, and metabolic control immediately before and 3 months after the programme. Patients were reported to have improved their scores on all measures, and the authors concluded these results 'suggest that outpatient education offers a significant inprovement in diabetic control'. Our own studies (7-9) of similar variables in 209 patients attending a two-day programme showed a 25% increase in diabetes knowledge, a significant normalization of diabetes attitudes, and an improvement in HbA_{1c} from 11.3% (average 1 month before) to 9.0% (average 6 months after). However, we also found a substantial rise in HbA_{1c} levels during the 3 months immediately preceding the programme, suggesting that many patients may have been referred to the programme during a period of deteriorating control; thus, subsequent improvement included a bias due to the 'Hawthorne effect', with compliance improving simply because patients were aware that their behaviour was under scrutiny.

Editors of diabetes-specific journals have tended lately to adopt a more rigorous approach to the design of evaluation studies, and the number of controlled trials of diabetes education has increased exponentially. The results have not been entirely supportive. Korhonen et al (10) were among the first to present strong evidence that diabetes education by itself had no effect on metabolic control. Their study elicited the very cogent criticism from Pichert (11) and Anderson (12) that diabetes education programmes vary widely on many dimensions, and any research publication must include a detailed description of the intervention under scrutiny.

Terrent et al (13) in Sweden randomly allocated 37 adult insulin-dependent diabetes mellitus (IDDM) patients to 1 of 4 conditions involving education and/or self-monitoring of blood glucose (SMBG) and found that SMBG, but not education, improved HbA_{1c} to a certain degree. A study in Indianapolis of 532 patients, predominantly elderly, black women with non-insulin-dependent diabetes mellitus (NIDDM) of long duration, used random assignment to experimental and control groups (14). The experimental intervention included didactic instruction, skill exercises and behavioural modification techniques, and 275 patients (52%) were followed for up to 4 years. Differences in knowledge between experimental and control subjects 11-14 months after instruction were minimal, but self-care skills and compliance were significantly higher in the experimental group. Experimental group patients also experienced greater reductions in fasting blood glucose and glycosylated haemoglobin, and in body weight, blood pressure and serum creatinine.

In a Nebraska study of a home diabetes education programme, a total of 373 diabetic inpatients were randomly allocated to intervention and control groups (15). The authors provided comprehensive details on the nature of the intervention, which was tailored to each patient's needs as identified by an (unpublished) Needs Assessment instrument. After 6 months, the intervention group scored an average 19% higher than the control group on diabetes knowledge and 1% higher on a skills assessment (both instruments unpublished). There were no differences in the number of preventable diabetes-related hospitalizations at 6 months, or in a smaller number of patients followed to 12 months. Like Korhonen and co-workers, these authors concluded that educational intervention alone, in the absence of concurrent changes in the health-care delivery system, was ineffective. Experimentally controlled trials have certainly resulted in a reduction in the size of programme effects compared with the earlier uncontrolled studies.

Refinements in outcome measurement   Many of the studies cited above have continued the common practice of using unstandardized measurement instruments to assess diabetes knowledge, attitudes and behavioural skills, and no data are reported on the validity or reliability of these measures. The expanding catalogue of psychosocial outcome measures now in print should make this practice obsolete.

Assal and Aufseesser-Stein (1) have reviewed several of the published questionnaires of diabetes knowledge. The latest range of attitude assessment instruments have focussed on the cognitive component in terms of diabetes-specific health beliefs and perceived control of diabetes (16, 17), while our own research has concentrated on developing a norm-referenced measure of emotional adjustment (18). Wing et al (19) confirmed, with their objective measure of compliance to SMBG, that subjects' self-reports significantly overestimated actual compliance rates.

The publication of well-researched measures of psychosocial and behavioural outcomes is paralleled by refinements in the selection and assessment of biomedical outcomes for educational research. Blood glucose levels have steadily been replaced in the literature by glycosylated haemoglobin, and assays for this measure have undergone considerable modification (20), making comparisons among studies sometimes misleading.

A number of studies suggest that the use of single biomedical outcomes, such as glycosylated haemoglobin alone, may disguise genuine effects of a more subtle nature, especially since the evidence linking diabetes control with macrovascular, and possibly microvascular, complications does not support the predominant role of blood glucose (21). Thus, Stevens et al (22), in a controlled trial of patient education designed to increase dietary carbohydrate and fibre intake, reported that increased intake was associated with reductions in fasting plasma glucose levels, cholesterol and high-density lipoprotein (HDL), but were unrelated to changes in weight, serum insulin levels, or HbA_{1c} levels over the study period.

Hospitalization rates continue to be used as a measure of programme effectiveness in reducing diabetes-related morbidity. Fishbein (23) reported a reduction in hospitalizations following an outpatient education programme in Rhode Island, with potential cost savings over the 4 years of the study of US $674,400. Hospitalization rates, and the reasons for hospitalization, were assessed by record review and physician interview. However, in the absence of a control group who do not receive the educational intervention, it is difficult to exclude the possibility that the reduction in hospitalizations was a consequence of secular effects or of referral bias, since physicians are unlikely to refer patients to an outpatient education programme for no reason.

A study by Zaremba et al (24) advises caution in the use of hospitalization data based on self-report. These authors compared self-reported rates with the Maine Blue Cross/Blue Shield inpatient claims file and found a reliability ratio of 0.77, with 16% of patients over-reporting and 7% under-reporting their hospitalizations prior to attending the education programme. Patients younger than 45 years were responsible for significantly fewer errors in reporting. More cogent criticisms of heavy reliance on hospitalization rates, as measures of intervention effect, are their sensitivity to alterations in referral patterns which may coincide with the introduction of programmes, and the fact that they omit all potential outcomes which intervene.

Clarifying the role of diabetes education

Specification of the target population   Awareness of the scope and limitations of the available outcome measures, and of the advantages of experimental controls, has contributed substantially to the improved standard of educational research published in the past 2-3 years. As knowledge of educational processes develops, educational interventions have responded by becoming increasingly specific with respect to target populations and the assessed needs of those populations.

Problems of the young, intractable patient continue to be a major concern. A range of psychological issues involved in the treatment of severe non-compliance were reviewed by Boehnert and Popkin (25), and Golden et al (26) described the effectiveness of a hierarchical set of medical, educational and psychosocial interventions in reducing recurrent ketoacidosis in a paediatric sample.

Research at the Joslin Diabetes Center (27) addresses the difficult and sensitive area of the special needs of patients with established complications of diabetes: they suggested that the onset of proliferative retinopathy portends a life crisis which renders metabolic control more sensitive to additional life stress, and that this association is not found among patients whose diabetes is more stable. The special needs of the low socioeconomic status (SES) patient have been the focus of Hopper's research for some years (28); her results indicate a number of activities, available to diabetes educators, which may positively influence diabetes control and decrease negative utilization patterns. A recent Canadian study (29) suggests that risk factors for cardiovascular disease are higher among men than women in this low SES group.

Sexual dysfunction in association with diabetes has traditionally been identified with male impotence. A Danish group (30) explored the sexual relationships in 51 couples where one partner has IDDM and reported that the couple's acceptance of diabetes was a better predictor of sexual dysfunction than was the presence of peripheral neuropathy in the diabetic partner; sexual dysfunction in women was also predicted by indices of psychological adjustment to diabetes.

Extension of the range of interventions   Educational approaches still follow the tenets of traditional attitude change theory, which views attitude in terms of cognitive, emotional and behavioural components. However, the exclusively knowledge-based programme is now almost extinct (if it ever existed in practice), and the range of activities encompassed by the term 'diabetes education' has expanded to include all manner of interventions, from one-to-one behaviour modification, through traditional didactic instruction, to group psychotherapy and community-based programmes.

The cross-fertilization of developed concepts among diverse fields of health education, including diabetes education, has been beneficial to each. Thus, Glanz (31) reviewed studies of nutrition education for weight reduction, diabetes, cancer, low-fat diets, sodium-restricted diets, and diets for patients with renal disease; her synthesis of this literature concentrated on the importance of problem diagnosis, the use of behavioural and biological measures of programme effectiveness, and issues involved in the maintenance of behaviour change.

Behavioural interventions aimed at self-care behaviours in diabetes were reviewed by Wing et al (32), who conceptualized the diabetic regimen in terms of a behavioural self-regulation model based on a negative feedback control system. The 4 components of this system are: (a) blood glucose monitoring behaviour; (b) corrective responses (such as insulin administration or sugar ingestion); (c) modification of diet, exercise and stress; and (d) self-reinforcement of self-regulatory behaviour. The authors reviewed intervention studies separately for IDDM and NIDDM within the framework provided by this model, and provided positive recommendations for future research in this important area.

The related area of blood glucose discrimination training is being investigated intensively. Gross et al (33) showed that a small sample of patients could improve the accuracy of their blood glucose estimation substantially, although no effects were shown on metabolic control. Cox et al (34) used factor analytical techniques to examine the differential effects of different stressors on diabetic control; their continuing research programme has highlighted the complex and idiosyncratic nature of these effects. Another area for behavioural intervention which continues to attract research interest is self-monitoring of blood glucose. A simple, controlled trial of educational effectiveness in learning SMBG reported 22-37% error in the 'self-instruction' group compared with 9% in the 'educator-instruction' group (35). Mazze and colleagues, in their research with glucose monitoring equipment containing a memory chip, have demonstrated the unreliability of patient-generated data using SMBG (36), and shown that this performance may be improved by appropriately designed intervention (37).

Interventions involving groups offer the dual benefits of more cost-effective use of available resources, and enhancement of attitude change through group interaction (9, 38). Tattersall et al (39) reviewed the need for psychosocial support in the treatment of diabetes and proposed group psychotherapy as a neglected alternative. Kaplan et al (40) reported that teenagers randomly assigned to a social skills learning group had significantly lower HbA_1 than a control group.

A developing area for diabetes education, and a logical extension of the activities of diabetes educators, is the multidisciplinary coordination of diabetes care within the hospital and its wider community. Wylie-Rosett et al (41) conducted a chart audit, staff interviews, and observations to evaluate care standards at a large teaching hospital in New York. Their assessment indicated major discrepancies in the evaluation of patient needs, a failure to implement current diagnostic criteria for diabetes, and inadequate urine testing procedures. The authors then implemented a multidisciplinary teaching programme which was followed by overall improvement in all 8 measures of standards of care. The intervention was estimated to represent a net annual saving of US $50,000 for each individual discharged and receiving home health-care assistance.

Community activities are a major target of the diabetes Education and Control Program reported recently by Gifford and Zimmet in Australia (42). This programme is evaluating several implementation models which seek to integrate ambulatory diabetes education programmes into community health care centres. Primary preventive education aimed at the prevention of diabetes in at-risk populations (characterised by family history, HLA-DR3 or HLA-DR4 antigens, and excess obesity) represents a challenging role for diabetes education in the future (43).

Programme evaluation in the context of diabetes management

Evaluation models for diabetes education

Diabetes education is evolving rapidly in the 1980s. Problem diagnosis has established a clearer perspective on the needs of specific patient groups, and the range of potential interventions has expanded well beyond that expressed in the simplistic educational dogma that 'knowledge equals action'. Educational evaluation has developed to a point where it is now quite rare to find published reports which do not contain details of the intervention itself and at least an attempt at summative evaluation. More commonly, evaluation is being built into programme development from its inception.

In response to this increasingly scientific approach to diabetes education, a number of authors have proposed theoretical models which seek: (a) to integrate the results of research from disparate sources; (b) to integrate diabetes education within the broader context of diabetes care; and (c) to provide a framework for ongoing research and evaluation.

The health programme evaluation model proposed by Green et al (44) has been adapted to the specific case of diabetes education by Dunn et al (8, 9). According to this model, changes in predisposing factors like knowledge, attitudes and beliefs, which are caused by the intervention, lead to changes in behaviour in respect of daily diabetes management. This improved compliance is then suppposed to produce improved control of diabetes, measured by blood glucose, glycosylated haemoglobin etc., which in turn results in reduced morbidity and mortality from the disease in the long term. The model emphasises that the strict evaluation of programme impact ceases with our demonstration of its effect on the predisposing variables. From that point on, we are testing the hypothesis, based on clinical and epidemiological evidence (which is by no means conclusive), that these changes lead to improved control and reduced risk of complications. Many of these changes may require months or years to take effect. Thus, any evaluation which omits the intervening steps is seriously prejudicing its chances of detecting real programme effects.

Specific models have also been proposed to describe educational effects in terms which are extensively grounded within the empirical literature of related disciplines. The Health Belief Model continues to generate data suggesting that diabetes-specific beliefs and cognitions are a potent influence on compliance, and (possibly) directly on metabolic control (16, 17). Rosenstock (45) reviewed studies on patient compliance and proposed a comprehensive framework based on the Health Belief Model expanded to include the learning theory concept of perceived self-efficacy. Long-term maintenance of changed behaviour, in this framework, is addressed in terms of the relapse prevention model derived from social learning theory.

The number and complexity of theoretical models is perhaps somewhat daunting to the uninitiated, though it is an accurate indication of the state of the art in diabetes education, where the accelerated rate of published scientific data has tended to outstrip conceptual rigour and appropriate experimental design. Preoccupation with theoretical models reflects healthy activity and a concern to redress this imbalance.

Process evaluation and the integration of diabetes care

Assal et al (46) have argued that diabetes care in general has remained poor, despite the advent of insulin and sophisticated technologies to augment medical management. The prime reason for this situation, the authors believe, is 'the widespread failure... to recognize the fundamental importance of diabetes education as an integral part of diabetes care'. Whilst physicians may resist education for the variety of personal and political reasons Assal and associates suggest, it remains incumbent on diabetes education itself to provide the scientific evidence supporting the integration of education within a global approach to diabetes, combining biomedical, psychosocial, and educational elements.

In addition to its demonstrated effectiveness in the multidisciplinary coordination of inpatient care (41), diabetes education has an important role to play in the trend to outpatient management of diabetes. Hamman et al (47) examined patterns of medical care use and the prognosis for acute complications after diagnosis for children with newly diagnosed IDDM over a 4-year period in Colorado. Their exploratory, uncontrolled study concluded that a 42% reduction in total nights hospitalized could occur if children with 'mild' or 'normal' severity were treated largely in the outpatient setting. Hoskins et al (48) reported a significant improvement in glycosylated haemoglobin in patients commenced on insulin, or re-stabilized, in an outpatient paramedical diabetes care centre. Results were similar to those for patients admitted to hospital for stabilization during the same period. Ling et al (49) suggest that the diabetic day care unit will ultimately replace the diabetes clinic, just as the latter has increasingly replaced inpatient management as the regimen of choice.

Direct benefits of educational intervention in outpatient management practice were reported in Adamson and Gullion's study (50) of a diabetes professional education programme in a rural/suburban community. Medical record and survey data on 397 patients, collected before and after the programme, showed increased frequencies of recommending SMBG and foot examination by the physicians, and in ketone testing by patients. However, no improvements were noted in the monitoring of other complications of diabetes, or in blood glucose levels or hospitalization rates.

A controlled trial of an intervention to increase adherence to prescribed office visits, conducted by Smith et al (51) in Indianapolis, stratified 859 patients by risk of hospitalization and randomly assigned them within strata to control and intervention groups. The interventions included mailed information on phone numbers, early warning signs, educational booklets, and appointment reminders. The results showed a 14% improvement in keeping scheduled visits relative to the control group, and the effects were greatest in the high-risk patients.

The future for diabetes education

Studies addressing this integration of educational activities within a 'global approach' to diabetes (46) must acknowledge the important differences in referral practices and cost structures which operate within the health care systems of different countries. Scott et al (52), from their scrutiny of a computerized discharge system in a New Zealand general hospital, concluded that admission rates were substantially lower among patients who were *'sufficiently motivated'* to attend diabetes education programmes. Whilst reimbursement issues continue to preoccupy those committed to diabetes education, there is a tendency to overlook the poignant fact that much of the 'evidence' supporting the effectiveness of education comes from programmes which attract only the motivated, higher SES patient, particularly where substantial costs are involved. The low-SES patient, who may well be at higher risk for the complications of diabetes (28, 29), frequently remains ignorant of or indifferent to the potential for increased self-management.

These issues are particularly critical in the United States, where third-party reimbursement for diabetes education is well established in some states, and is pursued nationally through a recent policy statement from the American Diabetes Associates (53). The policy is not without its critics: Kaplan and Davis (54) observed that only 2 of the 13 studies cited in support of the policy statement used experimental controls, and both of these failed to assign subjects randomly to treatment condition. Moreover, there was no accounting for costs or attrition rates in the majority of programmes, and it appeared that some programmes actually increased health care expenditure. Where attrition rates were reported, they were high.

The fact that some hospitals and third-party payers in the United States are prepared to reimburse institutions for the cost of providing preventive-oriented patient education programmes represents a significant change in philosophy —

one which has profound implications for public health care policy in respect of other chronic diseases, and for health-promotion programmes in the general population (55). Diabetes education has played a significant role in this movement towards greater recognition of quality of life as a justifiable target for health care intervention. If diabetes education is to continue this contribution, it must maintain the current initiatives in respect of: (a) clear identification of the target population; (b) appropriate integration within the global concept of diabetes care; and (c) scientifically based research and evaluation of all its activities.

References

1. Assal J-P, Aufseesser-Stein M (1986): Patient education in diabetes therapy. In: Alberti KGMM, Krall LP (Eds) *The Diabetes Annual/2*, p. 156. Elsevier, Amsterdam.
2. Bradley C (1985): Psychological aspects of diabetes. In: Alberti KGMM, Krall LP (Eds), *The Diabetes Annual 1*, p. 374. Elsevier, Amsterdam.
3. *Practical Diabetes* (Editor: AK Baksi. Asgood Publishing, Petersfield, Hants. UK) uses a network of regional advisers as consultants to educators and other health professionals intending to publish research studies.
4. National Diabetes Advisory Board (1983): *The Prevention and Treatment of Five Complications of Diabetes*. HHS 83-8392, US Government Printing Office.
5. National Diabetes Advisory Board (1984): National standards for patients diabetes education programs. *Diabetes Care, 7*, 31.
6. Paulozzi LJ, Norman JE, McMahon P, Connell FA (1985): Outcomes of a diabetes education program. *Public Health Rep., 99*, 575.
7. Dunn SM, Turtle JR (1982): Assessment techniques and the limitations of diabetes education. *Diabetes, 31, Suppl. 2*, 452.
8. Dunn SM (1985): The Psychological Impact of Diabetes Education: Implications for Metabolic Control. Unpublished doctoral dissertation, Faculty of Medicine, University of Sydney.
9. Dunn SM (1986): Reactions to educational techniques: coping strategies for diabetes and learning. *Diabetic Med., 3*, 419.
10. Korhonen T, Huttunen JK, Aro A et al (1983): A controlled trial on the effects of patient education in the treatment of insulin-dependent diabetes. *Diabetes Care, 6*, 256.
11. Pichert JW (1983): Not all medicines (or patient education programs) are the same. *Diabetes Care, 6*, 618.
12. Anderson RM (1983): Defining and evaluating diabetic patient education. *Diabetes Care, 6*, 619.
13. Terrent A, Hagfall O, Cederholm U (1985): The effect of education and self-monitoring of blood glucose on glycosylated hemoglobin in type 1 diabetes: a controlled 18-month trial in a representative population. *Acta Med. Scand., 217*, 47.
14. Mazzuca SA, Moorman NH, Wheeler ML et al (1986): The Diabetes Education Study: a controlled trial of the effects of diabetes patient education. *Diabetes Care, 9*, 1.
15. Rettig BA, Shrauger DG, Recker RR et al (1986): A randomized study of the effects of a home diabetes education program. *Diabetes Care, 9*, 173.
16. Bradley C, Brewin C, Gamsu DS, Moses JL (1984): Development of scales to measure perceived control of diabetes mellitus and diabetes-related health beliefs. *Diabetic Med., 1*, 213.

17. Harris R, Linn MW (1985): Health beliefs, compliance, and control of diabetes mellitus. *South. Med. J., 78,* 162.
18. Dunn SM, Smartt HH, Beeney LJ, Turtle JR (1986): The measurement of emotional adjustment in diabetic patients: validity and reliability of the ATT39. *Diabetes Care, 9,* 480.
19. Wing RR, Epstein LH, Nowalk MP et al (1985): Compliance to self-monitoring of blood glucose: a marked-item technique compared with self-report. *Diabetes Care, 8,* 456.
20. Eross J, Kreutzman D, Jiminez M et al (1984): Colorimetric measurement of glycosylated protein in whole blood, red blood cells, plasma and dried blood. *Ann. Clin. Biochem., 21,* 477.
21. Rodger NW (1985): Multicenter study of effect (of insulin pump therapy) on microvascular disease. *Diabetes, 34, Suppl. 1,* 331.
22. Stevens J, Burgess MB, Kaiser DL, Sheppa CM (1985): Outpatient management of diabetes mellitus with patient education to increase dietary carbohydrate and fiber. *Diabetes Care, 8,* 359.
23. Fishbein HA (1985): Precipitants of hospitalization in insulin-dependent diabetes mellitus (IDDM): a statewide perspective. *Diabetes Care, 8, Suppl. 1,* 61.
24. Zaremba MM, Willhoite B, Ra K (1985): Self-reported data: reliability and role in determining program effectiveness. *Diabetes Care, 8,* 486.
25. Boehnert CE, Popkin MK (1986): Psychological issues in treatment of severely non-compliant diabetics. *Psychosomatics, 27,* 11.
26. Golden MP, Herrold AJ, Orr DP (1985): An approach to prevention of recurrent diabetic ketoacidosis in the pediatric population. *J. Pediatr., 107,* 195.
27. Jacobson AM, Rand LI, Hauser ST (1985): Psychologic stress and glycemic control: a comparison of patients with and without proliferative retinopathy. *Psychosom. Med., 47,* 372.
28. Hopper SV, Schechtman KB (1985): Factors associated with diabetic control and utilization patterns in a low-income, older adult population. *Patient Educ. Couns., 7,* 275.
29. Millar WJ, Wigle DT (1986): Socioeconomic disparities in risk factors for cardiovascular disease. *Can. Med. Assoc. J., 134,* 127.
30. Jensen SB (1986): The natural history of sexual dysfunction in diabetic women: a 6-year follow-up study. *Acta Med. Scand., 219,* 73.
31. Glanz K (1985): Nutrition counselling for risk factor reduction and patient education: a review. *Prev. Med., 14,* 721.
32. Wing RR, Epstein LH, Nowalk MP, Lamparski DM (1986): Behavioral self-regulation in the treatment of patients with diabetes mellitus. *Psychol. Bull., 99,* 78.
33. Gross AM, Magalnick LJ, Delcher HK (1985): Blood glucose discrimination training and metabolic control in insulin-dependent diabetics. *Behav. Res. Ther., 23,* 507.
34. Cox DJ, Taylor AG, Nowacek G et al (1984): The relationship between psychological stress and insulin-dependent diabetic blood glucose control: preliminary investigations. *Health Psychol., 3,* 63.
35. Ward WK, Haas LB, Beard JC (1985): A randomized, controlled comparison of instruction by a diabetes educator versus self-instruction in self-monitoring of blood glucose. *Diabetes Care, 8,* 284.
36. Mazze RS, Shamoon H, Pasmantier R et al (1984): Reliability of blood glucose monitoring by patients with diabetes mellitus. *Am. J. Med., 77,* 211.
37. Mazze RS, Pasmantier R, Murphy JA, Shamoon H (1986): Self-monitoring of capillary blood glucose: changing the performance of individuals with diabetes. *Diabetes Care, 8,* 207.
38. Dunn SM, Hoskins PL, Alford JB, Turtle JR (1982): Cost-benefit analysis of audiovisual techniques in diabetes education. In: Mngola EN (Ed.), *Proceedings, 11th Congress, International Diabetes Federation, Nairobi 1982,* p. 17. Excerpta Medica, Amsterdam.

39. Tattersall RB, McCulloch DK, Aveline M (1985): Group therapy in the treatment of diabetes. *Diabetes Care, 8,* 180.
40. Kaplan RM, Chadwick MW, Schimmel LE (1985): Social learning intervention to promote metabolic control in type I diabetes mellitus: pilot experiment results. *Diabetes Care, 8,* 152.
41. Wylie-Rosett J, Villeneuve M, Mazze R (1985): Professional education in a long-term-care facility: program development in diabetes. *Diabetes Care, 8,* 481.
42. Gifford S, Zimmet P (1986): A community approach to diabetes education in Australia — the Region 8 (Victoria) Diabetes Education and Control Program. *Diabetes Res. Clin. Pract., 2,* 105.
43. Mazze RS, Sinnock P, Deeb L, Brimberry JL (1985): An epidemiological model for diabetes mellitus in the United States: five major complications. *Diabetes Res. Clin. Pract., 1,* 185.
44. Green LW, Levine DM, Deeds S (1975): Clinical trials of health education for hypertensive outpatients: design and baseline data. *Prev. Med., 4,* 417.
45. Rosenstock IM (1985): Understanding and enhancing patient compliance with diabetic regimens. *Diabetes Care, 8,* 610.
46. Assal JP, Mühlhauser I, Pernet A et al (1985): Patient education as the basis for diabetes care in clinical practice and research. *Diabetologia, 28,* 602.
47. Hamman RF, Cook M, Keefer S et al (1985): Medical care patterns at the onset of insulin-dependent diabetes mellitus: association with severity and subsequent complications. *Diabetes Care, 8, Suppl. 1,* 94.
48. Hoskins P, Alford J, Fowler P et al (1985): Outpatient stabilization programme — an innovative approach in the management of diabetes. *Diabetes Res, 2,* 85.
49. Ling P, Lovesay JM, Mayon-White VA et al (1985): The diabetic clinic dinosaur is dying: will diabetic day units evolve? *Diabetic Med., 2,* 163.
50. Adamson TE, Gullion DS (1986): Assessment of diabetes continuing medical education. *Diabetes Care, 9,* 11.
51. Smith DM, Norton JA, Weinberger M, McDonald CJ et al (1986): Increasing prescribed office visits: a controlled trial in patients with diabetes mellitus. *Med. Care, 24,* 189.
52. Scott RS, Brown LJ, Clifford P (1985): Use of health services by diabetic persons. II. Hospital admissions. *Diabetes Care, 8,* 43.
53. Sinnock P, Deeb LC (1986): ADA policy on third-party reimbursement for outpatient education: a reply. *Diabetes Care, 9,* 93.
54. Kaplan RM, Davis WK (1986): Evaluating the costs and benefits of outpatient diabetes education and nutrition counselling. *Diabetes Care, 9,* 81.
55. Schwartz R, Zaremba M, Ra K (1985): Third-party coverage for diabetes education program. *Qual. Rev. Bull., 11,* 213.

The Diabetes Annual/3
K.G.M.M. Alberti and L.P. Krall, editors
© 1987 Elsevier Science Publishers, B.V.

14 Pregnancy and diabetes: gestational diabetes

CLAUS KÜHL AND LARS MØLSTED-PEDERSEN

Introduction

Recently published work on diabetes and pregnancy continues to stress the importance of careful and meticulous control of maternal glycaemia during pregnancy for the continued reduction of the incidence of adverse fetal and neonatal outcome (1-6). This highly important issue was also discussed in the first two volumes of *The Diabetes Annual*.

Whereas many clinicians used to believe that good glycaemic control in diabetic pregnancy is only achievable by means of continuous subcutaneous insulin infusion, there is now evidence that equally excellent control may be accomplished by use of multiple insulin injections (1, 2, 7). It is generally agreed that glycaemic control should be optimalized already before conception (4, 7), but there is still controversy about the desired level of diabetic control. It thus remains to be seen how tight the glycaemic control of maternal diabetes has to be, both before and after conception, in order to diminish (or prevent?) the incidence of congenital malformations. It is also unknown whether 'too good' glycaemic control, leading to maternal hypoglycaemia, can be deleterious to the embryo during the period of organogenesis (8). Current clinical studies in Copenhagen and elsewhere will hopefully provide answers to these important questions in the next few years.

Problems pertaining to pregnancy in patients with insulin-dependent diabetes mellitus (IDDM) will undoubtedly continue to attract a lot of attention in the future. This should not, however, lead us to forget an equally important condition relevant to pregnancy: gestational diabetes. In June, 1985, the summary and recommendations of the second International Workshop-Conference on Gestational Diabetes Mellitus was published (9), and in July-August, 1986, the American Diabetes Association's endorsement of these recommendations became public (10). An abbreviated version of the recommendations was subsequently published by the American College of Physicians (11).

Since there is still a lot of controversy about the definition, treatment and control of gestational diabetes mellitus, we have chosen to make this year's chapter of the *Annual* a review of this disorder.

Gestational diabetes

Gestational diabetes mellitus is defined as carbohydrate intolerance of variable severity with onset or first recognition during the present pregnancy (9). This definition, which was unanimously endorsed by the participants of the Second International Workshop-Conference on Gestational Diabetes Mellitus, is now widely accepted by clinicians involved in this field. It differs from previous definitions which also required a normal fasting blood glucose concentration in pregnancy and a return to normal glucose tolerance after delivery (12, 13). Furthermore, according to most previous definitions, only dietary treatment was needed for the treatment of gestational diabetes (12). The new definition is considerably more operational and it will undoubtedly make easier comparison of clinical research studies in gestational diabetes in the future.

Aetiology and pathophysiology

Gestational diabetes mellitus is a heterogeneous disorder that complicates 2-3% of all pregnancies in the Western world (14, 15) and it is usually diagnosed in the second half of pregnancy. The mean age of women with gestational diabetes is normally higher and the pre-pregnancy weight is also higher than that of pregnant women who retain a normal glucose tolerance in pregnancy (14, 15). Freinkel et al (16) found in a survey of 199 gestational diabetic women that HLA-DR3 and HLA-DR4 antigens were more often present than in a control group of 148 consecutive gravidae with normal glucose tolerance. Moreover, at the time of diagnosis, cytoplasmic islet cell antibodies (ICA) were significantly more common in women with gestational diabetes than in controls (16). The 'positive' tissue types and the presence of ICA were, however, found predominantly in gestational diabetes associated with a high (i.e. ≥ 7.2 mmol/l) fasting plasma glucose concentration. Such cases would be classified in many centres as IDDM with onset during pregnancy. Thus, at the Copenhagen centre for diabetes in pregnancy, tissue-typing of gestational diabetic women has never disclosed any similarity to IDDM, and ICA-positive sera have not been found with any greater frequency than in healthy controls (unpublished results). There is little doubt that the incidence of newly diagnosed IDDM is significantly increased in pregnant women (17) and these cases should clearly be distinguished from 'true' gestational diabetes.

Why pregnancy is capable of inducing gestational diabetes is still partly unknown (18). The insulin response to oral glucose and mixed meals are equally large in gestational diabetic and healthy pregnant women, but the insulin response per unit of glycaemic stimulus (the 'insulinogenic index') is significantly lower in gestational diabetic women than in controls (19, 20). Diabetes-like changes in glucagon secretion are not observed in gestational diabetes nor is insulin degradation increased (19, 20). No difference in insulin binding (at tracer insulin concentrations) to monocytes from healthy pregnant controls and gestational diabetic subjects is found and insulin receptor binding is largely unaffected by pregnancy in both groups (21). The cause of gestational diabetes could therefore be a relative lack of circulating insulin combined with one or more postreceptor defect(s). The cellular basis for the insulin resistance in pregnancy and how it is brought about are not yet fully understood, but it seems that the hypercortisolaemia found in pregnancy could play a significant pathogenic role (22). Most women are able to counteract the insulin resistance of pregnancy by increasing their insulin secretion. However, when the capacity of insulin secretion is not sufficiently large to meet the requirement, glucose intolerance develops and the woman develops gestational diabetes.

Screening for gestational diabetes

The glucose intolerance of gestational diabetes is usually mild, but nevertheless it is associated with a higher incidence of complications during pregnancy and, in some cases, an increased perinatal mortality and infant morbidity (15). Since proper treatment of the mother seems to improve the prognosis for the fetus (15), it is important to screen for gestational diabetes so that treatment of the patient can be instituted as early in pregnancy as possible.

There is no general agreement about how one should screen for gestational diabetes mellitus. In the past, screening was always selective, i.e. based on either clinical risk factors including a family history of diabetes or presence of obesity, hypertension and glycosuria, or on a past obstetric history such as delivery of a macrosomic infant, an infant with malformation or an unexplained stillbirth. However, even though large-scale selective screening is feasible (23), it is not always adequate. Thus, up to 50% of women who go on to develop gestational diabetes will fail to manifest these screening criteria (24). Glycosuria is a poor screening criterion since it is found in about 50% of normal healthy pregnant women (25). Therefore, *all* pregnant women should be screened at approximately 24-28 weeks' gestation, at which stage the diabetogenic stress of pregnancy is most pronounced (18). Selected high-risk patients, those with gestational diabetes in a previous pregnancy or women with carbohydrate intolerance while treated with corticosteroids may be screened earlier in pregnancy. Similarly, if the initial screen at 24-28 weeks' gestation is negative but the patient is thought to be at great risk for gestational diabetes, a repeat test should be scheduled at 32 weeks.

How should the screening then be performed? It is obvious that the screening test has to be simple in order to be universally applicable to pregnant women as part of routine antenatal care. Lind (26) advocates such a simple screening system based on the determination of a random venous whole blood glucose concentration. Screening all antenatal patients by this method does not inconvenience the patients, but it seems to be considerably less efficient in identifying gestational diabetic subjects than the more traditional systems. Thus, out of a total of 2403 consecutive antenatal patients only 4 (0.2%) were found to have unequivocal diabetes mellitus. Similarly, screening by a single determination of glycosylated haemoglobin is not a valid method (27).

Based on the shortcomings of selective screening and the above-mentioned principles of non-selective screening, the American Diabetes Association (ADA) now recommends (10) that all pregnant women who have not been identified as having glucose intolerance before the 24th week should be given 50 g of oral glucose between the 24th and 28th week. This is given without regard to time of the last meal or time of day. Venous plasma glucose should be measured 1 hour later and if this value equals or exceeds 140 mg/100 ml (7.8 mmol/l), then the woman should have a full diagnostic oral glucose tolerance test (OGTT). This screening test has recently been validated (28) and it is now implemented in many places throughout the United States, whereas most European centres still favour selective screening methods. There is little doubt, however, that the American system will become more universally implemented, also because it is the easiest system to follow. Outpatient screening using the American system and a reflectance meter might be feasible but can at present not be recommended since the meter read-out may differ by as much as 22% from the value of the central laboratory chemistry analyser (29).

With regard to the diagnostic OGTT, there is also a lack of universal agreement. The Americans recommend a 100-g OGTT, the outcome of which should be interpreted according to the diagnostic criteria of O'Sullivan and Mahan (30). This means that an OGTT is considered diabetic if two or more of the venous plasma glucose concentrations are equal to or exceed: fasting, 105 mg/100 ml (5.8 mmol/l); 1 hour, 190 mg/100 ml (10.6 mmol/l); 2 hours, 165 mg/ 100 ml (9.2 mmol/l); 3 hours, 145 mg/100 ml (8.1 mmol/l). Many European centres still use 50-g OGTTs and, naturally, other cut-off points, whereas only a few centres use an intravenous glucose tolerance test or a meal test. The Diabetic Pregnancy Study Group (DPSG) of the European Association for the Study of Diabetes has decided to follow the recent WHO recommendations (31) according to which one should try to establish the diagnosis for gestational diabetes based on a 75-g OGTT. A subgroup of DPSG members is currently collecting such data which will hopefully be made generally available within a year or two.

Treatment

Once the diagnosis of gestational diabetes mellitus has been established, patients are started on a diet that excludes simple sugars, but, again, there is some disagreement between Americans and Europeans with regard to the caloric content of the diet. Since gestational diabetes frequently occurs in obese women, many Europeans would chose to institute a hypocaloric diet consisting of 1200-1500 kcal whereas the Americans, following the ADA's recommendations (10), generally prescribe an isocaloric diet (i.e. 35-38 kcal/kg of pre-pregnancy ideal body weight). The Americans are reluctant to prescribe hypocaloric diets because they fear that the gestational diabetic, due to her relative insulin resistance (19), is prone to develop hyperketonaemia. The fear is that the ketone bodies might impair fetal brain development, and hence the IQ score of the infant later in life (32).

Studies in vitro have demonstrated that ketone bodies inhibit the biosynthesis of pyrimidines in the fetal rat brain (33). This could lead to impaired cell replication since pyrimidines are necessary for the synthesis of both RNA and DNA. Recent animal experiments also indicate that hyperketonaemia leads to a significant decrease in fetal arterial oxygen tension and oxygen content concomitant with increases in fetal lactate levels and fetal heart rate (34). Since similar changes were observed in normoglycaemic and hyperglycaemic fetuses (34), the adverse effect of maternal hyperketonaemia on the fetus is also relevant to gestational diabetes. The view that maternal hyperketonaemia might exert a harmful influence on fetal cerebral development is not unanimously accepted. Thus, in a carefully conducted Swedish study, Persson (35) reports the 5-year morbidity experience of a group of 73 children born to diabetic and gestational diabetic mothers in one institution. No severe neurological defect was found and intellectual performance was normal (35). Acetonuria was present in 24 of the mothers, whose infants all had a normal IQ score at follow-up (35).

Glycaemic control is evaluated every 1-2 weeks until delivery by measuring fasting and postprandial glucose levels. The therapeutic goals are fasting plasma glucose levels below 6 mmol/l and postprandial plasma glucose below 7 mmol/l. Recent studies indicate that tight metabolic control, as defined by these plasma glucose levels, will reduce the incidence of fetal macrosomia significantly (36-38).

Approximately 10-15% of all gestational diabetic women will demonstrate fasting or postprandial hyperglycaemia (15), and in these cases insulin treatment must be initiated. Insulin can be given either as intermediate-acting insulin or as a mixture of short- and intermediate-acting insulin twice daily. Multiple insulin injections are only rarely needed. Insulin treatment should be discontinued after delivery; since insulin treatment might be needed in a subsequent pregnancy or during intercurrent illness, one should preferably prescribe human insulin to decrease the likelihood of antibody formation. Insulin treatment of gestational diabetes is feasible (38, 39) and it seems also capable of normalizing plasma 3-hydroxybutyrate levels, a result which is not always achievable by dietary treatment alone (40). Insulin treatment is most easily controlled by home glucose monitoring (41), despite the fact that many patients report incorrect, i.e. too low, values (42).

A recent article by Tallarigo et al (43) focuses on the importance of even minor degrees of carbohydrate intolerance. The authors investigated a large group of apparently healthy pregnant women who were subjected to an OGTT in the 3rd trimester of pregnancy. All OGTTs were normal according to the O'Sullivan and Mahan criteria (30) but, irrespective of this, it was possible to demonstrate a correlation between the mother's 2-hour OGTT plasma glucose value and the incidence of macrosomia and congenital anomalies of the infants, as well as toxaemia and the frequency of caesarean section in the mothers (43). The study underlines the importance of adequate control of even minor disturbances of carbohydrate metabolism in pregnancy and it questions the correctness of O'Sullivan and Mahan's diagnostic criteria.

In the very large Copenhagen series of diabetic pregnancies no increased frequency of congenital malformations was found in infants of gestational diabetic mothers (44) and the same is true for another large Danish series from the city of Aarhus (45). The explanation for Tallarigo and co-workers' finding of up to 5% congenital anomalies in infants of mothers with normal glucose tolerance is obscure. It is important to note that the congenital anomalies were clearly minor and that it is also necessary to study a much larger number of patients to evaluate the possibility of a relationship between 'subdiabetic' plasma glucose levels and the frequency of congenital anomalies.

Antepartum fetal surveillance and delivery

Gestational diabetic patients may be allowed to continue pregnancy safely until 40 weeks. Especially in women with an unreliable menstrual history, it is recommended that an ultrasound examination with assessment of fetal age be performed as soon as gestational diabetes is diagnosed. Patient management throughout the remainder of pregnancy, including antepartum fetal surveillance which is feasible in gestational diabetic pregnancy (46), and definition of the optimum date of delivery, should, in case of discrepancy, rather be guided by the ultrasound-estimated age than by the menstrual age. When evaluating the ultrasound scan in early pregnancy, one should, however, bear in mind that some fetuses of gestational diabetic women, as in pregnant women with IDDM (47), are smaller than normal in early pregnancy as judged by the crown-rump length (48). If labour cannot be safely induced at 40 weeks, fetal surveillance should be intensified (46).

Postpartum control

Women with gestational diabetes should be subjected to an OGTT approximately 2 months after delivery to evaluate whether they are still glucose-intolerant. If this is the case, dietary treatment, which is normally discontinued at the time of delivery, should be re-instituted together with metabolic control at regular intervals. Even if the postpartum OGTT is normal, yearly control OGTTs should be arranged since gestational diabetic subjects have a considerably increased risk of developing manifest diabetes later in life (49). These well-known results from O'Sullivan's series from Boston have recently been questioned, however, by Stowers et al in Aberdeen (50). They followed 112 women with impaired glucose tolerance diagnosed after pregnancy, and who therefore are assumed to have had gestational diabetes, for a period of up to 22 years. About one-third of the women had been treated with chlorpropamide and the others by diet only. At the final assessment, approximately 35% had abnormal glucose tolerance and less than 7% overt diabetes. Chlorpropamide did not prove significantly more effective in preventing the development of overt diabetes than did diet alone. The prevalence of impaired glucose tolerance and overt diabetes at follow-up was significantly less in the Aberdeen series than in O'Sullivan's study (49). This difference might be attributable to the fact that, in Aberdeen, patients were treated in the follow-up period, whereas the Boston cases were treated only during pregnancy.

Contraception

Family planning and contraception must be reviewed with the patient during the postpartum period. Intrauterine devices are safe and effective in diabetic women (51) and a recent study from Copenhagen (52) showed that a low-dose triphasic oral contraceptive (ethinyloestradiol and levonorgestrel) did not adversely affect important parameters of lipid and carbohydrate metabolism in a group of 16 women with previous gestational diabetes who were treated during a 6-month period. Even though it seems safe to prescribe this kind of oral contraceptive to previous gestational diabetic women, sterilization should be discussed with the patient when she has completed her family.

Follow-up of offspring

Whereas all women with previous gestational diabetes should be followed up at yearly intervals, it is less certain whether their offspring should also be regularly controlled. The outcome of the above-mentioned Swedish follow-up study of 73 children born to diabetic and gestational diabetic mothers (35) hardly justifies regular follow-up. In contrast, Pettitt et al (53) recently reported that children of women with abnormal glucose tolerance during pregnancy, aged 15-19 years at follow-up, had a higher mean post-challenge plasma glucose concentration than did children of women with normal glucose tolerance. Even though it is questionable whether these findings obtained in the Pima Indian tribe are relevant to other ethnic groups, it is worth noting that the offspring (12-45 years old) of NIDDM women, who metabolically bear a close resemblance to gestational diabetics, can show extensive metabolic changes including impaired glucose tolerance (54).

References

1. Carta Q, Meriggi E, Trossarelli GF et al (1986): Continuous subcutaneous insulin infusion versus intensive conventional insulin therapy in type I and type II diabetic pregnancy. *Diabète Métab., 12,* 121.
2. Coustan DR, Reece EA, Sherwin RS et al (1986): A randomized clinical trial of the insulin pump *vs* intensive conventional therapy in diabetic pregnancies. *J.Am. Med. Assoc., 255,* 631.
3. Kitzmiller JL, Younger MD, Hare JW et al (1985): Continuous subcutaneous insulin therapy during early pregnancy. *Obstet. Gynecol., 66,* 606.
4. Hadden DR (1986): Diabetes in pregnancy 1985. *Diabetologia, 29,* 1.
5. Mølsted-Pedersen L, Kühl C (1986): Obstetrical management in diabetic pregnancy: the Copenhagen experience. *Diabetologia, 29,* 13.
6. Skyler JS (1986): Control of diabetes during pregnancy: 1985. *J.Am. Med. Assoc., 255,* 647.
7. Møller Jensen B, Kühl C, Mølsted-Pedersen L et al (1986): Preconceptional treatment with insulin infusion pumps in insulin-dependent diabetic women with particular reference to prevention of congenital malformations. *Acta Endocrinol., 112, Suppl. 277,* 81.
8. Freinkel N, Dooley SL, Metzger BE (1985): Care of the pregnant woman with insulin-dependent diabetes mellitus. *N. Engl. J. Med., 313,* 96.
9. Beard R, Bennett P, Coustan D et al (1985): Summary and recommendations of the Second International Workshop-Conference on Gestational Diabetes Mellitus. *Diabetes, 34, Suppl. 2,* 123.
10. American Diabetes Association (1986): Position statement: gestational diabetes mellitus. *Diabetes Care, 9,* 430.
11. Leading article (1986): Gestational diabetes mellitus. *Ann. Intern. Med., 105,* 461.
12. Pedersen J (1977): *The Pregnant Diabetic and Her Newborn.* Munksgaard, Copenhagen.
13. Kühl C, Holst JJ (1976): Plasma glucagon and the insulin: glucagon ratio in gestational diabetes. *Diabetes, 25,* 752.
14. Sepe SJ, Connell FA, Geiss LS, Teutsch SM (1985): Gestational diabetes: incidence, maternal characteristics, and perinatal outcome. *Diabetes, 34,* 13.
15. Gabbe SG (1986): Gestational diabetes mellitus. *N. Engl. J. Med., 315,* 1025.
16. Freinkel N, Metzger BE, Phelps RL et al (1986): Gestational diabetes mellitus: a syndrome with phenotypic and genotypic heterogeneity. *Horm. Metab. Res., 18,* 427.
17. Buschard K, Buch I, Mølsted-Pedersen L et al (1987): Increased incidence of true type I diabetes acquired during pregnancy. *Br. Med. J., 294,* 275.
18. Kühl C (1984): Islet responsiveness in I.G.D.M.s. In: Sutherland HW, Stowers JM (Eds), *Carbohydrate Metabolism in Pregnancy and the Newborn,* pp 187-189. Churchill/Livingstone, Edinburgh.

19. Kühl C, Hornnes PJ, Andersen O (1985): Etiology and pathophysiology of gestational diabetes mellitus. *Diabetes, 34, Suppl. 2,* 66.
20. Kühl C, Hornnes PJ (1986): Endocrine pancreatic function in women with gestational diabetes. *Acta Endocrinol., 112, Suppl. 277,* 19.
21. Andersen O, Kühl C, Buch I (1986): Insulin receptors in normal pregnant women and women with gestational diabetes. *Acta Endocrinol., 112, Suppl. 277,* 27.
22. Hornnes PJ, Kühl C (1984): Cortisol and glucose tolerance in pregnancy. *Diabète Métab., 10,* 1.
23. Mortensen HB, Mølsted-Pedersen L, Kühl C, Backer P (1985): A screening procedure for diabetes in pregnancy. *Diabète Métab., 11,* 249.
24. Marquette GP, Klein WR, Niebyl JR (1985): Efficacy of screening for gestational diabetes. *Am. J. Perinatol., 2,* 7.
25. Lind T, Hytten FE (1972): The excretion of glucose during normal pregnancy. *J. Obstet. Gynaecol. Br. Cwlth, 79,* 961.
26. Lind T (1985): Antenatal screening using random blood glucose values. *Diabetes, 34, Suppl. 2,* 17.
27. Cousins L, Dattel B, Hollingsworth D et al (1985): Screening for carbohydrate intolerance in pregnancy: a comparison of two tests and reassessment of a common approach. *Am. J. Obstet. Gynecol., 153,* 381.
28. Weiner CP, Fraser MM, Burns JM et al (1986): Cost efficacy of routine screening for diabetes in pregnancy: 1-h versus 2-h specimen. *Diabetes Care, 9,* 255.
29. Landon MB, Cembrowski GS, Gabbe SG (1986): Capillary blood glucose screening for gestational diabetes: a preliminary investigation. *Am. J. Obstet. Gynecol., 155,* 717.
30. O'Sullivan JB, Mahan CM (1964): Criteria for the oral glucose tolerance test in pregnancy. *Diabetes, 13,* 278.
31. WHO Study Group (1985): Diabetes mellitus. *WHO Techn. Rep. Ser., 727.*
32. Churchill JA, Berendes HW, Nemore J (1969): Neuropsychological deficits in children of diabetic mothers. *Am. J. Obstet. Gynecol., 105,* 257.
33. Bhasin S, Shambough GE (1982): Fetal fuels. V. Ketone bodies inhibit pyrimidine biosynthesis in fetal rat brain. *Am. J. Physiol., 243,* E234.
34. Miodovnik M, Skillman CA, Hertzberg V et al (1986): Effect of maternal hyperketonemia in hyperglycemic pregnant ewes and their fetuses. *Am. J. Obstet. Gynecol., 154,* 394.
35. Persson B (1986): Longterm morbidity in infants of diabetic mothers. *Acta Endocrinol., 112, Suppl. 277,* 156.
36. Lin C-C, River J, River P et al (1986): Good diabetic control early in pregnancy and favorable fetal outcome. *Obstet. Gynecol., 67,* 51.
37. Willman SP, Leveno KJ, Guzick DS et al (1986): Glucose threshold for macrosomia in pregnancy complicated by diabetes. *Am. J. Obstet. Gynecol., 154,* 470.
38. Berne C, Wibell L, Lindmark G (1985): Ten-year experience of insulin treatment in gestational diabetes. *Acta Paediatr. Scand., Suppl. 320,* 85.
39. Bellmann O (1986): Therapy of gestational diabetes. *Acta Endocrinol., 112, Suppl. 277,* 50.
40. Maresh M, Gillmer MDG, Beard RW et al (1985): The effect of diet and insulin on metabolic profiles of women with gestational diabetes mellitus. *Diabetes, 34, Suppl. 2,* 88.
41. Goldberg JD, Franklin B, Lasser D et al (1986): Gestational diabetes: impact of home glucose monitoring on neonatal birth weight. *Am. J. Obstet. Gynecol., 154,* 546.
42. Langer OD, Mazze RS (1986): Diabetes in pregnancy: evaluating self-monitoring performance and glycemic control with memory-based reflectance meters. *Am. J. Obstet. Gynecol. 155,* 635.
43. Tallarigo L, Giampietro O, Penno G et al (1986): Relation of glucose tolerance to complications of pregnancy in nondiabetic women. *N. Engl. J. Med., 315,* 989.

44. Mølsted-Pedersen L, Fog Pedersen J (1985): Congenital malformations in diabetic pregnancies. *Acta Paediatr. Scand., Suppl. 320*, 79.
45. Klebe JG, Espersen T, Allen J (1986): Diabetes mellitus and pregnancy. *Acta Obstet. Gynaecol. Scand., 65*, 235.
46. Landon MB, Gabbe SG (1985): Antepartum fetal surveillance in gestational diabetes mellitus. *Diabetes, 34, Suppl. 2*, 50.
47. Pedersen JF, Mølsted-Pedersen L (1981): Early fetal growth delay detected by ultrasound marks increased risk of congenital malformation in diabetic pregnancy. *Br. Med. J., 283*, 269.
48. Fog Pedersen J, Mølsted-Pedersen L (1985): The possibility of an early growth delay in White's class A diabetic pregnancy. *Diabetes, 34, Suppl. 2*, 47.
49. O'Sullivan JB (1978): Gestational diabetes: factors influencing the rates of subsequent diabetes. In: Sutherland HW, Stowers JM (Eds), *Carbohydrate Metabolism in Pregnancy and the Newborn*, pp. 425-435. Springer, New York.
50. Stowers JM, Sutherland HW, Kerridge DF (1985): Long-range implications for the mother: the Aberdeen experience. *Diabetes, 34, Suppl. 2*, 106.
51. Skouby SO, Mølsted-Pedersen L, Kühl C (1986): Contraception in diabetic women. *Acta Endocrinol., 112, Suppl. 277*, 125.
52. Skouby SO, Kühl C, Mølsted-Pedersen L et al (1985): Triphasic oral contraception: metabolic effects in normal women and those with previous gestational diabetes. *Am. J. Obstet. Gynecol., 153*, 495.
53. Pettit DJ, Bennett PH, Knowler WC et al (1985): Gestational diabetes mellitus and impaired glucose tolerance during pregnancy. *Diabetes, 34, Suppl. 2*, 119.
54. Leslie RDG, Volkmann HP, Poncher M et al (1986): Metabolic abnormalities in children of non-insulin dependent diabetics. *Br. Med. J., 293*, 840.

The Diabetes Annual/3
K.G.M.M. Alberti and L.P. Krall, editors
© 1987 Elsevier Science Publishers, B.V.

15   Diabetic retinopathy

EVA M. KOHNER AND P.S. SHARP

Introduction

Two years ago when the first review of diabetic retinopathy appeared, photo-coagulation was already accepted universally as a form of treatment, but was still relatively new. It was anticipated that with the improvement of technology and the considerable amount of research invested in the treatment and pathogenesis of diabetic retinopathy major advances would have been made by now. What progress has there been in these last two years? There were over 800 publications concerned with diabetic retinopathy, often repetitive, often contradictory and only occasionally advancing understanding or management of the disease process. The problems we face today are similar to those faced two years ago: the assessment of diabetic retinopathy; which functional changes are important; and the importance of genetic factors. The effect of diabetic control has still not been clearly established and new forms of treatment are still on trial. Diabetic maculopathy remains a problem at present, apparently far from solution.

The pathogenic mechanisms in the evolution of retinopathy are not understood, and there are no suitable animal models. We can say, with Dr Faust, who after all the years of study had to admit: 'Hier steh ich nun, ich armer Tor, und bin so klug als wie zuvor!' ('Here I stand, I poor fool, and am as wise as when I started' — Goethe).

Assessment of severity of diabetic retinopathy

Assessment of severity of lesions can be based on clinical examination, on grading of retinal photographs and fluorescein angiograms.

Photographic assessment

Since the adaptation of the Airlie House system of photographic assessment (1) by the Wisconsin Group (2) this method of grading has become the 'gold standard' of photographic assessment. It is based on trained readers assessing 7 stereo pairs of retinal photographs for individual lesions in comparison with standard photographs, allowing for 3 grades of severity of lesions. The lesions are then grouped by prognostic importance and enable the graders to assign a retinopathy level to each eye. The main advantage of the system is its flexibility. Thus, using the same grading system, various levels can be assigned according to the degree of sensitivity required. The original Wisconsin system was used for the Diabetic Retinopathy Study (DRS) (3), which involved proliferative and severe non-proliferative retinopathy, and few levels were sufficient. For the Early Treatment of Diabetic Retinopathy Study (ETDRS) the levels were extended (4) as they were for the Kroc Insulin Pump Study (5). However, even these levels were insufficient for the very earliest forms of retinopathy, as in the Diabetic Control and Complications Trial (DCCT) where the number of levels, especially in the early lesions, was expanded (6). The scheme will need further modification for the United Kingdom Prospective Diabetic Study of 'maturity-onset' diabetes, where only 4 fields are photographed, especially as in this group of patients hard exudates (HE) in the macular field are extremely important.

The Wisconsin system is undoubtedly useful for research and allows comparison of treatment effects in different centres. The disadvantage is that it is very expensive, requiring highly trained staff. It is clearly not necessary for the management of patients. Clinical assessment of retinopathy for management is usually sufficient in all but the milder forms of diabetic maculopathy. Thus in a study comparing ophthalmoscopy and fundus photography in 1949 persons, Moss et al (7) found an 86% agreement between ophthalmologists and retinal photographs for presence or absence of retinopathy, non-proliferative and proliferative lesions. The disagreement was mainly in the milder forms of retinopathy, although there were 4 cases where proliferative lesions were missed by ophthalmologists (out of a total of 170). This appears to be an important discrepancy, but it must be remembered that only direct ophthalmoscopy was included, and the group as a whole was more used to looking at retinal photographs, though they were all highly trained. Ophthalmoscopy through undilated pupils is less satisfactory, and Klein et al (8) found only just over 54% agreement.

When comparing the relatively newly available non-mydriatic 45° single-field cameras with observations by untrained examiners, the non-mydriatic camera recorded 4 times as many patients having retinopathy as did the physicians (9, 10). By contrast, when a trained ophthalmologist examined through dilated pupils the fundi of 62 patients (selected randomly) from the diabetic and diabetic eye clinic, agreement between camera and doctor was 96% (11). In this study even the diabetic clinic physicians showed a 93% agreement with the photographic recording. Agreement between non-mydriatic and mydriatic cameras taking seven 30° fields showed an agreement of over 82% (8). Therefore the non-mydriatic camera is certainly satisfactory for epidemiological studies, where non-insulin-dependent diabetes is the more common disease. However, in these patients diabetic maculopathy is the common form of retinopathy and macular oedema cannot be diagnosed from the pictures obtained. It will also miss those who have peripheral new vessels only. Using non-mydriatic cameras for screening for retinopathy in developed countries is advocated by some (9, 11). It is an expensive method of screening and does not solve the problem of the number of middle-aged and elderly in whom satisfactory pictures cannot be obtained. Thus, in the Klein study (8) nearly a third of the photographs through undilated pupils were 'lost'.

For any method of assessment, adequately trained staff are needed. Thus in a Canadian study (12) eyes were not examined or examined inadequately in 62 out of 123 diabetic patients admitted to hospital for intercurrent disease. In well-trained groups there is little difference between the pick-up rate of ophthalmologists and diabetic clinic physicians (11, 13).

Fluorescein angiograms

Fluorescein angiograms are of particular value in research, and most centres dealing with diabetic retinopathy will use them at least in the management of diabetic maculopathy. Patients do not like the procedure because some feel sick and all are yellow afterwards. In the United States considerable difficulty has been experienced in quantitatively assessing early lesions, mainly because the photographers do not receive the same training as they receive in colour photography.

The procedure is safe. Thus in a large study of side effects reported during 1984 Yannuzzi et al (14) found mild reactions, such as nausea, vomiting and sneezing in 1:6.3 patients, more severe reactions, such as urticaria, syncope and thrombophlebitis, in 1:77 to 1:115 cases. Severe reactions occurred in 1:19,000 cases, while deaths occurring within 24 hours of the fluorescein angiogram was in 1:222,000, a very occasional, not necessarily related, occurrence.

On analysing angiograms the most commonly seen abnormality is hyperpermeability. It is common even in normal eyes, although it is much more common in diabetic subjects (15) and there is good reproducibility of assessment (16). Careful studies of angiograms are useful in understanding the evolution of lesions, and in this respect the wide-angled cameras can be really useful.

Niki et al (17) noted that the site of original non-perfusion (peripheral, mid-peripheral, central or generalised) was important prognostically, the generalised and central types having the worst prognosis. More recently Fryler (18) noted that even in diabetic maculopathy there was significant non-perfusion in the retinal periphery. Occasionally revascularisation of non-perfused areas occurs. This is most commonly a precursor to neovascularisation (19) but it may be recanalisation of basement membrane tubes and represent a reparative process (19, 20).

Quantitative assessment of fluorescein angiograms is time-consuming even with computer-assisted methods (21). Microaneurysm-counting, previously reported as a reproducible method of assessing early retinopathy (22, 23), has been shown in such cases to correlate well with retinopathy levels and very well with the most commonly found lesions, using the modified Airlie House grading system (24). Strong correlations with microaneurysms, haemorrhages and cotton-wool spots were present, while the relationship was weaker with hard exudates (as they are less common in early retinopathy of insulin-dependent patients), and there was none with venous abnormalities. The next step in quantifying angiograms is that of non-perfusion areas. Bresnick et al (25) measured the circumference of the perifoveal avascular zone as well as its longest diameter. He found that in diabetic subjects the foveal avascular zone (FAZ) was enlarged; the largest diameter of over 1 mm was seen almost exclusively in those with proliferative retinopathy. The FAZ size correlated with peripheral nonperfusion. In a more detailed study Sleightholm et al (26) found that the measurement of both the FAZ and the intercapillary distance in the perifoveal area was reproducible between technician and doctor, with the within-observer reproducibility also being good. Investigating early retinopathy in insulin-dependent patients using continuous subcutaneous insulin infusion (CSII), they found that in those patients, who all remained non-proliferative, the FAZ was similar to that of normal subjects, and remained so during the period of study. On the other hand, the peripheral (2-5°) intercapillary distances increased in those whose retinopathy deteriorated significantly, indicating that deterioration of retinopathy is associated with the development of areas of non-perfusion (27).

Functional abnormalities in diabetic retinopathy

In the review in *The Diabetes Annual/1*, functional abnormalities were included in the assessment of retinopathy. This is no longer done, because functional abnormalities, although common and important and thought by some to be of prognostic importance, are now known not to replace adequate examination of the fundus. In addition, with improved technology and more investigators using similar techniques there is now often more disagreement than agreement about the findings and their importance. This is particularly so with vitreous fluorophotometry, measuring blood-retinal barrier (BRB) integrity, with blood flow and autoregulation and to a lesser extent with electrodiagnostic tests.

Visual acuity

Of all the functional tests this is the only one which really matters to the patient. The assessment of visual acuity is reproducible when standard methods are used

(28). Klein et al (29) reported on visual impairment in their large epidemiological studies of South Wisconsin diabetic patients in which they examined 996 patients diagnosed under the age of 30 years and 1370 diagnosed after that age. In the younger age group even after 30 years of diabetes 80% had a visual acuity of 6/12 or better in at least one eye, and after 22 years about 10% were legally blind. The overall visual loss was 1.4% with moderate impairment and 3.6% with blindness. In 86% of these patients diabetic retinopathy was the cause of severe visual defect. In the older age group 70% had a visual acuity of 6/12 or better after 20 years of diabetes. Legal blindness occurred in 1.6%, the great majority being over 60 years of age. In these patients diabetic retinopathy was the cause of blindness in only 33% of patients. These findings agree with those of other studies; good vision in insulin-dependent diabetes mellitus (IDDM) is usual until the complications of proliferative retinopathy cause severe visual loss. This can be prevented to a large extent by photocoagulation or treated by vitrectomy. Diabetic maculopathy causes visual loss in the older age group, but this rarely causes complete blindness as the navigational vision in the peripheral retina is maintained. Other causes of visual loss, such as glaucoma and disciform degeneration of the macula, are more common in the elderly than diabetic retinopathy.

Even when visual acuity is normal, visual impairment can be detected in patients by testing low-contrast sensitivity. This is not a specific test, as impairment is also noted in ocular hypertension, glaucoma and Parkinson's disease (30). In diabetic patients it is noted already before the presence of retinopathy (31), although there is no uniform agreement about this as Sokol et al found normal contrast sensitivity in IDDM patients without retinopathy (32).

Appreciation of colour and ability to discriminate between colours is important for diabetic patients who test urine or use blood glucose sticks. Again there is no agreement between observers. In a detailed study Bresnick et al (33) found that using the 100-hue test diabetic subjects had marked impairment in the blue-yellow region. This impairment correlated with severity of retinopathy and macular oedema. Green et al (34), while agreeing that colour discrimination defects were related to severity of retinopathy, thought it was not a sufficiently specific test for screening purposes. Roy et al (35, 36) found far fewer abnormalities. In an unpublished study at Hammersmith Hospital, blue-yellow defects were common in those with retinopathy, but were rarely severe, even in severe retinopathy. The colour defect did not interfere with estimating blood glucose values using BM Glycemie 1-44® test-strips. Indeed the blue-yellow of the BM strips was estimated more accurately by all groups of patients and controls than the red-green of Visidex® test-strips, probably because when colours are compared, it is not only the colour but lightness and darkness, i.e. contrast in hue. This is more marked on BM Glycemie than Visidex test-strips.

Electrodiagnostic tests

Electrodiagnostic tests give an overall estimate of retinal function. Whether this is of value in diabetic patients in whom examination of the fundus is possible, is doubtful.

The macular recovery time after exposure to high-intensity light (nyctometry) had been used by Frost-Larsen and Larsen (37) as a predictor of proliferative retinopathy. This work beautifully illustrates the pitfalls of much reported research. Thus, delayed recovery time at the initial examination occurred in 40 patients, 36 of whom had severe or moderate background retinopathy. It was normal in 114 patients, of whom only 21 had similar degrees of retinal change. In the other 93 there was either no retinopathy or only a few microaneurysms. Little wonder that more of the abnormal recovery time patients developed proliferative lesions after 5 or more years. More remarkable is the deterioration of the normal group. Those who developed proliferative retinopathy also had a longer duration of diabetes and poorer diabetic control. To relate deterioration to macular recovery time without taking the other aspects into account is unsatisfactory.

Frost-Larsen and co-workers even related macular recovery time to Simonsen's oscillatory potentials (38). Oscillatory potentials have been shown in 1980 by Simonsen (39) and in 1984 by Bresnick et al (40) to have predictive value for the development of proliferative retinopathy. However, in both these studies those who had the more markedly reduced oscillatory potentials also had the more severe retinopathy. Certainly, Arden et al (41) using Bresnick's technique could not repeat his results; their retinopathy patients had gradually decreasing oscillatory potentials with increasing retinopathy, but it was not felt that the test was prognostically reliable for individuals. In contrast pattern electroretinographic (ERG) changes were only slightly different in patients with no retinopathy, those with few MA only, and mild diabetic retinopathy. However, when preproliferative lesions developed, even in the absence of macular oedema, the pattern ERG became markedly abnormal. Since this test is abnormal in macular disease, it is of interest that in preproliferative retinopathy where the lesions are most marked in the mid- and far periphery, abnormalities are seen. This suggests a marked abnormality of capillary perfusion even in the central retina. It would be expected that photocoagulation, a basically destructive procedure, will reduce ERG waves, as found by Perlman et al (42). These findings confirm that laser treatment affects pigment epithelium and the photoreceptors. In contrast, Hennekes and Deschner (43) found that the markedly abnormal and reduced oscillatory potentials of proliferative retinopathy sometimes increase after panretinal or focal photocoagulation, suggesting improved retional function.

While the role of ERG is doubtful, flash visual-evoked potentials (VEP) were found to be of use in predicting visual outcome of vitrectomy when fundus examination was not possible due to vitreous opacities. Patients with a VEP latency of 100 ms or less showed marked improvement after surgery while those with longer latency showed either no change in visual acuity or a deterioration (44). By contrast, in a group of 59 patients of whom 30 improved and 29 did not after surgery, neither ERG nor VEP were thought to be helpful in predicting outcome (45). In conclusion, electrodiagnostic tests remain tools of research and there is no clear clinical indication for their use in diabetic retinopathy as a routine test. They may be helpful in localising lesions when poor visual acuity cannot be explained by retinal appearance.

Vitreous fluorophotometry

Vitreous fluorophotometry measures the penetration of fluorescein into the vitreous following intravenous or oral administration. When first introduced (46), it was thought to give an accurate quantitative evaluation of breakdown of the BRB. Since this was thought to occur already at a time when clinical retinopathy was not present, it was hailed as a predictor of impending retinopathy. Since some animal studies (47, 48) and studies on patients (49-51) suggested that improved metabolic control reduced leakage and by implication improved BRB integrity, it was hoped that improved control in the pre-retinopathic stage would prevent the appearance of clinical diabetic retinopathy. Differences between observers was thought to be due to different equipment and different methods of usage of the equipment (52). The appearance of commercially available equipment with a standardised protocol was expected to overcome these problems, but it did not. Cunha-Vaz et al (53) still found that posterior vitreous fluorophotometric readings in 20 eyes of 12 normal subjects had lower readings 3 mm from the chorioretinal peak than 16 eyes of 9 patients with no retinal lesions. In a detailed study, Chahal et al (54) looked at permeability coefficient and index and diffusion coefficient in 19 normal eyes of 14 normal subjects on two separate occasions using plasma-free fluorescein concentrations as well as the vitreous concentrations. The method gave reproducible results in normal subjects using a mathematical model for the vitreous fluorescein scan and the plasma-free fluorescein curves. When diabetic patients with no or minimal retinopathy were studied, no difference from normal subjects was found (55). The findings in diabetic patients in Chahal's work for the 3 mm from the retinal peak were similar to those of Cunha-Vaz, and it was the normal data which were significantly lower in Cunha-Vaz's studies. Since that time a communication from the NEI concerning normal subjects (56) suggests that the findings of Chahal are probably correct.

Studying permeability and inward and outward diffusion of fluorescein from the vitreous, Ogura et al (57) also found similar results and felt that outward permeability, which is greater than inward permeability of fluorescein in the vitreous, is not really important in the early stages of fluorophotometry. Fluorescein monoglucuronide, which may also be present in the vitreous by the end of 60 min, also does not contribute significantly to fluorophotometric readings because of its low fluorescence (58).

The best scientific work on the subject comes from Lund-Anderson's group. These workers first applied a mathematical model of the eye to quantitate fluorescein permeability into and diffusion in the vitreous (59, 60). They have used their technique in 20 eyes of normal volunteers and 20 eyes of IDDM patients and found no difference between the two groups (61). In 29 healthy subjects Kjaergaard found that there was some leakage of fluorescein into the posterior vitreous which increased with increasing eye and blood pressure, but was not affected by serum glucose level (62). CSII, which was previously thought to improve leakage (51), was not found to have any effect when the more careful measurements of Lund-Anderson were used (63).

It is to be hoped that vitreous fluorophotometry results in experimental animals will give the answer. Many centres used animal models, but unfortunately almost all used rats (64-66). Because of the small volume of the vitreous, in the region of the resolving power of the equipment, the measurements are not really valid, since anterior vitreous fluorescence from ciliary body leakage is included in the measurements. More interesting is the study, again in rats, of the effects of pH on fluorescein transfer (67). Significant effects of pH were noted only in pH ranges not seen in human subjects. Grimes (68), in an excellent study, used quantitative fluorescein microscopy in control and streptozotocin-diabetic rats. She also measured both free and bound fluorescein glucuronide in the plasma of these animals. Initial fluorescein entry into the retina and vitreous occurred from the choroid by diffusion, creating a steep intensity gradient from outer to inner retina. The diabetic rats had higher fluorescein concentrations at 2 min after injection than had normal animals, but this was related to the transiently higher free fluorescein concentrations. The retinal fluorescence returned to normal levels with the return to normal of plasma free fluorescein. Grimes did not think there was any BRB dysfunction in the diabetic rats. Grimes' results correspond to those of Wallow (69) who, using horseradish peroxidase, also found no difference in BRB function between diabetic and normal rats.

There is now little doubt that vitreous fluorophotometry cannot reliably identify a preretinopathic state. It is however useful in studies of early retinopathy where it gives a quantitative evaluation of a particularly important lesion in diabetic retinopathy, namely leakage. Thus, Plehwe et al (70) were able to show in patients treated with CSII that significant deterioration of retinopathy is associated with increased leakage, while no or minor changes do not alter vitreous fluorophotometric readings. Indeed, it confirms earlier observations that microaneurysms on the whole only leak slightly or not at all; leakage of fluorescein comes from generalised leaking capillaries.

Retinal blood flow and autoregulation

Since ischaemia is one of the predisposing factors for the development of proliferative retinopathy, reduction in blood flow in early diabetes and early retinopathy would be expected. However, studies in the past, relying mainly on mean transit times of fluorescein (71-73), suggested that flow in early diabetes and in early retinopathy was increased. Further support for this possibility was raised by work in experimental animals (74, 75), which indicated that a sudden rise in blood glucose to above 20 mmol/l increased retinal and choroidal flow significantly. In Atherton's work (74), this was shown to be related to glucose itself and not to osmotic changes, as iso-osmolar mannitol did not cause the same changes in blood flow. Indeed, so convinced were most investigators of the increased blood flow that McMillan (76) even suggested that this increased blood flow could damage the endothelial cells and thus act as a pathogenic mechanism in the development of vascular occlusion.

Undoubtedly there are flow changes in diabetic retinopathy, but in the light of more recent work their exact nature is now no longer clear. During the last few years fluorescein angiographic determination of blood flow, although still in use in some countries, and even adapted to video recording (77, 78), has been replaced by two non-invasive techniques: the blue light entoptic phenomenon and laser doppler velocimetry. Both these techniques have been developed by Riva and co-workers (79-81), and both have been used extensively.

The blue-light entoptic phenomenon allows visualisation of the patient's own white cells (WBC) in the perifoveal capillaries and by comparing their speed with that of simulated WBC on a video screen, flow velocity can be established. By measuring the vessel diameters supplying and draining the capillaries an estimate of retinal blood flow can be achieved. The method is subjective, but in most patients, reproducible to above 80% (82); in many younger patients it is as high as 90%. The disadvantage is the great variation of WBC speed between normal individuals, ranging from 0.3 to 1.1 mm/s. Using this technique, diabetic patients without retinopathy had a blood flow similar to normal subjects. Those with early retinopathy had a wide variation of blood flow, a third of all being above the upper limit of the non-diabetic controls, so that the 'mean' flow velocity was increased. In patients with preproliferative and proliferative retinopathy, flow was decreased and photocoagulation made very little difference to this (82).

The blue-light entoptic technique was also used to study the effect of increasing blood glucose levels in normal controls, and in diabetic patients on CSII and therefore with near-normal glucose levels at the start of the experiment (83).

Blood glucose was raised in the normal subjects to 11 mmol/l and in diabetics to 17.5 mmol/l. There was a variable response in blood flow, but the changes were small, some showing an increase and some showing a decrease in blood flow. It is possible that the difference between human subjects and experimental animals is due to the lower rate of increase in blood glucose and the lower level achieved. It is also possible, however, that autoregulation maintains macular blood flow at near-normal levels; in the experimental animals flow in large vessels was measured which also supply the peripheral retina.

Using the Laser Doppler Velocimeter (LDV), Grunwald (84) found a reduced flow velocity in diabetic patients even when there was only background retinopathy. This flow was reduced even more with increasing retinopathy, as well as after photocoagulation when volume flow was also reduced (presumably because there was less viable retinal tissue) (85). Feke and co-workers also used the LVD (86), although based on a slit lamp rather than a retinal camera, and measured both pulsatility and flow velocity. These workers thought that both measurements were reduced in mild retinopathy and increased with increasing severity of retinal lesions. The difference between Riva's group and Feke's results is difficult to explain, but taking all available evidence it appears that flow is *decreased* with increasing severity of retinopathy. In mild retinopathy and no retinopathy there is at present no consensus of opinion, nor is the relationship of blood flow, as measured by LDV, and the blue-light entoptoscope really known.

Why should blood flow be altered in diabetes? It would be expected that if there is widespread capillary occlusion or destruction of retina by photocoagulation, flow would be reduced. However, the reason why perifoveal flow should be involved when this area is left relatively normal cannot be explained.

Abnormalities in the retinal circulation in diabetes are further demonstrated by abnormalities of autoregulation. Using the blue-light entoptic phenomenon, Fallon (87) found that in normal subjects breathing 60% oxygen, flow velocity was markedly reduced (by 46% of that at room air), and markedly increased with 10% oxygen (by 36%). In diabetic subjects there were some changes but they were small and not significant, with the exception of patients with proliferative retinopathy. In these patients hypoxia produced almost no change (3%), while they were still able to respond to hyperoxia by reducing blood flow (88). These results differ significantly from those of Grunwald et al (89), who found that the response to hyperoxia decreased gradually from 61% in normal subjects to 24% in patients with proliferative lesions and this was restored to 54% by panretinal photocoagulation, an improvement not noted by Fallon in his study.

While there are variations between findings, it appears that hypoxia is already present in diabetic patients with proliferative retinopathy, causing maximal dilatation and flow. Improvement following photocoagulation could modify this by more healthy retinal oxygenation. In the present state of knowledge, however, it can only be stated that there is an association between flow and autoregulation changes and diabetic retinopathy. Their pathogenic or aetiological importance remains unknown.

The treatment of diabetic retinopathy

At present there is no treatment known which will prevent the development of retinopathy or prevent the progression of mild retinopathy to more severe forms. Photocoagulation, although often effective, cannot guarantee maintenance or return of good vision, especially in patients with diabetic macular oedema. Vitrectomies are often helpful in restoring vision in patients who have already lost it, improved techniques improving the results. Nevertheless, when the retina is severely damaged, the ability of surgical intervention to influence visual recovery must be limited. There is therefore a constant search for new and better methods of treatment; not least of these are improved methods of achieving good control of diabetes.

Diabetic control

The hypothesis that microvascular complications of diabetes, in particular retinopathy, are related to poor glycaemic control has been suggested for a long time, but could not be tested adequately until reliable methods were available for assessing diabetic control, such as glycosylated haemoglobin and home monitoring of blood glucose. It was also essential to have methods of insulin therapy which could achieve near-to-normal glucose levels. The latter can be achieved by intensified insulin therapy using multiple injections and probably even better using CSII, or other infusion routes such as the intraperitoneal one, perhaps using implanted devices (90, 91).

Evidence for importance of glycaemic control Hyperglycaemia is the hallmark of diabetes, but it is always associated with other metabolic abnormalities. While in diabetic dogs prevention of retinopathy by 'good control' was achieved (92) this has not been possible in human subjects. The observation of a 'diabetes-like' retinopathy in hypergalactosaemic dogs, who have none of the other metabolic changes of hyperglycaemia, suggests that hexose sugars by themselves can cause retinopathy (93, 94).

A number of epidemiological and cross-sectional studies show that HbA_1 or mean blood glucose levels are higher in those with retinopathy that those without. Most studies have looked at IDDM (95-100), but there are a number which looked at non-insulin-dependent diabetes mellitus (NIDDM) patients only, or both IDDM and NIDDM (101-106). Most reports compare only patients with and without retinopathy, but two Scandinavian studies (98, 105) also found that patients with proliferative retinopathy had higher HbA_1 values than those without.

Klein et al (102) studied macular oedema in both diabetic patients diagnosed under 30 years of age and those diagnosed after 30 years. In both groups duration of diabetes was the most important factor, but in both the HbA_1 levels were higher in those with macular oedema than in those without. The study by Nathan et al (104), which has many shortcomings, is interesting because it shows the increasing prevalence of retinopathy with increasing HbA_{1c}. Thus, there was about a 10% incidence in those with an HbA_{1c} of 6% or less, rising steadily to over 60% in those with an HbA_{1c} of 12% or more. In the Scandinavian study an HbA_{1c} of 8.5% or less was associated with retinopathy in 9% of patients, and above that value over 20% had lesions. It made no difference (for presence or absence of retinopathy) whether HbA_{1c} was under 10.5% or above (105). It is also important to note that a normal HbA_{1c} did not protect completely from retinopathy. The other important point is that even in the studies where there is a significant difference between the HbA_1 levels, the differences are small. Thus, in the Klein study of macular oedema in those over 30 years old at time of diagnosis the difference is only 0.7% after 0-14 years diabetes duration and 0.9% over 15 years (102). The difference is similarly small in those under 30 years at diagnosis. In the study by Doft et al (95), the difference was about 1%, as it was also in the total Wisconsin study (101). All these studies therefore indicate that poor metabolic control is not necessarily associated with retinopathy or with its more severe forms, nor does good control always protect.

Is there then a level of HbA_1 that one should aim at to prevent or improve retinopathy? The Diabetic Control and Complications Trial in the United States may eventually answer this question, although the poorly controlled group there is run at glucose and HbA_1 levels above that which is generally aimed for in the United Kingdom. In the meantime a number of longitudinal studies, all of only 1-3 years' duration, using CSII are available in patients with a wide range of retinopathy.

Continuous subcutaneous insulin infusion (CSII) and retinopathy   The initial enthusiasm for CSII in early retinopathy was fired by two case-reports (107, 108) of marked improvement of retinopathy with improved control. The enthusiasm was followed by disappointment, if not despair, when the many reports of deteriorating retinopathy with improved control were noted (109-113). Most importantly, the 3 randomised controlled clinical studies of Oslo, Steno and Kroc (114-116) also found initial deterioration of retinopathy. These 3 groups all studied IDDM patients with mild or minimal retinopathy and in all 3 studies there was a control group, randomly assigned to remain on conventional treatment. The Oslo investigators also had a group with intensified conventional treatment.

The findings were that in the first 6-12 months the retinopathy deteriorated more in the CSII than the conventionally treated patients. More patients had developed more severe lesions, in particular cotton-wool spots (soft exudates) and intraretinal microvascular abnormalities (IRMA). In the Kroc study, alone among all the studies, those with the mildest retinopathy showed the most deterioration (117, 118). The Oslo group (114) as well as the Kroc study (118) were able to show that the most severe deterioration of retinopathy occurred in those who also showed the greatest fall and lowest levels of blood glucose and HbA_1. The suggestion was that improving control more gradually would prevent this deterioration of retinopathy. It was thought that the rapid normalisation of blood glucose reduces blood flow drastically and this causes both hypoxia and ischaemia in the already damaged vascular bed, causing the cotton-wool spots and IRMA, both manifestations of ischaemic retinae.

A study by Sleightholm and co-workers does not seem to support this theory (119). In a small study, 14 patients with mild retinopathy (Wisconsin Grade 20-40) were randomly allocated to rapid or slow reduction of blood glucose (in 1 or 4 months) by CSII. Retinal blood flow was measured at entry, 2 days, 1 months and 4 months after CSII using the blue-light entoptic phenomenon. By 1-4 months 8 of the 14 patients showed significant deterioration of their retinopathy, while the other 6 remained at the same retinopathy level. The rate of blood glucose fall had little effect (although the 2 with the greatest fall were among those who deteriorated more). Blood flow at 2 days seemed to be the most relevant. A marked increase was seen in 4 out of 5 patients who did not deteriorate (1 was not measured at 2 days), while those who did show deterioration had a small but definite fall in flow velocity in the foveal capillaries. By 1 and 4 months flow speed was similar in both groups, and generally lower than pre-CSII.

There have been many other studies with mixed populations of proliferative and mild retinopathies (120-122), and mild, minimal and no retinopathies (123-126). Of these, only Mogensen's study had an adequate randomised control group and adequate follow-up. These workers did not observe real benefit from the pump, but they also failed to observe development of IRMA and cotton-wool spots. In the Belfast patients the short duration of CSII had no significant effect (125). The other studies are difficult to evaluate. Kelly, for example, used the same patients as controls followed by treatment (not a randomised crossover study) and diabetic control of these patients did not improve to near-normal HbA_1 levels. Friberg et al (121) had a conventionally treated group but it was not randomly allocated and, as reported in 1985, their method of microaneurysm counting was rather cavalier. In other studies, since patients with proliferative retinopathy were treated by photocoagulation, the effect of CSII was impossible to evaluate adequately (120).

After 1 year of therapy there was therefore a real clinical dilemma, whether the treatment should continue. The Oslo group already noted improvement among their patients between 6 and 12 months. The Steno group explained the situation to their patients and were thus able to continue with their study for a second year (127). The results showed a marked change from that of the first year. In the first year of the study some CSII and conventionally treated patients improved; 10 CSII but only 5 conventionally treated patients deteriorated. By 2 years, 7 CSII and only 2 conventionally treated patients had milder retinopathy and 6 versus 10 patients deteriorated. The results of the Oslo study were similar (128). When the 2 studies were combined, the deterioration was significantly less in the CSII patients than in the conventionally treated group with a P-value of <0.03 (129).

In the Kroc study one-third of the patients in each group changed their therapy, but there was no difference from those who agreed to stay on their original treatment. An analysis of those who stayed on the original treatment (23 CSII and 24 conventional treatment) was therefore possible. Analysis was also performed comparing patients by original assessment (130). Both analyses showed that the conventionally treated patients continued to deteriorate gradually from 0 to 8-24 months. There was a significant difference between the mean retinopathy levels between 0 and 24 months. In the CSII patients there was a more marked deterioration form 0 to 8 months, but this was reversed between 8 and 24 months, so that the initial and 2-year retinopathy levels were similar. Identical results were present in the microaneurysm studies. The studies therefore suggest that good control has to be prolonged to be really efficacious and, unless new vessels develop, one should not resort to photocoagulation in these patients. Even 2 years is a short period of time for arrest or reversal of lesions which have taken over 10 years to develop. Thus, while a definite conclusion cannot be reached on the role of good control in reducing retinopathy, the results of the Diabetes Control and Complications Study will hopefully confirm that it is worth making an effort to keep good glycaemic control.

Drug therapy in diabetic retinopathy

Because the beneficial effect of good control had not been definitely proven and because many patients would rather take drugs than make the required effort to maintain good blood glucose control, several new drugs have been tried, all with slight or no adequately proven effect.

Antiplatelet agents The Early Treatment of Diabetic Retinopathy Study treated some of their 3000 patients with aspirin; the allocation to the aspirin group was by a randomisation procedure. After many years there are no published results, implying that as yet they have not shown statistically acceptable benefit or damage. One other aspirin study has been reported from two French and two British centres. Patients (n = 475) were stratified by treatment into insulin-treated and tablet- or diet-treated groups and were randomly allocated to aspirin alone (1 g/d) or aspirin and dipyridamole (aspirin 1 g, dipyridamole 235 mg/d) or placebo (131). All patients had mild or minimal retinopathy and the severity was determined by counting microaneurysms on fluorescein angiograms (132). All patients were studied for 3 years. The results were disappointing. The actively treated group developed significantly fewer new microaneurysms each year than the placebo group. There was no difference between the two active treatment groups. While the results reached statistical significance, the clinical importance of this difference was small, if any, in the region of one microaneurysm each year in the macular field (113). It is therefore not advised that aspirin should be given for the treatment of retinopathy alone. These results are not really unexpected. At the time of starting the study the abnormalities known to exist in in-vitro platelet studies of diabetic patients were thought to be a key factor in capillary occlusion, the essential abnormality of diabetic retinopathy. This theory was not really proven and most workers now believe that many of the platelet abnormalities (which undoubtedly do exist) are secondary to disease of the endothelial cells and may represent a reparative process.

Other drugs Of other drugs affecting viscosity or coagulation are two which have reached the literature. Glipizide even convinced the reviewers of the *New England Journal of Medicine* (134), showing reduced basement membrane thickness in muscle capillary in treated chemical diabetics. It did not convince this reviewer.

Calcium dobesilate was reported to reduce viscosity, fibrinogen and cholesterol levels (135, 136), and improve retinopathy (135-137). The studies were unsatisfactory and calcium dobesilate is probably totally ineffective in diabetic retinopathy despite its widespread use on the continent of Europe.

Aldose reductase inhibitors The finding that galactosaemic retinopathy in dogs was similar to diabetic retinopathy was a strong stimulus for the study of these drugs (93). The theory is that high glucose in the blood enters cells lining the vessel wall. In the presence of aldose reductase rapid conversion of glucose to sorbitol occurs, the sorbitol being broken down only slowly by sorbitol dehydrogenase to fructose. High concentrations of sorbitol in cells would exert a harmful osmotic effect. In galactosaemic rats, basement membrane thickening was prevented by sorbinil (138) and by tolrestat (139), both being aldose reductase inhibitors. Such drugs were also effective in reducing pericyte loss, increased capillary tortuosity and basement membrane thickening of streptozoto-cin-diabetic rats fed on a high-fructose diet (140). Matchinsky's group (141), who studied sorbitol and myoinositol levels in pigment-epithelium of strep-tozotocin-diabetic rats, found the former increased and the latter decreased. The associated abnormalities of the C-wave of the electroretinogram were pre-vented by sorbinil. While Matchinsky thought that the pigment epithelium might be useful in the study of the pathogenesis of the complications of dia-betes, this is doubtful as the pigment epithelium is not obviously involved in diabetic retinopathy.

There are at present two major studies of aldose reductase inhibitors in pro-gress. The sorbinil study in the United States has 600 patients with no or mini-mal retinopathy. This study has been in progress for some 3 years without any significant effect being reported. In the United Kingdom and France, Statil, another drug with similar action but fewer side effects, is on trial. The study is still in the recruiting phase. Thus, several more years will be needed to decide whether aldose reductase and sorbitol have an important role in the prevention and development, respectively, of retinopathy. Certainly the strong statement by Cogan et al (142) that '... diabetic retinopathy is related to sorbitol accumula-tion!!' is not yet warranted.

Photocoagulation

The value of photocoagulation in the treatment of sight-threatening re-tinopathy has been clearly established by the Diabetic Retinopathy Research Study (DRS) (3, 143, 144), and by the British Multicentre Study (145) for pro-liferative lesions and by the British Study (146) for diabetic maculopathy. More recent work is concerned with techniques and complications, and only few deal with important advances in management.

Diabetic maculopathy The British Multicentre Study using the xenon arc found significant benefit from treatment of macular oedema (146). That study also showed that blindness was most effectively prevented when the treatment was given early, when visual acuity was still good (6/6-6/9) and the treatment effect was not significant in those whose visual acuity at entry was 6/36 or worse.

The large Early Treatment of Diabetic Retinopathy Study reported their findings in 1985 (147). The question asked was: 'Is photocoagulation effective in the treatment of macular oedema?' After a complex randomisation proce-dure patients with macular oedema and mild to moderate retinopathy either had immediate or deferred photocoagulation. There were 754 eyes treated immediately focally and 1490 eyes deferred. The assessment of visual acuity was by the ETDRS chart, and the evaluation is complex. Nevertheless, the results were as expected from the British Study. Obviously they were more detailed and more significant, because the large number of patients enabled more subgroups, and laser treatment allowed more precise aiming of the light beam. A significantly lower number of eyes lost 3 or more lines of visual acuity in the early treatment group if the visual acuity was 20/20-20/25, 20/30-20/40 or 20/40-20/60, the difference was only significant at two time-points (16 and 20 mth) if it was worse than 20/60 (approx. 6/12). Immediate treatment was also significantly better than deferred treatment at all time-intervals after 8 months in allowing a gain of one or more lines of visual acuity. The results are important because they now emphasise without doubt the value of early treatment of macular oedema. The study also defines 'clinically important macular oedema' as any of the following characteristics: (a) thickening of the retina at or within 500 microns of the centre of the macula; (b) hard exudates at or within 500 microns of the centre of the macula, if associated with thickening of adjacent retina; (c) a zone or zones of thickening one disc area or larger, any part of which is within one disc diameter from the centre of the macula. They also defined treatable lesions, such as focal leakage, diffuse leakage and avascular areas of the retina.

While there is little doubt the focal leakage and circinate hard exudates respond well to treatment, results are less satisfactory in cystoid and ischaemic oedema. Thus the French Group (148) found that although photocoagulation improved cystoid macular oedema, the visual acuity in such patients did not improve.

Clearly, focal treatment is only useful if the lesions are focal. More extensive treatment is required for diffuse macular oedema. Thus, grid photocoagulation has been used for some time. McDonald and Schatz, reviewing retrospectively patients treated by this method (149), found that 67% of eyes improved; 15 also showed improvement of visual acuity. In only 5 eyes did the visual acuity decrease by two or more lines. The authors felt that poor results were associated with foveal exudates or ischaemia, and poor preoperative visual acuity. Segal and Ducasse also found that treatment of early macular oedema was effective in 84% of 129 eyes (150). Summarising the results, one must agree with Patz et al (151) that early treatment is most effective and delay may cause significant visual loss.

Proliferative retinopathy   The DRS study clearly showed the great advantage of photocoagulation compared with no treatment in proliferative retinopathy (143). This treatment seems to remain effective even after long periods of follow-up (152).

In the DRS study the results of argon laser therapy were considerably better than that of the xenon arc with fewer patients showing severe visual loss. It is therefore interesting to look at the study of Okun et al (153). This group of ophthalmologists did not join the DRS because they were convinced that photocoagulation is effective and that the xenon arc was a good instrument. They also felt that if the DRS came out unfavourably the cause would have been the inexperience of the treaters. In 1984, they therefore surveyed 2688 consecutive eyes treated by xenon arc who had lesions which would have enabled them to join the DRS study. They showed that the cumulative event rates of severe visual loss per 100 eyes was less after 3 years in their patients (8.8) compared with the DRS argon-treated eyes (10.2). The difference grew with time, so that after 6 years it was only 13.3, while the DRS xenon-treated eyes had a rise of 15.9, and the argon-treated patients 17.5. The percent of eyes with severe visual loss of 5 lines or more was also less than in either xenon- or argon-treated patients in the DRS, although two lines were lost by more than in the DRS study. Thus it appears that it is the user and not the equipment which is important. It is of course possible that the DRS patients had somewhat more severe retinopathy, as Rand et al (154) demonstrated that there are certain features, primarily disc new vessels but also haemorrhages and severity of micro-aneurysms which are associated with severe visual loss. Even systemic characteristics, especially urinary protein, is associated with visual loss.

Nevertheless, xenon arc is still used at both Moorfields Eye Hospital and Hammersmith Hospital to treat persistent new vessels which cause recurrent vitreous haemorrhage when argon has been used 'adequately'. The rare cases of florid retinopathy also seem to respond better to xenon arc than argon laser. These are patients with rapidly advancing lesions which have to be treated almost as an emergency. There is little doubt that argon causes less visual field loss than xenon, but Liang and colleagues found the ERG did not differ in the two eyes when one was treated with xenon and one with argon, until the area burned by the xenon was twice that of the argon-treated eye (155).

In most instances after the original treatment series of 1500-3000 burns, the retinopathy improves, but in some patients new vessels persist. Doft and Blankenship (156) found that in 72% of eyes with DRS high-risk characteristic these decreased by 3 weeks after treatment. Those which did not improve by this time tended to remain at high risk even after 6 months. This may have been due to inadequate treatment. Indeed, Vine (157) found that in 12 out of 23 eyes, which did not initially respond to argon laser therapy, did so when further treatment was applied to an average of 7550 burns. More would have responded had xenon been used.

Complications of photocoagulation   No effective treatment is without its complications. In photocoagulation this is common, although usually they are minor and do not interfere with normal life. Thus, Higgins and colleagues found reduced contrast sensitivity after panretinal photocoagulation when visual acuity remained normal (158). More important is the possibility of induction of cataract which, however, is uncommon (159). Subretinal, chorioretinal and choriovitreal neovascularisation is not uncommon and usually indicates too heavy burns. Only one such case was examined histologically (160), but most regular treaters have observed such patients, especially of the krypton laser is used. Abnormalities of the pupil following laser therapy were examined in 22 patients by Lobes and Bourgon (161). They found sector palsies, accommodative paresis and cholinergic supersensitivity and concluded that laser therapy damaged parasympathetic innervation of the iris.

McDonald and Schatz (162) analysed the causes of 2 or more lines visual loss in patients following photocoagulation. By far the commonest cause was chronic macular oedema which occurred in 14 out of 44 eyes which lost vision.

It is important to remember that complications can occur especially in patients with proliferative retinopathy who are often asymptomatic at the time of treatment. Nevertheless, the benefits of treatment are such that they far outweigh any possible complications.

Vitrectomy

The importance of the vitreous as a scaffold for the development of proliferative retinopathy has been well documented (163). It has also been documented by histology and electron microscopy. Recent work by Schepens' group (164) indicates that dense vitreoretinal adhesions may cause traction in the macular area even in the absence of posterior vitreous detachment (PVD) and thus cause macular oedema. For the vitreous to detach with increasing age is expected. Tagawa et al (165) examined 1021 eyes of 570 patients with diabetic retinopathy. They found complete PVD as part of the ageing process. In younger patients without proliferative retinopathy but following photocoagulation, it was also common. Proliferative retinopathy interfered with complete but was associated with partial PVD. It is this partial detachment which may damage retinal vessels and cause haemorrhage.

Vitrectomies are used for the clearance of vitreous (intragel) haemorrhage, traction detachment and more recently, with improved techniques, for removal of epiretinal membranes. Elevated (forward) new vessels with or without haemorrhage give the best results, as it can prevent the tractional complications of retinopathy (166). Michels' group (167) treated 365 cases of retinal detachment secondary to proliferative diabetic retinopathy. Of these, 245 (67%) obtained a satisfactory anatomical result (reattachment of the retina) although the final visual outcome of 5/200 or better was lower at 227 (62%).

Of the features which indicated favourable outcome, the important ones were: visual acuity preoperatively better than 5/200, retinal detachment not exceeding 1/4 of the fundus and limited to the posterior pole, retaining at the crystalline lens, absence of macular detachment, and absence of iatrogenic retinal breaks. More recently, Rice et al (168) analysed 264 consecutive cases where they removed macular epiretinal membranes. Two factors — preoperative visual acuity and duration of blurred vision before surgery — could predict good visual acuity with 69% accuracy; eyes showing significant improvement could be predicted with 80% accuracy. While visual acuity of 20/100 or better was associated with the best visual outcome, greatest improvement occurred with poorer vision. Prolonged blurring of vision indicated a poor result.

Vitreous haemorrhage is a not uncommon complication of vitrectomy. Novak et al (169) found that 63% 596 consecutive patients had a haemorrhage in the first 24 hours after operation. This haemorrhage cleared slowly over 9.1 weeks in phakic, but in 3.4 weeks in aphakic, eyes. Later, vitreous haemorrhage occurred in 88 (23%) of eyes, again clearing more rapidly in aphakic eyes. Ficker et al (170) also found phakic eyes to have more vitreous haemorrhage, but found that endophotocoagulation could prevent this. Similarly, endocoagulation (or adequate photocoagulation prior to vitrectomy) reduced the frequency of postoperative haemorrhage and rubeosis iridis, the latter occurring mostly in aphakic eyes. The Baltimore group experimented with ε-aminocaproic acid (171) and intravitreal thrombin (172). Both these drugs were effective in reducing intraoperative and immediate postoperative bleeding, although they had little influence on later changes.

Vitreous haemorrhage with severe reduction of vision (to less than light perception at 1.5 meters) had a poor visual outcome. Best results were obtained in those with better acuity preoperatively (171). Thompson et al (172) found that prognosis for vitrectomy was worse in those who had a visual acuity preoperatively of less than 5/200, iris neovascularisation and traction or rhegmatous retinal detachment. They also found that the need for fluid or gas exchange during operation and iatrogenic breaks were associated with a 1.5-3.9 times greater risk of poor final visual acuity. Kramptz-Glass and Laqua (173) obtained up to 82% success rate in their vitrectomy cases when this was for just vitreous haemorrhage; this decreased to 63% when haemorrhage and traction detachment were both present. For rhegmatogenous detachment the outlook was poorer, being only 55%. Similarly, intraoperative complications were least at 1% in those with vitreous haemorrhage only.

It is clear that while vitrectomy is a most useful addition to the treatment possibilities in diabetic retinopathy, early adequate photocoagulation will avoid its need in most, though unfortunately not all, patients.

Risk factors for diabetic retinopathy

Genetic factors

While there is ample evidence for an HLA antigen association for IDDM, there is very little to relate them to retinopathy. This is not unexpected, since 97% of these patients develop diabetic retinopathy (174). It has been suggested that proliferative retinopathy may be related to HLA antigens, but this was not confirmed by Middleton et al (175) or Saari (176). Scheinin et al (177) found increased B15 in patients with proliferative retinopathy, compared with non-retinopathic patients, but HLA-DR4 and DR1 were both decreased. In the large study of the Joslin Clinic, Rand et al (178) found proliferative retinopathy to be associated with DR 3/0, 4/0 and x/x. This finding was only true in the absence of myopia. DR3 and DR4 in combination were found in those whose disease progressed over a period of 4 years (179). Another genetic component C4,B3 was thought to be associated with diabetic microangiopathy by Mijovic et al (180), suggesting an immunological basis for diabetic retinopathy. However, there is really inadequate evidence for the importance of *known* genetic determinants to be firmly associated with either retinopathy in general or even severe diabetic retinopathy.

Blood pressure

Among the more recent observations of risk factors, blood pressure appears to be the most important in the epidemiological studies of Klein (181) and constable et al (182). Klein's study is particularly interesting because of the very thorough protocol used. They defined hypertension as systolic ≥160 mmHg and diastolic ≥95 mmHg in those aged 25 years and over at the time of measurement, and in younger persons ≥140/≥90 mmHg. Patients on hypotensive therapy were considered to be hypertensive whatever their blood pressure. Using this method, hypertension was present in 21.9% of patients diagnosed before their 30th year, and 58.1% in the older age group. In the younger age group severity of retinopathy was only associated with diastolic pressure after 10 years' duration of diabetes (174), while it was related to proliferative retinopathy in all in whom diabetes was diagnosed after the age of 30 (101). In the study by Walker et al (183), retinopathy was weakly related to blood pressure in women only. Vigstrup and Mogensen (184) examined 29 patients 7 years apart and found that those whose retinopathy progressed had a higher blood pressure both initially and at the end of the study than those in whom it did not progress. Sjolie (185) found that patients with retinopathy had higher blood pressure than those without, but there was no difference between those with background and proliferative retinopathy. Chahal et al (186) found in NIDDM patients that those with systolic blood pressure over 160 mmHg had significantly more severe retinopathy than those with systolic pressure under 140 mmHg. There was no relation between progression of retinopathy and blood pressure levels, probably because those with elevated pressure were treated.

Other risk factors

Among the known risk factors, Klein et al (187) looked at gravidity and found that when corrected for duration of diabetes, previous gravidity was no longer a risk factor for retinopathy. In a small study from Chicago, Phelps et al (188) found that retinopathy deterioration during pregnancy was related not only to initial retinopathy status and initial HbA_1, but also to rate and degree of fall in blood glucose. They suggested that the retinopathy deterioration is related to good control as suggested before by the pump studies. Soubrane et al (189) found retinopathy to deteriorate during pregnancy, while the Belfast group found that vision was maintained (190) even in the most severe cases.

Another factor of possible importance is smoking; this is supported in males only by Walker et al (183) and negated by the much more comprehensive study of Klein (191). Rather unexpectedly, Young et al (192) found heavy alcohol consumption a prognostic predictor of retinopathy. More expectedly, proliferative retinopathy was related to impaired renal function (184). Of particular interest is the study of the Steno Group who found that the incidence of proliferative retinopathy is greatly increased in those who develop microalbuminuria, indicating that all microvascular complications tend to progress together (193).

Finally, presence of cataract seems to be associated with diabetic retinopathy (194). The other risk factors of control and duration do not require any further evaluation.

Pathogenic mechanisms

Of the many pathogenic mechanisms proposed really new work has been restricted to the possible role of growth hormone and growth factors, and only these are being considered here.

The role of growth hormone

Re-assessment of pituitary ablation in the treatment of diabetic retinopathy A long-term follow-up of patients with proliferative retinopathy, treated by yttrium-90 (^{90}Y) pituitary implantation has recently been carried out (195) to re-assess the effect of pituitary ablation on diabetic microvascular disease. Medical aspects were assessed in 117 consecutive patients who underwent pituitary ablation between 1960 and 1976. The 5-year mortality in these patients was 17.6%, and the 10-year mortality was 51%, figures lower than generally reported in patients with proliferative retinopathy. Ophthalmological follow-up was carried out in 100 of these patients operated on between 1965 and 1976. Of these patients, the visual acuity in the better eye at the time of operation was 6/12 or more in 84% of patients, and this percentage remained unchanged at the time of the 5- and 10-year follow-up. By 5 years, new vessels on the disc had improved from an initial grading of 2.7 ± 1.6 to 0.8 ± 1.2 (mean $\pm$ SD, $P < 0.001$); by 10 years, there was no disc neovascularisation in any eye. There was similar improvement in peripheral new vessels, hard exudates, microaneurysms and haemorrhages. This improvement is remarkable when it is considered that spontaneous regression of proliferative retinopathy is uncommon, and it is concluded that pituitary ablation had a beneficial effect on the course of diabetic microvascular complications.

The cause of growth hormone hypersecretion in diabetes Improvement in diabetic retinopathy after pituitary ablation has traditionally been ascribed to removal of abnormally high 24-hour growth hormone (GH) levels in diabetic subjects. This hypothesis was first proposed by Lundbaek et al (196), and although the idea has found its way into the major textbooks, it has not been the subject of objective scrutiny since. There has recently been renewed interest in the hypothesis in view of the development of long-acting analogues of somatostatin which have the potential to suppress 24-hour GH levels, but it would first be relevant here to review the cause of GH hypersecretion in diabetes in order to understand better the logic behind pharmacological GH suppression.

As a fundamental point, it is worth pointing out that GH in the only pituitary hormone which is produced in excessive quantities in diabetic subjects. It is therefore possible that the abnormality does not lie at the pituitary level since any defect at this level would be unlikely to affect GH alone. The defect is therefore more likely to lie in the GH regulatory mechanisms. Due to a peculiarity of human physiology, GH secretion in man is more closely related to circulating glucose levels than in other animal species. Since diabetic rats do not demontrate GH hypersecretion (197), it is possible that GH hypersecretion in diabetic man is mediated by the elevated glucose levels acting on the hypothalamic glucose-sensitive cells. Certainly improvement in glycaemic control is known to lead to improvement in abnormal GH secretion in diabetes.

Beyond these basic observations, little more can be said regarding the cause of GH hypersecretion in diabetes. Various stimuli, such as thyrotrophin-releasing hormone (TRH), arginine and dopamine have been found to stimulate GH release in diabetic but not in normal subjects; however, the significance of these observations is obscure since the mechanism of action of these stimuli is not known. It has been suggested that the GH response to TRH in diabetic subjects is caused by oversensitivity of a normal pathway (198), and the same may apply to the other stimuli. In other respects, GH regulation in diabetes is normal. Bromocriptine has a GH-stimulatory effect as in normal subjects (119), and a normal response to hypoglycaemia (200) indicates that the feedback loop is intact.

Further work into the cause of abnormal GH secretion in diabetes was made possible with the availability of GH-releasing factor (GRF). It was first demonstrated that, in normal subjects, hyperglycaemia leads to suppression of GRF-mediated GH secretion (201). It has subsequently been shown that the same is not true of diabetic subjects (202). This suggests that the GH suppressive mechanism initiated by hyperglycaemia in normal man is defective in diabetes. This mechanism is mediated by production of hypothalamic somatostatin, and it is therefore possible that hyperglycaemia in diabetic subjects either fails to stimulate somatostatin release, or diabetic subjects are resistant to the somatostatin produced. Certainly, chronic hyperglycaemia would be expected to cause chronic overproduction of hypothalamic somatostatin, which in turn would lead to pituitary somatostatin resistance. This possibility would provide a possible cause for all the described abnormalities of GH hypersecretion in diabetes.

A further possible cause for excessive GH production in diabetes is the presence of a defect of glucose transport across the blood-brain barrier (BBB) in diabetic subjects, leading to central neuroglycopaenia in the presence of a normal peripheral blood glucose. The phenomenon of 'relative hypoglycaemia' has been well described (203) and, if proven, would lead to elevated GH levels in normoglycaemic diabetic subjects. A recent study of transport of ^{11}C-3-*O*-methyl-D-glucose across the BBB studied using positron emission tomography in diabetic subjects, including those with microvascular disease, has failed to demonstrate any defect of hexose transport across the BBB in diabetes (204). There is therefore no explanation for GH hypersecretion in diabetes at this level.

Finally, at the tissue level, a further cause for GH hypersecretion in diabetes exists. There has been considerable interest in the GH-dependent growth factor, insulin-like growth factor I (IGF-I) in diabetes. Certain workers have demonstrated a negative correlation between serum levels of IGF-I and glycaemic control assessed by glycosylated HbA_1 (205, 206). We have confirmed this in patients with diabetic retinopathy (unpublished observations). This suggests that poor glycaemic control leads to a failure of IGF-I generation in response to GH, a finding akin to that observed in starvation (207). This has been demonstrated more directly with the observation that children with good glycaemic control have a greater IGF-I response to exogenous GH administration than do children with poor control (208). Such a condition of GH resistance in poorly controlled diabetes would lead to elevation of GH levels by negative feedback. Precisely what impact this phenomenon has on diurnal levels of GH in diabetes is not known, but hopefully the glycaemic control of most treated diabetic subjects is not sufficiently poor to make this 'starvation phenomenon' a major contributor to elevated GH levels. In conclusion, there is cause for excessive GH production in diabetes at both central and tissue levels. The abnormality of GH regulation at central level, mediated by lack of, or resistance to, hypothalamic somatostatin is probably the major defect.

Long-acting somatostatin analogues in diabetes The development of long-acting analogues of somatostatin (209) has raised the possibility of suppression of both GH and gut hormones in diabetic subjects with potentially beneficial effect on both glycaemic control and diabetic microvascular disease. Initial results with bolus doses of SMS 201-995 (Sandoz) in IDDM subjects were promising (210), but a recent study of long-term therapy has demonstrated that GH secretion is not completely suppressed by subcutaneous injection twice daily (211). The Hammersmith group has been able to confirm this in patients with proliferative diabetic retinopathy. SMS 201-995, 500 µg 3 times daily, led to only a modest decrease in serum IGF-I, and no change in 24-hour GH levels. By contrast, gastrointestinal side effects and hypoglycaemia were a problem. This suggests that although the analogue is suppressing gut hormones, it is not having the desired effect at central level. Administration by continuous subcutaneous infusion did not overcome this problem, and this somatostatin analogue is therefore unlikely to be useful in treatment of diabetic retinopathy. Although disappointing, this result allows further speculation on the cause of GH hypersecretion in diabetes. From the discussion in the previous section, it follows that administration of somatostatin analogue will not cause GH suppression in diabetes. Thus, a somatostatin analogue is not a logical pharmacological method of GH suppression in diabetes, and other methods will need to be sought.

Growth factors and diabetic retinopathy

Ischaemia plays a prominent role in the natural history of proliferative diabetic retinopathy. The precise mechanisms leading to microvascular damage and closure are not clear, and various clinical studies have not provided a good correlation between glycaemic control in diabetic subjects and the severity of microvascular disease. However, the fact remains that on fluorescein angiography in patients with all grades of diabetic retinopathy, areas of capillary non-perfusion are a prominent feature. As a general concept, it is easy to imagine that such retinal ischaemia might lead to new vessel production in an attempt to improve retinal perfusion. In more concrete terms, the link between retinal ischaemia and new vessel production is hard to define. As long ago as 1948, it was proposed that retinal ischaemia leads to the production of a vasoproliferative factor (212), but, to date, this putative factor has escaped identification.

Two observations can be interpreted as providing indirect evidence for the presence of a tissue growth factor which plays a significant role in the development of proliferative retinopathy. Firstly, panretinal photocoagulation causes regression of new vessels, direct treatment to the vessels not being necessary to produce this effect. This suggests that photocoagulation produces its beneficial effect in proliferative retinopathy, not by directly sealing the abnormal vessels, but rather by suppression of production of a vasoproliferative factor by the retina as a whole. Secondly, in tissue culture, it has been shown that retinal endothelial cell growth is enhanced by a medium which has first been used to support the growth of pericytes (unpublished observations). This suggests that ordered retinal endothelial growth is dependent upon some factor produced by the supporting intramural pericytes, these cells being reduced in number early in the natural history of diabetic retinopathy.

At present, the specific nature and number of tissue growth factors present in man is uncertain, but it is likely that with further characterisation of the various factors so far identified, most will in fact prove to be identical to the few factors presently known and sequenced (such as the insulin-like growth factors, platelet-derived growth factor, endothelial growth factor and nerve growth factor). In the context of diabetic retinopathy, IGF-I (also known as somatomedin-C) has received most attention. The reason for this interest stems from the fact that IGF-I is the major circulating growth factor in man, and was one of the first for which reliable bioassays and radioimmunoassays were developed. Furthermore, IGF-I is known to be GH-dependent (213).

A few workers have measured serum IGF-I specifically in patients with diabetic retinopathy. Merimee et al (214) were the first to suggest that IGF-I levels are higher in patients with proliferative retinopathy than in other diabetics, and this is the work which has received most publicity. However, it should be pointed out that there was no significant difference between IGF-I levels in patients with and without retinopathy in this study. The investigators then identified 7 patients out of the total study group of 80 patients with what was termed 'rapidly progressive' retinopathy, and these subjects were found to have IGF-I values significantly greater than the mean value. The ages of the subjects with active retinopathy were not stated, and since this type of retinopathy is most commonly found in patients in their early twenties, and serum IGF-I levels are age-dependent, it is not clear whether these patients simply represent a younger subgroup of the whole.

Other investigators, measuring IGF-I bioassay in a small group, have found IGF-I to be higher than normal in patients with proliferative retinopathy (215), but this was not confirmed by others in a larger study group measuring IGF-I by radioimmunoassay (216). Certainly the experience of the authors is that there is a significant correlation between serum IGF-I and activity of diabetic retinopathy, but even in patients with proliferative retinopathy, the values are not significantly higher than in normal subjects. Further, values fall toward normal with the regression of new vessels after photocoagulation, suggesting that eleva-

tion in serum IGF-I is a transitory phenomenon at the time of vascular proliferation. It is therefore not possible to ascribe a definite role to IGF-I in the
pathogenesis of proliferative retinopathy since it must first be documented that
the rise in IGF-I antedates the onset of proliferation. Further, in view of the
paracrine model proposed for the production of IGF-I (217), more information
on IGF-I levels in the eyes of patients with proliferative retinopathy is required
since serum levels are probably not the important component. In an attempt to
overcome this problem, Grant and co-workers have measured IGF-I values in
the vitreous of patients with proliferative retinopathy, and found these to be
higher than in a non-diabetic control group (218). While of interest, such information is difficult to interpret since elevated levels may represent vascular leakage into the vitreous in patients with proliferative retinopathy. We are thus
some way from attributing the onset of vascular proliferation in diabetes to a
rise in IGF-I, but there is a correlation of interest in this context in that sudden
improvement in glycaemic control is known to lead to both a deterioration in retinopathy (116) and a rise in IGF-I (219). This suggests that IGF-I is worthy of
further investigation as the link between ischaemia and proliferation in diabetic
retinopathy.

The other major growth factor which has been the object of some interest in
the context of retinopathy is fibroblast growth factor (FGF). Basic FGF has
been isolated from various tissues, including brain, pituitary and retina, and
causes an increase in extracellular matrix as well as causing proliferation of both
vascular and fibrous tissue (220). These sites of origin together with the actions
of this factor make it an attractive contender for the proposed vasculogenic
factor in diabetic retinopathy. The fact that FGF causes production of extracellular matrix is important in view of the basement membrane thickening which
is an early feature of diabetic retinopathy. Production of this factor by the retina
is obviously important, but production by the pituitary gland may provide the
link between pituitary ablation and improvement in proliferative retinopathy.
A short report has recently suggested that FGF is elevated in the vitreous of patients with proliferative retinopathy (221), although confirmation in larger
numbers is needed.

Thus far, absolute identification or even confirmation of the presence of a
growth factor which provides the stimulus to proliferation in an ischaemic
diabetic retina has not been demonstrated. However, in view of the recent upsurge of interest in tissue growth factors, more are likely to come under scrutiny
with regard to diabetic retinopathy. From the above account, it can be seen that
the information to date is slim, but this is likely to change in the near future.

References

1. Davis MD, Norton EWD, Myers FL (1968): Airlie clarification of diabetic retinopathy. In: Goldberg MF, Fine SL (Eds), *Treatment of Diabetic Retinopathy*, p. 7. Department of Health, Education and Welfare, Bethesda, MD.
2. Klein BE, Davis MD, Segal P et al (1984): Diabetic retinopathy: assessment of severity and progression. *Ophthalmology, 91,* 10.
3. Diabetic Retinopathy Study Research Group (1981): Modification of the Airlie House clarification of diabetic retinopathy. *Invest. Ophthalmol. Vis. Sci., 21,* 210.
4. Early Treatment of Diabetic Retinopathy Research Group (1980): *Manual of Operations.* Department of Health, Education and Welfare, Bethesda, MD.
5. Davis MD, Hubbard LD, Trautman J, Klein R for the Kroc Collaborative Study Group (1985): Studies of retinopathy: methodology for assessment and clarification with fundus photographs. *Diabetes, 34, Suppl. 3,* 42.
6. Diabetic Control and Complications Study (1985): *Manual of Operations.* Department of Health, Education and Welfare, Bethesda, MD.
7. Moss SE, Klein R, Kessler SD, Richie KH (1985): Comparison between ophthalmoscopy and fundus photography in determining severity of diabetic retinopathy. *Ophthalmology, 92,* 62.
8. Klein R, Klein BEK, Neider MW et al (1985): Diabetic retinopathy as detected using ophthalmoscopy: a non-mydriatic camera and a standard fundus camera. *Ophthalmology, 92,* 485.
9. Ryder REJ, Vora JP, Akica JA et al (1985): Possible new method to improve detection of diabetic retinopathy. *Br. Med. J., 291,* 1256.
10. Ryder REJ, Young S, Vora JP et al (1985): Practical diabetes: screening for diabetic retinopathy using polaroid retinal photography through undilated pupils. *Prac. Diabetes, 2,* 34.
11. Williams R, Nussey S, Humphrey R, Thompson G (1986): Assessment of non-mydriatic fundus photography in detection of diabetic retinopathy. *Br. Med. J., 293,* 1140.
12. Edwards AL (1986): Fundoscopic examination of patients with diabetes who are admitted to hospital. *Can. Med. Assoc. J., 134,* 1236.
13. Scobie IN, MacCuish AC, Barrie T et al (1981): Serious retinopathy in a diabetic clinic: prevalence and therapeutic implications. *Lancet, 2,* 520.
14. Yannuzi LA, Rohrer KT, Tindel LJ et al (1986): Fluorescein angiography, complication survey. *Ophthalmology, 93,* 611.
15. Nielsen NV (1985): The normal fundus angiogram. IV. *Acta Ophthalmol., 63,* 459.
16. Nielsen NV (1985): The normal fundus angiogram. V. Intraobserver, interobserver and interocular variation of the fundus fluorescein angiogram. *Acta Ophthalmol., 63,* 463.
17. Niki T, Muraoka K, Shimizu K (1984): Distribution of capillary nonperfusion in early-stage diabetic retinopathy. *Ophthalmology, 91,* 1431.
18. Freyler H (1985): Das periphere Fluoreszenzangiogramm bei diabetischer Retinopathie. *Klin. Mbl. Augenheilkd., 186,* 184.
19. Muraoka K, Shimizu K (1984): Intraretinal neovascularisation in diabetic retinopathy. *Ophthalmology, 91,* 1440.
20. Mohan R Kohner EM (1986): Retinal revascularisation in diabetic retinopathy. *Br. J. Ophthalmol., 70,* 114.
21. Sleightholm MA, Arnold J, Aldington SJ, Kohner EM (1984): Computer aided digitisation of fundus photographs. *Clin. Phys. Physiol. Meas., 5,* 295.
22. Baudoin C, Maneschi F, Quentel G et al (1983): Quantitative evaluation of fluorescein angiograms. *Diabetes, 32, Suppl. 2,* 8.

23. Kohner EM, Lawson P, Ghosh G, Testa M (1985): Assessment of fluorescein angiograms. *Diabetes, 34, Suppl. 3,* 56.
24. Kohner EM, Sleightholm MA (1986): Does microaneurysm count reflect the severity of diabetic retinopathy? *Ophthalmology, 93,* 586.
25. Bresnick GH, Condit R, Syrjala S et al (1984): Abnormalities of the foveal avascular zone in diabetic retinopathy. *Arch. Ophthalmol., 102,* 1286.
26. Sleightholm MA, Arnold J, Kohner EM (1987): Diabetic retinopathy: assessment of non-perfused areas on fluorescein angiograms. Submitted for publication.
27. Sleightholm MA, Aldington SJ, Arnold J, Kohner EM (1987): Diabetic retinopathy: assessment of severity and progression from fluorescein angiograms. Submitted for publication.
28. Klein R, Klein BEK, Moss SE, DeMets D (1983): Inter-observer variation in refraction and visual acuity measurement using a standardized protocol. *Ophthalmology, 90,* 1357.
29. Klein R, Klein BEK, Moss SE (1984): Visual impairment in diabetes. *Ophthalmology, 91,* 1.
30. Regan D, Neima D (1984): Low-contrast letter charts in early diabetic retinopathy, ocular hypertension, glaucoma, and Parkinson's disease. *Br. J. Ophthalmol., 68,* 885.
31. Della Sala S, Bertoni G, Somazzi L et al (1985): Impaired contrast sensitivity in diabetic patients with and without retinopathy: a new technique for rapid assessment. *Br. J. Ophthalmol., 69,* 136.
32. Sokol S, Moskowitz A, Skarf B et al (1985): Contrast sensitivity in diabetics with and without background retinopathy. *Arch. Ophthalmol., 103,* 51.
33. Bresnick GH, Condit RS, Palta M et al (1985): Association of hue discrimination loss and diabetic retinopathy. *Arch. Ophthalmol., 103,* 1317.
34. Green FD, Ghafour IM, Allan D et al (1985): Colour vision of diabetics. *Br. J. Ophthalmol., 69,* 533.
35. Roy MS, McCulloch C, Hanna AK, Mortimer C (1984): Colour vision in long standing diabetes mellitus. *Br. J. Ophthalmol., 68,* 215.
36. Roy MS, Gunkel RD, Podgor MJ (1986): Colour vision defects in early diabetic retinopathy. *Arch. Ophthalmol., 104,* 225.
37. Frost-Larsen K, Larsen H-W (1985): Macular recovery time recorded by nyctometry, a screening method for selection of patients who are at risk of developing proliferative diabetic retinopathy. *Acta Ophthalmol., 63, Suppl. 173,* 39.
38. Frost-Larsen K, Larsen H-W, Simonsen SE (1980): Oscillatory potential and nyctometry in insulin dependent diabetics. *Acta Ophthalmol., 58,* 879.
39. Simonsen SE (1980): The value of oscillatory potential in selecting juvenile diabetics at risk of developing proliferative retinopathy. *Acta Ophthalmol., 58,* 865.
40. Bresnick GH, Korth K, Groo A, Palta M (1984): Electroretinographic oscillatory potentials predict progression of diabetic retinopathy: preliminary report. *Arch. Ophthalmol., 102,* 1307.
41. Arden GB, Hamilton AMP, Wilson-Holt J et al (1986): Pattern electroretinograms become abnormal when background retinopathy deteriorates to a preproliferative stage: possible use as a screening test. *Br. J. Ophthalmol., 70,* 330.
42. Perlman I, Gdal-on M, Miller B, Zonis S (1985): Retinal function of the diabetic retina after argon laser photocoagulation assessed electroretinographically. *Br. J. Ophthalmol., 69,* 240.
43. Hennekes R, Deschner R (1984): Alteration of oscillatory potentials in diabetics induced by photocoagulation of the retina. *Graefe's Arch. Clin. Exp. Ophthalmol., 221,* 230.
44. Scherfig E, Edmund J, Tinning S, Trojaborg W (1984): Flash visual evoked potential as a prognostic factor for vitreous operations in diabetic eyes. *Ophthalmology, 91,* 1475.

45. Algvere P, Persson HE, Wanger P (1985): Preoperative electroretinograms and visual evoked cortical potentials for predicting outcome of vitrectomy in diabetics. *Retina, 5,* 179.
46. Cunha-Vaz JG, De Abreau F, Campos AJ, Figo GN (1975): Early breakdown of the blood retinal barrier in diabetes. *Br. J. Ophthalmol., 59,* 649.
47. Kernell A, Arnguist H (1983): Effect of insulin treatment of the blood-retinal barrier in rats with streptozotocin induced diabetes. *Arch. Ophthalmol., 101,* 968.
48. Krupin T, Waltman SR, Szewczyk P et al (1982): Fluorophotometric studies on the blood retinal barrier in experimental animals. *Arch. Ophthalmol., 100,* 63.
49. Cunha-Vaz JG, Zeimer R, Wong WP, Kiani RP (1982): Kinetic vitreous fluorophotometry in normals and non insulin dependent diabetics. *Ophthalmology, 89,* 751.
50. White NH, Waltman SR, Krupin T, Santiago JV (1982): Reversal of abnormalities in ocular fluorophotometry in insulin dependent diabetes after 5 to 9 months of improved diabetic control. *Diabetes, 31,* 80.
51. Lauritzen T, Frost-Larsen K, Larson HW, Deckert T (1983): Effect of one year normal blood glucose levels on retinopathy in insulin dependent diabetics. *Lancet, 1,* 200.
52. Kohner EM, Alderson AR (1981): Vitreous fluorophotometry. *Trans. Ophthalmol. Soc. UK, 101,* 446.
53. Cunha-Vaz JG, Gray JR, Zeimer RC et al (1985): Characterisation of the early stages of diabetic retinopathy by vitreous fluorophotometry. *Diabetes, 34,* 53.
54. Chahal PS, Chowienczyk PJ, Kohner EM (1985): Measurement of blood-retinal barrier permeability: a reproducibility study in normal eyes. *Invest. Ophthalmol. Visual Sci., 26,* 977.
55. Chahal PS, Fallon T, Jennings SJ et al (1986): Vitreous fluorophotometry in patients with no or minimal diabetic retinopathy. *Diabetes Care, 9,* 134.
56. Roy MS, Bonner RF, Bungay PM et al (1986): Posterior vitreous fluorophotometry in normal subjects. *Arch. Ophthalmol., 104,* 1004.
57. Ogura Y, Tsukahara Y, Saito I, Kondo T (1985): Estimation of the permeability of the blood-retinal barrier in normal individuals. *Invest. Ophthalmol. Visual Sci., 26,* 969.
58. Chahal PS, Neal MJ, Kohner EM (1985): Rapid metabolism of fluorescein after intravenous administration. *Invest. Ophthalmol. Visual Sci., 26,* 764.
59. Lund-Andersen H, Krogsaa B, La Cour M, Larsen J (1985): Quantitative vitreous fluorophotometry applying a mathematical model of the eye. *Invest. Ophthalmol. Visual Sci., 26,* 698.
60. Lund-Andersen H, Krogsaa B, Larsen J (1985): Calculation of the permeability of the blood-retinal barrier to fluorescein. *Graefe's Arch. Clin. Exp. Ophthalmol., 222,* 173.
61. Krogsaa B, Lund-Andersen H, Mehlsen J, Sestoft L (1986): The blood-retinal barrier permeability to fluorescein in normal subjects and in juvenile diabetics without retinopathy. *Acta Ophthalmol., 64,* 173.
62. Kjaergaard JJ (1985): Fluorophotometric studies of twenty-nine healthy subjects. *Graefe's Arch. Clin. Exp. Ophthalmol., 222,* 267.
63. Krogsaa B, Lund-Andersen H, Lauritzen T et al (1985): The blood-retinal barrier permeability to fluorescein in juvenile diabetics treated with continuous subcutaneous insulin infusion. *Acta Ophthalmol., 63, Suppl. 173,* 104.
64. Kernell A, Dahlkvist H, Arnqvist H, Ludvigsson J (1985): Influence of metabolic control on the blood-retinal barrier in streptozocin diabetic rats. *Graefe's Arch. Clin. Exp. Ophthalmol., 222,* 179.
65. Blair NP, Jones CW, Rusin MM (1984): Pathophysiology of the blood-retinal barrier in experimental diabetes: vitreous fluorophotometry using carboxyfluorescein and fluorescein. *Arch. Ophthalmol., 102,* 1808.
66. Vine AK, Kisley AM, Betz AL, Howatt WF (1984): Vitreous fluorophotometry in rats with streptozotocin-induced diabetes. *Arch. Ophthalmol., 102,* 1083.

67. Blair NP, Rusin MM, Shakin E (1985): The effect of pH on the transfer of fluorescein across the blood-retinal barrier. *Invest. Ophthalmol. Visual Sci., 26,* 1133.
68. Grimes PA (1985): Fluorescein distribution in retinas of normal and diabetic rats. *Exp. Eye Res., 41,* 227.
69. Wallow IHL (1983): Posterior and anterior permeability defects? Morphologic observations on streptozotocin-treated rats. *Invest. Ophthalmol. Visual Sci., 24,* 1259.
70. Plehwe W, Sleightholm MA, Kohner EM (1986): Vitreous fluorophotometry may predict deterioration of diabetic retinopathy in patients commencing subcutaneous insulin infusion. *Diabetologia, 29,* 583A.
71. Kohner EM, Hamilton AM, Saunders SJ et al (1975): The retinal blood flow in diabetes. *Diabetologia, 11,* 27.
72. Kohner EM (1976): The problems of retinal blood flow in diabetes. *Diabetes, 25, Suppl. 2,* 839.
73. Riva CE, Roberts WP, McMeel JW, BenSira I (1976): Arteriovenous mean circulation time in the human retina. In: De Lacy JJ (Ed.), *Fluorescein Angiography,* p. 113. Junk, The Hague.
74. Atherton A, Hill DW, Keen H et al (1980): The effect of acute hyperglycaemia on the retinal circulation in the normal rat. *Diabetologia, 18,* 233.
75. Goldstick TK, Ernest JF (1982): The effect of glucose, oxygen and carbon dioxide on choroidal blood flow. *Invest. Ophthalmol. Visual Sci., 23,* 194.
76. McMillan DE (1978): Rheological and related factors in diabetic retinopathy. In: Kohner EM (Ed.), *International Ophthalmology Clinics, 1978,* p. 35. Little, Brown, Boston.
77. Preussner PR, Richard G, Darrelmann OG et al (1983): Quantitative measurement of retinal blood flow in human beings by application of digital image processing methods to television fluorescein angiograms. *Graefe's Arch. Clin. Exp. Ophthalmol., 221,* 110.
78. Richard G, Darrelmann OGr, Kreissig I et al (1984): Videoangiografische Unterteilung der Netzhautkreislaufzeit: Ihre Bedeutung für die Diagnostik von Durchblutungsstörungen der Netzhaut. *Fortschr. Ophthalmol., 81,* 592.
79. Riva CE, Feke GT (1981): Laser Doppler velocimetry in the measurement of retinal blood flow. In: Goldman (Ed.), *The Biomedical Laser,* p. 135. Springer, New York.
80. Feke GT, Riva CE (1978): Laser doppler measurements of blood velocity in human retinal vessels. *J. Optom. Soc. Am., 68,* 526.
81. Riva CE, Petrig B (1980): Blue field entoptic phenomenon and blood velocity in retinal capillaries. *J. Optom. Soc. Am., 70,* 1234.
82. Fallon TJ, Chowienczyk P, Kohner EM (1986): Measurement of retinal blood flow in diabetes by the blue light entoptic phenomenon. *Br. J. Ophthalmol., 70,* 43.
83. Fallon TJ, Sleightholm MA, Chahal P, Kohner EM (1987): The effect of acute hyperglycaemia on flow velocity in the macular capillaries. *Invest. Ophthalmol. Visual Sci.,* in press.
84. Grunwald JE, Riva CE, Bruckner AJ et al (1984): Retinal blood flow in diabetes mellitus. *Invest. Ophthalmol. Visual Sci., 25, Suppl. 8.*
85. Grunwald JE, Riva CE, Bruckner AJ et al (1986): Effect of panretinal photocoagulation on retinal blood flow in proliferative diabetic retinopathy. *Ophthalmology, 93,* 590.
86. Feke GT, Tagawa H, Yoshida A et al (1985): Retinal circulatory changes related to retinopathy progression in insulin dependent diabetes mellitus. *Ophthalmology, 92,* 1517.
87. Fallon TJ, Maxwell D, Kohner EM (1985): Retinal vascular autoregulation in conditions of hypoxia and hyperoxia using the blue light entoptic phenomenon. *Ophthalmology, 92,* 701.
88. Fallon TJ, Maxwell D, Kohner EM (1985): Autoregulation of retinal blood flow in diabetic retinopathy under hypoxia and hyperoxia. *Invest. Ophthalmol. Visual Sci., 26, Suppl.,* 244.
89. Grunwald JE, Riva CE, Bruckner AJ et al (1984): Altered vascular response to 100% oxygen breathing in diabetes mellitus. *Ophthalmology, 91,* 1447.

90. Irsiglcr K, Kritz H, Hagmueller G et al (1983). In: Irsigler K, Kritz H (Eds), *Diabetes treatment with Implantable Insulin Infusion Systems*, p. 52. Urban and Schwarzenberg, Munich.
91. Irsigler K, Knatterud G, Lovett R (1986): Pump treatment for diabetic patients. *Paediatr. Adolesc. Endocrinol.*, *15*, 204.
92. Engerman R, Bloodworth JMB, Nelson S (1977): Relationship of microvascular disease in diabetes to metabolic control. *Diabetes*, *26*, 760.
93. Engerman R, Kern TS (1984): Experimental galactosaemia produces a diabetes-like retinopathy. *Diabetes*, *33*, 92.
94. Engerman R, Kern TS (1986): Hyperglycaemia as a cause of diabetic retinopathy. *Metab. Clin. Exp.*, *35*, *Suppl. 4*, 20.
95. Doft BH, Kingsley LA, Orchard TF et al (1984): The association between long term diabetic control and early retinopathy. *Ophthalmology*, *91*, 763.
96. Weber B, Burger W, Hartmann R et al (1986): Risk factors for the development of retinopathy in children and adolescents with type I diabetes mellitus. *Diabetologia*, *29*, 23.
97. Klein R, Klein BEK, Moss SE et al (1984): The Wisconsin epidemiologic study of diabetic retinopathy. II. Prevalence and risk of diabetic retinopathy when age at diagnosis less than 30 years. *Arch. Ophthalmol.*, *102*, 520.
98. Sjolie AK (1985): Ocular complications in insulin treated diabetes mellitus. *Acta Ophthalmol.*, *63*, *Suppl. 172.*
99. Rand LI, Krolewski AS, Aiello LM et al (1985): Multiple factors in the prediction of risk in proliferative diabetic retinopathy. *N. Engl. J. Med.*, *313*, 1433.
100. Ide CH, Goldstein DE, Wilson RJ (1984): Beziehungen zwischen Blutzuckerkontrollwerten und der Entwicklung der diabetischen Retinopathie (Langzeituntersuchung). *Klin. Monatsbl. Augenheilkd.*, *185*, 373.
101. Klein R, Klein BEK, Moss SE et al (1984): The Wisconsin epidemiologic study of diabetic retinopathy: prevalence and risk of diabetic retinopathy when age at diagnosis is 30 or more years. *Arch. Ophthalmol.*, *102*, 527.
102. Klein R, Klein BEK, Moss SE et al (1984): The Wisconsin epidemiologic study of diabetic retinopathy. IV Macular oedema. *Ophthalmology*, *91*, 1464.
103. Howard-Williams J, Patel P, Jelfs R et al (1985): Polyunsaturated fatty acids and diabetic retinopathy. *Br. J. Ophthalmol.*, *69*, 15.
104. Nathan DM, Singer DE, Hodgson-Harrington C, Perlmuter LC (1986): Retinopathy in older type II diabetics. *Diabetes*, *35*, 797.
105. Jerneld B, Ngvere P (1985): Prevalence of retinopathy in diabetes treated with oral hypoglycaemic agent. *Acta Ophthalmol.*, *63*, 535.
106. Monson JP, Koios G, Toms GC et al (1986): Relationship between retinopathy and glycaemic control in insulin dependent and non insulin dependent diabetes. *J. R. Soc. Med.*, *79*, 274.
107. Irsigler K, Knitz H, Najemnik C, Freiger H (1979): Reversal of florid retinopathy. *Lancet*, *2*, 1068.
108. White MC, Kohner EM, Pickup FC, Keen H (1981): Reversal of diabetic retinopathy by continuous subcutaneous insulin infusion. *Br. J. Ophthalmol.*, *65*, 307.
109. Lawson PM, Champion MC, Canny LLB et al (1982): Continuous subcutaneous insulin infusion does not prevent progression of proliferative and pre-proliferative retinopathy. *Br. J. Ophthalmol.*, *66*, 762.
110. Puklin JE, Tamborlane WV, Felig P et al (1982): Influence of long term insulin infusion pump treatment of type I diabetic retinopathy. *Ophthalmology*, *89*, 735.
111. Bernsmeier H, Sonnenberg GE (1984): Die diabetische Retinopathie unter der kontinuierlichen subkutanen Insulininfusionstherapie. *Fortschr. Ophthalmol.*, *81*, 267.
112. Van Ballegooie E, Hooymans JMM, Timmerman Z et al (1984): Rapid deterioration of

diabetic retinopathy during treatment with continuous subcutaneous insulin infusion. *Diabetes Care, 7,* 236.

113. Waldhäusl W, Fryler H, Bratusch-Marrain P et al (1983): Kontinuierliche subkutane Insulininfusion. *Dtsch. Med. Wochenschr., 108,* 570.
114. Dahl-Jorgensen K, Brinchmann-Hansen O, Hanssen KF, Bjoro T (1985): Rapid tightening of blood glucose control leads to transient deterioration of retinopathy in insulin dependent diabetes mellitus: The Oslo Study. *Br. Med. J., 290,* 811.
115. Lauritzen T, Deckert T, and Steno Study Group (1982): One year's experience of insulin pumps in diabetes. *Nord. Med., 97,* 130.
116. Kroc Collaborative Study Group (1985): Blood glucose control and the evolution of diabetic retinopathy and albuminuria. *N. Engl. J. Med., 311,* 365.
117. Canny CLB, Kohner EM, Trautman J et al (1985): Comparison of stereo fundus photographs in patients with insulin dependent diabetes during conventional insulin treatment or continuous subcutaneous insulin infusion. *Diabetes, 34, Suppl. 3,* 50.
118. Testa MA, Puklin J, Sherwin R, Simonson DC, for the Kroc Collaborative Study Group (1985): Clinical predictors of retinopathy and its progression in patients with type I diabetes during CSII or conventional insulin treatment. *Diabetes, 34, Suppl. 3,* 61.
119. Sleightholm MA, Aldington S, Kohner EM (1987): Retinal blood flow is important in deterioration of retinopathy on CSII. Submitted for publication.
120. Hooymans JMM (1986): *The Course of Diabetic Retinopathy during Treatment with Continuous Subcutaneous Insulin Infusion,* Thesis. Van Denderen, Groningen.
121. Friberg TR, Rosenstock J, Sanborn G et al (1985): The effect of long-term near normal glycemic control on mild diabetic retinopathy. *Ophthalmology, 92,* 1051.
122. Zaluski S, Millet P, Selam JL (1985): Améliorations de la rétinopathie du diabétique traité par pompe à insuline intrapéritonéale. *J. Fr. Ophthalmol., 8,* 449.
123. Beck-Nielsen H, Richelsen B, Mogensen CE et al (1985): Effect of insulin pump treatment for one year on retinal function and retinal morphology in patients with IDDM. *Diabetes Care, 8,* 585.
124. Olsen T, Ehlers N, Nielsen CB, Beck-Nielsen H (1985): Diabetic retinopathy after one year of improved metabolic control obtained by continuous subcutaneous insulin infusion (CSII). *Acta Ophthalmol., 63,* 315.
125. Bell PM, Hayes GR, Hadden DR, Archer DB (1985): The effect of plasma glucose control by continuous subcutaneous insulin infusion or conventional therapy on retinal morphology and urinary albumin excretion. *Diabète Métab., 11,* 254.
126. Kelly TM, Sanborn GE, Haug PJ, Edwards CQ (1984): Effect of insulin infusion pump use on diabetic retinopathy. *Arch. Ophthalmol., 102,* 1156.
127. Lauritzen T, Frost-Larsen K, Larsen H-W, Deckert T, and The Steno Study Group (1985): Two years experience with continuous subcutaneous insulin infusion in relation to retinopathy and nephropathy. *Diabetes, 34, Suppl. 3,* 74.
128. Dahl-Jorgensen K, Brinchmann-Hansen O, Hanssen K et al (1986): Effect of near normoglycaemia for two years on progression of early diabetic retinopathy, nephropathy and neuropathy: The Oslo Study. *Br. Med. J., 293,* 1195.
129. Hanssen K, Dahl-Jorgensen K, Lauritzen T et al (1986): Diabetic control and microvascular complications: the near normoglycaemic experience. *Diabetologia, 29,* 677.
130. The Kroc Collaborative Study Group (1985): Effect of diabetic control on retinopathy: follow-up report of the Kroc randomised clinical trial. *Invest. Ophthalmol. Visual Sci., 26, Suppl. 1,* 85.
131. Group d'Etude DAMAD (1982): Protocol général. *Diabète Métab., 8,* 91.
132. Group d'Etude DAMAD (1982): Protocol ophtalmologique. *Diabète Métab., 8,* 307.
133. The DAMAD Study Group (1987): The effect of aspirin alone and aspirin and di-

pyridamole in early diabetic retinopathy: a randomised controlled clinical study. In preparation.

134. Camerini-Davalos RA, Velasco C, Glasser M, Bloodworth Jr JMB (1983): Drug-induced reversal of early diabetic microangiopathy. *N. Engl. J. Med., 309,* 1551.
135. Benarroch IS, Brodsky M, Rubenstein A (1985): Treatment of blood hyperviscosity with calcium dobesilate in patients with diabetic retinopathy. *Ophthalmic Res., 17,* 131.
136. Vojnikovic B (1984): Hyperviscosity in whole blood, plasma, and aqueous humor decreased by doxium (calcium dobesilate) in diabetics with retinopathy and glaucoma: a double-blind controlled study. *Ophthalmic Res., 16,* 150.
137. Adank C, Koerner F (1985): Calcium dobesilate in diabetic retinopathy: a retrospective controlled study. *Ophthalmologica, 190,* 102.
138. Robinson Jr WG, Kador PF, Kinoshita JH (1983): Retinal capillaries: basement membrane thickening by galactosemia prevented with aldose reductase inhibitor. *Science, 221,* 1177.
139. Robinson Jr WG, Kador PF, Akagi Y (1986): Prevention of basement membrane thickening in retinal capillaries by a novel inhibitor of aldose reductase, tolrestat. *Diabetes, 35,* 295.
140. Kojima K, Matsubara H, Harada T (1985): Effects of aldose reductase inhibitor on retinal microangiopathy in streptozotocin-diabetic rats. *Jpn. J. Ophthalmol., 29,* 99.
141. MacGregor LC, Matschinsky FM (1985): Treatment with aldose reductase inhibitor or with myoinositol arrests deterioration of the electroretinogram of diabetic rats. *J. Clin. Invest., 76,* 887.
142. Cogan DG, Kinoshita JH, Kador PF (1984): Aldose reductase and complications of diabetes. *Ann. Intern. Med., 101,* 82.
143. The Diabetic Retinopathy Study Research Groups (1976): Preliminary report on effects of photocoagulation therapy. *Am. J. Ophthalmol., 81,* 383.
144. The Diabetic Retinopathy Study Research Group (1979): Four risk factors for severe visual loss in diabetic retinopathy. *Arch. Ophthalmol., 97,* 654.
145. British Multicentre Study Group (1984): Photocoagulation for proliferative diabetic retinopathy: randomised controlled clinical trial using the xenon arc. *Diabetologia, 26,* 109.
146. British Multicentre Study Group (1983): Photocoagulation for diabetic maculopathy: a randomised controlled clinical trial using the xenon arc. *Diabetes, 32,* 1010.
147. Early Treatment of Diabetic Retinopathy Study Research Group (1985): Photocoagulation for diabetic macular oedema. *Arch. Ophthalmol., 103,* 1796.
148. Gaudric A, Ramioul E, Chaine G, Coscas G (1984): Traitement de l'oedème maculaire cystoïde diabétique par photocoagulation au laser à argon. *J. Fr. Ophtalmol., 7,*
149. McDonald HR, Schatz H (1985): Grid photocoagulation for diffuse macular oedema. *Retina, 5,* 65.
150. Segal A, Ducasse A (1985): Evaluation of argon laser photocoagulation of the posterior pole in oedematous diabetic retinopathy. *Ophthalmologica, 191,* 139.
151. Patz A, Rice TA, Murphy RP et al (1985): Photocoagulation for diabetic macular oedema. *Arch. Ophthalmol., 103,* 1796.
152. Little HL (1985): Treatment of proliferative diabetic retinopathy: long-term results of argon laser photocoagulation. *Ophthalmology, 92,* 279.
153. Okun E, Johnston P, Boniuk I, et al (1984): Xenon arc photocoagulation of proliferative diabetic retinopathy: a review of 2688 consecutive eyes in the format of the Diabetic Retinopathy Study. *Ophthalmology, 91,* 1458.
154. Rand LI, Prud'homme GJ, Ederer F, Canner PL (1985): Factors influencing the development of visual loss in advanced diabetic retinopathy: Diabetic Retinopathy Study (DRS) report No. 10. *Invest. Ophthalmol. Visual Sci., 26,* 983.
155. Liang JC, Fishman GA, Huamonte FU, Anderson RJ (1983): Comparative electroretinograms in argon laser and xenon arc panretinal photocoagulation. *Br. J. Ophthalmol., 67,* 520.

156. Doft BH, Blankenship G (1984): Retinopathy risk factor regression after laser panretinal photocoagulation for proliferative diabetic retinopathy. *Ophthalmology, 91,* 1453.
157. Vine AK (1985): The efficacy of additional argon laser photocoagulation for the persistent, severe proliferative diabetic retinopathy. *Ophthalmology, 92,* 1532.
158. Higgins KE, Myers SM, Jaffe MJ et al (1986): Temporary loss of foveal contrast sensitivity associated with panretinal photocoagulation. *Arch. Ophthalmol., 104,* 997.
159. Shapiro A, Tso MOM, Goldberg MF (1984): Argon laser-induced cataract: a clinicopathologic study. *Arch. Ophthalmol., 102,* 579.
160. Wallow I, Johns K, Barrie P et al (1985): Chorioretinal and choriovitreal neovascularisation after photocoagulation for proliferative diabetic retinopathy: clinicopathologic correlation. *Ophthalmology, 92,* 523.
161. Lobes Jr LA, Bourgon P (1985): Pupillary abnormalities induced by argon laser photo-coagulation. *Ophthalmology, 92,* 234.
162. McDonald HR, Schatz H (1985): Visual loss following panretinal photocoagulation for proliferative diabetic retinopathy. *Ophthalmology, 92,* 388.
163. Kohner EM, McLeod D, Marshall J (1982): Diabetic eye disease. In: Keen H, Jarrett J (Eds), Arnold, London. *Complications of Diabetes,* p. 19.
164. Schepens CL, Avila MP, Jalkh AE, Trempe CL (1984): Role of the vitreous in cystoid macular oedema. *Surv. Ophthalmol., 28,* 499.
165. Tagawa H, McMeel W, Furukawa H et al (1986): Vitreous changes in diabetic retinopathy and physiologic ageing. *Ophthalmology, 93,* 596.
166. Shea M (1983): Early vitrectomy in proliferative diabetic retinopathy. *Arch. Ophthalmol., 101,* 1204.
167. Ratner CM, Michels RG, Auer C, Rice CA (1983): Pars plana vitrectomy for complicated retinal detachments. *Ophthalmology, 90,* 1323.
168. Rice TA, De Bustros S, Michels RG et al (1986): Prognostic factors in vitrectomy for epiretinal membranes of the macula. *Ophthalmology, 93,* 602.
169. Novak MA, Rice TA, Michels RG, Auer C (1984): Vitreous haemorrhage after vitrectomy for diabetic retinopathy. *Ophthalmology, 91,* 1485.
170. Ficher LA, Passani P, Leaver PK, McLeod D (1986): Xenon arc endophotocoagulation during vitrectomy for diabetic vitreous haemorrhage. *Graefe's Arch. Clin. Exp. Ophthalmol., 224,* 423.
171. De Bustros S, Glaser BM, Michels RG, Auer C (1985): Effect of epsilon-aminocaproic acid on postvitrectomy haemorrhage. *Arch. Ophthalmol., 103,* 219.
172. Thompson JT, Glaser BM, Michels RG, De Bustros S (1986): The use of intravitreal thrombin to control haemorrhage during vitrectomy. *Ophthalmology, 93,* 279.
173. Kramptz-Glass G, Laqua H (1986): Pars-plana-Vitrectomie bei der proliferativen diabetischen Retinopathie. *Klin. Mbl. Augenheilkd., 188,* 283.
174. Klein R, Klein BEK, Moss SE et al (1984): The Wisconsin epidemiologic study of diabetic retinopathy: Prevalence and risk of diabetic retinopathy when age at diagnosis is less than 30 years. *Arch. Ophthalmol., 102,* 520.
175. Middleton D, Johnston PB, Gillespie EL (1985): HLA-DR antigen association with proliferative diabetic retinopathy. *Int. Ophthalmol., 8,* 33.
176. Saari KM (1984): Diabetes mellitus and diabetic retinopathy. *Acta Ophthalmol., 62,* 98.
177. Scheinin T, Groop L, Teir H (1985): HLA-types and insulin responses in insulin dependent diabetics with or without proliferative retinopathy. *J. Clin. Lab. Immunol., 18,* 17.
178. Rand LI, Krolewuski AS, Aiello LM (1985): Multiple factors in the prediction of risk of proliferative diabetic retinopathy. *N. Engl. J. Med., 313,* 1433.
179. Malone JI, Grizzard WS, Espinoza LR et al (1984): Risk factors for diabetic retinopathy in youth. *Pediatrics, 73,* 756.

180. Mijovic C, Fletcher J, Bradwell AR et al (1985): Relation of gene expression (allotypes) of the fourth component of complement to insulin dependent diabetes and its microangiopathic complications. *Br. Med. J., 291,* 9.
181. Klein R, Klein BEK, Moss SE, DeMets DL (1985): Blood pressure and hypertension in diabetes. *Am. J. Epidemiol., 122,* 75.
182. Constable IJ, Knuiman MW, Welborn TA (1984): Assessing the risk of diabetic retinopathy. *Am. J. Ophthalmol., 97,* 53.
183. Walker JM, Cove DH, Beevers DG (1985): Cigarette smoking, blood pressure and the control of blood glucose in the development of diabetic retinopathy. *Diabetes Res., 2,* 183.
184. Vigstrup J, Mogensen CE (1985): Proliferative diabetic retinopathy: at risk patients identified by early detection of microalbuminuria. *Acta Ophthalmol., 63,* 530.
185. Sjolie AK (1985): Blood pressure and retinopathy in insulin treated diabetic patients with early onset: an epidemiological study. *Acta Ophthalmol., 63, Suppl. 173,* 48.
186. Chahal PS, Ingelsby DV, Sleightholm MA, Kohner EM (1985): The effect of blood pressure on the progression of diabetic retinopathy. *Hypertension, 7, Suppl. 2,* 1.
187. Klein BEK, Klein R (1984): Gravidity and diabetic retinopathy. *Am. J. Epidemiol., 119,* 564.
188. Phelps RL, Sakol P, Metzger BE et al (1986): Changes in diabetic retinopathy during pregnancy: correlation with regulation of hyperglycaemia. *Arch. Ophthalmol., 104,* 1806.
189. Soubrane G, Canivet J, Coscas G (1985): Influence of pregnancy on the evolution of background retinopathy: preliminary results of a prospective fluorescein angiography study. *Int. Ophthalmol., 8,* 249.
190. Price JH, Hadden DR, Archer DB, Harley JMcDG (1984): Diabetic retinopathy in pregnancy. *Br. J. Obstet. Gynaecol., 91,* 11.
191. Klein R, Klein BEK, Davis MD (1983): Is cigarette smoking associated with diabetic retinopathy? *Am. J. Epidemiol., 118,* 228.
192. Young RJ, McGulloch DK, Prescott RJ, Clarke BF (1984): Alcohol: another risk factor for diabetic retinopathy? *Br. Med. J., 288,* 1035.
193. Deckert T (1986): Personal communication.
194. Klein BEK, Klein R, Moss SE (1985): Prevalence of cataracts in a population-based study of persons with diabetes mellitus. *Ophthalmology, 92,* 1191.
195. Sharp PS, Fallon TJ, Kohner EM et al (1987): Long term follow up of patients with proliferative retinopathy who were treated with ^{90}Y pituitary implantation. *Diabetologia,* in press.
196. Lundbaek K, Christensen NJ, Jensen Va et al (1970): Diabetes diabetic angiopathy and growth hormone. *Lancet, 2,* 131.
197. Imaki T, Shibasaki T, Masuda A et al (1986): The effect of glucose and free fatty acids on growth hormone (GH releasing factor mediated GH secretion in rats). *J. Clin. Endocrinol. Metab., 63,* 2390.
198. Chiodera P, Coiro V, Speroni G et al (1984): The growth hormone response to TRH in insulin dependent diabetics involves a cholinergic mechanism. *J. Clin. Endocrinol. Metab., 59,* 794.
199. Cassar J, Edwards R, Mashiter K, Kohner EM (1975): Bromocriptine and serum growth hormone levels in diabetes mellitus. *Lancet, 2,* 181.
200. Sonksen P, Srivastava MC, Tompkins CV, Nabarro JDN (1972): Growth hormone and cortisol responses to insulin infusion in patients with diabetes mellitus. *Lancet, 2,* 155.
201. Sharp PS, Foley K, Chahal P, Kohner EM (1984): The effect of plasma glucose on the growth hormone releasing factor in normal subjects. *Clin. Endocrinol., 20,* 497.
202. Sharp PS, Foley K, Kohner EM (1984): Evidence for a central abnormality in the regulation of growth hormone secretion in insulin dependent diabetes. *Diabetic Med., 1,* 205.

203. Harris M, Prout BJ (1970): Relative hypoglycaemia. *Lancet, 2,* 317.
204. Brooks DJ, Gibbs JSR, Sharp HS et al (1986): Regional cerebral glucose transport in insulin dependent diabetic subjects studied using ^{11}C-3-O-methyl-d-glucose and positron emission tomography. *J. Cereb. Blood Flow Metab., 6,* 240.
205. Winter RJ, Phillips LS, Klein MN et al (1979): Somatomedin activity and diabetic control in children with insulin-dependent diabetes. *Diabetes, 28,* 952.
206. Blethen SL, Sargeant DT, Whitlow MG, Santiago JV (1981): Effect of pubertal stage and recent blood glucose control on plasma somatomedin-C in children with insulin dependent diabetes mellitus. *Diabetes, 30,* 868.
207. Clemmons DR, Klibanski A, Underwood LE et al (1981): Reduction of plasma immunoreactive somatomedin-C during fasting in humans. *J. Clin. Endocrinol. Metab., 53,* 1247.
208. Lanes R, Recker B, Fort B, Lifshitz F (1985): Impaired somatomedin generation test in children with insulin-dependent diabetes mellitus. *Diabetes, 34,* 156.
209. Bauer W, Briner U, Doepfner W et al (1982): SMS 201-995: a very potent and selective octapeptide analogue of somatostatin with prolonged action. *Life Sci., 31,* 1133.
210. Spinas GA, Bock A, Weller U (1985): Reduced post prandial hyperglycaemia after subcutaneous injection of somatostatin analogue (SMS 201-995) in insulin dependent diabetes mellitus. *Diabetes Care, 8,* 429.
211. Davies RR, Miller M, Turner SJ et al (1986): Effects of somatostatin analogue SMS 201-995 in insulin dependent diabetes. *Clin. Endocrinol., 25,* 739.
212. Michaelson IC (1948): The mode of development of the vascular system of the retina. *Trans. Ophthal. Soc. UK, 68,* 137.
213. Copeland KC, Underwood LE, Van Wyk JJ (1980): Modulation of immunoreactive somatomedin-C in human serum by growth hormone: dose, response, relationships and effect on chromatographic profiles. *J. Clin. Endocrinol. Metab., 50,* 690.
214. Merimee TJ, Zapf J, Froesch ER (1983): Insulin-like growth factors: studies in diabetics with and without retinopathy. *N. Engl. J. Med., 309,* 527.
215. Ashton IK, Dornan TL, Pocock AF et al (1983): Plasma somatomedin activity and diabetic retinopathy. *Clin. Endocrinol., 19,* 105.
216. Lamberton PR, Goodman AD, Kasoff A et al (1984): Von Willebrand factor, fibronectin and insulin-like growth factors I and II in diabetic retinopathy and nephropathy. *Diabetes, 33,* 125.
217. Underwood LE, D'Ercole AJ, Clemmons DR, Van Wyk JJ (1986): Paracrine functions of the somatomedins. *Clin. Endocrinol. Metab., 15,* 59.
218. Grant M, Russel B, Fitzgerald C, Merimee TJ (1986): Insulin-like growth factors in the vitreous: studies in control and diabetic subjects with neovascularisation. *Diabetes, 35,* 416.
219. Tamborlane WV, Hintz RL, Bergman M et al (1981): Insulin infusion pump treatment of diabetics: influence of improved metabolic control on plasma somatomedin levels. *N. Engl. J. Med , 305,* 303.
220. Gospodarowicz D (1984): Brain and pituitary fibroblast growth factors. In: Li CH (Ed.), In: *Hormonal Proteins and Peptides: Growth Factors, Vol. 12,* p. 205. Academic Press, London-New York.
221. Baird A, Culler F, Jones KL, Guillemin R (1985): Angiogenic factor in human ocular fluid. *Lancet, 2,* 563.

The Diabetes Annual/3
K.G.M.M. Alberti and L.P. Krall, editors
© 1987 Elsevier Science Publishers, B.V.

16 Autonomic neuropathy

D.J. HOSKING

Introduction

In the last few years the introduction of new techniques has considerably expanded the scope for the investigation of autonomic function. As a consequence a clearer picture is emerging of the pathophysiological basis of the
major clinical syndromes. This is of great importance because it offers the possibility of more rationally based therapy in an area where too often treatment is
empirical and ineffective.

The well-established cardiovascular reflexes remain ever popular and while a
few continue to reanalyse their growing experience or search for the Holy Grail
of the 'best test', others have been more imaginative. In particular their use as
a standard by which to evaluate new tests of previously inaccessible sites in the
autonomic nervous system has been widely utilised and has made it possible to
build up a picture of the pattern in which the autonomic nervous system becomes affected by diabetes. In addition, these tests lend themselves to the preliminary assessment of newer therapies for diabetic neuropathy.

Natural history of diabetic autonomic neuropathy

It has been known for some time that the autonomic nervous system is involved
early in the course of diabetes. A recent study (1) showing that parasympathetic
cardiovascular reflexes were abnormal in 9 out of 12 patients with Type I diabetes (IDDM) within 2 years of diagnosis and in 12 out of 17 patients who had
Type II diabetes (NIDDM) for 1 year was primarily of interest because of the
picture it gave of the pattern of damage in early autonomic neuropathy. Pupillary reflexes were also studied in the same patients and because the mean value
was decreased it was suggested that there was a diffuse involvement of the autonomic nervous system. Since over half the patients had normal pupillary reflexes (but most would have had abnormal cardiovascular reflexes), the main
message seemed to be that such involvement is very patchy.

The use of cardiovascular reflexes as a 'gold standard' by which to assess
other aspects of autonomic function was illustrated by a study of neuroendo-

crine function in diabetic patients (2). Use was made of the observation that the first 15-20 minutes of the pancreatic polypeptide (PP) response to a meal is dependent on the presence of an intact vagus. In addition, the noradrenaline response to intravenous edrophonium, which is dependent on sympathetic integrity, was also tested. In normal subjects or diabetic patients with intact cardiovascular reflexes (heart rate response to deep breathing, standing and the Valsalva manoeuvre and the blood pressure response to posture and sustained hand grip) (3), noradrenaline increased by 70% within 2-6 minutes after 10 mg of edrophonium (Tensilon). A similar response was seen in the 4 diabetic subjects with parasympathetic damage, but there was no rise in those with sympathetic (and parasympathetic) dysfunction. Conversely, those diabetic patients with parasympathetic damage ($\pm$sympathetic neuropathy) failed to show an increase in PP after a standard meal. The normal subjects and the diabetic patients without neuropathy showed increases of up to 400% within 6 minutes of eating.

These tests are useful indicators of autonomic neuropathy extending beyond the cardiovascular system. While this may be due to the diffuse nature of diabetic neuropathy as the authors suggested, this can only be proved by more extensive testing. However, the range of potential tests is now so vast that it is difficult to imagine anyone with enough stamina to be so investigated.

That the autonomic nervous system may not be uniformly involved by neuropathy was shown by a study (also from the Edinburgh group) where diabetic subjects with varying degrees of peripheral neuropathy (new painful, chronic painful and recurrent foot ulcers) were compared with a group without clinical evidence of neuropathy (4). Each group was similar with respect to age, duration and type of diabetes. Although sensory nerve conduction velocities showed a progressively more severe impairment (new painful < chronic painful < foot ulcers), each of these groups had a comparable degree of autonomic neuropathy. This suggested that large-fibre (myelinated) sensorimotor neuropathy may not necessarily occur in parallel with small-fibre (unmyelinated) damage and that different factors may be involved in determining the site and extent of the neuropathy. Another function of cardiovascular reflexes is to try to use them to predict who will progress to symptomatic autonomic neuropathy. In a re-assessment of patients after a 6-year interval, the initial mean values for heart rate variability and the response to tilting were lower in those who subsequently developed symptoms (5). Unfortunately, the degree of overlap between those who did and those who did not progress to a symptomatic stage was so great that measurements in an individual have no predictive value.

There does seem, however, to be general agreement that spontaneous improvement in autonomic neuropathy is uncommon. Sequential testing (3) showed that most subjects either remain static (71%) or get worse (26%). The relative proportion of these groups depends on the interval between testing. The preponderance of the former probably reflects the relatively short (about 3 months) interval between tests in some patients in this particular study. Abnormalities of those tests which measure heart rate responses (parasympathetic function) antedate those which measure blood pressure (sympathetic function) and this has been general experience. Again the patchy nature of the involvement, or alternatively the lack of quantitative relationships between individual tests, was shown by the failure of heart rate variability to distinguish between those with different degrees of severity of cardiovascular neuropathy.

Pathology

Characterisation of the pathological basis of autonomic neuropathy is severely limited by the lack of availability of human material, particularly during the early phase of damage and by the paucity of reproducible findings at autopsy. The spontaneously diabetic BB rat provides a good model for IDDM and has the added advantage that it develops symptomatic autonomic neuropathy (diarrhoea, colonic dilatation and urinary retention).

In the vagus nerve (predominantly unmyelinated preganglionic fibres) and the penile nerve (myelinated postganglionic, cholinergic and VIP-containing fibres) degenerative changes develop in axons which increase in frequency with the duration of diabetes (6). The main features include glycogenosome accumulation and sequestration of membrane-bound axonal material and are indicative of a primary axonal process with secondary changes in myelin and Schwann cells. Thes changes were similar to those seen in the peripheral nervous system (7) but different from the dystrophic axons of sympathetic paravertebral ganglia (8). Here the axons were swollen and contained densely packed branching tubular networks (20-40 nm diameter) while others showed stacks or whorls of multilayered membranes or accumulations of electron-dense material mixed with vesicles and filaments. A previously undescribed appearance was that of a branching tubular network with a diameter of 80-100 nm which often enclosed electron-dense material. Again the frequency of these changes increased with the duration of diabetes while their distribution, in close proximity to cells of the sympathetic ganglia, suggested a preganglionic origin. The ganglion cells themselves showed no qualitative change, but there was a decrease in synapse number which correlated with the increasing severity of axonal dystrophy. Postganglionic fibres of the grey ramus showed accumulation of glycogenosomes and axonal sequestration similar to those seen in the parasympathetic nerves. Abnormalities were most prevalent in the prevertebral coeliac ganglion followed, in order, by the mesenteric nerve, the superior cervical ganglion and the paravertebral ganglion (9). The heterogeneity of the parasympathetic and sympathetic axonal changes may indicate a difference in their pathogenesis and might also account for the variation in the time course of appearance of functional abnormality.

Wistar rats after a year of streptozotocin-induced diabetes showed both similarities and differences to the changes seen in the BB rat (10). Neuropathy was most marked in the preganglionic sympathetic axons, although glycogen deposits were seen in all fibre types. The presence of Schwann cell degeneration with a relatively normal axonal appearance implies that the former was the site of primary damage and in this respect resembles the sequence seen in peripheral nerves but differs from that seen in the BB rat. Intracellular abnormalities included changes in the Golgi apparatus, mitochondria and smooth endoplasmic reticulum and are reminiscent of the changes seen in hypoxia.

Response to treatment

Cardiovascular reflexes have been of particular value in the assessment of new forms of treatment for autonomic neuropathy. Much current interest centres on the aldose reductase inhibitors, although other modalities including continuous subcutaneous insulin infusion, somatostatin analogues and acupuncture have also been investigated.

The aldose reductive inhibitor, sorbinil, 250 mg daily for 6 weeks, improved vagal function in a double-blind, placebo-controlled randomised non-crossover trial in diabetic subjects with symptomatic polyneuropathy (11). Autonomic function was assessed from the E/I ratio (longest RR interval after expiration : shortest RR interval after corresponding inspiration) after deep breathing (6 breaths per minute) and from the minimum resting heart rate. Improvement was obtained despite unchanged glycaemic control (assessed from HBA_1), but was poorest in those with the most abnormal cardiovascular reflexes, although isolated cases with symptomatic autonomic neuropathy showed clinical amelioration.

A similar, but longer (6 months), study used sorbinil in the same dosage and found only a small, although significant, benefit (12). No major clinical response was obtained in the sorbinil-treated patients nor was there any improvement in sensory threshold. In 3 of the 9 neurophysiological tests (motor nerve conduction velocity of the posterior tibial nerve, F-wave latency and sensory distal latency of the ulnar nerve) and 1 of 5 autonomic function tests (heart rate variability during deep breathing) there was a significant improvement in the treatment group. However, there was no evidence of a progressive improvement during the treatment period and the benefits were no greater than those reported from shorter trials. As with the previous study, diabetic control remained unchanged (and poor) during sorbinil treatment.

It may be that there is a reversible element to autonomic neuropathy which can be corrected by sorbinil while persistent abnormality reflects the presence of an irreversible component. Alternatively, other factors, e.g. glycosylation of myelin proteins or axonal hypoxia unaffected by sorbinil, may account for the relatively slight improvement to be obtained with this form of treatment.

Animal studies also show evidence of reversible damage in autonomic nerve fibres (13). Using a different aldose reductase inhibitor (Statil; ICI-128436) in rats with 3 weeks of streptozotocin-induced diabetes the defective axonal transport of choline acetyltransferase activity proximal to short-term constrictions in the vagus and sciatic nerves was prevented. Accumulation of sorbitol and fructose was either prevented or reduced, as was the depletion of myoinositol. It may be that this aldose reductase inhibitor corrected abnormal $(Na^+ + K^+)$-ATPase activity which predisposed to impaired myoinositol uptake by the nerve. Although supportive, the relevance of these acute studies to the chronic autonomic neuropathy of man remains uncertain.

CSII has also been used to improve autonomic neuropathy, although the benefit has only been shown with respect to cardiovascular reflexes rather than symptoms. After only 10 days of near-normal blood glucose profiles there was an increase in the Valsalva ratio (14). After a longer period (4-8 months) there was evidence of more widespread benefit as measured by the heart rate response to the Valsalva manoeuvre, posture and deep breathing. However, the improvements were not progressive with prolonged treatment, suggesting that better control had produced a function/metabolic rather than a structural change in the autonomic nervous system.

Another interesting development has been the use of a somatostatin analogue (SMS-201-995) to treat symptomatic autonomic neuropathy (15). In 4 IDDM patients with multiple complications, the drug prevented postprandial hypotension when given in a dose of 0.2-0.4 µg/kg, which has little or no hyperglycaemic effect. Standing blood pressure was also raised, although at this dose 2 patients with gastroparesis experienced abdominal cramps and nausea. The mode of action is uncertain. Insulin is known to reduce blood pressure, but the pressor response was not offset by insulin administration to non-diabetic subjects with postural hypotension. Although an effect mediated through gut peptides remains a possibility, no likely candidate has been identified. Somatostatin and SMS-201-995 decrease splanchnic blood flow (but have no effect on systemic vasoconstriction) and this seems the most plausible explanation for these observations.

Other examples of agents which have been used with success to control specific autonomic symptoms are given in the following sections. Often they are also of theoretical interest because of the insight that they give into possible pathogenetic mechanisms.

Clinical testing of autonomic function

It is now possible to test autonomic function in a wide range of organs and the main problem is to decide what some of these findings mean. Areas of particular importance are the description of the pattern of spread autonomic neuropathy and the mechanism by which the main clinical syndromes are produced.

Gastrointestinal tract

Oesophagus Disordered oesophageal motility is usually asymptomatic (16), but improved manometric techniques have identified changes which appear more specific for diabetic neuropathy (17) than those described in the past. Patients with diabetic neuropathy show multiphasic, multipeaked peristaltic waves which differ from those seen in non-diabetic or diabetic subjects without neuropathy by being more frequently and widely distributed throughout the smooth muscle of the oesophagus as well as being of greater amplitude. Their enhancement by the cholinesterase inhibitor, edrophonium, and abolition by atropine point to the role of vagal denervation. An interesting observation was that depression and anxiety were 4 times more common in patients with disordered oesophageal motility than in those in whom it was normal (18). Moreover, the correlation between disordered motility and the presence of peripheral neuropathy was improved if those with psychiatric symptoms were excluded from analysis. Psychiatric illness may effect autonomic function tests and may make it difficult to identify pathogenetic interrelationships.

Stomach There are still a few reports of gastric secretory activity in diabetics, such as that showing impaired acid and pancreatic polypeptide secretion following sham feeding (19). Most current research, however, centres around the measurement of upper gastrointestinal motility.

A widely used technique is to record the pattern of fasting motility which shows a characteristic appearance termed the 'migrating motor complex' (MMC). This has 4 components, the most important of which is termed 'Phase III activity' which seems to be concerned with emptying the stomach of undigested debris. The MMC seems to be initiated by a surge in the plasma motilin concentration and this relationship has recently been studied in diabetic patients with gastroparesis (20). In these patients plasma motilin levels were increased but showed the expected oscillations in concentration seen in normal subjects. However, antral Phase III activity was absent. Infusion of metoclopramide (10 mg) initiated Phase III activity in both normal subjects and the diabetic patients with gastroparesis. Although plasma motilin level rose in the normal subjects, they fell in the diabetic subjects, raising a question about the relationship between motilin and motility. One explanation for this apparent discrepancy may be that metoclopramide has both cholinergic agonist and dopamine antagonist effects. The former may be more important in normal subjects in stimulating motilin release which then initiates antral Phase III activity. In contrast, in the diabetic patients with gastroparesis the direct dopamine antagonist effect may be the stimulus to Phase III activity which, by emptying the stomach, may relieve gastric distension which is known to be a stimulus to motilin release (21). Isotopic measurements of the solid and liquid components of gastric emptying (22) provide ample evidence of the delay which occurs in gastroparesis and of the acute improvement to be obtained with metoclopramide (23-25) and domperidone (26, 27). The response to long-term therapy is much less consistent in that the acute improvement in solid emptying was reported to be retained at 14 days (25) but lost at 35-51 days (27), although both groups of workers found that the improvement in liquid emptying was sustained. Conversely, the short-term correction of delayed liquid emptying was lost when the patients were retested at 28 days (23), although the emptying of a semisolid meal was still improved at 21 days (24). The techniques used in these studies were very similar and these discrepancies may reflect individual variations in response and severity of the underlying gastroparesis. It is interesting that symptomatic improvement persisted in all studies and this raises the possibility that at least part of the therapeutic benefit from these agents relates to a central effect. However, domperidone was ineffective in improving either objective or subjective features of delayed oesophageal emptying (28).

Intestine   The disordered motility seen in patients with gastroparesis may not be confined to the stomach. It may also involve the upper small intestine (29) where there may be a reduction in the frequency of Phase III activity and long bursts of powerful but non-propagated contractions. The presence of unco-ordinated intestinal motility raises the possibility that there may be an underlying disturbance of both parasympathetic and sympathetic innervation. This is of particular interest because the presence of disordered intestinal motility correlates poorly with the severity of symptoms such as diarrhoea. However, if it was the sympathetic component which was important in the production of diabetic diarrhoea, then this would fit in with the observation that α_2-adrenergic receptors are important in the regulation of fluid and electrolyte transport across the enterocyte (30). It would also be consistent with reports that clonidine (31) and lidamidine (32) which have α_2-adrenergic receptor agonist activity decrease the number of bowel movements and improve the consistency of the stools in diabetic diarrhoea.

   Animal models of diabetic diarrhoea have been particularly useful in identifying possible pathogenetic mechanisms. In chronically diabetic rats with diarrhoea there is impaired fluid and electrolyte absorption in the ileum and colon (but not in jejunum) associated with a decreased noradrenaline content of the mucosa (30). The light-microscopic appearance of the mucosa is normal and these changes, which were not seen in insulin-treated chronically diabetic rats or untreated acute diabetes, could be reproduced in non-diabetic rats by sympathetic denervation with 6-hydroxydopamine, suggesting an important role of impaired enterocyte noradrenergic innervation.

The difference between acute and chronic diabetes in this study raises a question mark over the significance of gut peptide changes in acutely diabetic animals. Rats with diabetes of 10 weeks duration showed increased concentrations of gastric somatostatin and jejunal vasoactive intestinal polypeptide (VIP), while substance P was reduced at both sites (33). In rats which had been diabetic for 8 weeks immunohistochemical studies showed increased amounts of VIP in the nerve fibres and cell bodies of the myenteric plexus of the ileum, and in the circular muscle layer of ileum and proximal colon (34). Total hormone content measured biochemically was also increased at these sites, but substance P appeared histochemically to be unchanged by comparison with control non-diabetic animals. Unfortunately, in these two latter studies intestinal motility was not measured and none of the animals developed diarrhoea. Thus, the pathogenetic significance of these findings is uncertain, particularly when seen in the context of acute rather than chronic diabetes.

Genitourinary system

The range of diagnostic techniques available for the investigation of impotence continues to improve and increase in specificity.

Reduced conduction velocity in the dorsal nerve of the penis, a terminal branch of the pudendal nerve, appears to be an early marker of pelvic neuropathy in IDDM patients with impotence (35). Abnormal conduction can be made more obvious by gently stretching the penis, the dorsal nerve normally being coiled in the flaccid state. In this particular study the latency of the bulbocavernosus reflex was normal, suggesting that this is a later feature of neuropathy which, however, antedated abnormalities of the pudendal-evoked response (36).

Both these studies compared impotent diabetic subjects with potent non-diabetic controls, making it impossible to identify specific neuropathic mechanisms causing diabetic impotence. The inappropriate choice of controls is a recurrent problem in this field.

The multifactorial nature of impotence was illustrated by a study of vascular, neuropathic and psychological function in diabetic subjects with and without impotence (37). Vascular and neuropathic tests were commonly abnormal but failed to discriminate between those with and without impotence. Only the psychological tests (Minnesota Multiphasic Personality Inventory) proved useful in this respect.

In an attempt to make a more physiological assessment of the factors affecting erectile function (38) Bancroft et al (39) in a well-controlled study examined the response to sexual fantasy and erotic films. Changes in penile diameter and penile pulse amplitude in response to sexual fantasy failed to distinguish between organic and psychogenic subgroups. However, the response to film provided good discrimination. As a group, the diabetic patients showed a poorer response than the non-diabetic subjects and this was most obvious in those with other evidence of autonomic neuropathy (abnormal cardiovascular reflexes). Although many of the patients with retinopathy also had neuropathy, the presence of microangiopathy correlated most closely with the impairment of penile blood flow rather than with erectile ability. A comparison with responses obtained during sleep is awaited. This type of study also opens the possibility of its use as the therapeutic manoeuvre in diabetic patients with psychogenic impotence.

Over the last few years there have been several attempts to improve erectile ability by pharmacological means in those who either failed to respond to psychotherapy or in whom organic factors cannot be rectified. The most recent of these (40) describes the use of papaverine (30 mg) and phentolamine (0.5-1.0 mg) injected into the corpus cavernosum. Significant erections were obtained within 10 minutes which increased further during foreplay and intercourse. Satisfactory results were achieved by 59 of 62 patients, many of whom had a significant organic component to their impotence. The erections last about 2 hours and a small subgroup of patients were taught self-injection. Priapism remains an ever-present worry but only developed in 1 case. It does however limit the use of this technique to those with facilities for the management of this complication.

The cost advantage of this approach is very attractive given the considerable expense of penile prostheses. It might also be useful in the preoperative assessment and counselling of those referred for surgery. Postoperatively most patients are satisfied with the result and feel that their preoperative expectations had been fulfilled (41). However, a significant proportion (14%) are disappointed by the operation, perhaps because of unrealistic expectations both by themselves and their partners. This might be avoided by a trial period during which erections are achieved pharmacologically.

Sexual dysfunction in women has received very much less attention than male impotence. Unlike men, sexual dysfunction is not more common in diabetic women (42). Decreased libido is the commonest manifestation while chronic tiredness is the main somatic complaint. In a 6-year study, 64% of IDDM females showed no evidence of sexual dysfunction while 43% of those with symptoms at the outset improved spontaneously (43). The main determinant of sexual problems seemed to be the degree to which diabetes had been accepted. There was no correlation with objective measurements of the severity of diabetes or with the presence of neuropathic or vascular complications. Interesting sidelines of this study were that, not surprisingly, diabetic patients show more emotional disturbances than their non-diabetic spouses, but also underestimate the stress experienced by their non-diabetic partner.

Cardiovascular system

Blood pressure regulation   Hypertension in diabetic patients involves both sodium accumulation and increased cardiovascular reactivity (44). Exchangeable, and by inference total body, sodium is increased by about 10% in diabetic patients with and without hypertension. This is due to enhancement by insulin of renal tubular sodium reabsorption. Since plasma and blood volumes are generally normal or low in diabetic subjects, this suggests that the excess sodium is distributed either in the interstitial space or intracellularly. This may be relevant to the enhanced pressor response to noradrenaline and angiotensin II which occurs in both normotensive and hypertensive diabetic patients. This increased responsiveness appears independent of age, type of antidiabetic treatment or the presence of retinopathy and neuropathy. Its cause is uncertain. Sodium retention increases angiotensin II receptor affinity and although thiazide diuretics reduce both exchangeable sodium and blood pressure, they do not diminish the sensitivity to angiotensin II. Other possible explanations include thickening of blood vessels, particularly resistance vessels or changes in the efferent renal arterioles and juxtaglomerular apparatus. The development of sodium retention and cardiovascular hyperreactivity in normotensive diabetic patients may be an important factor in predisposing them to the subsequent development of hypertension.

Although insulin increases cell potassium and the $ICF/ECF\ K^+$, thus potentially altering vascular reactivity, this change appears too transient to affect blood pressure (45). Similarly the interrelationship between insulin administration, catecholamine release and sympathetic nervous system activity is complex but is altered by diabetic neuropathy. Insulin administration increases plasma noradrenaline, which although causing vasoconstriction also leads to venoconstriction, an increase in capillary pressure and a reduction in plasma volume. A fall in blood pressure is prevented by increased sympathetic activity which results in a rate-mediated increase in cardiac output. In diabetic patients with sympathetic neuropathy the attenuated vasoconstrictor response leads to hypotension even though heart rate increases. These changes are exacerbated if the insulin leads to hypoglycaemia because adrenaline secretion will be enhanced with consequent vasodilatation. Although these mechanisms have been extensively described in the past, they are well reviewed in a recent supplement to *Hypertension* (46).

The role of dopaminergic receptors in blood pressure control has recently been explored using the dopamine receptor antagonist, metoclopramide (47). A dose of 20 mg i.v. given to diabetic patients with postural hypotension improved the degree of tilt which could be tolerated and reduced the fall in mean arterial pressure which had previously accompanied this manoeuvre. This improvement was due to an increase in total peripheral resistance and not cardiac output. Metoclopramide also produced a modest improvement in the plasma renin activity in response to tilting (consistent with the known action of dopamine to inhibit renin release), although plasma aldosterone levels were unchanged. Vasoconstriction and heart rate responses to the cold pressor test were also improved in these diabetic patients. Metoclopramide may improve vasoconstrictor tone by an effect on the specific parasympathetic dopamine receptors which inhibit noradrenaline output by nerve terminals. The fact that increments in plasma catecholamine activity have not been found under these circumstances may not exclude this hypothesis since plasma levels are a small and variable reflection of total sympathetic activity.

Another interesting facet of blood pressure regulation affected by autonomic neuropathy is the antidiuretic hormone (ADH) response to volume contraction (48). In diabetic patients with abnormal heart rate responses (to deep breathing, the Valsalva manoeuvre and posture) who were acutely volume-depleted with intravenous frusemide, ADH release was not stimulated in response to tilting as it was in diabetic patients with intact cardiovascular reflexes. An intact renin-angiotensin system is needed for the maximum ADH response to volume depletion. However, this was not the explanation for the abnormal responses in this study because both groups of diabetic patients achieved similar levels of plasma renin activity and aldosterone after tilting. The findings are consistent with a diabetic vagal neuropathy impairing the role of low pressure cardiac (atrial) receptors in modulating the ADH response to volume depletion.

All these studies fit nicely together and give a reasonably consistent picture of the complex set of neuroendocrine changes which are involved in blood pressure regulation and which may be threatened by the development of diabetic autonomic neuropathy.

Counterregulation (see also The Diabetes Annual/2, Chapter 18)

Hypoglycaemia stimulates both neural and humoural defense mechanisms, but the relative importance of these two components is uncertain. Glucagon secretion and β-adrenergic stimulation are known to be important and their roles were assessed in baboons with 2-deoxy-D-glucose induced hypoglycaemia (49). The glucagon response was blocked by a somatostatin infusion while β-adrenergic blockade was maintained with propranolol. Use of either of these agents alone did not prevent the recovery of plasma glucose from hypoglycaemia. However, their use in combination had a profound effect in reducing the recovery of glucose to 15% of that seen in control experiments.

These observations are, of course, consistent with clinical experience which shows that most insulin-dependent diabetic patients have impaired or absent glucagon responses to hypoglycaemia even after prolonged optimal treatment. As a consequence, their recovery from hypoglycaemia depends upon β-adrenergic mechanisms which are easily opposed by β-blocker therapy for angina or hypertension. Moreover, catecholamine responses to hypoglycaemia may assume a greater importance under these circumstances, but may themselves be significantly impaired by autonomic neuropathy. In a study comparing normal with diabetic subjects both with and without abnormal cardiovascular reflexes, the latter group showed greatly reduced adrenaline and noradrenaline responses to insulin-induced hypoglycaemia (50). The changes in adrenaline secretion were quite striking and were associated with a delayed blood glucose recovery. As expected, the glucagon responses were subnormal in both diabetic groups, although growth hormone and cortisol increased to the same level as that seen in control subjects. Thus, not only will blood sugar recovery be slowed by the presence of autonomic neuropathy but the warning clinical manifestations are also likely to be absent. In such studies it is important to take care over age-matching (as was done in the above study) because noradrenaline, but not adrenaline, responses to stress are increased in the elderly. Essentially similar findings were reported from a more recent study (51), with the additional information that somatostatin responses to hypoglycaemia were lost in diabetic patients with a sympathetic autonomic neuropathy. Strangely, the blood glucose responses were no different between those with and without neuropathy.

Pupillary reflexes

The great attraction of pupillary reflexes is that they are easily accessible. Since dilatation is a sympathetic function, they usefully complement cardiovascular reflexes such as heart rate variability which are parasympathetically mediated. Measurement is relatively easy and one option is to use a polaroid camera with a hood over the patient's head to achieve total darkness (52). This both dilates the pupils and avoids any element of pupillary contraction due to accommodation. Measurements are unaffected by different degrees of light adaption due to variations in illumination of the surroundings. Pupil and iris diameters are both functions of age, but expressing the former as a percentage of the latter reduces the variance and also makes the measurement independent of photographic magnification. Age is still an important variable, but it is relatively easy to construct a normal range.

It is interesting that in the pupil damage to sympathetic fibres precedes that to the parasympathetic fibres and as such is the reverse of that generally seen in the cardiovascular system and elsewhere. Nerve terminals innervating the dilator muscle showed mitochondrial abnormalies, dense bodies and lamellar accumulations while no such changes were seen in the corresponding nerve terminals to the sphincter muscle (53). The mechanism responsible for this damage is disputed. The observation of an association between iritis and autonomic neuropathy was used to suggest an autoimmune basis for the nerve damage

(54). However, this was refuted by another large survey which found no predisposition of diabetic patients with autonomic neuropathy to develop iritis (55). There may be something special about the pupil and this may be a useful area of future investigation.

The eye also allows direct evaluation of the effect of sympathetic stimulation on the retinal vasculature. Using a non-invasive ophthalmodynamometric technique to measure changes in retinal artery blood pressure in response to the cold pressor test, a recent study raised intriguing questions about the relationship between autonomic neuropathy and retinopathy (56). In IDDM patients, retinal artery pressure rose after cold pressor testing. This was not seen in non-diabetic controls or in 4 diabetic subjects with autonomic neuropathy, none of whom had retinopathy. However, there was one diabetic with both autonomic neuropathy and retinopathy and in this patient retinal artery pressures did rise after the cold pressor test. Hypertension and raised retinal artery pressure are known to be contributors to the development of diabetic retinopathy and these findings raise the interesting question as to whether autonomic neuropathy, in some circumstances, may be protective by limiting retinal artery hypertension.

Breathing

Ventilatory reflexes have also aroused considerable attention both because they are relatively easy to measure and because they may be implicated in the sudden death which may occur in those with advanced autonomic neuropathy.

In the last year two studies have compared the ventilatory response to hypercapnia and hypoxia in normal control subjects and diabetic patients with and without autonomic neuropathy. In the earlier study, impaired responses to hypoxia and hypercapnia were found in both diabetic groups, although these abnormalities were more marked in those with neuropathy (57). In a later study the responses to hyperoxic hypercapnia were normal in both diabetic groups, although the hypoxic drive to breathing was impaired in those with autonomic neuropathy (58). In fact, 5 of the 8 diabetics in this group had lost their ventilatory drive and responses to hypoxia. These findings complement a third study which examined breathing patterns during sleep, which is the time when sudden death may occur. Abnormalities which included central or obstructive sleep apnoea and brief breathing irregularities during Stage III and IV non-REM sleep were more common in IDDM patients with abnormal cardiovascular reflexes (59). A worrying practical implication of these finding was that those with abnormal breathing patterns during sleep could not be identified by their ventilatory responses while awake.

Conclusions

Several encouraging trends are apparent in the study of autonomic neuropathy. Investigation of the pathophysiological basis of the major clinical syndromes has received a considerable boost by technological advances. This has been coupled with a growing appreciation of the relationship between the autonomic nervous system and a wide range of neuroendocrine responses. Not only does this expand the breadth of investigation, but it also allows replacement of older invasive tests by ones which are both more acceptable to patients while being more specific. Unfortunately this does bring new problems to the fore. The ramifications of this system are so complex that great care must be exercised to avoid triggering homeostatic responses which distort apparently straightforward experiments.

Asked why he always robbed banks, the American Sutton was reputed to answer 'because that's where the money is'. A combination of heart rate variability and supposition is no substitute for a vigorous application of Sutton's Law in terms of specific investigations in the study of symptomatic autonomic neuropathy.

References

1. Pfeifer MA, Weinberg CR, Cook DL et al (1984): Autonomic neural dysfunction in recently diagnosed diabetic subjects. *Diabetes Care, 7,* 447.
2. Ewing DJ, Bellavere F, Espi E et al (1986): Correlation of cardiovascular and neuroendocrine tests of autonomic function in diabetes. *Metab. Clin. Exp., 35,* 349.
3. Ewing DJ, Martyn CN, Young RJ et al (1985): The value of cardiovascular autonomic function tests: 10 years experience in diabetes. *Diabetes Care, 8,* 491.
4. Young RJ, Zhou YO, Rodriguez E et al (1986): Variable relationship between peripheral somatic and autonomic neuropathy in patients with different syndromes of diabetic polyneuropathy. *Diabetes, 35,* 192.
5. Sundkvist G, Lilja B (1985): Autonomic neuropathy in diabetes mellitus: a follow up study. *Diabetes Care, 8,* 129.
6. Yagihashi S, Sima AAF (1986): Diabetic autonomic neuropathy in the BB rat: ultrastructural and morphometric changes in parasympathetic nerves. *Diabetes, 35,* 733.
7. Sima AAF, Bouchier M, Christensen H (1983): Axonal atrophy in sensory nerves of the diabetic BB Wistar rat: a possible early correlate to human diabetic neuropathy. *Ann. Neurol., 13,* 264.
8. Yagihashi S, Sima AAF (1985): Diabetic autonomic neuropathy in the BB rat: ultrastructural and morphometric changes in the sympathetic nerves. *Diabetes, 34,* 558.
9. Yagihashi S, Sima AAF (1985): Diabetic autonomic neuropathy: the distribution of structural changes in sympathetic nerves in the BB rat. *Am. J. Pathol., 121,* 138.
10. Kneil PC, Junker U, Perrin IV et al (1986): Varied effects of experimental diabetes on the autonomic nervous system of the rat. *Lab. Invest., 54,* 523.
11. Jaspan JB, Towle VL, Maselli R et al (1986): Clinical studies with an aldose reductase inhibitor in the autonomic and somatic neuropathies of diabetes. *Metab. Clin. Exp., 35, Suppl.,* 83.

12. Fagius J, Brattenberg A, Jameson S et al (1985): Limited benefit of treatment of diabetic polyneuropathy with an aldose reductase inhibitor: a 24 week controlled trial. *Diabetologica, 28,* 323.
13. Tomlinson DR, Townsend J, Fretten P (1985): Prevention of defective axonal transport in streptozotocin diabetic rats by treatment with 'Statil' (ICI 128436), an aldose reductase inhibitor. *Diabetes, 34,* 970.
14. Fedele D, Bellavere F, Cardone C et al (1985): Improvement of cardiovascular autonomic reflexes after amelioration of metabolic control in insulin dependent diabetic subjects with severe autonomic neuropathy. *Horm. Metab. Res., 17,* 410.
15. Hoeldtke RD, O'Dorisio TM, Boden G (1986): Treatment of autonomic neuropathy with a somatostatin analogue SMS-201-995. *Lancet, 2,* 602.
16. Channer KS, Jackson PC, O'Brien I et al (1985): Oesophageal function in diabetes mellitus and its association with autonomic neuropathy. *Diabetic Med., 2,* 378.
17. Loo FD, Dodds WJ, Soergel KH et al (1985): Multipeaked oesophageal peristaltic pressure waves in patients with diabetic neuropathy. *Gastroenterology, 88,* 485.
18. Clouse RE, Lustman PJ, Reidel WL (1986): Correlation of oesophageal motility abnormalities with neuropsychiatric status in diabetics. *Gastroenterology, 90,* 1146.
19. Buysschaert M, Donckier J, Dive A et al (1985): Gastric acid and pancreatic polypeptide responses to sham feeding are impaired in diabetic subjects with autonomic neuropathy. *Diabetes, 34,* 1181.
20. Achem-Karam SR, Funakoshi A, Vinik AI et al (1985): Plasma motilin concentration and interdigestive migrating motorcomplex in diabetic gastroparesis: effect of metoclopramide. *Gastroenterology, 88,* 492.
21. Christofides ND, Sarson DL, Albuquerque RH et al (1979): Release of gastrointestinal hormones following an oral water load. *Experientia, 35,* 1521.
22. Horowitz M, Collins PJ, Shearman DJC (1985): Disorders of gastric emptying in humans and the use of radionuclide techniques. *Arch. Intern. Med., 145,* 1467.
23. Schade RR, Dugas MC, Lhotsky DM et al (1985): Effect of metoclopramide on gastric liquid emptying in patients with diabetic gastroparesis. *Dig. Dis. Sci., 30,* 10.
24. Ricci DA, Saltzman MB, Meyer C. et al (1985): Effect of metoclopramide in diabetic gastroparesis. *J. Clin. Gastroenterol., 7,* 25.
25 Wright RA, Clemente R, Wathen R (1985): Diabetic gastroparesis: an abnormality of gastric emptying of solids. *Am. J. Med. Sci., 289,* 240.
26. Watts GF, Armitage M, Sinclair J et al (1985): Treatment of diabetic gastroparesis with oral domperidone. *Diabetic Med., 2,* 491.
27. Horowitz M, Harding PE, Chatterton BE et al (1985): Acute and chronic effects of domperidone on gastric emptying in diabetic autonomic neuropathy. *Dig. Dis. Sci., 30,* 1.
28. Maddern GJ, Horowitz M, Jamieson GG (1985): The effect of domperidone on oesophageal emptying in diabetic autonomic neuropathy. *Br. J. Clin. Pharmacol., 19,* 441.
29. Camilleri M, Malagelada JR (1984): Abnormal intestinal motility in diabetics with the gastroparesis syndrome. *Eur. J. Clin. Invest., 14,* 420.
30. Chang EB, Bergenstal RM, Field M (1985): Diarrhoea in streptozotocin treated rats. *J. Clin. Invest., 75,* 1666.
31. Fedorak RN, Field M, Chang EB (1985): Treatment of diabetic diarrhoea with clonidine. *Ann. Intern. Med., 102,* 97.
32. Goff JS (1984) Diabetic diarrhoea and lidamidine. *Ann. Intern. Med., 101,* 874.
33. Ballman M, Conlon JM (1985): Changes in the somatostatin, substance P and vasoactive intestinal polypeptide content of the gastrointestinal tract following streptozotocin induced diabetes in the rat. *Diabetologia, 28,* 355.
34. Belai A, Lincoln J, Milner P et al (1985): Enteric nerves in diabetic rats: increase in vasoac-

tive intestinal polypeptide but not substance P. *Gastroenterology, 89,* 967.

35. Lin JT, Bradley WE (1985): Penile neuropathy in insulin dependent diabetes mellitus. *J. Urol., 133,* 213.

36. Ertekin C., Akyurekli O, Gurses AN et al (1985): The value of somatosensory evoked potentials and bulbocavernosus reflex in patients with impotence. *Acta Neurol. Scand., 71,* 48.

37. Buvat J., Lemaire A., Buvat-Herbaut M et al (1985): Comparative investigations in 26 impotent and 26 non-impotent diabetic patients. *J. Urol., 133,* 34.

38. Bancroft J, Bell C (1985): Simultaneous recording of penile diameter and penile arterial pulse during laboratory based erotic stimulation in normal subjects. *J. Psychosom. Res., 29,* 303.

39. Bancroft J, Bell C, Ewing DJ et al (1985): Assessment of erectile function in diabetic and non-diabetic impotence by simultaneous recording of penile diameter and penile arterial pulse. *J. Psychosom. Res., 29,* 315.

40. Zorgniotti AW, Lefleur RS (1985): Autoinjection of the corpus cavernosum with a vasoactive drug combination for vasculogenic impotence. *J. Urol., 133,* 39.

41. Peterson HR, Best JD, Berger R et al (1985): Attitudes of diabetic men after implantation of a semi-rigid penile prosthesis. *Diabetes Care, 8,* 156.

42. Jensen SB (1985): Sexual dysfunction in younger insulin treated diabetic females: a comparative study. *Diabète Métabol., 11,* 278.

43. Jensen SB (1986): The natural history of sexual dysfunction in diabetic women: a 6 year follow up study. *Acta Med. Scand., 219,* 73.

44. Weidmann P, Beretta-Piccoli C, Trost BN (1985): Pressure factors and responsiveness in hypertension accompanying diabetes mellitus. *Hypertension, 7, Suppl. II,* 33.

45. Vierhapper H (1985): Effect of exogenous insulin on blood pressure regulation in healthy and diabetic subjects. *Hypertension, 7, Suppl. II,* 49.

46. Weidmann P, Mogensen CE, Ritz E (Eds) (1985) *Diabetes and Hypertension. Proceedings, I International Symposium on Hypertension Associated with Diabetes Mellitus.*

47. Bessa AM, Zanella MT, Saragoca MA et al (1984) Acute haemodynamic and humoral effects of metoclopramide on blood pressure control: improvement in subjects with diabetic orthostatic hypotension. *Clin. Pharmacol. Ther., 36,* 738.

48. Grimaldi A, Pruszczynski W, Thervet F et al (1985) Antidiuretic hormone response to volume depletion in diabetic patients with cardiac autonomic dysfunction. *Clin. Sci., 68,* 545.

49. Asplin CM, Raghu PK, Koerker DJ et al (1985) Glucose counterregulation during recovery from neuroglycopenia: which mechanism is important? *Metab. Clin. Exp., 34,* 15.

50. Horie H, Hanafusa T, Matsuyama T et al (1984) Decreased response of epinephrine and norepinephrine to insulin induced hypoglycaemia in diabetic autonomic neuropathy. *Horm. Metabol. Res., 16,* 398.

51. Fernandez-Castaner M, Webb S, Levy I et al (1985) Somatostatin and counterregulatory hormone responses to hypoglycaemia in diabetics with and without autonomic neuropathy. *Diabète Métabol., 11,* 81.

52. Smith SA, Dewhirst RR (1986) A simple diagnostic test for pupillary abnormality in diabetic autonomic neuropathy. *Diabetic Med., 3,* 38.

53. Ishikawa S, Bensaoula T, Uga S et al (1985) Electron microscopic study of iris nerves and muscles in diabetes. *Ophthalmologica, 191,* 172.

54. Guy RJC, Richards F, Edmonds ME et al (1984) Diabetic autonomic neuropathy and iritis: an association suggesting an immunological cause. *Br. Med. J., 289,* 343.

55. Martyn CN, Young RJ, Ewing DJ (1986) Is there a link between iritis and diabetic autonomic neuropathy? *Br. Med. J., 292,* 934.

56. Osei K, Fields PG, Cataland S et al (1985) Abnormal retinal artery responses to stress in patients with Type I diabetes. *Am. J. Med.*, *78*, 595.
57. Montserrat JM, Cochrane GM, Wolf C et al (1985) Ventilatory control in diabetes mellitus. *Eur. J. Respir. Dis.*, *67*, 112.
58. Sobotka PA, Liss HP, Vinik AI (1986) Impaired hypoxic ventilatory drive in diabetic patients with autonomic neuropathy. *J. Clin. Endocrinol. Metab.*, *62*, 658.
59. Mondini S, Guilleminault C (1985) Abnormal breathing patterns during sleep in diabetes. *Ann. Neurol.*, *17*, 391.

The Diabetes Annual/3
K.G.M.M. Alberti and L.P. Krall, editors
© 1987 Elsevier Science Publishers, B.V.

17 Early diabetic renal involvement and nephropathy

Can treatment modalities be predicted from identification of risk factors?

C.E. MOGENSEN

Introduction

End-stage renal failure due to the metabolic and hormonal aberrations of diabetes is now the most common single renal disease in dialysis and transplantation units throughout the Western world (1). Moreover, proteinuria in diabetic patients is the main marker of the profound overmortality seen in these patients, non-proteinuric diabetic patients showing only a borderline increase in mortality compared with the background population (2). These facts were also discussed in *The Diabetes Annual/1* (1). In the last few years only a few centers have been engaged in research on early changes in the diabetic kidney, attempting to define risk factors in order to find a basis for new treatment modalities. The present review will be selective, focussing mainly on the following important clinical aspects of insulin-dependent diabetes: Can patients at risk for nephropathy be defined, and, once identified, can these patients be offered treatment that may postpone or even prevent late diabetic nephropathy? A number of reviews on early or incipient diabetic nephropathy are already available (3-6).

Identifying a risk factor does not necessarily imply that eliminating the risk factor in question will postpone the disease. The risk factor may only be a marker of the disease, an innocent bystander, not necessarily involved in the pathogenesis of glomerular and renal damage. Hence, clinical intervention trials are needed when risk factors are established on the basis of clinical studies.

Classification of renal involvement and nephropathy in diabetes

The concept of microalbuminuria

It is now well documented that microalbuminuria, defined as abnormally raised

albumin excretion without clinical proteinuria, is an excellent marker of subsequent overt diabetic nephropathy. Similar results have appeared from 3 centers (7-10). It is hardly surprising, however, that the level of raised urinary
albumin excretion (UAE) which predicts diabetic nephropathy varies from
center to center (Table 1). The studies in question have all been retrospective
and not specifically planned for long-term follow-up, although the data appeared to be suitable for evaluation. The procedures for urine collection, patient composition and follow-up period varies between the studies, and these
differences are likely to explain the different discriminatory levels of UAE.
Table 1 provides a summary of studies on the development of overt diabetic
nephropathy on the basis of early detection of microalbuminuria.

Urinary albumin excretion in young normal persons, males and females, is
about 5 µg/min and the excretion rate very seldom exceeds 12-15 µg/min. The
variability of UAE is considerable in both diabetic and non-diabetic subjects,
with a coefficient of variation of 25-40% (11, 12). Multiple collections are therefore advisable.

TABLE 1   *Summary of studies of development of overt diabetic nephropathy (DN) based on
early microalbuminuria*

	London*	Copenhagen**	Aarhus***
Female/male	22/41	42/29	0/43
Follow-up (%)	75	100	98
Mean age at screening	40	30	25
(yr)	(17-60)	(13-50)	(18-31)
Mean duration of diabetes	10	12	12
at screening (yr)	(1-41)	(2-36)	(7-20)
Follow-up period (yr)	14	6 (mean)	10 (mean)
Proposed discrimination	30	70	15
value (µg/min)			
Development of DN above	7/8	7/7	12/14
discrimination value			
Development of DN below	2/55	3/64	0/29
discrimination value			
Urine sample	overnight	24-hour	short-term at hospital
No. of urine samples	≥ 1	≥ 3	≥ 3
Methods	RIA	radial immune diffusion	RIA

　* From Viberti et al (8).
　** From Mathiesen et al (10).
*** From Mogensen et al (9).
RIA = radioimmunoassay.

TABLE 2   Microalbuminuria and diabetic nephropathy (DN): stages in diabetic renal involvement and nephropathy

Stage	Designation	Main characteristics	Main structural changes	GFR (ml/min)	Albumin excretion (UAE)	Blood pressure	Suggested main pathophysiological change
Stage 1	Hyperfunction and hypertrophy stage*	Large kidneys and glomerular hyperfiltration	Glomerular hypertrophy; normal basement membrane and mesangium	≈ 150	May be increased	N	Glomerular volume expansion and increased intraglomerular pressure
Stage 2 In short-term diabetes (7-15 yr)	'Silent' stage with normal UAE but structural lesion present	Normal UAE	Increasing basal membrane (BM) thickness and mesangial expansion	With or without hyperfiltration*	N (often increased in stress situations)	N	Changes as indicated above but quite variable (dependent on metabolic control?); in addition, increased accumulation of BM and BM-like material
In long-term diabetes			No or few studies	With or without hyperfiltration**	N (often in stress situations)	N or slightly elevated	
Stage 3 Early	Incipient DN (or 'at-risk patient')	Persistently elevated UAE (20-200 µg/min)	Severity probably in between stage 2 and 4	≈ 160	20-70 µg/min	Often elevated compared with healthy subjects increasing by 3.5% per year Also blood pressure elevated during exercise	Glomerular closure probably starts in this stage In some patients high intraglomerular pressure
Late				≈ 130	70-200 µg/min		

				GFR	UAE	Blood pressure	
Stage 4			Further increase in basement membrane thickening and mesangial expansion				
Early	Overt DN	Clinical proteinuria or UAE >200 µg/min	Increasing rate of glomerular closure	≈ 130-70	> 200 µg/min	Often frank hypertension	High rate of glomerular closure and advancing mesangial expansion
Intermediate			Hypertrophy of remaining glomeruli	≈ 70-30		Hypertension almost ubiquitous	
Advanced				≈ 30-10		Hypertension almost ubiquitous	Hyperfiltration in remaining glomeruli (deleterious)
Stage 5							
Uremia	End-stage renal failure		Generalized glomerular closure	0-10	Decreasing (due to nephron closure)	High but often controlled by dialysis treatment	Advanced lesions and glomerular closure

* Changes present probably in all stages when control imperfect.
** Possible marker of future nephropathy (if GFR > 150 ml/min).
GFR = glomerular filtration rate; N = normal; UAE = urinary albumin excretion.

A new classification system

The recognition of the importance of microalbuminuria as a predictor of renal disease in diabetes and also the description of glomerular hyperfiltration and hypertrophy in diabetes, already present at diagnosis, have underlined the need for a redefinition of diabetic nephropathy which takes these new developments into account (3, 4, 13-15). Redefinition is most easily made by defining new stages in the development of renal changes in insulin-dependent diabetes.

These stages, as well as their main characteristics, are outlined in Table 2. The following stages can be defined:

Stage 1: Glomerular hyperfunction and hypertrophy stage present at diagnosis. It should be mentioned that certain features at this stage will accompany diabetes also of longer duration when metabolic control is imperfect.

Stage 2: The silent stage with normal albumin excretion but with structural lesions present. This stage may last for many years; in fact, some patients will continue in this stage throughout their life. Occasionally, in stress situations, e.g. during episodes of very poor metabolic control or during moderate exercise, albumin excretion rate may increase, but this is a readily reversible phenomenon.

Stage 3: Incipient diabetic nephropathy is characterized by persisting microalbuminuria. Patients with microalbuminuria have a very high risk of subsequent development of overt diabetic nephropathy. However, intervention may certainly be possible at this stage, reversing both structural and functional changes.

Stage 4: Overt diabetic nephropathy is characterized by proteinuria, hypertension and subsequent fall in glomerular filtration rate (GFR).

Stage 5: End-stage renal failure is the clinical syndrome of uremia, with generalized nephron closure and very low GFR.

Quantitative definition of microalbuminuria and incipient diabetic nephropathy

In 1985 a consensus was reached among research workers from diabetes centers in Belgium, Denmark and England regarding the definition of microalbuminuria and incipient diabetic nephropathy (16): microalbuminuria is considered to be present when UAE is greater than 20 μg/min and less or equal to 200 μg/min. This level corresponds approximately to 30-300 mg/24 h. Incipient diabetic nephropathy (Stage 3) is considered to be present when microalbuminuria is found in at least 2 of 3 urine samples collected consecutively, preferably within a period of 6 months. If more than 3 are available, the mean UAE should be within the microalbuminuria range of 20-200 μg/min. Urine should be sterile and obtained in the non-ketotic state. The best possible control of diabetes should be achieved prior to determination of UAE. Other causes of increased albumin excretion rate should be excluded, especially if diabetes has been present for less than 6 years. Overt diabetic nephropathy (Stage 4) is considered to be present when UAE is greater than 200 µg/min in at least 2 of 3 samples collected within 6 months or when the mean value of UAE of multiple collections exceeds 200 µg/min. As in the case of incipient diabetic nephropathy, urine samples should be sterile and obtained in non-ketotic patients; again, other causes of increased UAE should be excluded. According to this definition, the dip-stick tests for urine protein should not be applied when classifying diabetic renal disease. The use of dip-stick tests may indeed confuse research workers because it is very likely that a heterogeneous patient sample will be obtained (17).

Definition of risk factors

Parameters associated with progression to end-stage renal failure

The process of identifying risk factors requires that the progression of diabetic renal disease should be monitored. The following parameters have been proposed in the longitudinal follow-up of patients: hyperfiltration, micro-albuminuria/macroalbuminuria, and fall in GFR (Table 3).
Hyperfiltration Abnormally high GFR is a characteristic feature in early diabetes. If hyperfiltration is pronounced (>150 ml/min, corrected to 1.73 m^2 body surface) and it is present for many years, it is associated with a considerable risk of subsequent diabetic nephropathy (9, 18, 19). A reduction in GFR from the supranormal level could therefore be considered beneficial if it is not associated

TABLE 3   *Insulin-dependent diabetes mellitus: prediction, pathogenesis and markers of diabetic nephropathy*

Stages		Marker of future progression	Involved in pathogenesis	Marker of already established disease
1+2	Hyperfiltration	likely	likely	not likely
3	Microalbuminuria	certain	suggested	likely
4	Proteinuria	certain	suggested	certain
4	Rate of decline in GFR	certain	—	certain

GFR = glomerular filtration rate.

with an increase in UAE. Thus, normalization of high GFR may be an appropriate test parameter in normoalbuminuric patients, i.e. Stage 2 patients.

Changes in UAE Increase in UAE might also be used in normoalbuminuric patients, but according to recent follow-up studies (7, 8-10) only a few normoalbuminuric patients will develop increased values in a 10-year follow-up period. A change in UAE is therefore not very appropriate for use as a test in normoalbuminuric patients. If it is used, very long-term follow-up is necessary, probably 12-20 years.

In patients with persistent microalbuminuria an increase in UAE is a major test parameter. It has been shown that progression of UAE is rather slow: the transition from low microalbuminuria to macroalbuminuria may last for 8-10 years (12, 20). In patients with overt diabetic nephropathy, clinical proteinuria must also be considered as an important test parameter in the evaluation of progression of renal disease (21, 22).

Fall rate of GFR GFR probably starts to fall in patients with incipient diabetic nephropathy (9). In patients with overt diabetic nephropathy, the rate of decline in GFR is most often linear with time, at least when exact clearance techniques are used, e.g. constant infusion technique with insulin, labelled iothalamate clearance or a single-shut procedure with ^{51}Cr-EDTA (21, 22).The reciprocal of serum creatinine may also decline in a linear fashion, but this is a less well defined parameter (23).

Renal ultrastructure So far, there are no long-term follow-up studies of the predictive power of abnormal glomerular ultrastructure in patients with early diabetic nephropathy. Relevant test parameters, to be evaluated in repeated biopsies, would be basement membrane thickening, mesangial expansion and also the number of occluded glomeruli. Some authors recommend that renal biopsies be included in follow-up of patients (24, 25).

Studies of the structural and biochemical correlates of microalbuminuria (versus normoalbuminuria in diabetic patients), using biopsy procedures, are clearly needed. The designation 'microalbuminuria' is likely to cover a spectrum of patients with regard to the severity of underlying renal lesions. Thus, the predictive power of microalbuminuria can undoubtedly be considerably enforced by such measures. Efforts to intervene are likely to be much more successful when the structural counterpart to function is well defined (1, 24, 25).

Period of follow-up

It is important to note that progression of nephropathy in the incipient phase is rather slow, the annual mean increase rate in UAE being 15-20%. Also, it should be considered that a given treatment modality may be difficult to sustain for a prolonged period without any other intervention. Thus, can optimized insulin treatment be given without considering blood pressure elevation? To have clinical relevance, studies of the spontaneous course as well as studies on the effect of intervention should be sufficiently long: at least 2-3 years. Of course, the final end-point would be development of end-stage renal failure. However, since in many patients under study the development of renal failure may last for decades, end-stage renal failure is not really a feasible test parameter. Hence, investigators should be satisfied to consider intermediate end-points related to end-stage renal failure. These include increasing microalbuminuria, increasing macroproteinuria or the rate of decline in GFR, or the development of overt nephropathy. Of course, an ultrastructural evaluation of glomeruli could be extremely useful in such studies, but so far no data are available in man.

The role of blood glucose control or the metabolic risk factor(s)

Normoalbuminuria Clinical evidence suggests that the quality of metabolic control is related to the development of long-term diabetic nephropathy. However, there are no prospective long-term follow-up studies on the relationship of metabolic control and the subsequent development of nephropathy in normoalbuminuric patients. Very long-term follow-up is necessary and close assessment of metabolic control is also required e.g. by multiple measurements of HbA_{1c} over a decade or even for a longer period. Such studies have so far not been performed.

The GFR is positively correlated to HbA_{1c}. Since a very high GFR predicts future nephropathy, there is now indirect evidence that poor control is associated with future nephropathy, possibly mediated via hyperfiltration (26). Interestingly, patients respond to the same degree of long-term hyperglycemia with different degrees of hyperfiltration (26).

Incipient diabetic nephropathy The rate of increase in UAE has been shown to be associated with HbA_{1c} in a 2-year follow-up study in patients with incipient diabetic nephropathy (20).

Overt diabetic nephropathy. An association between the rate of decline in GFR and HbA_{1c} has also been documented in overt diabetic nephropathy (27, 28).

It can be concluded that the rate of progression of nephropathy, in both the incipient and the overt phase, seems to be correlated with the quality of metabolic control.

Elevated blood pressure as a risk factor

At the clinical diagnosis of diabetes (Stage 1) in insulin-dependent diabetes there is no evidence of blood pressure elevation (19).

In normoalbuminuric patients (Stage 2) blood pressure is also generally quite normal. If blood pressure is clearly elevated in such patients, (> 160/95 mmHg) and if there is normoalbuminuria, it is likely that the patients have two coexisting diseases, namely diabetes mellitus and essential hypertension (29). The long-term effect of essential hypertension on structural lesions in the diabetic kidney is unknown. Patients with normoalbuminuria generally remain normotensive, despite an additional decade of diabetes (9, 19).

Incipient diabetic nephropathy (Stage 3) In a longitudinal study it was documented that an increased rate of UAE in incipient diabetic nephropathy was closely correlated with the blood pressure level (12). This observation, which may have important clinical implications, has recently been confirmed in a controlled clinical study using the insulin pump versus conventional treatment (20). It appeared from this study that a high rate of increase in UAE was closely associated with an increase in blood pressure over a 2-year period. In cross-sectional studies blood pressure was shown to be elevated by about 10% in microalbuminuria patients, when compared with those having normoalbuminuria (10, 30, 31).

Overt diabetic nephropathy In patients with overt diabetic nephropathy an association between blood pressure elevation and the rate of progression of nephropathy, as measured by the rate of decline in GFR, has been found in two recent studies (32, 33).

In summary, blood pressure elevation is closely associated with impairment of renal function. Even patients with microalbuminuria show an increase in blood pressure and progression of early nephropathy also seems to be related to blood pressure. It is probable that early structural lesions in the kidney cause blood pressure elevation as well as microalbuminuria. Blood pressure elevation is likely to accelerate renal damage.

High protein intake in the diet: a potential risk factor

It is known that a high protein intake induces some degree of hyperfiltration in normal man (5). An association between the level of GFR and protein intake has also been documented recently, although there is considerable overlap between groups with different protein intakes (34). Since hyperfiltration is likely to be involved in the pathogenesis of diabetic nephropathy, a high protein intake over many years may be a risk factor for diabetic nephropathy. However, long-term studies are not available. In overt diabetic nephropathy, no association was found between the rate of decline in GFR and the protein intake (35). It should be emphasized that other factors that may have a greater influence on progression were carefully controlled, e.g. level of blood pressure as well as

TABLE 4 *Insulin-dependent diabetes mellitus: association between relevant predictive test parameters and blood glucose control, blood pressure level and protein content of diet*

Stage		Long-term blood glucose control	Blood pressure level	Protein content of diet
1+2	Degree of hyperfiltration	associated with HbA$_{1c}$	not correlated	probably associated
3	Yearly increase in microalbuminuria	associated with HbA$_{1c}$	associated with MABP or yearly rise in MABP	?
4	Rate of decline in GFR	associated with HbA$_{1c}$	associated with MABP	not associated

GFR = glomerular filtration rate; MABP = mean arterial blood pressure.

metabolic control. The issue regarding dietary intervention in diabetes and renal disease is still not settled (36, 37).

Table 4 summarizes the association between major risk factors (blood glucose control, blood pressure and protein content of diet) and test parameters for progression, as discussed above.

Early hyperfiltration: a risk factor for late nephropathy?

There have been only a few long-term studies on the role of glomerular hyperfiltration in the long-term genesis of late diabetic nephropathy (9, 18, 19). Exact measurements of GFR have been performed in only a few centers. In fact, 3 studies with slightly different entrance criteria, from the same center (9, 18, 19), document that hyperfiltration is closely associated with late nephropathy, also compared with the predictive factor of microalbuminuria for late nephropathy (19). However, it cannot be ruled out that both hyperfiltration and late nephropathy are caused by another factor that determines both hyperfiltration and nephropathy, namely long-term poor metabolic control. There is now strong evidence from animal experiments that hyperfiltration is involved in the pathogenesis of diabetic nephropathy. Also, it is suggested that amelioration of hyperfiltration by dietary or pharmacological means will prevent renal lesions in the experimental animal (38, 39).

The perspective of intervention, on the basis of risk factors

Metabolic control

There is now evidence to indicate that the quality of metabolic control plays a central role in both the initiation and progression of nephropathy in insulin-dependent patients, although modulating or permissive factors may exist (4, 5). The next question is therefore whether improvement in metabolic control has a beneficial effect on renal involvement or nephropathy in diabetic patients. Several studies have been undertaken during the last few years to clarify whether optimized treatment, in most cases using insulin pumps, would influence the progression of renal disease or modify renal function.

Normoalbuminuric patients The only functional abnormality to be detected at this stage is glomerular hyperfiltration. Since hyperfiltration seems to be associated with the development of late nephropathy, a reduction in hyperfiltration may be beneficial by preventing future deterioration of renal function. It has been shown that insulin pump treatment is able to reverse hyperfiltration in selected diabetic patients with normal albumin excretion (40, 41). However, the long-term effect is not impressive, which may be explained by the fact that, at least in some studies, patients were not poorly controlled prior to entry to the study (42). The most dramatic effect is seen early after institution of pump treatment; after long-term treatment the effect is less pronounced. There may be a small decline also in renal plasma flow, but so far no change has been seen in kidney size (41-43), in contrast with the reduction in size seen after the start of insulin treatment in newly diagnosed patients (41). It is very difficult to conduct such studies over a sufficient number of years (decades?) to establish whether development of microalbuminuria or overt nephropathy can be prevented in these patients.

Studies with a heterogeneous patient population A number of studies had been started before the concept of microalbuminuria was widely accepted (44-46). In these studies, therefore, patients with normo- and microalbuminuria are mixed, and microalbuminuria or normoalbuminuria is not used as entrance criterion. Also, multiple collection of urine samples (at least 3) was not performed; rather, a single value was used. In these preliminary studies, patients were apparently classified after results were obtained which may have given rise to a bias in the interpretation of data (44), especially when patients with only a borderline increase in UAE (13-20 µg/min) were included as being microalbuminuric. However, there seems to be a reduction in UAE with months of optimized treatment in microalbuminuria patients, i.e. a beneficial effect.

It is even more difficult to evaluate studies which include patients with normo-, micro- and macroalbuminuria, especially when the number of patients is small (17). A reduction in GFR may be induced by better metabolic control in those with normoalbuminuria or slightly raised microalbuminuria (46). Patients with overt nephropathy may show a reduction in GFR due to progressive renal damage with glomerular occlusion or mesangial expansion. Firm interpretation of results from such studies with mixed patient populations are not possible (47).

Incipient diabetic nephropathy   In a newly published prospective study (20) 36 insulin-dependent patients with persistently elevated urinary albumin excretion rate (incipient diabetic nephropathy) were randomized to conventional treatment or insulin pump treatment. At 1 year kidney size was reduced, but no significant changes in GFR or urinary albumin excretion rate were observed (48). However, after 2 years' observation, using a more sensitive technique for following urinary albumin excretion rate in individual patients (using longitudinal regression lines), the progressive increase in UAE continued in the conventionally treated group but was arrested or even reversed in insulin-pump-treated patients (20). A significant reduction in HbA_{1c} and also in mean blood glucose levels was obtained in the pump-treated patients, no change being seen in the conventionally treated patients. GFR was reduced significantly in the pump-treated patients, probably as a result of better metabolic control. No change was seen in GFR in the conventionally treated group with unchanged HbA_{1c}. In addition, after 2 years, 5 patients in the conventionally treated group had developed overt nephropathy versus none in the pump-treated group. These results are encouraging and strongly suggest a beneficial effect of improved metabolic control in these patients. However, future research is necessary to provide decisive evidence that a reduction in microalbuminuria will also in the long-term prevent nephropathy and excess mortality (20). Of great interest, it appeared that blood pressure increased in the observation period only in patients on conventional treatment.

Overt nephropathy   No large-scale controlled studies have been conducted on the influence of improved metabolic control on the progression of overt nephropathy, as measured by the rate of decline in GFR. A study from the Guy's Hospital group on a limited number of patients (49) concluded that no effect could be detected by optimized control of these patients. However, due to the small number involved in the study, poorly documented control of blood pressure and the inclusion of patients in different phases of renal disease, even important effects of metabolic control may have gone undetected. The mean progression rate was in fact lower in the pump group, but under the circumstances of the study the change was not statistically significant. New studies would therefore be of interest to clarify whether improved metabolic control is able to retard the progression of overt nephropathy. Such studies, on a large scale, would be difficult to conduct, however. In the meantime it would seem prudent for the clinician to try to obtain the best possible metabolic control, even in these patients. It is not unreasonable to suggest that hyperglycemia will continue to be deleterious to kidneys even when already damaged. Cross-sectional studies suggest that progression is more rapid in patients who are poorly controlled (27, 28).

Antihypertensive treatment

Normoalbuminuric patients   Blood pressure elevation is first seen in patients with incipient diabetic nephropathy, generally not in normoalbuminuric patients. Nevertheless, it would be of interest to assess the effect of angiotensin-converting-enzyme (ACE) inhibitors in hyperfiltering normoalbuminuric patients. A reduction in hyperfiltration by ACE inhibition, or other non-glycemic intervention, would certainly be an interesting approach to early treatment. Such studies are in progress in some centers.

Incipient diabetic nephropathy   Blood pressure is significantly elevated in incipient diabetic nephropathy and progression is more rapid in patients with elevated or increasing blood pressure (12, 20, 30, 31). One longitudinal study, comprising only 6 patients (50) and using cardioselective beta-blockers and diuretics as antihypertensive agents, suggests that the rate of progression can be reversed in these patients by lowering the blood pressure. In this study, the increase in the rate of UAE was 18% per year before treatment in patients followed for an average of 5 years without intervention. During antihypertensive treatment the change in UAE was significantly reversed with a rate of *decline* in UAE of 17% per year in patients followed for an average of 3 years during treatment. No significant change was seen in renal hemodynamics and GFR was very well preserved, being even in the hyperfiltering range. Blood pressure was reduced by about 10%; before treatment the blood pressure averaged 135/93 mmHg and during treatment 124/84 mmHg, i.e. it fell to nearly normal levels. Antihypertensive treatment in the stage of incipient diabetic nephropathy may therefore have a more beneficial effect on the progression of renal disease than treatment started at the stage of overt diabetic nephropathy. It would be of interest to see whether this effect could be reproduced in large-scale randomized double-blind case-control studies. In the study mentioned above, patients were used as their own internal controls, probably a very sensitive method to detect an effect (21, 22). However, it may be difficult to exclude other factors involved in the regression of microalbuminuria. Importantly, no change was seen in blood glucose control, and dietary protein remained unchanged during the study (50).

Overt diabetic nephropathy New studies have shown that GFR decreases linearly with time in insulin-dependent patients with nephropathy (21, 22). The rate of decline in GFR varies considerably from patient to patient, but in each patient the rate of decline is fairly linear, with a decline rate of approximately 0.9 ml/min/mth on average in the untreated situation. Two studies have shown that effective antihypertensive treatment is able to decrease the rate of decline in renal function in these patients. The reduction in the rate of progression is rather dramatic, being about 60% (21, 22). Assuming the continuous linear fall rate of GFR, end-stage renal failure can be postponed for many years by this treatment modality. In these studies a combination of cardioselective beta-blockers, diuretics and vasodilators was used as antihypertensive therapy.

In addition to the above two studies, using internal controls, a case-control study of 16 insulin-dependent patients with nephropathy has also been carried out (51). The patients were matched carefully for sex, age, duration of diabetes, retinopathy, albuminuria, GFR and level of blood pressure. Also in this study the rate of decline in GFR could be decreased considerably; albuminuria was also significantly reduced by antihypertensive treatment, when comparing the two groups.

The effect of ACE inhibitors has been evaluated in patients with advanced overt diabetic nephropathy. During ACE inhibition there was a slowing in the progression of the renal disease in these patients (52). Recently it has been shown that monotherapy with captopril for 12 weeks diminished albuminuria in diabetic patients with overt nephropathy (53).

It can be concluded that arterial blood pressure seems to have a complex relationship with renal disease in diabetes. It is likely that renal damage raises blood pressure in a complex way. On the other hand, increased blood pressure accelerates the course of nephropathy and intrarenal hypertension may be an important factor in the genesis of progression of renal disease. This vicious circle seems to be broken by antihypertensive treatment and it can be concluded that effective normalization of blood pressure not only reduces proteinuria, but that end-stage renal failure is also considerably postponed (54).

Protein restriction

There are few studies on protein restriction using a modern classification of renal involvement in diabetes. Some of the studies have so far only been published as abstracts and are therefore difficult to analyze in detail (56, 57).

Normoalbuminuria or near-normal albuminuria GFR can be decreased considerably by lowering the protein content of the diet in both diabetic and non-diabetic subjects and thus a potential risk factor can be eliminated (55). The study concluded that increased renal function in diabetes may be related in part to the excessive protein content in commonly prescribed diabetic diets. Moderate dietary protein restriction is an additional approach to the correction of diabetic hyperfiltration.

Microalbuminuria patients   In microalbuminuric patients a clear reduction in UAE on an isocaloric low-protein diet has been reported (56). In these patients no changes in blood pressure or in glycemic control were recorded. It can be concluded that short-term restriction of dietary proteins (over 3 weeks) reduces microalbuminuria and also GFR, independent of glycemia and arterial pressure changes. Long-term studies are needed.

TABLE 5   *Insulin-dependent diabetes mellitus: effect of intervention on relevant test parameters in the stages of diabetic renal disease*

Stage	Test parameter	Effect of optimized insulin treatment	Effect of antihypertensive treatment	Effect of low-protein diet
(1)2	Hyperfiltration	↓	unknown	↓
3	Microalbuminuria	↓	↓	↓
4	Rate of decline in GFR + macroproteinuria	Not documented in a small material	↓	↓
Goal of treatment	All parameters:	HbA$_{1c}$ <7.5%	≤125/85 mmHg	< ? (45-60 g/70 kg)**

  * In young patients.
** Under investigation.
GFR = glomerular filtration rate.

Overt nephropathy   The effect of a low-protein diet (40 g/24 h) was studied in insulin-dependent patients with overt nephropathy (57). The rate of decline in renal function was studied before and during 12 months on a low-protein diet. The authors observed a fall in total protein excretion. More importantly, the rate of decline in GFR was reduced in many patients during the low-protein diet, although there was a variable response.

   Table 5 summarizes the effect of intervention (optimized insulin treatment, antihypertensive treatment and low-protein diet) on relevant test parameters associated with eventual end-stage renal failure.

Conclusions

There is now circumstantial evidence to indicate that the initiation and progression of renal disease in diabetes is associated with the degree of metabolic control, although there are important modifying factors such as blood pressure elevation and possibly dietary protein intake. It is likely that unknown permissive factors also exist and further studies are clearly needed to clarify, for example, why some patients develop nephropathy and others do not, despite similar metabolic control over the years.

It is likely that metabolic control, blood pressure level and protein intake are not only risk factors, but are also involved in the pathogenesis of diabetic nephropathy. Intervention using optimized glycemic control, optimized blood pressure treatment and a low-protein diet seem promising as treatment modalities. Long-term studies have so far been carried out only with respect to antihypertensive treatment and clinicians are anxiously awaiting long-term results of the other treatment modalities. In addition to optimized control and a low-protein diet, there are other perspectives of non-glycemic intervention that should be evaluated (58), such as the long-term effect of aldose reductase inhibition, platelet-active drugs, and the effect of somatostatin analogues in inhibiting growth hormone hypersecretion in diabetes. Combined intervention, for example, with optimized glycemic control, antihypertensive treatment, and maybe a reduced protein diet (at least not a high-protein diet) already seems a prudent policy in our treatment program.

Early detection of patients at risk for late nephropathy is already good clinical practice. Easy, rapid and inexpensive methods for detection of microalbuminuria in the clinical setting are now available (59-63). The nephelometric method is rapid and sufficiently sensitive and is probably best suited for clinical purpose (60, 61).

References

1. Ellis EN, Mauer SM (1985): Diabetic nephropathy. In: Alberti KGMM, Krall LP (Eds), *The Diabetes Annual/1*, p. 309. Elsevier, Amsterdam.
2. Borch-Johnsen K, Kragh Andersen P, Deckert T (1985): The impact of proteinuria on the relative mortality in patients with type I (insulin-dependent) diabetes mellitus. *Diabetologia, 28,* 590.
3. Rosenstock J, Raskin P (1986): Early diabetic nephropathy - assessment and potential interventions. *Diabetes Care, 9,* 529.
4. Mogensen CE (1987): Microalbuminuria as a predictor of clinical diabetic nephropathy. *Kidney Int., 31,* 673.
5. Viberti GC, Wiseman MJ (1986): The kidney in diabetes: significance of the early abnormalities. *Clin. Endocrinol. Metab., 15,* 753.
6. Hanssen KF, Dahl-Jørgensen K, Lauritzen T et al (1986): Diabetic control and microvascular complications: the near-normoglycaemic experience. *Diabetologia, 29,* 677.
7. Parving HH, Oxenbøll B, Svendsen PA et al (1982): Early detection of patients at risk of developing diabetic nephropathy: a longitudinal study of urinary albumin excretion. *Acta Endocrinol., 100,* 500.

8. Viberti GC, Jarrett RJ, Mahmud U et al (1982): Microalbuminuria as a predictor of clinical nephropathy in insulin-dependent diabetes mellitus. *Lancet, 1,* 1430.
9. Mogensen CE, Christensen CK (1984): Predicting diabetic nephropathy in insulin-dependent patients. *N. Engl. J. Med., 311,* 89.
10. Mathiesen ER, Oxenbøll B, Johansen K et al (1984): Incipient nephropathy in type I (insulin-dependent) diabetes. *Diabetologia, 26,* 406.
11. Feldt-Rasmussen B, Mathiesen ER (1984): Variability of urinary albumin excretion in incipient diabetic nephropathy. *Diabetic Nephropathy, 3,* 101.
12. Christensen CK, Mogensen CE (1985): The course of incipient diabetic nephropathy: studies of albumin excretion and blood pressure. *Diabetic Med., 2,* 97.
13. Mogensen CE, Christensen CK, Vittinghus E (1983): The stages in diabetic renal disease: with emphasis on the stage of incipient diabetic nephropathy. *Diabetes, 32,* 64.
14. Christensen CK (1984): Abnormal albuminuria and blood pressure rise in incipient diabetic nephropathy induced by exercise. *Kidney Int., 25,* 819.
15. Christiansen JS (1985): Glomerular hyperfiltration in diabetes. *Diabetic Med., 2,* 235.
16. Mogensen CE, Chachati A, Christensen CK et al (1985/1986): Microalbuminuria: an early marker of renal involvement in diabetes. *Uremia Invest., 9,* 85.
17. Bending JJ, Viberti GC, Watkins PJ, Keen H (1986): Intermittent clinical proteinuria and renal function in diabetes: evolution and effect of glycaemic control. *Br. Med. J., 292,* 83.
18. Mogensen CE (1986): Early glomerular hyperfiltration in insulin-dependent diabetics and late nephropathy. *Scand. J. Clin. Lab. Invest., 46,* 201.
19. Mogensen CE, Christensen CK (1985): Blood pressure changes and renal function changes in incipient and overt diabetic nephropathy. *Hypertension, 7,* 11-64.
20. Feldt-Rasmussen B, Mathiesen E, Deckert T (1986): Effect of two years of strict metabolic control on the progression of incipient nephropathy in insulin-dependent diabetes. *Lancet, 2,* 1300.
21. Mogensen CE (1982): Long-term antihypertensive treatment inhibiting progression of diabetic nephropathy. *Br. Med. J., 285,* 685.
22. Parving H-H, Andersen AR, Smidt UM, Svendsen PAA (1983): Early aggressive antihypertensive treatment reduces rate of decline in kidney function in diabetic nephropathy. *Lancet, 1,* 1175.
23. Tchobroutsky G, Altman JJ, Bazot M et al (1986): Beneficial effect of tight control of glycaemia and blood pressure in 37 patients with severe diabetic nephropathy. *Diabetologia, 29,* 599A.
24. Steffes MW, Ellis EN, Mauer SM (1986): Complications of diabetes mellitus and factors affecting their progression.*Clin. Chem., 32,* B54.
25. Østerby R (1986): Structural changes in the diabetic kidney. *Clin. Endocrinol. Metab., 15,* 733.
26. Mogensen CE, Christensen CK, Christiansen JS et al (1987): Early hyperfiltration and late renal damage in insulin-dependent diabetes. In: *Proceedings, International Workshop on Diabetic Angiopathy in Children, Berlin, 1986.* In press.
27. Nyberg G, Blomé G, Nordén G (1986): Constant glomerular filtration rate in diabetic nephropathy: correlation to blood pressure and blood glucose control. *Acta Med. Scand., 219,* 67.
28. Nyberg G, Blohmé G, Nordén G (1987): Impact of metabolic control on progression of clinical diabetic nephropathy. Submitted for publication.
29. Christensen CK, Krusell LR, Mogensen CE (1986): Increased blood pressure in diabetes: essential hypertension or diabetic nephropathy? *Diabetologia, 29,* 527A.
30. Wiseman M, Viberti GC, Mackintosh D et al (1984): Glycaemia, arterial pressure and micro-albuminuria in type 1 (insulin-dependent) diabetes mellitus. *Diabetologia, 26,* 401.

31. Christensen CK (1984): Abnormal albuminuria and blood pressure rise in incipient diabetic nephropathy induced by exercise. *Kidney Int.*, *25*, 819.
32. Berglund J, Lins L-E, Lins P-E (1985): Metabolic and blood pressure monitoring in diabetic renal failure. *Acta Med. Scand.*, *218*, 401.
33. Hasslacher Ch, Stech W, Wahl P, Ritz E (1985): Blood pressure and metabolic control as risk factors for nephropathy in type 1 (insulin-dependent) diabetes. *Diabetologia, 28,* 6.
34. Wiseman MJ, Hunt RE, Goodwin A et al (1987): Dietary composition and renal function in healthy subjects. *Nephron*, in press.
35. Nyberg G, Nordén G, Attman PO et al (1987): Diabetic nephropathy - is protein harmful? *J. Diabetic Complicat.*, in press.
36. Wood FC, Bierman EL (1986): Is diet the cornerstone in management of diabetes? *N. Engl. J. Med., 315,* 1224.
37. El Nahas AM, Coles GA (1986): Dietary treatment of chronic renal failure: ten unanswered questions. *Lancet, 1,* 597.
38. Zatz R, Dunn BR, Meyer TW et al (1986): Prevention of diabetic glomerulopathy by pharmacological amelioration of glomerular capillary hypertension. *J. Clin. Invest., 77,* 1925.
39. Anderson S, Rennke GH, Brenner BM (1986): Therapeutic advantage of converting enzyme inhibitors in arresting progressive renal disease associated with systemic hypertension in the rat. *J. Clin. Invest., 77,* 1993.
40. Beck-Nielsen H, Mogensen CE, Olsen T et al (1985): Effect of insulin pump treatment for 1 year on renal function and retinal morphology in patients with IDDM. *Diabetes Care, 8,* 585.
41. Christensen CK, Christiansen JS, Christensen T et al (1986): Effect of continuous subcutaneous insulin infusion during six months on kidney function and size in insulin-dependent diabetics. *Diabetic Med., 3,* 29.
42. Christensen CK, Christiansen JS, Schmitz A et al (1987): Effect of continuous subcutaneous insulin infusion on kidney function and size in IDDM patients - a two years controlled study. *J. Diabetic Complicat.*, in press.
43. Wiseman MJ, Saunders AJ, Keen H, Viberti GC (1985): Effect of blood glucose control on increased glomerular filtration rate and kidney size in insulin-dependent diabetes. *N. Engl. J. Med., 312,* 617.
44. Bending JJ, Viberti GC, Bilous RW, Keen H and The Kroc Collaborative Study Group (1985): Eight-month correction of hyperglycemia in insulin-dependent diabetes mellitus is associated with a significant and sustained reduction of urinary albumin excretion rates in patients with microalbuminuria. *Diabetes, 34, Suppl. 3,* 69.
45. Dahl-Jørgensen K, Brinchmann-Hansen O, Hanssen KF et al (1986): Effect of near normoglycaemia for two years on progression of early diabetic retinopathy, nephropathy, and neuropathy: the Oslo study. *Br. Med. J., 293,* 1195.
46. Bell PM, Hayes JR, Hadden DR, Archer DB (1985): The effect of plasma glucose control by continuous subcutaneous insulin infusion or conventional therapy on retinal morphology and urinary albumin excretion. *Diabète Métab., 11,* 254.
47. Parving H-H (1986): Letter. *Br. Med. J., 292,* 558.
48. Feldt-Rasmussen B, Mathiesen ER, Hegedüs L, Deckert T (1986): Kidney function during 12 months of strict metabolic control in insulin-dependent diabetic patients with incipient nephropathy. *N. Engl. J. Med., 314,* 665.
49. Viberti GC, Bilous RW, Mackintosh D et al (1983): Long term correction of hyperglycaemia and progression of renal failure in insulin dependent diabetes. *Br. Med. J., 286,* 598.
50. Christensen CK, Mogensen CE (1985): Effect of antihypertensive treatment on progression of disease in incipient diabetic nephropathy. *Hypertension, 7,* II-109.

51. Parving H-H, Andersen AR, Hommel E, Smidt UM (1985): Effects of long-term antihypertensive treatment on kidney function in diabetic nephropathy. *Hypertension, 7,* II-114.
52. Björck S, Nyberg G, Mulec H et al (1986): Beneficial effects of angiotensin converting enzyme inhibition on renal function in patients with diabetic nephropathy. *Br. Med. J., 293,* 471.
53. Hommel E, Parving H-H, Mathiesen E et al (1986): Effect of captopril on kidney function in insulin-dependent diabetic patients with nephropathy. *Br. Med. J., 293,* 467.
54. Parving H-H, Andersen AR, Smidt UM et al (1986): The effect of long-term antihypertensive treatment on kidney function in diabetic nephropathy (Abstract). *Diabetologia, 29,* 580.
55. Kupin WL, Cortes P, Dumler F et al (1987): Effect on renal function of a change from high to moderate protein intake in type I diabetic patients. *Diabetes, 36,* 73.
56. Cohen DL, Dodds RA, Viberti GC (1986): Reduction of microalbuminuria and glomerular filtration rate by dietary protein restriction in type 1 (insulin-dependent) diabetic patients: an effect independent of blood glucose control and arterial pressure changes. *Diabetologia, 29,* 528A.
57. Bending JJ, Dodds R, Keen H, Viberti GC (1986): Lowering protein intake and the progression of diabetic renal failure. *Diabetologia, 29,* 516A.
58. Mogensen CE, Østerby R (1987): Structural and functional alterations in the diabetic kidney. *Front. Diabetes, 8,* 67.
59. Feldt-Rasmussen B, Dinesen B, Deckert M (1985): Enzyme immunoassay: an improved determination of urinary albumin in diabetics with incipient nephropathy. *Scand. J. Clin. Lab. Invest., 45,* 539.
60. Marre M, Claudel J-P, Ciret P et al (1987): A laser immunonephelometry method for routine quantification of urinary albumin excretion. *Clin. Chem., 33,* 209.
61. Harmoinen A, Ala-Houhala I, Vuorinen P (1985): Rapid and sensitive immunoassay for albumin determination in urine. *Clin. Chim. Acta, 149,* 269.
62. Watts GF, Bennett JE, Rowe DJ et al (1986): Assessment of immunochemical methods for determining low concentrations of albumin in urine. *Clin. Chem., 32,* 1544.
63. Christensen CK, Ørskov C (1984): Rapid screening PEG radioimmunoassay for quantification of pathological microalbuminuria. *Diabetic Nephropathy, 3,* 92.

The Diabetes Annual/3
K.G.M.M. Alberti and L.P. Krall, editors
© 1987 Elsevier Science Publishers, B.V.

18   Atherosclerosis in diabetes mellitus*

JOHN A. COLWELL

Introduction

Accelerated atherosclerosis of most of the major arteries is characteristic of diabetes mellitus. This is true in both insulin-dependent (IDDM) and non-insulin-dependent (NIDDM) diabetic subjects, and contributes an increased risk 1.2-6 times that of control subjects for peripheral vascular, coronary artery, or cerebrovascular disease (1-3). It is also true in monkeys with spontaneous diabetes (4). These and other vascular complications contribute greatly to morbidity and exceptionally high yearly health-care costs (estimated at $11 billion/year in the United States) in subjects with diabetes mellitus.

In view of these facts, and with the development of improved techniques for the study of disease, there has been an upsurge of interest in factors which may be of importance in diabetes in accelerating the atherosclerotic process (5, 6). Obviously, if the pathogenesis of the disorder is understood, preventive measures can be tried logically and techniques to deal with existing arterial disease in diabetes can be developed or improved.

There are new concepts about the pathophysiology of atherosclerosis in non-diabetic models which can be used to construct a hypothetical scheme for diabetic as well as non-diabetic subjects. The roles of the endothelium, platelets, and lipids/lipoproteins have received considerable attention. Review articles have considered the subject in depth, and should be consulted for details and for older references (7-9). It is the purpose of this Chapter to provide an updated review of the factors which may accelerate atherosclerosis in diabetes, and which creates a pathogenetic scheme which builds upon current knowledge of the development of atherosclerosis in the non-diabetic state. Key review articles will be cited, as well as epidemiologic studies, new information on genetic factors, and therapeutic approaches which are based upon sound pathophysiologic principles.

---

*Supported by Veterans Administration Research Funds.

Epidemiology

A number of factors interact to produce atherosclerosis. The process is a complex one which is influenced by primary and secondary risk factors. The classic primary risk factors, which arise external to the vascular wall, are hypertension, cigarette smoking, increased blood cholesterol levels, and diabetes mellitus. Thus, although diabetes is a primary risk factor, its effects are clearly modulated by the presence of other risk factors (5). This fact means that it may be difficult to separate out the independent effects of diabetes on the process from other factors which interact with it to accelerate atherosclerosis. Thus, Jarrett has pointed out that since there is a poor correlation between duration of diabetes and atherosclerosis in NIDDM subjects, and since individuals with impaired glucose tolerance have an increased risk to develop coronary heart disease, it is likely that diabetes (NIDDM) develops in individuals who already possess characteristics which increase the risk of atherosclerosis in addition to the risk of developing diabetes (10).

In the past few years, there has been an explosion of information on the epidemiology of vascular disease in different populations with diabetes. Since West's classic volume (11) and a few major prospective studies, there had been only limited information until recent years. Updated information from older studies is now available as well as new data from populations that had received little attention in the past. The net result of these newer reports is to confirm and extend older observations defining diabetes as a primary risk factor for atherosclerosis.

The Framingham population was studied after 27 years to determine the relationship of disability to cardiovascular risk factors (12). A cumulative disability index was assigned to 2021 persons free from diagnosed cardiovascular disease. Diabetes, hypertension and body mass index were associated with disability in women. This raises the question of the contribution of subclinical atherosclerosis to disability in such diabetic subjects. New information from two other classical studies — the Whitehall and Tecumseh studies (13, 14) — has also been presented. In the Whitehall study of 18,403 male civil servants, aged 40-64 years, the 10-year mortality rates from coronary heart disease (CHD) and stroke showed a non-linear relationship to 2-hour blood glucose values. There was a significantly increased risk for glucose-intolerant subjects (2-hour values 96-199 mg/100 ml; 5.3-11.1 mM) and for diabetic subjects (2-hour value over 199 mg/100 ml; 11.1 mM). Age and blood pressure were the two factors most strongly related to subsequent death from coronary heart disease in the glucose-intolerant and diabetic groups. This study confirmed the importance of hypertension as an associated risk factor in these types of diabetic subjects. In a 12-20 year follow-up of 921 men and 937 women, aged 40 years or older, who were free from coronary heart disease at entry, the Tecumseh group found that previously diagnosed diabetes was a significant risk factor for coronary heart disease mortality in males and in females (14). This was true even after adjusting for systolic blood pressure, serum cholesterol, relative weight, and cigarette smoking.

New population studies were added to these older studies. In Scandinavia, 464 individuals were followed for 22 years in the Kockum study (15). Important risk factors for CHD included diabetes mellitus, heredity, smoking, hypertension, hypercholesterolemia, and hypertriglyceridemia. In Western Australia, a cross-sectional study of 1084 rural Caucasoid diabetic subjects revealed a high rate of clinical macrovascular disease, including CHD (13%), stroke (8%), and peripheral vascular disease (38%) (16). Age was the major contributing factor for total macrovascular disease in both IDDM (179 patients) and NIDDM (905 patients). In the latter group, other contributing factors were plasma glucose, high-density lipoprotein cholesterol, and total cholesterol levels. In Southern California, a prospective population-based study of men and women aged 40-79 years was reported after 7 years of follow-up (17). When the 212 men and 131 women who had diabetes were compared to the 2104 non-diabetic subjects, the age-adjusted relative risk of death in diabetes attributed to CHD was 2.5 for diabetic men and 3.4 for diabetic women. In a separate report on this population (18), these authors documented a large and significant interaction between cigarette smoking and diabetes, such that about 65% of the CHD deaths among diabetic subjects could be attributed to this interaction.

Studies were also reported in other, more homogeneous populations. In the San Antonio Study, Mexican Americans comprised the study group (19). Such obesity-related risk factors as diabetes, hypertension, hypertriglyceridemia, and low low-density lipoprotein (LDL) cholesterol levels tended to approach normal when socioeconomic states rose. This study underscores the importance of cultural and socioeconomic factors on risk factor development in this population. In a study of 503 Mexican NIDDM subjects, 49% had peripheral vascular disease, and 22% CHD (20). High lipid levels and increased blood pressure were seen in those with CHD, and the presence of peripheral vascular disease was related to smoking. In Puerto Rico, a total of 2585 rural and 6208 urban men, aged 45-64, were studied for 8 years for development of CHD (21). The prevalence of diabetes in the urban population was double that in the rural population, and elevated blood glucose at baseline (over 139 mg/100 ml; 7.7 mM) was significantly associated with CHD death in urban men. In another study of urban men, it was found that urban American Indians in Minneapolis had a high risk for heart disease and stroke and that a higher prevalence of diabetes, smoking and obesity was found in this population than in Caucasians in the region (22).

On can conclude from these epidemiologic studies that diabetes continues to be identified as a primary risk factor for CHD in a variety of populations.

Interaction of diabetes with other risk factors to accelerate atherosclerosis of coronary and peripheral vessels is also confirmed.

Genetics

Advances in the techniques of molecular biology have aided the definition of genetic factors which may be important in atherosclerosis. In one study, the proportion of subjects homozygous for DNA restriction fragments (U-alleles) in the polymorphic region flanking the 5′-end of the insulin gene of chromosome 11 was higher in a group of NIDDM patients than in normal controls (23). The U-alleles were found to be strongly associated with macrovascular disease in diabetic and non-diabetic subjects.

A promising approach has been to look for genetic markers near the sites of genes that are known to be involved in lipid metabolism as well as sites near the insulin gene. In a study of 500 patients in West Germany who had coronary angiopathy, 3 markers near the apolipoprotein genes A-I, C-III, and A-IV were associated with an increased risk for CHD, while one marker near the insulin gene was also associated (24). Other studies have related insulin and apolipoprotein A-I and C-III gene polymorphism to hypertriglyceridemia and diabetes mellitus (25-27).

Eventually, it should be possible to define genetic markers which will predict which patients are at high risk for vascular disease and to institute preventive measures early in life in such individuals.

Pathogenesis

Ross and co-workers have developed a hypothetical scheme of the pathogenesis of atherosclerosis which is supported by work in animal models (28, 29). Based on cholesterol-feeding experiments in monkeys, these workers suggest that the initial lesion in atherosclerosis, which leads to the development of the fatty streak, is adherence of circulating monocytes to the endothelium. Following this, there is subendothelial migration of the monocyte/macrophage, and release of growth factors into this area. These growth factors, which may also be released by endothelium, cause growth and migration of arterial smooth muscle cells. Retraction of endothelium over areas of macrophage accumulation may then be seen, caused by superoxides or by other toxic products released by the activated cells. At this site of endothelial damage, platelets may adhere, aggregate, and release potent intracellular materials, including platelet-derived growth factor and products of the arachidonic acid pathway, such as thromboxane and other eicosanoids.

Lipid accumulation is a classical lesion of atherosclerosis, and is seen as intracellular and extracellular cholesterol in macrophages to produce foam cells, or in smooth muscle cells and connective tissue. Low-density lipoproteins and remnants may deliver cholesterol to atherosclerotic lesions and high-density lipoproteins may act to prevent cholesterol deposition. Depending upon endothelial and other counterregulatory forces, this process could contribute to fibrosis, lipid accumulation, and/or thrombosis. Alterations in the vascular wall could be involved, as could a variety of factors extrinsic to the blood vessel itself, such as cigarette smoking, hypertension and infections.

Whatever the precise sequence of events, it is clear that an understanding of the atherosclerotic process could emerge from studies of the various factors extrinsic to and intrinsically part of the arterial wall. In order to determine the effect of a disease state such as diabetes mellitus, it is logical to examine how diabetes may alter these pathogenetic processes. The effects of diabetes on endothelium, monocyte/macrophages, platelets, smooth muscle cells, lipids/lipoproteins, blood coagulation and flow will be reviewed. How accelerated atherosclerosis in diabetes affects various target organs will also be considered, as will new studies which have been directed at preventive therapy for atherosclerosis.

Endothelium

Since endothelial damage is an early event in atherosclerosis, it is appropriate to consider how this may occur in diabetes mellitus and what the evidence is that it is present in diabetes. Endothelial damage may occur by a variety of mechanisms. Two, which may be operative in diabetes, are physical and biochemical influences. Hypertension is present in diabetes more often than in control subjects, and is a probable cause of endothelial damage. Cigarette smoking may exert a major effect on the vascular system by endothelial damage. It has been postulated that the increased vascular wall stiffening present in diabetes may contribute to endothelial damage, particularly at areas of great stress by impairing the usual resilient response of the endothelial cells to arterial wall distention and relaxation.

Local flow conditions also play a role in atherogenesis, possibly via endothelial damage. Plaques are characteristically found in areas of separated flow, at branch points of vessels. The pattern of the separated flow is influenced by pulsatility of arterial flow and by the angular momentum of blood, which combine to produce shear stress which may affect the endothelial cells adversely (30).

Several studies have indicated that glucose may be toxic to human endothelial cells, and lead to delayed replication, disturbed cell cycles, increased release of Von Willebrand factor activity (31), and accelerated death in in-vitro systems (32). Cholesterol feeding in animals results in fatty streak accumulation at areas of monocyte attachment to damaged endothelium (29). Elevated levels of very-low-density lipoprotein (VLDL) in diabetes have been shown to cause endothelial damage (33). Under certain conditions, free fatty acids may also cause endothelial damage. There is limited information on the effects of other metabolites and/or nutrients which are altered in the diabetic state, but additional studies on individual amino acids, fatty acids, and/or lipoproteins would be of great interest.

Evidence that endothelial damage is present in diabetes mellitus has been extensively reviewed (7-9). Studies have generally focused on plasma levels or endothelial release in vitro or in vivo of materials which can serve as endothelial markers. These include Von Willebrand factor activity, prostaglandins, fibrinolytic activity, and fibronectin.

Von Willebrand factor

There were at least 15 reports of Von Willebrand factor activity in diabetes mellitus between 1964 and 1983 (8, 9). In the majority of these reports, elevated plasma levels of either VIIIR:WF (ristocetin co-factor activity) or VIII:Ag (Von Willebrand factor antigenic activity) were found in diabetes mellitus. Since Von Willebrand factor is produced mainly by endothelium, increases in plasma levels may indicate altered endothelial function. Increased levels may be found before clinically apparent vascular disease and in animal models shortly after induction of diabetes, suggesting that endothelial damage is a very early event in diabetes. More recent studies in patients with diabetic macroangiopathy confirmed the observation that, in this situation, endothelial cells increase in size and store increased amounts of Von Willebrand factor. However, a suggestion which appeared in older studies (34) that growth hormone may modulate Von Willebrand factor release was not confirmed by growth hormone infusion studies in normal and NIDDM subjects (35). Short-term metabolic control with insulin did not return to normal the elevated plasma Von Willebrand factor in diabetic human subjects or rats with streptozotocin-induced diabetes.

The functional significance of altered Von Willebrand factor levels in diabetes mellitus is not clear. However, since Von Willebrand factor is a molecule that is critical for normal platelet adhesiveness and since its relative absence in pig models appears to protect against cholesterol feeding-induced atherosclerosis (36), it is accepted as a co-factor in the pathogenesis of atherosclerosis. In any case, the consistent findings of elevated plasma levels in diabetes mellitus indicate that endothelial damage may occur early in the course of that disorder, and one can postulate that this could predispose such individuals to acceleration of the atherosclerotic process as a result of this damage.

Prostacyclin

Prostacyclin (PGI_2) is a product of arachidonic acid metabolism and can be synthesized and released by vascular endothelium. It is a potent vasodilator and platelet antiaggregatory substance; as such, it has been postulated to have a protective role in the development of atherosclerosis. Prostacyclin synthesis and release from vascular tissues in diabetes has received extensive study (7-9). Between 1978 and 1986, there were at least 32 reports of prostacyclin levels in animal models of diabetes mellitus (9) (rat, swine guinea-pigs, mice), and decreased synthesis and/or release of prostacyclin has generally been found. Chronic insulin treatment can restore values to normal. There are certain vascular beds, however, in which increased prostacyclin synthesis is seen in diabetic animals. Thus, renal mesangial cells (37) and the coronary circulation (38, 39) synthesize increased quantities of prostacyclin in diabetic animals when compared with controls.

There are also many studies of prostacyclin levels in human subjects with diabetes mellitus. Between 1979 and 1986, there were at least 17 reports of prostacyclin release by vasculature obtained as surgical specimens or estimations of prostacyclin levels by the measurement of its metabolite, 6-keto-$PGF_{1\alpha}$ in subjects with diabetes mellitus (9). Generally, the levels of these eicosanoids have been found to be low in diabetic patients (9).

There are intriguing aspects of the prostacyclin story which require further study, however. Analysis of prostacyclin by measuring its metabolite, 6-keto-$PGF_{1\alpha}$, is subject to error (40). The level of the defect in the synthetic scheme is not clear; presumably, it is proximal to prostacyclin synthetase, since this activity is not decreased in venous tissue obtained from diabetic subjects (41). Human diabetic umbilical arteries will synthesize increased quantities of 15-hydroxy-5,8,11,13-eicosatetraenoic acid (15-HETE), an arachidonic acid metabolite which may inhibit cyclo-oxygenase (42). Thus, this is one possible biochemical explanation for the decreased synthesis of prostacyclin in diabetes, since its synthesis is dependent on the cyclo-oxygenase pathway. Red blood cells obtained from diabetic subjects stimulate normal endothelium to release increased quantities of prostacyclin (43).

Thus, prostacyclin release is often depressed in diabetes, but there are differences in various vascular cells, and release may be increased under certain circumstances. As with Von Willebrand factor, these findings can be interpreted as evidence of endothelial damage in diabetes, and further work is needed to define the role of prostacyclin in atherosclerosis.

Fibrinolytic activity

Plasminogen activator is produced by the endothelium and acts as the enzyme in the system which converts plasminogen to plasmin. Plasmin is a limiting factor in the growth and dissolution of thrombi, since it is responsible for the degradation of the fibrin clot. Thus, plasminogen activator activity has been assessed with great interest in diabetes, both as an index of endothelial activity and also as an indicator of an altered coagulation system in this disease. Activity has generally been assessed in plasma, with or without stimulation by venous compression or other means. It has also been estimated in vascular tissue taken from diabetic subjects. In the majority of studies, the action of a euglobulin precipitate of plasma on fibrin plates in vitro, the euglobulin lysis time is measured. The euglobulin precipitation step removes most, but not all, plasma inhibitors of fibrinolytic activity. In a few studies, dilute whole-blood clot lysis time is measured. More recently, studies using solid-phase radioassay techniques or plasminogen activator antigenic activity (t-PA) have been used.

A summary of 22 reports in the medical literature has been published (9). In view of the many methods used and the heterogeneous nature of the subjects studied, it is difficult to generalize about the results of these studies. Thus, either decreased, normal or increased levels of fibrinolytic activity have been reported in diabetes. It is likely that much of the confusion is caused by the fact that assays which are dependent upon fibrinolytic activity in vitro represent a balance between activators and inhibitors in plasma. Recent evidence supports this view in diabetes mellitus, where an excess of inhibitors has been found in the presence of normal levels of a t-PA antigenic activity (44, 45). Of interest is the report that 24 hours of normoglycemia induced by insulin therapy in IDDM will depress euglobulin lysis time and t-PA activity (46), suggesting a means by which insulin may contribute to thrombogenesis in diabetes. Clearly, more research is needed in this interesting area of investigation.

Fibronectin

Fibronectin is a high-molecular-weight protein which is produced by endothelium, fibroblasts and other mesenchymal cells. It interacts with cell surfaces and extracellular matrix components, and binds with collagen and heparin. In view of the interest in endothelial function in diabetes, and with the availability of sensitive assays, there have appeared a few reports of its activity in diabetes mellitus. In patients with IDDM, resting plasma fibronectin levels are normal. However, after endothelial stimulation by venous compression, plasma fibronectin levels rise more in IDDM subjects than in normal controls (47). Non-enzymatic glycation of fibronectin is increased more than two-fold in diabetic dogs and is proportional to plasma glucose levels (48). It has been shown that non-enzymatic glycosylation of fibronectin will inhibit its binding to connective tissue components (49). This, in turn, could contribute to faulty integrity of extracellular matrices in diabetes. Elevated plasma levels of fibronectin have been found in NIDDM, particularly those with enhanced platelet aggregation (50). Thus, elevated fibronectin may be related to the altered platelet function and vascular wall integrity in diabetes, and may be viewed as another piece of non-specific evidence of endothelial damage in the disease.

Platelets

For almost 20 years, investigators have been intrigued by the possibility that altered platelet behavior in diabetes mellitus may play a role in diabetic vascular disease.

A summary of altered platelet functions which have been reported in diabetes mellitus is given in Table 1. The evidence from the older literature which underlies this table can be found in a number of recent review articles (7-9), and will not be summarized here. New observations on platelet function in diabetes which have appeared in the past few years will be reviewed below.

TABLE 1. *Altered platelet function in diabetes mellitus*

↑ Adhesiveness		
↑ Aggregation		
Platelet-plasma interactions		
Von Willebrand factor	Immune complexes	Lipoproteins
Fibrinogen		
↑ Arachidonic acid metabolism		
↑ Phospholipase activity		
↑ Thromboxane A_2, prostaglandin E_2		
↑ Plasma β-thromboglobulin, platelet Factor 4, platelet-derived growth factors		
↓ Platelet survival		

Platelet adhesion

Older studies of platelet adhesion in diabetes generally used techniques which did not distinguish platelet adhesion from platelet aggregation (9). More recently, a newer method using a rotating-probe device has been used, and the adhesiveness of washed platelets from diabetic rats was studied (51, 52). In this system, no difference between platelets from diabetic and control rats was seen, suggesting that previous reports of increased adhesiveness in diabetes may have been due to increased aggregability of platelets, which would not affect this system. On the other hand, elevated levels of plasma proteins which increase platelet adhesiveness (Von Willebrand factor and fibrinogen) are found in diabetes mellitus, and earlier studies may have been correct, when platelet-rich plasma was used. Further, new studies which have shown increased adhesiveness of washed platelets from IDDM patients to cultured bovine endothelium (53) lend support to the idea that platelet adhesiveness is increased in subjects with diabetes mellitus.

Platelet aggregation

There are over 50 studies of platelet aggregation in diabetic animals and in man which have been reported in the scientific literature, and the majority of these have reported increased sensitivity to platelet-aggregating agents in platelet-rich plasma or in whole blood in diabetes mellitus (7-9, 54-56). The presence of this phenomenon in platelets from newly diagnosed diabetic subjects (9) and in washed platelets from rats shortly after the induction of streptozotocin-induced diabetes (51, 57) suggests that the altered platelet function is a manifestation of the abnormal metabolic state of diabetes, rather than merely the result of established vascular disease. However, species differences exist. Increased platelet sensitivity to aggregating agents could not be shown in experimentally induced diabetes in dogs. Since these animals developed retinopathy, the role of altered platelet behavior in this form of microangiopathy was questioned (58).

Platelet-plasma interactions

Early studies demonstrated that plasma from diabetic subjects could enhance ADP-induced platelet aggregation in vitro (7-9). The nature of plasma-platelet interactions has received further study in recent years. Platelet-activity factor (PAF) stimulation of platelets from IDDM subjects caused more release of thromboxane and hydroxytryptamine than did stimulation of control platelets (59). Fibrinogen binding to platelets from diabetic subjects is increased, correlates with hyperaggregability, and is suppressed by aspirin. This suggests that increased fibrinogen binding is mediated by increased formation of endoperoxides and/or thromboxane (60). Involvement of other plasma factors in the hypersensitivity of platelets to aggregating agents was suggested by studies in IDDM children, which showed a positive correlation of aggregation with apolipoprotein A1 and a negative correlation with plasma triglyceride levels (61). Immune complexes from IDDM subjects were shown to accentuate ADP-induced platelet aggregation in earlier studies (62). Thus, in vivo, it is likely that platelet-plasma interactions play a role in altered platelet behavior in diabetes (Table 1).

Platelet metabolism of arachidonic acid

Since the seminal observations by Halushka and associates of increased production of prostaglandin E_2 by platelets from diabetic subjects (63), there have been many additional observations of arachidonic acid metabolism in diabetes mellitus. These have been the subject of several recent reviews (7-9, 64). These studies have generally reported increased synthesis of thromboxane B_2 and of other eicosanoids from platelets from animals and human subjects with diabetes mellitus. Increased thromboxane synthesis presumably plays a role in the increased aggregation in diabetes, since both are blocked by thromboxane synthetase inhibitors and by a thromboxane receptor antagonist (65).

The exact sites responsible for the increased thromboxane synthesis are not completely defined. There may be multiple sites. Thus, there is evidence of increased arachidonic acid incorporation into platelet phospholipids in NIDDM subjects (66), but no evidence of increased platelet arachidonic acid stores (67). The activity of fatty acid cyclo-oxygenase and/or thromboxane synthetase in platelets in diabetes mellitus has not yet been determined. A low platelet vitamin E content may be a contributory factor to the increased thromboxane synthesis seen in platelets from IDDM subjects (68).

Platelet-specific proteins

Many previous studies have shown elevated plasma levels of the platelet-specific proteins, β-thromboglobulin (BTG) and platelet Factor 4 (PF4) (7-9). This is particularly apparent in diabetic subjects with existing vascular disease, and is generally interpreted as reflecting in vivo platelet aggregation and release. In one recent study, BTG levels were positively correlated with plasma triglycerides, cholesterol, phospholipids, and total plasma lipids in IDDM subject (69). Plasma BTG levels were also correlated positively with platelet adhesiveness to bovine endothelium in IDDM patients in another study (53). PF4 levels within platelets were found to be lower in diabetic subjects than in controls, but the release of PF4 after heparin was increased in diabetes mellitus (70).

An exciting area of platelet research, and one which may relate directly to atherosclerosis, according to Ross (28, 29), is that of platelet-derived growth factors. Studies from at least two different laboratories have now indicated that growth factors released by platelets may be found in excess in diabetic subjects. Umeda and co-workers found that a platelet lysate prepared from IDDM patients caused increased DNA synthesis in cultured vascular smooth muscle cells (71). Koschinsky and co-workers found that serum growth factors were present in NIDDM patients which would cause growth stimulation of human arterial smooth muscle cells (72, 73). A serum fraction of molecular weight

<3500 was found to have growth-promoting activity 2-10 times that of growth hormone or insulin on arterial smooth muscle cells or fibroblasts. In view of the potential importance of platelet-derived and other growth factors in atherosclerosis, further research in this critical area is awaited with interest.

Platelet survival

There are many studies showing a decreased platelet survival in subjects with diabetes mellitus (7-9). In general, there is reduced platelet survival when vascular disease is present in diabetes mellitus. Since such findings could be merely the result of the vascular disease and not be related to the diabetic state, recent studies have been done in streptozotocin-induced diabetes in rats — an animal model that is presumably free from vascular disease. Platelet survival was reduced shortly after the induction of diabetes (2 weeks), and then was prolonged after 4 weeks of diabetes (74). Cross-transfusion experiments showed that platelet alterations caused the diminished survival in the acute state, while factors independent of platelets were involved in chronically diabetic animals. Platelet survival was also prolonged in spontaneously diabetic BB Wistar rats with diabetes of 3-5 months (75).

These studies illustrate the importance of carefully defining the type and duration of diabetes when platelet survival studies are done. They support the view that both diabetes and vascular disease can shorten platelet survival, but that chronic diabetes without vascular disease is associated with counter-regulatory processes that normalize or prolong platelet survival.

Effect of therapy

Interest in the 'platelet story' has led to attempts to modify platelet function by therapy with insulin, sulfonylureas, lipid-lowering drugs, or drugs which affect platelet behavior.

Several studies have reported on the effect of intensive treatment with insulin on altered platelet function in diabetes mellitus. Insulin treatment of rats with streptozotocin-induced diabetes for 7 days returned ADP-induced, but not thrombin-induced, aggregation of washed platelets to normal (76). Short-term (24-hour) treatment of IDDM subjects by Biostator was reported to reduce plasma BTG and PF4 levels (77). In studies of longer duration, Mayfield and colleagues reported that intensive insulin therapy for several weeks would lower platelet thromboxane release and decrease aggregation to arachidonic acid, but not to ADP (78). In a longer-term study of 16 weeks in diabetic subjects with neuropathy, Jackson and co-workers reported that near-normal metabolic control reduced collagen-induced thromboxane release, but did not normalize aggregation to ADP, collagen or arachidonic acid (79). In another study, no effect of intensive insulin therapy on ADP-induced aggregation, BTG, PF4 or clotting factors was observed in IDDM patients (80). It is clear from these studies that variable effects of insulin therapy on platelet function have been reported from different laboratories and in different populations. While species and patient differences may account for some of the disparity, it also appears that while insulin therapy may suppress thromboxane release, it has no consistent effects on platelet aggregation.

In one study in NIDDM patients, glibenclamide therapy was observed to lower glucose, BTG and thromboxane levels (81).

One large-scale study of the effects of aspirin (325 mg t.i.d.) plus dipyridamole (75 mg t.i.d.) (versus placebo) on major vascular events in patients with NIDDM after amputation for gangrene was reported (82, 83). No effects of antiplatelet therapy were seen on major end-points of opposite side amputations and vascular deaths. There also was no effect with secondary end-points of myocardial infarction, total deaths, or total amputations. A protective effect on the secondary end-point of strokes and transient ischemic atrophy was observed. This finding was like that seen in other antiplatelet studies, suggesting that the cerebral circulation is particularly sensitive to the protective effects of antiplatelet drugs.

There are several other studies on antiplatelet drugs in diabetic vascular disease. The largest is the NIH-sponsored Early Treatment in Diabetic Retinopathy Study (ETDRS), where the effects of aspirin (650 mg once daily) versus placebo on diabetic retinopathy are being studied (84). In this study, the effects of aspirin on major vascular events were also monitored.

Conclusion

It is clear that altered platelet function is found in diabetes mellitus. Thus, increased platelet adhesiveness and aggregation can be found in patients with or without vascular disease and in animal models of diabetes. Platelet interactions with plasma constituents, including platelet-activating factor(s), Von Willebrand factor, immune complexes, fibrinogen, lipoproteins, and (possibly) glucose have been shown to be accentuated in diabetes mellitus. One metabolic explanation is increased production of thromboxane, probably via increased phospholipase activity and possibly related to increased arachidonic acid transfer from circulating lipoproteins into platelet membrane stores. Other non-arachidonic-acid-mediated causes of platelet hyperaggregability exist, and require further study. Evidence in vivo of platelet activation in diabetes exists, as shown by accelerated platelet turnover, increased plasma levels of platelet-specific proteins, BTG and PF4, and increase in circulating platelet aggregates. A role of altered platelet function in atherosclerosis is suggested by studies showing increased activity of platelet-derived growth factor in diabetic subjects.

However, in spite of this strong background of altered platelet function in diabetes, there is no direct (or indirect) evidence to show conclusively that it contributes to the accelerated atherosclerosis characteristic of diabetes. It is likely that the best clinical evidence will come from antiplatelet studies in patients with diabetes. If such studies should show a protective effect of antiplatelet agents on major vascular end-points in diabetic subjects, this would be compelling evidence supporting a role of altered platelet behavior in the pathogenesis of vascular disease of diabetes mellitus.

Red blood cells

Alterations of red blood cells (RBC) in diabetes mellitus have long been recognized. In diabetes, RBC may have decreased deformability, an increased tendency to aggregate, and may cause increased shear stress, particularly at branch points of vessels (30). Increased RBC cholesterol content was found in diabetes in one study, and was related to decreased RBC deformability and to HbA_{1c} levels (85). In another study in IDDM, no changes in membrane fluid or membrane cholesterol levels were found (86). A possible reconciliation of these findings was reported by Goebel et al (87). These investigators found that only old RBC from NIDDM subjects displayed decreased deformability, while young cells had normal deformability. In another study, short-term treatment with insulin altered RBC membrane lipids, suggesting another reason for variability between studies (88). These findings, along with earlier studies, suggest that altered RBC deformability, perhaps related to changes in RBC membrane lipid content, are present in some subjects with diabetes, but not in all patients. These changes may contribute to atherosclerosis at areas of shear stress.

Insulin

Some older studies have suggested that hyperinsulinemia may contribute to accelerated atherosclerosis in diabetes. This postulate has been the subject of a number of review articles, and a symposium was recently held which analyzed this subject in depth (89). This symposium concluded that while there was suggestive epidemiological and basic research information to support the hypothesis, much more research was needed before one could determine the precise role of insulin as an atherogenic factor.

In one prospective study, 247 NIDDM patients were followed with electrocardiograms (ECG) for 5 years (90). At baseline, subjects with abnormal ECG had higher fasting and post-glucose insulin levels than did those with normal ECG. Patients who developed ECG abnormalities in 5 years had higher fasting insulin levels before and after development of the abnormalities. This is another correlative study between plasma insulin levels and cardiac events which lends support to the idea that endogenous hyperinsulinemia may contribute to atherosclerosis of the coronary arteries.

In a study of first-degree relatives of IDDM patients who had oral glucose tolerance tests, positive correlations between insulin response and levels of the atherogenic lipids cholesterol, LDL-cholesterol, and triglycerides were seen (91). In a separate study, an inverse relationship between C-peptide responses to glucose and HDL-cholesterol levels were seen in a group of insulin-treated diabetic subjects (92). These studies suggest that lipid/lipoprotein disorders associated with endogenous hyperinsulinemia may help account for accelerated atherosclerosis seen in some diabetic subjects. One mechanism by which insulin may act was provided by a study of aortic metabolism in pigs with peripheral hyperinsulinemia (93). Pigs were immunized with crystalline insulin and showed impaired glucose tolerance, increased fasting serum-free insulin and C-peptide ratios, and increased postprandial insulin/glucose ratios. In these pigs, elevation of aortic triglycerides was found when compared with control pigs.

Other hormones

A correlation between high serum estrogen levels and myocardial infarction in men prompted a study of the ratio of serum estradiol to testosterone levels in NIDDM subjects (94). An elevated ratio was found, suggesting to the authors that hyperestrogenemia may contribute to accelerated atherosclerosis in diabetes. In a study of 83 IDDM and NIDDM subjects, 32% were found to have increased levels of angiotensin-converting enzyme activity; however, no correlation with diabetic vascular disease was found (95).

The vascular wall

It has been postulated that the vascular wall stiffness that occurs in diabetes mellitus may result from non-enzymatic glycosylation of vascular wall proteins. Cerami and co-workers have pointed out that glucose-protein adducts could form in diabetes which would be similar to the Maillard reaction which occurs in stored food (96, 97). Cross-linking of these products would result in decreased protein solubility and altered mechanical properties. In support of this hypothesis, these investigators showed that incubation of tendon collagen with reducing sugars results in increased breaking time which correlates with the appearance of cross-linked browning products. Studies of dura mater collagen in IDDM patients showed findings characteristic of increased browning (96, 97).

Increased glycosylation of lens-capsule basement membrane in diabetes, compatible with that seen in premature aging, was observed in another study (98).

These findings are of great interest. Results with vascular wall collagen from individuals or animals with diabetes are needed. However, the hypothesis is a very attractive one to help explain the vascular wall stiffening seen in diabetes mellitus. Further, since there is evidence that such vascular wall products can trap circulating lipids (99), this provides an additional mechanism by which these changes could contribute to atherosclerosis.

Lipids and lipoproteins

The hypothesis that altered lipid/lipoprotein metabolism is a major contributor to atherosclerosis receives support in non-diabetic as well as diabetic individuals. Elevated plasma cholesterol levels are recognized as a major risk factor for coronary artery disease and for other major vascular events. It is therefore critical that careful attention be given to alterations of the lipid/lipoprotein levels which may occur in diabetes to help explain accelerated atherosclerosis in that disorder. This problem will be explored from 3 points of view: (a) plasma levels of lipids/lipoproteins; (b) lipid/lipoprotein cell interactions; and (3) therapy.

Plasma levels of lipids/lipoproteins (see also Chapter 25)

A relatively clear picture of plasma levels of lipids/lipoproteins in subjects with IDDM and NIDDM has now emerged (7-9). In those who are in poor metabolic control, plasma levels of cholesterol and triglycerides are usually high, as are plasma low-density lipoprotein (LDL) and very-low-density lipoprotein (VLDL) levels. While these levels may be easily returned to normal with insulin therapy in IDDM, they are often more resistant to such therapy in NIDDM. In the latter group, a combination of elevated cholesterol and triglyceride levels, reflecting increased hepatic VLDL production as well as poor peripheral clearance, is frequently the case. HDL-cholesterol levels are often depressed in NIDDM subjects, while they are frequently normal or elevated in IDDM.

These studies have been confirmed by observations from a variety of populations and centers. In a study of the Pima Indians, elevation of plasma VLDL and LDL triglycerides with depression of HDL-cholesterol were seen in men and women, while elevation of LDL-cholesterol was seen only in women (100). In Japan, 57% of NIDDM subjects studied had high VLDL and LDL levels, and a correlation with obesity was seen (101). In France, elevated total cholesterol and triglycerides with depressed HDL-cholesterol were reported in NIDDM patients (102). In the United States, it was found that NIDDM had a greater effect on triglyceride and lipoprotein cholesterol levels in women than in men (103), suggesting an explanation for the increased risk of atherosclerosis in diabetic women.

In IDDM patients, the influence of metabolic control with insulin on lipid/lipoprotein levels was re-emphasized. A direct correlation between glycosylated hemoglobin and triglycerides and an indirect correlation between glucosylated hemoglobin and HDL-cholesterol was noted (104). Increased HDL-cholesterol levels in IDDM children were found, and were postulated to be related to insulin therapy (105). Race was shown to influence HDL-cholesterol levels in a survey of Blacks and Whites in the United States (106). Finally, IDDM subjects with albuminuria (over 150 mg/d) showed elevated total and LDL-cholesterol, triglycerides, and apolipoprotein B (apo-B) levels, while HDL-cholesterol levels were low (107).

Several mechanisms have been suggested to explain these alterations in plasma lipid/lipoprotein levels in NIDDM. In a series of ingenious studies, Fielding and associates have explored altered reverse cholesterol transport in NIDDM (108). They found that VLDL and LDL from NIDDM had an increased ratio of cholesterol to phospholipid, and that this increased free cholesterol content would block cholesterol ester transfer to these lipoproteins by HDL cholesterol. In another study of apoproteins in NIDDM, increased levels of apo-C-III and decreased levels of apo-E were found (109). It was suggested that diabetes might alter these apolipoproteins, perhaps through sialation, and thereby inhibit the VLDL catabolism which is accelerated by these co-factors. Thus, mechanisms by which diabetes alters lipoprotein metabolism were suggested, and studies of lipoprotein-cell interactions gave information on how and why atherosclerosis might be accelerated in the diabetic state.

Lipid/lipoprotein cell interactions

VLDL and remnant particles that are loaded with triglyceride may accumulate in diabetic patients. These particles are preferentially taken up by macrophages, leading to intracellular accumulation of cholesterol esters and/or triglycerides (110, 111). Changes in the relative proportions of apo-C and apo-E which occur in diabetes may facilitate this process (112, 113). Non-enzymatic glycosylation of the VLDL apolipoprotein moiety in diabetes may also play a role in the recognition of these particles by macrophages. Glycosylated apo-E and apo-C may be transferred from HDL to chylomicra and to VLDL in diabetes and contribute to this process (114). It is possible that glycosylation of these particles may alter macrophage recognition (115). It has been reported that VLDL isolated from patients with NIDDM will result in greater accumulation of triglycerides and cholesterol esters by macrophages than will VLDL from non-diabetic individuals (116, 117).

Alterations in the LDL molecule in diabetes mellitus may also alter cellular recognition. LDL isolated from IDDM subjects in poor metabolic control are taken up and degraded less efficiently by human fibroblasts than are LDL taken from normal controls or from the same subjects after control of hyperglycemia by insulin (118). These LDL particles are rich in triglyceride, and it has been shown that triglyceride-enriched LDL from non-diabetic individuals are poorly recognized by fibroblasts (120). However, non-enzymatic glycosylation of LDL in vitro will alter their biological activity, leading to a reduced degradation of glycosylated LDL by fibroblasts (120). Antibodies specific for glycosylated LDL have been demonstrated in diabetes, and it is suggested that glycosylation may have rendered these lipoproteins immunogenic. It is possible that this may help account for high immune complex levels in diabetes and atherosclerosis (121).

Since macrophages are cells which are critical to the atherosclerotic process, it is of interest to explore studies of LDL-macrophage interactions in diabetes mellitus. Interaction of LDL glycosylated in vitro with mouse peritoneal macrophages suggested that glycosylated LDL were not recognized by these cells (122, 123). Recently, however, an increase in cholesterol ester synthesis in human macrophages exposed to LDL isolated from IDDM patients has been shown (116, 117). A significant correlation between the degree of LDL glycosylation and cholesterol ester synthesis was observed, and similar results were obtained with LDL glycosylated in vitro (124). There is also enhanced degradation of glycosylated LDL by macrophages, which occurs by a process independent of the classic LDL receptor pathway (124). Insulin therapy will increase LDL degradation by macrophages and will increase LDL clearance (125). These studies suggest a mechanism by which foam cells may accumulate in diabetes mellitus.

When LDL is modified in vitro by incubation with VLDL and lipid transfer proteins, to yield particles like those seen in diabetic subjects with hypertriglyceridemia, the uptake and degradation of LDL by cultured fibroblasts are reduced (126). Non-enzymatic glycosylation of LDL by incubation with glucose will inhibit uptake and degradation by endothelial cells (127).

As noted above, HDL levels and composition may be affected in diabetes. Cholesterol efflux from fibroblasts is inhibited when the cells are incubated in plasma from poorly controlled NIDDM subjects (108). This may be due to altered reverse cholesterol transport, i.e. a transfer of free cholesterol from VLDL and LDL to HDL in diabetes which inhibits uptake by HDL of free cholesterol from cells (108). Studies are needed on the effects of triglyceride enrichment and/or glycosylation of HDL on the function of HDL to remove cholesterol from cholesterol-overloaded cells.

Therapy

In view of the probable importance of altered lipid/lipoprotein levels in atherosclerosis in diabetes, there have been many studies of the effect of therapy for diabetes on these changes. Earlier studies had shown a correlation between HbA_{1c} levels and plasma LDL and HDL-cholesterol levels, with a return towards normal with intensive insulin therapy in IDDM patients (128). These studies have now been confirmed with insulin therapy in IDDM children and adolescents (129), diabetic ketoacidosis (130), and other IDDM populations (131). In one study, plasma apo-B levels were particularly responsive to insulin therapy in IDDM (132); in another study, there were minimal changes observed if the patients had mild or moderate hyperglycemia (133). One study explored the effect of diet therapy on lipid/lipoprotein levels in IDDM (134). In this study, it was clearly established that a high-carbohydrate, low-fat, cholesterol-restricted diet would result in a significant fall in serum cholesterol, LDL-cholesterol, and apo-B concentrations. HDL-cholesterol levels also fell, but the LDL-cholesterol/HDL-cholesterol levels were unchanged.

The effects of caloric restriction and weight loss on atherosclerotic risk factors were once again demonstrated in subjects with NIDDM. In Australia, there was a loss of weight, and a fall in plasma glucose, insulin, triglycerides, and VLDL triglycerides in Aborigines with NIDDM who were tested while leading an urban existence and 7 weeks of living as hunter-gatherers (135). In obese NIDDM subjects given a protein-sparing fast and/or gastric bypass surgery, glycemic control improved and significant improvement in all atherosclerotic risk factors occurred (136). In another population of NIDDM patients, 3 months of a hypocaloric (200 kcal/d) diet resulted in a fall in VLDL triglycerides and a rise in HDL-cholesterol with no change in lipoprotein lipase activity, suggesting that decreased synthesis, rather than increased clearance, accounted for the fall in VLDL triglyceride (137). In another study, improved metabolic control in NIDDM patients with marked hypertriglyceridemia lowered triglyceride levels by decreasing VLDL triglyceride overproduction in the majority of patients (138). However, responses were not uniform, and in two patients the effect was primarily an increased fractional clearance rate of VLDL triglyceride.

Several new studies examined the effect of high-fiber, high-carbohydrate diets in NIDDM patients. As had been reported in earlier studies, these diets will result in lowering of serum cholesterol, triglycerides, VLDL-cholesterol, and LDL-cholesterol levels (139). One study showed that these effects are due to the high fiber, rather than the high carbohydrate, content of the diet (140).

Finally, the influences of thiazides and beta-blockers on serum lipid levels were analyzed in diabetic patients. Subjects with insulin-treated diabetes who were taking thiazides were found to have higher LDL-cholesterol and HbA_{1c}

levels than did those on furosemide or no diuretic (141). Beta-blockers were found to cause elevations in serum triglycerides in 48%, to increase LDL-cholesterol in 31%, and to decrease HDL-cholesterol in 43%, of a mixed group of diabetic and non-diabetic subjects (142). No differences between cardioselective and non-selective beta-blockers were seen.

Therapy of diabetes, therefore, should consist of vigorous attempts to modify the major risk factors associated with atherosclerosis. These include stopping smoking, treatment of hypertension (with avoidance of thiazides and beta-blockers, if possible), glycemic control by diet, sulfonylureas, or insulin, and diets designed to cause weight reduction in the obese. Major goals are to change atherosclerosis-inducing lipid and lipoprotein levels, elevated plasma glucose, high blood pressure levels, and return excess weight to normal. It is likely that an exercise program is also beneficial; however, there are limited studies of this in diabetic subjects.

Conclusions

In this Chapter, we have attempted to review recent evidence on the epidemiology, genetics, pathogenesis and therapy of atherosclerosis in diabetes mellitus. First, the pathogenesis in non-diabetic individuals is a subject of active research, and therefore is open to changing views. Extrapolation from current postulates to a disease state as complicated and heterogeneous as diabetes mellitus could be inaccurate and misleading. Investigators are limited by a variety of factors in their search to delineate mechanisms involved in the atherosclerotic process in man. Thus, there has been limited access to normal arterial tissue for studies in vitro, and non-invasive techniques for assessing the degree and extent of early lesions of atherosclerosis in vivo are limited. Longitudinal studies are compromised by these limitations of technique and by the slow progression of the process. Investigators have therefore often relied upon correlative relationships and/or studies using cell systems which may not be directly transferable to the atherosclerotic process in man. Animal models are also limited, leading to the result that much of the work in animals has been done in species in which atherosclerosis is a difficult lesion to produce. Clinical trials in diabetes, which could provide useful indirect information, have been sparse in number, and usually have been secondary prevention trials in patients with very advanced vascular disease. Primary prevention of atherosclerosis is of greatest importance.

Nevertheless, the situation is improving. Advances in surgical techniques in man, with close co-ordination of investigators from various disciplines, have led to the availability of fresh human tissue from coronary bypass patients and other individuals who undergo major surgery. Tissue culture techniques allow investigators to study directly the metabolism and function of critical components of the human arterial tree, and to manipulate objectively variables involved in the atherosclerotic process. Non-invasive techniques for assessing the vascular system in man are undergoing refinement, and are becoming more available to clinical investigators. Techniques of molecular biology are opening up new approaches to the genetic influences on atherosclerosis. There has been an explosion of biochemical and physiological information about prostaglandins and their derivatives and about lipids, lipoproteins and apolipoproteins in recent years. Improved animal models of atherosclerosis and diabetes mellitus exist, and work using such animals as monkeys and pigs is beginning to appear. Clinical trials are moving in the direction of primary, rather than secondary, prevention trials, and are directed at processes such as lipids/lipoproteins and/or platelets/prostaglandins which are postulated to be operative as early events in the process of atherosclerosis in diabetes mellitus.

With this background and perspective, it is useful to provide an overview which reflects current knowledge of the pathogenesis of atherosclerosis in diabetes mellitus. Endothelial injury appears to be an early event in the pathogenesis of atherosclerosis in diabetes, as it is in the non-diabetic individual. Endothelial damage might occur from hypertension, cigarette smoking, elevated LDL and/or free fatty acids, hyperglycemia, advanced glycosylation end-products, and immunologic or infectious causes. Direct evidence to support these postulates is needed in diabetes. However, evidence that endothelial damage is present in diabetes clearly exists, and includes elevation of plasma Von Willebrand factor and fibronectin levels, decreased prostacyclin release, and altered fibrinolytic activity. Platelets are more adherent in diabetes, and aggregate more readily in response to aggregating agents in vitro, releasing thromboxane, a powerful vasoconstrictor and proaggregatory agent. Other evidence of altered platelet function in diabetes includes platelet-plasma interactions, elevated plasma levels of platelet-specific proteins, and decreased platelet survival. There may also be increased release of platelet-derived growth factors, but more research is needed in this critical area in diabetes mellitus. Presumably, this process could activate the intrinsic coagulation scheme; however, studies in this area are conflicting. Although it is an attractive hypothesis, it is not clear whether a hypercoagulable state accounts for a thrombotic tendency in diabetes.

Recent studies implicating the macrophage as an important cell in atherosclerosis have stimulated new investigations directed at the effects of diabetes on macrophage function. There is now evidence that foam cells may result from many alterations of lipoproteins which are characteristic of the diabetic state, including increased production and/or decreased clearance of chylomicron and VLDL remnants, triglyceride enrichment of LDL and VLDL, glycosylation of VLDL and LDL, and glycosylation of apolipoproteins which affect particle recognition by macrophages. The role of HDL as a protective lipoprotein has stimulated interest in its alterations in the diabetic state. Low plasma levels are often found in diabetes, and it appears that glycosylation and/ or triglyceride enrichment of HDL in diabetes may occur and may modify its role in reverse cholesterol transport. Thus, the net effect of these and other lipid/lipoprotein alterations would be to promote atherosclerosis in diabetes.

It must be recognized that this model is arbitrary and simplistic. It virtually ignores the important variables of blood flow, altered white and red blood cell function, increased blood coagulation, medial wall changes, glycosylation of other proteins, small vessel disease, neuropathy, and genetic factors — all of which presumably contribute to atherosclerosis in the diabetic state. Nevertheless, it is hoped that the scheme we have presented in this review reflects the state of current knowledge in the areas emphasized, and that it can provide a stimulus for further research work on this critically important medical problem.

References

1. Barrett-Conner E, Orchard T (1985): Diabetes and heart disease. In: Harris MI, Hamman RF (Eds), *National Diabetes Data Group, Diabetes in America, Diabetes Data Compiled 1984*, Ch. XVI, pp. 1-41. NIH Publ. No. 85-1468. US Department of Health and Human Services, Public Health Service, Bethesda, MD.
2. Palumbo PJ, Melton LJ (1985): Peripheral vascular disease and diabetes. In: Harris MI, Hamman RF (Eds), *National Diabetes Data Group, Diabetes in America, Diabetes Data Compiled 1984*, Ch. XV, pp. 1-21. NIH Publ. No 85-1468, US Department of Health and Human Services, Public Health Service, Bethesda, MD.
3. Kuller LH, Dorman JS, Wolf PA (1985): Cerebrovascular disease and diabetes. In: Harris MI, Hamman RF (Eds), *National Diabetes Data Group, Diabetes in America, Diabetes Data Compiled 1984*, Ch. XVIII, pp. 1-18. NIH Publ. No. 85-1468, US Department of Health and Human Services, Public Health Service, Bethesda, MD.
4. Grundy SM (1984): Correlations of aortic histology with gross aortic atherosclerosis and metabolic measurements in diabetic and nondiabetic *Macaca nigra. Atherosclerosis, 52*, 85.
5. Grundy SM (1983): Atherosclerosis: pathology, pathogenesis, and role of risk factors. *Dis. Mon., 29*, 58.
6. Ruderman NB, Haudenschild C (1984): Diabetes as an atherogenic factor. *Prog. Cardiovasc. Dis., 26*, 373.
7. Colwell JA, Lopes-Virella ML, Halushka PV (1981): Pathogenesis of atherosclerosis in diabetes mellitus. *Diabetes Care, 4*, 121.
8. Colwell JA, Winocour PD, Lopes-Virella M, Halushka PV (1983): New concepts about the pathogenesis of atherosclerosis in diabetes mellitus. *Am. J. Med., 75*, 67.
9. Colwell JA, Lopes-Virella MF, Winocour PD, Halushka PV (1987): New concepts about the pathogenesis of atherosclerosis in diabetes mellitus. In: Levin ME, O'Neal LW (Eds), *The Diabetic Foot, 4th ed.* Mosby, St Louis, MS. In press.
10. Jarrett RJ (1984): Type 2 (non-insulin-dependent) diabetes mellitus and coronary heart disease — chicken, egg or neither? *Diabetologia, 26*, 99.
11. West KM (Ed.) (1978): *Epidemiology of Diabetes and Its Vascular Lesions, 1st ed,*. pp. 1-579. Elsevier, New York.

12. Pinsky JL, Branch LG, Jette AM et al (1985): Framingham disability study: relationship of disability to cardiovascular risk factors among persons free of diagnosed cardiovascular disease. *Am. J. Epidemiol., 122,* 644.

13. Fuller JH, Shipley MJ, Rose G et al (1983): Mortality from coronary heart disease and stroke in relation to degree of glycaemia: The Whitehall Study. *Br. Med. J., 287,* 867.

14. Butler WJ, Ostrander Jr LD, Carman WJ, Lamphiear DE (1985): Mortality from coronary heart disease in the Tecumseh study: long-term effect of diabetes mellitus, glucose tolerance and other risk factors. *Am. J. Epidemiol., 121,* 541.

15. Persson B, Johannson BW (1984): The Kockum study: twenty-two year follow-up. *Acta Med. Scand., 216,* 485.

16. Welborn TA, Knuiman M, McCann V et al (1984): Clinical macrovascular disease in Caucasoid diabetic subjects: logistic regression analysis of risk variables. *Diabetologia, 27,* 568.

17. Barrett-Connor E, Wingard DL (1983): Sex differential in ischemic heart disease mortality in diabetics: a prospective population-based study. *Am. J. Epidemiol., 118,* 489.

18. Suarez L, Barrett-Connor E (1984): Interaction between cigarette smoking and diabetes mellitus in the prediction of death attributed to cardiovascular disease. *Am. J. Epidemiol., 120,* 670.

19. Stern MP, Rosenthal M, Haffner SM et al (1984): Sex difference in the effects of socio-cultural status on diabetes and cardiovascular risk factors in Mexican Americans: The San Antonio Heart Study. *Am. J. Epidemiol., 120,* 834.

20. Paisey RB, Arredondo G, Villalobus A et al (1984): Association of differing dietary, metabolic, and clinical risk factors with macrovascular complications of diabetes: a prevalence study of 503 Mexican type II diabetic subjects. *Diabetic Care, 7,* 421.

21. Cruz Vidal M, Garcia Palmieri MR, Costas Jr R et al (1983): Abnormal blood glucose and coronary heart disease: The Puerto Rico Heart Health Program. *Diabetes Care, 6,* 556.

22. Gillum RF, Gillum BS, Smith N (1984): Cardiovascular risk factors among urban American Indians: blood pressure, serum lipids, smoking, diabetes, health knowledge, and behavior. *Am. Heart J., 107,* 765.

23. Owerbach D, Johansen K, Billesbolle P et al (1982): Possible associations between DNA sequences flanking the insulin gene and atherosclerosis. *Lancet, 2,* 1291.

24. Kolata G (1986): Reducing risk: a change of heart? *Science, 231,* 669.

25. Josett NI, Rees A, Williams LG et al (1984): Insulin and apolipoprotein A-I/C-III gene polymorphisms relating to hypertriglyceridaemia and diabetes mellitus. *Diabetologia, 27,* 180.

26. Josett NI, Williams LG, Hitman GA, Galton DJ (1984): Diabetic hypertriglyceridaemia and related 5' flanking polymorphism of the human insulin gene. *Br. Med. J., 288,* 96.

27. Baralle FE, Shoulders CC (1984): Lipoprotein genes and hyperlipidemia. *Schweiz. Med. Wochenschr., 114,* 1351.

28. Ross R, Glomset JA (1976): The pathogenesis of atherosclerosis. *N. Engl. J. Med., 295,* 369, 420.

29. Ross R (1986): The pathogenesis of atherosclerosis - an update. *N. Engl. J. Med., 3314,* 488.

30. McMillan DE (1985): Blood flow and the localization of atherosclerotic plaques. *Stroke, 16,* 582.

31. Mordes DB, Lazrachick J, Colwell JA, Sens DA (1983): Elevated glucose concentrations increase factor VIIIR:Ag levels in human umbilical vein endothelial cells. *Diabetes, 32,* 876.

32. Lorenzi M, Cagliero E, Toledo S (1985): Glucose toxicity for human endothelial cells in culture: delayed replication, disturbed cell cycle, and accelerated death. *Diabetes, 34,* 621.

33. Arbogast BW, Berry DL, Newell CL (1984): Injury of arterial endothelial cells in diabetic sucrose-fed and aged rats. *Atherosclerosis, 51,* 31.

34. Gonzalez J, Colwell JA, Sarji KE et al (1980): Effect of metabolic control with insulin on plasma von Willebrand Factor activity (9VIIIR:WF) in diabetes mellitus. *Thrombos. Res., 17,* 261.
35. Grecu EO, Sheikholislam BM, Abildgaard CF (1984): Lack of von Willebrand factor, factor VIII related antigen and factor VIII coagulant response to human growth hormone infusion in type 2 diabetes mellitus. *Am. J. Med. Sci., 287,* 3.
36. Fuster V, Bowie EJW, Lewis JC, Fass DN (1978): Resistance to arteriosclerosis in pigs with von Willebrand's disease. *J. Clin. Invest., 61,* 722.
37. Kreisberg JI, Patel PY (1983): The effects of insulin, glucose and diabetes on prostaglandin production by rat kidney glomeruli and cultured glomerular mesangial cells. *Prostaglandins Leukotrienes., Med., 11,* 431.
38. Rösen P, Senger W, Feuerstein J et al (1983): Influence of streptozotocin diabetes on myocardial lipids and prostaglandin release by the rat heart. *Biochem. Med., 30,* 19.
39. Roth DM, Reibel DK, Lefer AM (1983): Vascular responsiveness and eicosanoid production in diabetic rats. *Diabetologia, 24,* 372.
40. FitzGerald GA, Pedersen AK, Patrono C (1983): Analysis of prostacyclin and thromboxane biosynthesis in cardiovascular disease. *Circulation, 67,* 1174.
41. Saroyan RM, Kerstein MD, Kadowitz PJ et al (1984): Prostacyclin synthetase activity in diabetic human venous tissue. *Surgery, 96,* 179.
42. Setty Y, Stuart MJ (1986): 15-Hydroxy-5,8,11,13-eicosatetraenoic acid inhibits human vascular cyclooxygenase. *J. Clin. Invest., 77,* 202.
43. Wautier JL, Pintigny D, MacLouf J et al (1986): Release of prostacyclin after erythrocyte adhesion to cultured vascular endothelium. *J. Lab. Clin. Med., 107,* 210.
44. Gamba G, Perotti G, Grignani et al (1983): Activators and inhibitors of the fibrinolytic system in maturity-onset diabetes mellitus without thromboembolic manifestations. *Ric. Clin. Lab., 13,* 337.
45. Lipinska J, Lipinska B, Gurewich V (1979): Reversible inhibition of euglobulinic fibrinolytic activity in diabetes mellitus. *Thrombos. Haemostasis, 42,* 382.
46. Juhan-Vague I, Vague P, Poisson C et al (1984): Effect of 24 hours of normoglycaemia on tissue-type plasminogen activator plasma levels in insulin-dependent diabetes. *Thrombos. Haemostasis, 51,* 97.
47. Haitas B, Barnes AJ, Cederholm-Williams SA et al (1984): Abnormal endothelial release of fibrinolytic activity and fibronectin in diabetic microangiopathy. *Diabetologia, 27,* 493.
48. Tarsio JF, Wigness B, Rhode TD et al (1985): Nonenzymatic glycation of fibronectin and alterations in the molecular association of cell matrix and basement membrane components in diabetes mellitus. *Diabetes, 34,* 477.
49. Cohen MP, Ku L (1984): Inhibition of fibronectin binding to matrix components by non-enzymatic glycosylation. *Diabetes, 33,* 970.
50. Inoguchi T, Umeda F, Watanabe J et al (1986): Plasma fibronectin and platelet aggregation in diabetes mellitus. *Diabetes Res. Clin. Pract., 2,* 69.
51. Winocour PD, Kinlough-Rathbone RL, Mustard JF (1986): Pathways responsible for platelet hypersensitivity in rats with diabetes. I. Streptozotocin-induced diabetes. *J. Lab. Clin. Med., 107,* 148.
52. Winocour PD, Kinlough-Rathbone RL, Mustard JF (1986): Pathways responsible for platelet hypersensitivity in rats with diabetes. II. Spontaneous diabetes in BB Wistar rats. *J. Lab. Clin. Med., 107,* 154.
53. Rosove MH, Frank HJL, Harwig SSL, Berliner J (1985): Plasma beta-thromboglobulin is correlated with platelet adhesiveness to bovine endothelium in patients with diabetes mellitus. *Thrombos. Res., 37,* 251.
54. Mustard JF, Packham MA (1984): Platelets and diabetes mellitus. *N. Engl. J. Med., 311,* 665.

55. Paton RC, Passa Ph (1983): Platelets and diabetic vascular disease. *Diabète Métab.*, *9*, 306.
56. Jones RJ, Delamothe AP, Curtis LD et al (1985): Measurement of platelet aggregation in diabetics using the new electronic platelet aggregometer. *Diabetic Med.*, *2*, 105.
57. Winocour PD, Lopes-Virella M, Laimins M, Colwell JA (1983): Time course of changes in in vitro platelet function and plasma von Willebrand factor activity (VIIIR:WF) and factor VIII-related antigen (VIIIR:Ag) in the diabetic rat. *J. Lab. Clin. Med.*, *102*, 795.
58. Kern TS, Engerman RL (1984): Platelet aggregation in experimental diabetes and experimental galactosemia. *Diabetes*, *33*, 846.
59. Greco NJ, Arnold JH, O'Dorisio TM et al (1985): Action of platelet-activating factor on type 1 diabetic human platelets. *J. Lab. Clin. Med.*, *105*, 410.
60. DiMinno G, Silver MJ, Cerbone AM et al (1985): Increased binding of fibrinogen to platelets in diabetes: the role of prostaglandins and thromboxane. *Blood*, *65*, 156.
61. Ewald U, Kobbah N, Vessby B, Tuvemo T (1983): Increased platelet aggregability in diabetic children: relation to serum lipid and fatty acid composition. *Diabetologia*, *25*, 382.
62. Van Zile J, Kilpatrick M, Laimins M et al (1981): Platelet aggregation and release of ATP after incubation with soluble immune complexes purified from the serum of diabetic patients. *Diabetes*, *30*, 575.
63. Halushka PV, Lurie D, Colwell JA (1977): Increased synthesis of prostaglandin E-like material by platelets from patients with diabetes mellitus. *N. Engl. J. Med.*, *297*, 306.
64. Colwell JA, Halushka PV (1982): The role of prostaglandins in diabetes mellitus. In: Ellenberg M, Rifkin H, (Eds), *Diabetes Mellitus: Therapy and Practice, 3rd ed.*, pp. 295-308. McGraw-Hill, New York.
65. Watanabe J, Umeda F, Wakasugi H, Ibayashi H (1984): Effect of vitamin E on platelet aggregation in diabetes mellitus. *Tohoku J. Exp. Med.*, *143*, 161.
66. Takahashi R, Morita I, Saito Y et al (1984): Increased arachidonic acid incorporation into platelet phospholipids in Type 2 (non-insulin-dependent) diabetes. *Diabetologia*, *26*, 134.
67. Lopez-Espinoza I, Howard-Williams J, Mann JI et al (1984): Fatty acid composition of platelet phospholipids in non-insulin-dependent diabetics randomized for dietary advice. *Br. J. Nutr.*, *52*, 41.
68. Karpen CW, Cataland S, O'Dorisio TM, Panganamala RV (1984): Interrelation of platelet vitamin E and thromboxane synthesis in type I diabetes mellitus. *Diabetes*, *33*, 239.
69. Monnier LH, Chaintreuil JS, Colette C et al (1983): Plasma lipid fatty acids in platelet function in insulin-dependent diabetic patients. *Diabète Métab.*, *9*, 283.
70. O'Brien JR, Etherington MD, Pashley M (1984): Intra-platelet platelet factor 4 (IP.PF4) and the heparin-mobilisable pool of PF4 in health and atherosclerosis. *Thrombos. Haemostasis*, *51*, 354.
71. Umeda F, Franks DJ, Sugimoto H et al (1985): Effect of plasma, serum and platelets from diabetics on DNA synthesis in cultured vascular smooth muscle cells. *Clin. Invest. Med.*, *8*, 35.
72. Koschinsky T, Bunting CE, Rutter R, Gries FA (1985): Sera from Type 2 (non-insulin-dependent) diabetic and healthy subjects contain different amounts of a very low molecular weight growth peptide for vascular cells. *Diabetologia*, *28*, 223.
73. Koschinsky T (1984): Inborn and acquired metabolic disorders in human vascular cells in diabetes mellitus and hyperlipoproteinemias. *Fortschr. Med.*, *102*, 46.
74. Winocour PD, Laimins M, Colwell JA (1984): Platelet survival in streptozotocin-induced diabetic rats. *Thrombos. Haemostasis. 51*, 307.
75. Winocour PD, Kinlough-Rathbone RL, Mustard JF (1987): Platelet survival in rats with spontaneous diabetes mellitus. Submitted for publication.
76. Winocour PD, Lopes-Virella M, Laimins M, Colwell JA (1985): Effect of insulin treatment in diabetic rats on in vitro platelet function and plasma von Willebrand factor (VIIIR:WF) and factor VIII-related antigen (VIIIR/AG). *J. Lab. Clin. Med.*, *105*, 613.

77. Cucinotta D, Trifiletti A, Di Desare E et al (1985): The effect of a strict metabolic control on clotting factors and platelet function in diabetics with vascular disease. *G. Ital. Diabetol.*, 5, 311.

78. Mayfield RK, Halushka PV, Wohltmann HJ et al (1985): Platelet function during continuous insulin infusion treatment in insulin-dependent diabetic patients. *Diabetes, 34*, 1127.

79. Jackson CA, Greaves M, Boulton AJM et al (1984): Near-normal glycaemic control does not correct abnormal platelet reactivity in diabetes mellitus. *Clin. Sci., 67*, 551.

80. Rosove MH, Frank HJL, Harwig SSL (1984): Plasma beta-thromboglobulin, platelet factor 4, fibrinopeptide A, and other hemostatic functions during improved, short-term glycemic control in diabetes mellitus. *Diabetes Care, 7*, 174.

81. Brunner D, Klinger J, Weisbort J et al (1984): Thromboxane, prostacyclin, beta-thromboglobin, and diabetes mellitus. *Clin. Ther., 6*, 636.

82. Colwell JA, Bingham SF, Abraira C et al and The Cooperative Study Group (1984): V.A. Cooperative Study on Antiplatelet Agents in Diabetic Patients After Amputation for Gangrene. I. Design, methods, and baseline characteristics. *Controlled Clin. Trials, 5*, 165.

83. Colwell JA, Bingham SF, Abraira C et al and The Cooperative Study Group (1986): V.A. Cooperative Study on Antiplatelet Agents in Diabetic Patients After Amputation for Gangrene. II. Effects of aspirin and dipyridamole on atherosclerotic vascular disease rates. *Diabetes Care, 9*, 140.

84. Early Treatment Diabetic Retinopathy Study Research Group (1985): Photocoagulation for diabetic macular edema: Early Treatment Diabetic Retinopathy Study Report Number I. *Arch. Ophthalmol., 103*, 1796.

85. Cignarelli M, Blonda M, Cospite MR et al (1983): Alterations of erythrocyte lipid patterns and of some membrane related functions as a consequence of plasma lipid disorder in diabetes mellitus. *Diabète Métab., 9*. 272.

86. Hill MA, Court JM (1983): Erythrocyte membrane fluidity in type 1 diabetes mellitus. *Pathology, 15*, 449.

87. Goebel KM, Goebel FD, Lansser KG (1983): Pathologic fluidity, glycohemoglobin and metabolic disturbance of erythrocytes in Fontaine II diabetic microangiopathy. *Schweiz. Med. Wochenschr., 113*, 1936.

88. Juhan-Vague I, Driss F, Roul C et al (1984): Abnormalities of erythrocyte membrane lipids in insulin-dependent diabetics are improved by short term strict control of diabetes. *Clin. Hemorrheol., 4*, 455.

89. Colwell JA, Lopes-Virella ML, Mayfield R, Sens D (Eds) (1985): Proceedings, Workshop on Insulin and Atherogenesis. *Metabolism, 12, Suppl. 1*, 1.

90. Hillson RM, Hockaday TDR, Mann JI, Newton DJ (1984): Hyperinsulinaemia is associated with development of electrocardiographic abnormalities in diabetics. *Diabetes Res., 1*, 143.

91. Orchard TJ, Becker DJ, Bates M et al (1983): Plasma insulin and lipoprotein concentrations: an atherogenic association? *Am. J. Epidemiol., 118*, 326.

92. Laakso M, Voutilainen E, Sarlund H et al (1985): Inverse relationship of serum HDL and HDL_2 cholesterol to C-peptide level in middle-aged insulin-treated diabetics. *Metab. Clin. Exp., 34*, 715.

93. Falholt K, Alberti KGMM, Heding LG (1985): Aorta and muscle metabolism in pigs with peripheral hyperinsulinaemia. *Diabetologia, 28*, 32.

94. Phillips GB (1984): Evidence for hyperestrogenemia as the link between diabetes mellitus and myocardial infarction. *Am. J. Med., 76*, 1041.

95. Schernthaner G, Schwarzer Ch, Kuzmits R et al (1984): Increased angiotensin-converting enzyme activities in diabetes mellitus: analysis of diabetes type, state of metabolic control and occurrence of diabetic vascular disease. *J. Clin. Pathol., 37*, 307.

96. Monnier VM, Kohn RR, Cerami A (1984): Accelerated age-related browning of human collagen in diabetes mellitus. *Proc. Natl Acad. Sci. USA, 81,* 583.
97. Kohn RR, Cerami A, Monnier VM (1984): Collagen aging in vitro by nonenzymatic glycosylation and browning. *Diabetes, 33,* 57.
98. Cohen MP, Yu-Wu V (1983): Age-related changes in non-enzymatic glycosylation of human basement membranes. *Exp. Gerontol., 18,* 461.
99. Cerami A, Vlassara H, Brownlee M (1985): Protein glycosylation and the pathogenesis of atherosclerosis. *Metabolism, 34, Suppl. 1,* 37.
100. Howard BV, Knowler WC, Vasquez B et al (1984): Plasma and lipoprotein cholesterol and triglyceride in the Pima Indian population: comparison of diabetics and nondiabetics. *Arteriosclerosis, 4,* 462.
101. Hayashi K, Matsumoto H, Ito K, Ozono N (1984): The change of serum lipoproteins observed in noninsulin-dependent diabetic patients and a study of its mechanism. *Hiroshima J. Med. Sci., 33,* 619.
102. Beylot M, Garcia I, Temori SA et al (1983): Serum lipid levels in insulin-dependent and noninsulin-dependent diabetic patients: relation with control of diabetes and the presence of macroangiopathy. *Diabète Métab., 9,* 199.
103. Walden CE, Knopp RH, Wahl PW et al (1984): Sex differences in the effect of diabetes mellitus on lipoprotein triglyceride and cholesterol concentrations. *N. Engl. J. Med., 311,* 953.
104. Odetti P, Ansaldi E, Diara C et al (1983): Correlations between glycosylated haemoglobin and other metabolic parameters in insulin-dependent diabetics. *Diabète Métab., 9,* 26.
105. Ewald U, Gustafson S, Tuvemo T, Vessby B (1984): Increased high density lipoproteins in diabetic children. *Eur. J. Pediatr., 142,* 154.
106. Gartside PS, Khoury P, Glueck CJ (1984): Determinants of high-density lipoprotein cholesterol in blacks and whites: the second National Health and Nutrition Examination survey. *Am. Heart J., 108,* 641.
107. Vannini P, Ciavarella A, Flammini M et al (1984): Lipid abnormalities in insulin-dependent diabetic patients with albuminuria. *Diabetes Care, 7,* 151.
108. Fielding CJ, Reaven GM, Liu G, Fielding PE (1984): Increased free cholesterol in plasma low and very low density lipoproteins in non-insulin-dependent diabetes mellitus: its role in the inhibition of cholesteryl ester transfer. *Proc. Natl Acad. Sci. USA, 81,* 2512.
109. Takegoshi T, Haba T, Takeshita H et al (1985): Analysis of lipoprotein pattern and VLDL Apo C and E isoform of diabetic patients. *J. Jpn Diabetes Soc., 28,* 721.
110. Floren CH, Albers JJ, Bierman EL (1981): Uptake of chylomicron remnants causes cholesterol accumulation in cultured human arterial smooth muscle cells. *Biochim. Biophys. Acta, 663,* 336.
111. Gianturco SH, Bradley WA, Gotto Jr AM et al (1982): Hypertriglyceridemic very low density lipoproteins induce triglyceride synthesis and accumulation in mouse peritoneal macrophages. *J. Clin. Invest., 70,* 168.
112. Havel RJ, Chao Y, Windler EE et al (1980): Isoprotein specificity in the hepatic uptake of apolipoprotein E and the pathogenesis of familial dysbetalipoproteinemia. *Proc. Natl Acad. Sci. USA, 77,* 4349.
113. Shelburne F, Hanks J, Meyers W, Quarfordt SJ (1980): Effect of apoproteins on hepatic uptake of triglyceride emulsions in the rat. *J. Clin. Invest., 65,* 652.
114. Curtiss LK, Witztum JL (1985): Plasma apolipoproteins AI, AII, B, CI, and E are glucosylated in hyperglycemic diabetic subjects. *Diabetes, 34,* 452.
115. Kraemer FB, Chen YI, Lopez RD, Reaven GM (1985): Effects of noninsulin-dependent diabetes mellitus on the uptake of very low density lipoproteins by thioglycolate-elicited mouse peritoneal macrophages. *J. Clin. Endocrinol. Metab., 61,* 335.

116. Lyons TJ, Klein RL, Baynes J, Lopes-Virella MF (1986): VLDL and LDL from diabetic patients stimulate increased CE synthesis in human monocyte-derived macrophages. *Diabetes, 35,* 67A.

117. Lyons TJ, Klein RL, Baynes JW, Lopes-Virella MF (1986): Stimulation of CE synthesis in human monocyte-derived macrophages by LDL isolated from diabetic patients. *Clin. Res., 34,* 208A.

118. Lopes-Virella MF, Sherer GK, Lees AM et al (1982): Surface binding, internalization and degradation by cultured human fibroblasts of low density lipoproteins isolated from type I (insulin-independent) diabetic patients: changes with metabolic control. *Diabetologia, 22,* 430.

119. Hiramatsu K, Bierman EL, Chait A (1985): Metabolism of low-density lipoprotein from patients with diabetic hypertriglyceridemia by cultured human skin fibroblasts. *Diabetes, 34,* 8.

120. Steinbrecher UP, Witztum JL (1984): Glucosylation of low-density lipoproteins to an extent comparable to that seen in diabetes slows their catabolism. *Diabetes, 33,* 130.

121. Witztum JL, Steinbrecher UP, Kesaniemi YA, Fisher M (1984): Autoantibodies to glucosylated proteins in the plasma of patients with diabetes mellitus. *Proc. Natl Acad. Sci. USA, 81,* 3204.

122. Gonen B, Baenziger J, Schonfeld G et al (1981): Nonenzymatic glycosylation of low density lipoproteins in vitro. *Diabetes, 30,* 875.

123. Witztum JL, Mahoney EM, Ranks MJ et al (1982): Non-enzymatic glycosylation of LDL alters its biologic activity. *Diabetes, 31,* 283.

124. Lopes-Virella MF, Klein RL, Lyons T et al (1985): In vitro glucosylated LDL enhances CE synthesis in human monocyte-derived macrophages. *Circulation, 77,* 817.

125. Mazzone T, Foster D, Chait A (1984): In vivo stimulation of low-density lipoprotein degradation by insulin. *Diabetes, 33,* 333.

126. Chait A, Eisenberg S, Steinmetz A et al (1984): Low-density lipoproteins modified by lipid transfer protein have altered biological activity. *Biochim. Biophys. Acta, 795,* 314.

127. Lorenzi M, Cagliero E, Markey B et al (1984): Interaction of human endothelial cells with elevated glucose concentrations and native and glycosylated low density lipoproteins. *Diabetologia, 26,* 218.

128. Lopes-Virella MF, Wohltmann HJ, Loadholt CB, Buse MG (1981): Plasma lipids and lipoproteins in young insulin-dependent diabetic patients: relationship with control. *Diabetologia, 21,* 216.

129. Jos J, Thevenin M, Dumont G, Beyne P (1985): Effect of metabolic control on plasma lipids and lipoproteins in children and adolescents with insulin-dependent diabetes. *Diabète Métab., 11,* 174.

130. Joven J, Rubies-Prat J, De la Figuera M et al (1985): High density lipoprotein changes during treatment of diabetic ketoacidosis. *Diabète Métab., 11,* 102.

131. Lawson P, Trayner I, Rosenstock J, Kohner E (1984): The effect of continuous subcutaneous insulin infusion on serum lipids. *Diabète Métab., 10,* 239.

132. Gonen B, White N, Schonfeld G et al (1985): Plasma levels of apoprotein B in patients with diabetes mellitus: the effect of glycemic control. *Metab. Clin. Exp., 34,* 675.

133. Goldberg RB, Reeves ML, Seigler DE et al (1985): Lack of a persistent reduction in serum lipid and apoprotein levels in insulin-dependent diabetic patients receiving intensified insulin treatment. *Acta Diabetol. Lat., 22,* 93.

134. Hollenbeck CB, Connor WE, Riddle MC et al (1985): The effects of a high-carbohydrate low-fat cholesterol-restricted diet on plasma lipid, lipoprotein, and apoprotein concentrations in insulin-dependent (Type I) diabetes mellitus. *Metab. Clin. Exp., 34,* 559.

135. O'Dea K (1984): Marked improvement in carbohydrate and lipid metabolism in diabetic Australian Aborigines after temporary reversion to traditional lifestyles. *Diabetes, 33,* 596.
136. Hughes TA, Gwynne JT, Switzer BR et al (1984): Effects of caloric restriction and weight loss on glycemic control, insulin release and resistance, and atherosclerotic risk in obese patients with type II diabetes mellitus. *Am. J. Med., 77,* 7.
137. Vessby B, Selinus I, Lithel H (1985): Serum lipoprotein and lipoprotein lipase in over-weight, Type II diabetics during and after supplemented fasting. *Arteriosclerosis, 5,* 93.
138. Dunn FL, Raskin P, Bilheimer DW, Grundy SM (1984): The effect of diabetic control on very low-density lipoprotein - triglyceride metabolism in patients with type II diabetes mellitus and marked hypertriglyceridemia. *Metab. Clin. Exp., 33,* 117.
139. Pacy PJ, Dodson PM, Kubicki AJ et al (1984): Effect of a high fibre, high carbohydrate dietary regimen on serum lipids and lipoproteins in type II hypertensive diabetic patients. *Diabetes Res., 1,* 159.
140. Riccardi G, Rivellese A, Pacioni D et al (1984): Separate influence of dietary carbohydrate and fibre on the metabolic control in diabetes. *Diabetologia, 26,* 116.
141. Bloomgarden ZT, Ginsberg-Fellner F, Rayfield DJ et al (1984): Elevated hemoglobin A(1C) and low-density lipoprotein cholesterol levels in thiazide-treated diabetic patients. *Am. J. Med., 77,* 823.
142. Pittera A, Scalisi P, Sambataro L et al (1983): Comparison of the effects of cardioselective and non-cardioselective beta-blockers on serum lipids. *Curr. Ther. Res. Clin. Exp., 34,* 483.

The Diabetes Annual/3
K.G.M.M. Alberti and L.P. Krall, editors
© 1987 Elsevier Science Publishers, B.V.

19   Changes in blood, blood-related cells, and control of local blood flow in diabetes

DONALD E. McMILLAN

Introduction

In the last two years, previously fairly quiet investigative activity in this field has accelerated considerably, simultaneously broadening in scope. We shall start by reviewing the area of greatest activity, both previously and currently, namely platelet behavior in diabetic patients.

Platelets

A platelet is a cast-off cell projection able to attach itself to exposed sub-endothelium by adhesion or to another platelet by aggregation. During both processes, platelets usually change their shape in a pattern referred to as 'pseudopod formation'. They also discharge procoagulant proteins, including β-thromboglobulin. During their circulatory life, normally 9 days, platelets lose volume and become progressively less reactive, changing in chemical composition as well. Diabetic platelets are larger than normal when retinopathy is present (1). They are also low in density, especially in poor control (2). The large number of biochemical abnormalities detectable in platelet membranes require careful scrutiny because platelet survival is shortened and altered biochemical states can often be explained by the young age of the platelets.

Other platelet abnormalities in diabetes have been well documented in more than 80 studies since our last review. Increased sensitivity to thromboxane during poor control (3), reduced sensitivity to prostacyclin (3-5), and more exposed fibrinogen binding sites (6) were reported. Increased platelet aggregability is found in diabetic children (7) and in recent-onset diabetes (8), although it is less striking than in long-standing diabetes or diabetes complicated by vasculopathy (9) or proliferative retinopathy (10).

Platelet aggregability in diabetes is correlated with blood glucose and

354

glycosylated hemoglobin levels (11), is rapidly improved by glucose normalization using the artificial pancreas (12), but not normalized by near-normal glycemia (13). Exercise affects non-diabetic platelets by increasing the number of spontaneous aggregates present (14), but in diabetes no increase in platelet aggregability follows a period of exercise (15).

The actual role of the platelet in producing vascular disease is not clear. Endothelial cells can produce platelet-derived growth factor (PDGF) that promotes the migration of smooth muscle cells from the media to the intima (16). Therapeutic measures to reduce platelet aggregability in diabetes have produced only a modest improvement in outcome that is most strongly linked to reduced transient cerebral ischemia (17).

The coagulation propensity of diabetic subjects has been less frequently studied. The abnormality is improved by better control (12) and is greater in diabetics with retinopathy (10). Coagulation-promoting changes in blood from diabetic subjects include decreased antithrombin III activity; its increased glycosylation reduces adsorption of its heparin co-factor (18). Elevated levels of a large number of procoagulant plasma proteins including prekallikrein (19), β-thromboglobulin (20), and fibrinogen (21) have been reported. High fibrinopeptide A levels in diabetic vascular disease (20) demonstrated elevated intravascular fibrinogen disruption. This conclusion is further supported by the shortening of the circulatory half-life of fibrinogen in diabetic subjects, a change recently linked to hyperglycemia-associated increased plasma volume in individual diabetic patients (22).

Our expanding understanding of biochemical synthesis has shown that the quinone, vitamin K, acts as a co-factor in the formation of a new γ-carboxyl group adjacent to the carboxylic acid of the glutamic acid present at the amino terminus of procoagulant proteins. This post-synthesis modification, necessary for coagulation to occur, is blocked when dicoumarol-like anticoagulants are administered. Observation of accelerated thromboembolic events in a small number of patients receiving a dicoumarol-like anticoagulant led to the discovery of two vitamin-K-dependent *anticoagulant* proteins: protein C and protein S (23). Blood levels of protein C are decreased in diabetic subjects (24), favoring coagulation.

Leukocytes

Even though their glucose uptake is not influenced by insulin (25), leukocytes are affected by the diabetic state. Chemotaxis, phagocytosis (26), and bacterial destruction (27) are all impaired in poorly controlled diabetes. A number of metabolic activities are also altered, including decreased glutathione levels (28), impaired leukotriene synthesis (29), decreased glycogen synthase activity

(30), increased superoxide dismutase activity (31), and increased insulin-degrading activity (32).

Leukocytes may be involved in tissue infarction; they pass through the micro-circulation less easily than erythrocytes. When arterial pressure is marginal, leukocytes can become trapped in microvessels in large numbers. Later restoration of normal arterial pressure fails to dislodge the now adherent leukocytes, causing tissue perfusion to remain impaired (33). This 'no reflow' problem is made more likely by a high leukocyte count, a condition associated with amputation in diabetic patients with foot problems (34).

Erythrocytes and viscosity

Erythrocytes in diabetic subjects have received increasing attention. Several Nuclepore filtration studies have demonstrated reduced red-cell deformability in diabetic patients (35, 36), IDDM patients (37) and subjects with gestational diabetes (38). Leukocytes have been shown gradually to plug Nuclepore filters, affecting filtration results (39). Two studies in which leukocytes were removed by filtration through cotton fibers failed to show an abnormality of diabetic blood (39, 40). However, studies using other means to reduce leukocyte interference continue to show impaired red-cell filterability (41, 42). Evidence has been presented that both red and white blood cells are less readily filterable in diabetes (41). An improvement in red blood cell filtration by intravenous fructose-1,6-diphosphate appeared (43). Filtration studies of erythrocytes separated on the basis of density difference have given both positive (42) and negative (44) results.

Rheoscopy is a technique in which the degree of erythrocyte stretching and rate of tank-treading in high-shear flow are measured. Diabetic cells behaved normally in this situation in one study (45), whereas their performance was decreased by hyperglycemia and correlated with glycosylated hemoglobin level in another (42). Red cell filtration is reported to be normalized by cyclandelate, a vasoactive aldolase reductase inhibitor (46), but reversal by insulin administration even when hyperglycemia is maintained by a simultaneous glucose infusion (47) argues that sorbitol accumulation may not be directly involved.

Erythrocytes have been reported to be affected by insulin in vitro (47-49), but the observation has also been challenged (50). Mature red cells certainly have less than 100 insulin receptors. The actual count may be as low as 30. Any insulin effect implies considerable signal amplification, presumably enzymatically mediated. The red cell membrane is about 55% protein and 45% lipid. A number of reports have shown increased membrane protein glycosylation in diabetes, including the inner-surface network protein responsible for shape maintenance, spectrin (51). Several years ago we purified spectrin and studied its phosphorylation state in diabetes, but found no alteration. An erythrocyte membrane cholesterol/phospholipid ratio increase in diabetic red cells has been reported (52) that is compatible with reduced deformability, but the reported excess would be expected to change red cell morphology (53). Another study of cholesterol/phospholipid ratios failed to reveal any clear pattern (54). An unusual effect of insulin, an increase in vitro of erythrocyte magnesium counteracted by ouabain, was reported (55).

Reports continue to document elevation of low-shear-rate blood viscosity in diabetes (56) and to link it to the presence of diabetic retinopathy (57, 58). Several reports have examined the effect of therapeutic agents on blood viscosity. Two trials using calcium dobesilate (Doxium) had positive results (59, 60). Plasma exchange using Haemaccel (polygeline) lowered viscosity without improving claudication symptoms (61). Rutin (rutoside) was not effective in lowering viscosity (62) and reports on pentoxifylline (Trental) were equivocal (43, 63). Recent plasma protein studies revealed elevation of prekallikrein (19), C1-inhibitor (19), and fibronectin levels (64). Increase in the last was found to be correlated with blood viscosity (64). Reduced binding of acidic therapeutic agents was linked to both lowered albumin level and its increased glycosylation (65) in diabetes. Molecule for molecule, however, the ability of glycosylated albumin to bind phenobarbital (66) and the fatty acid anion, palmitate (67), was found to be normal.

Serum proteins

Measurement of glycosylated serum protein levels continues to be advocated as a means of monitoring changes in diabetic control over shorter periods than glycosylated hemoglobin (68, 69) even in gestational diabetes (70). But glycosylated serum protein was found not to be as accurate as glucose tolerance testing in detecting gestational diabetes (71). Insulin-mediated edema was reported as a rare side effect of intense management (72). Regular lowering of serum albumin in diabetic children during intense management is a disturbing aspect of tight control (73).

Plasma protein binding to glomerular, vascular and epithelial basement membranes continues to attract investigative interest. Immunoglobulin G_4 (IgG_4) binding to diabetic glomerular basement membrane was reported to have a binding affinity not seen for more alkaline IgG molecules (74).

Microcirculation

Increased protein and fluid leakage from diabetic blood vessels was again reported, manifested by entry of excessive fluorescein dye into nailfold tissue (75). A hypothesis linking increased vascular permeability to microangiopathy also appeared (76).

Evidence for an association between microangiopathy and reduced autoregulation of local blood flow has been extended in a series of reports (77-79). Glomerular filtration rate was found to be less effectively autoregulated in diabetic renal disease (80). Failure of dopamine to affect glomerular filtration unusually (81) was interpreted as evidence against an efferent vasoconstriction as the cause of elevated glomerular filtration in diabetes. Microscopical vital microcirculatory observations revealed poorly reactive vascular beds in the feet of diabetic patients (82). Auditory capillaries in diabetic subjects were found by direct measurement to be dilated (83) and local vascular changes were etiologically linked to neuropathy (84). Elevated endoneurial protein was also observed in biopsies from diabetic patients (85).

The vascular system is lined by endothelial cells that can proliferate in culture. Studies of endothelial cells in culture have led to a series of interesting conclusions. Hyperglycemia affects their replication and the integrity of their DNA (86). Endothelial cells of large vessels behave little differently in culture than microvascular cells, but an already low insulin degradation rate is even lower in the latter (87). Endothelial cells can be injured by very-low-density lipoprotein, the triglyceride-bearing lipoprotein fraction elevated in diabetic subjects (88). Endothelial cells have surface insulin receptors capable of contributing to the passage of insulin to the interstitium (89), even in brain capillaries (90).

Widening scientific interest and its potential for therapeutic intervention have interacted to expand activity in this area of diabetes research in the last two years.

References

1. Koneti RA, Goldberg RE, Walsh PN (1984): Platelet coagulant activities in diabetes mellitus: evidence for relationship between platelet coagulant hyperactivity and platelet volume. *J. Lab. Clin. Med., 103*, 82.
2. Collier A, Watson HHK, Matthews DM et al (1984): Platelet-density analysis and intraplatelet granule content in young insulin-dependent diabetics. *Diabetes, 35*, 1081.
3. Amado JA, Suarez M, Richard C, Sedano MC (1985): Influence of acetylsalicylic acid on bleeding time and serum thromboxane B_2 in diabetes mellitus type I. *Diabète Métab., 11*, 98.
4. Akai T, Naka K, Okuda K et al (1983): Decreased sensitivity of platelets to prostacyclin in patients with diabetes mellitus. *Horm. Metab. Res., 15*, 523.
5. Pillay PK, Pillay U, Balasubramaniam P, Lee KO (1985): Platelet sensitivity to prostacyclin in diabetes mellitus. *Ann. Acad. Med. Singapore, 14*, 229.
6. DiMinno G, Silver MJ, Cerbone AM et al (1985): Increased binding of fibrinogen to platelets in diabetes: the role of prostaglandins and thromboxane. *Blood, 65*, 156.

7. Ewald U, Kobbah M, Vessby B, Tuvemo T (1983): Increased platelet aggregability in diabetic children: relation to serum lipid and fatty acid composition. *Diabetologia, 25,* 382.

8. ·Coppola L, Misso L, Giugliano D et al (1984): Rapid decrease of platelet aggregation (ADP- and collagen-induced) and of platelet circulating aggregates by the artificial pancreas in insulin-dependent diabetics. *Diabète Métab., 10,* 31.

9. Fritschi J, Christe M, Marbet GA et al (1984): Platelet aggregation, beta-thromboglobulin and platelet factor 4 in diabetes mellitus and in patients with vasculopathy. *Thrombos. Haemostasis, 52,* 236.

10. Borsey DQ, Prowse CV, Gray RS et al (1984): Platelet and coagulation factors in proliferative diabetic retinopathy. *J.Clin. Pathol., 37,* 659.

11. Jones DB, Davis TME, Bown E et al (1986): Determinants of ADP-induced platelet aggregation in diabetes mellitus. *Diabetologia, 29,* 291.

12. Cucinotta D, Trifiletti A, Di Cesare E et al (1985): The effect of a strict metabolic control on clotting factors and platelet function in diabetics with vascular disease. *G. Ital. Diabetol., 5,* 311.

13. Jackson CA, Greaves M, Boulton AJM et al (1984): Near-normal glycaemic control does not correct abnormal platelet reactivity in diabetes mellitus. *Clin. Sci., 67,* 551.

14. Trovati M, Tamponi G, Schinco P et al (1984): Influence of submaximal muscular exercise on platelet aggregate ratio in healthy subjects and in insulin-dependent diabetic patients. *IRCS Med. Sci., 12,* 598.

15. Vicari AM, Margonato A, Petrelli P et al (1984): Plasma beta-thromboglobulin concentration at rest and after physical exercise in complicated and uncomplicated diabetes mellitus. *Diabète Métab., 10,* 235.

16. Ross R (1986): The pathogenesis atherosclerosis - an update. *N. Engl. J. Med., 314,* 488.

17. Colwell JA, Bingham SF, Abraira C et al (1986): Veterans administration cooperative study on antiplatelet agents in diabetic patients after amputation for gangrene. II. Effects of aspirin and dipyridamole on atherosclerotic vascular disease rates. *Diabetes Care, 9,* 140.

18. Brownlee M, Vlassara H, Cerami A (1984): Inhibition of heparin-catalyzed human antithrombin III activity by nonenzymatic glycosylation: possible role in fibrin deposition in diabetes. *Diabetes, 33,* 532.

19. Christie M, Gattlen P, Fritschi J et al (1984): The contact phase of blood coagulation in diabetes mellitus and in patients with vasculopathy. *Thrombos. Haemostasis, 52,* 221.

20. Librenti MC, D'Angelo A, Micossi P et al (1985): Beta-thromboglobulin and fibrinopeptide A in diabetes mellitus as markers of vascular damage. *Acta Diabetol. Lat., 22,* 39.

21. Fuller JH (1984): The haemocoagulation system and macroangiopathy in insulin dependent (type I) diabetes. *Ann. Clin. Res., 16,* 137.

22. Jones RL, Jovanovic L, Forman S, Peterson CM (1984): Time course of reversibility of accelerated fibrinogen disappearance in diabetes mellitus: association with intravascular volume shifts. *Blood, 63,* 22.

23. Clouse LH, Comp PC (1986): The regulation of hemostasis: the protein C system. *N. Engl. J. Med., 314,* 1298.

24. Vukovich TC, Schernthaner G (1986): Decreased protein C levels in patients with insulin-dependent type I diabetes mellitus. *Diabetes, 35,* 617.

25. Esmann V, Aarhus MD (1963): Effect of insulin on human leucocytes. *Diabetes, 12,* 545.

26. Davidson NJ, Sowden JM, Fletcher J (1984): Defective phagocytosis in insulin controlled diabetics: evidence for a reaction between glucose and opsonising proteins. *J. Clin. Pathol., 37,* 783.

27. Chhimpa I, Ramdeo IN, Solanki RL, Anand VK (1985): The bactericidal activity of polymorphonuclear neutrophilic leukocytes plasma suspension in diabetes mellitus. *Ind. J. Pathol. Microbiol., 28,* 91.

28. Chari SN, Nath N, Rathi AB (1984): Glutathione and its redox system in diabetic polymorphonuclear leukocytes. *Am. J. Med. Sci., 287,* 14.

29. Jubiz W, Draper RE, Gale J, Nolan G (1984): Decreased leukotriene B$_4$ synthesis of polymorphonuclear leukocytes from male patients with diabetes mellitus. *Prostaglandins Leukotrienes Med., 14,* 305.

30. Esmann V (1983): The polymorphonuclear leukocyte in diabetes mellitus. *J. Clin. Chem. Clin. Biochem., 21,* 561.

31. Nath N, Chari SN, Rathi AB (1984): Superoxide dismutase in diabetic polymorphonuclear leukocytes. *Diabetes, 33,* 586.

32. Theiss WC, Rupp GM, Varandani PT (1984): Insulin-degrading activity in mononuclear and polymorphonuclear circulating leukocytes of nondiabetic and diabetic subjects. *J. Clin. Endocrinol. Metab., 59,* 344.

33. Schmid-Schonbein GW, Engler RL (1983): Granulocytes as active participants in acute myocardial ischemia and infarction. *Am. J. Cardiovasc. Pathol., 1,* 15.

34. Wetter L, Lithner F, Hallmans G (1984): Is hemoglobin concentration a predictor for the outcome of distal gangrenous lesions in diabetics? *Acta Med. Scand., 216, Suppl.,* 29.

35. Barnikol WKR, Burkhard O (1984): The dependence of erythrocyte deformability on concentration of glucose in healthy people and in case of diabetes mellitus. *Funkt. Biol. Med., 3,* 249.

36. Hanss M, Attali JR, Helou C, Lemarie JC (1983): Erythrocyte deformability and diabetes. *Clin. Hemorrheol., 3,* 383.

37. Garcia Sanchez-Gabriel JA, Gaztambide Saenz S, Vazquez Garcia JA (1985): Study of erythrocyte deformability in type I diabetes mellitus. *Med. Clin., 85,* 827.

38. Kaibara M, Marumoto Y, Kobayashi T (1984): Blood viscosity and erythrocyte deformability in gestational diabetes. *Int. J. Gynaecol. Obstet., 22,* 221.

39. Stuart J, Stone PCW, Bareford D et al (1985): Evaluation of leucocyte removal methods for studies of erythrocyte deformability. *Clin. Hemorrheol., 5,* 137.

40. Ritchie DM (1985): Filtration of dilute erythrocyte suspension as a measure of erythrocyte deformability and its relationship to blood glucose control in diabetes mellitus. *Clin. Hemorrheol., 5,* 257.

41. Ernst E, Matrai A (1986): Altered red and white blood cell rheology in type II diabetes. *Diabetes, 35,* 1412.

42. Goebel KM, Goebel FD, Lanser KG (1983): Pathologic fluidity, glycohemoglobin and metabolic disturbance of erythrocytes in Fontaine II diabetic microangiopathy. *Schweiz. Med. Wochenschr., 113,* 1936.

43. Marsilii A, Petruzzi E, Di Noto C, Marini P (1984): Effects of fructose-1,6-diphosphate on the red cell deformability in diabetic patients. *Agressologie, 25,* 919.

44. Stone PCW, Bareford D, Keidan AJ et al (1986): Rheological study of density gradient fractionated erythrocytes in diabetes and atherosclerotic vascular disease. *Clin. Hemorrheol., 6,* 337.

45. Williamson JR, Gardner RA, Boylan CW et al (1985): Microrheologic investigation of erythrocyte deformability in diabetes mellitus. *Blood, 65,* 283.

46. Timmerman H (1984): Modes and mechanisms of action of vasoactive drugs and especially of cyclandelate. *Br. J. Clin. Pract., 38,* 10.

47. Juhan I, Buonocore M, Jouve R et al (1982): Abnormalities of erythrocyte deformability and platelet aggregation in insulin-dependent diabetics corrected by insulin in vivo and in vitro. *Lancet, 1,* 535.

48. McMillan DE (1983): Insulin, diabetes, and the cell membrane: an hypothesis. *Diabetologia, 24,* 308.

49. Dutta-Roy AK, Ray TK, Sinha AK (1985): Control of erythrocyte membrane microviscosity by insulin. *Biochim. Biophys. Acta, 816,* 187.

50. Sauerheber RD, Lewis UJ, Esgate JA, Gordon LM (1980): Effect of calcium, insulin and growth hormone on membrane fluidity: a spin label study of rat adipocyte and human erythrocyte ghosts. *Biochim. Biophys. Acta, 597,* 292.
51. McMillan DE, Brooks SM (1982): Erythrocyte spectrin glucosylation in diabetes. *Diabetes, 31,* 64.
52. Juhan-Vague I, Driss F, Roul C et al (1984): Abnormalities of erythrocyte membrane lipids in insulin-dependent diabetics are improved by short term strict control of diabetes. *Clinical Hemorrheol., 4,* 455.
53. Cooper RA, Durocher JR, Leslie MH (1977): Decreased fluidity of red cell membrane lipids in abetalipoproteinemia. *J. Clin. Invest., 60,* 115.
54. Otsuji S, Baba Y, Kamada T (1981): Erythrocyte membrane microviscosity in diabetes. *Horm. Metab. Res., 11,* 97.
55. Paolisso G, Sgambato S, Passariello N et al (1986): Insulin induces opposite changes in plasma and erythrocyte magnesium concentrations in normal man. *Diabetologia, 29,* 644.
56. Leiper JM, Lowe GDO, Anderson J et al (1984): Effects of diabetic control and biosynthetic human insulin on blood rheology in established diabetics. *Diabetes Res., 1,* 27.
57. Bode WA, Fonk T, Van der Veen EA, Van der Meer J (1985): Blood viscosity in diabetic retinopathy. *Neth. J. Med., 28,* 449.
58. Trope GE, Lowe GDO, Ghafour IM et al (1983): Blood viscosity in proliferative diabetic retinopathy and complicated retinal vein thrombosis. *Trans. Ophthalmol. Soci. UK, 103,* 108.
59. Vojnikovic B (1984): Hyperviscosity in whole blood, plasma, and aqueous humor decreased by doxium (calcium dobesilate) in diabetics with retinopathy and glaucoma: a double-blind controlled study. *Ophthalmic Res., 16,* 150.
60. Benarroch IS, Brodsky M, Rubinstein A et al (1985): Treatment of blood hyperviscosity with calcium dobesilate in patients with diabetic retinopathy. *Ophthalmic Res., 17,* 131.
61. Walker T, Matrai A, Flute PT, Dormandy JA (1985): Haemorrheological and functional changes in intermittent claudication following plasma exchange with Haemaccel. *Clin. Hemorrheol., 5,* 99.
62. Gallasch G, Dorfer CH, Schmitt TH, Stage A (1985): Efficacy of orally administered troxerutin on flow properties of human blood under defined conditions: a double-blind study in patients with diabetic and arteriosclerotic retinopathy. *Klin. Monatsbl. Augenheilk., 187,* 30.
63. Sternitzky R, Seige K (1985): Clinical investigation of the effects of pentoxifylline in patients with severe peripheral occlusive vascular disease. *Curr. Med. Res. Opin., 9,* 602.
64. Solerte SB, Piovella F, Viola C et al (1985): Plasma fibronectin, von Willebrand factor anti-gen, and blood rheology: association with diabetic microvascular disease. *Acta Diabetol. Lat., 22,* 239.
65. Ruiz-Cabello F, Erill S (1984): Abnormal serum protein binding of acidic drugs in diabetes mellitus. *Clin. Pharmacol. Ther., 36,* 691.
66. Danhof M, Hisaoka M, Levy G (1985): Kinetics of drug action in disease states. VI. Effect of experimental diabetes on phenobarbital concentration in rats at onset of loss of righting reflex. *J. Pharmacol. Exp. Ther., 232,* 435.
67. Murtiashaw MH, Winterhalter KH (1986): Non-enzymatic glycation of human albumin does not alter its palmitate binding. *Diabetologia, 29,* 366.
68. Lapolla A, Poli T, Valerio A, Fedele D (1985): Glycosylated serum proteins in diabetic patients and their relation to metabolic parameters. *Diabetes Res., 2,* 283.
69. Maudelonde T, Menez JF, Meskar A et al (1983): Glycosylated proteins and diabetic con-trol using subcutaneous continuous administration of insulin via a portable infusion pump. *Diabète Métab., 9,* 192.

70. Leiper JM, Talwar D, Robb DA et al (1985): Glycosylated albumin and glycosylated proteins: rapidly changing indices of glycemia in diabetic pregnancy. *Q. J. Med., 55*, 225.
71. McFarland KF, Murtiashaw M, Baynes JW (1984): Clinical value of glycosylated serum protein and glycosylated hemoglobin levels in the diagnosis of gestational diabetes. *Obstet. Gynecol., 64*, 516.
72. Wheatley T, Edwards OM (1985): Insulin edema and its clinical significance: metabolic studies in three cases. *Diabetic Med., 2*, 400.
73. Gebre-Medhin M, Ewald U, Tuvemo T (1985): Reduced serum proteins in diabetic children on a twice-daily insulin schedule. *Acta Paediatr. Scand., 74*, 961.
74. Melvin T, Kim Y, Michael AF (1984): Selective binding of IgG$_4$ and other negatively charged plasma proteins in normal and diabetic human kidneys. *Am. J. Pathol., 115*, 443.
75. Frey J, Furrer J, Bollinger A (1983): Transcapillary diffusion of NA-fluorescein in skin areas of the dorsum of the foot in juvenile diabetics. *Schweiz. Med. Wochenschr., 113*, 1964.
76. Viberti GC (1983): Increased capillary permeability in diabetes mellitus and its relationship to microvascular angiopathy. *Am. J. Med., 75*, 81.
77. Faris I, Vagn Nielsen H, Henriksen O et al (1983): Impaired autoregulation of blood flow in skeletal muscle and subcutaneous tissue in long-term type 1 (insulin-dependent) diabetic patients with microangiopathy. *Diabetologia, 25*, 486.
78. Henriksen O, Kastrup J, Parving H-H, Lassen NA (1984): Loss of autoregulation of blood flow in subcutaneous tissue in juvenile diabetes. *J. Cardiovasc. Pharmacol., 6*, S666.
79. Parving H-H, Kastrup J, Smidt UM (1985): Reduced transcapillary escape of albumin during acute blood pressure-lowering in Type 1 (insulin-dependent) diabetic patients with nephropathy. *Diabetologia, 28*, 797.
80. Parving H-H, Kastrup H, Smidt UM et al (1984): Impaired autoregulation of glomerular filtration rate in Type 1 (insulin-dependent) diabetic patients with nephropathy. *Diabetologia, 27*, 547.
81. Ter Wee PM, Van Ballegooie E, Rosman JB et al (1986): The effect of low-dose dopamine on renal haemodynamics in patients with Type 1 (insulin-dependent) diabetes does not differ from normal individuals. *Diabetologia, 29*, 78.
82. Fagrell B, Hermansson I-L, Karlander S-G, Ostergren J (1984): Vital capillary microscopy for assessment of skin viability and microangiopathy in patients with diabetes mellitus. *Acta Med. Scand., 687*, 25.
83. Myers SF, Ross MD, Jokelainen P et al (1985): Morphological evidence of vestibular pathology in long-term experimental diabetes mellitus. I. Microvascular changes? *Acta Otolaryngol., 100*, 351.
84. Powell HC, Myers RR (1984): Axonopathy and microangiopathy in chronic alloxan diabetes. *Acta Neuropathol., 65*, 128.
85. Ohi T, Poduslo JF, Dyck PJ (1985): Increased endoneurial albumin in diabetic polyneuropathy. *Neurology, 35*, 1790.
86. Lorenzi M, Cagliero E, Toledo S (1985): Glucose toxicity for human endothelial cells in culture: delayed replication, disturbed cell cycle, and accelerated death. *Diabetes, 34*, 621.
87. Dernovsek KD, Bar RS (1985): Processing of cell-bound insulin by capillary and macrovascular endothelial cells in culture. *Am. J. Physiol., 248*, E244.
88. Arbogast BW, Berry DL, Newell CL (1984): Injury of arterial endothelial cells in diabetic sucrose-fed and aged rats. *Atherosclerosis, 51*, 31.
89. King GL, Johnson SM (1985): Receptor-mediated transport of insulin across endothelial cells. *Science, 227*, 1583.
90. Frank HJL, Pardridge WM, Morris WL et al (1986): Binding and internalization of insulin and insulin-like growth factors by isolated brain microvessels. *Diabetes, 35*, 654.

The Diabetes Annual/3
K.G.M.M. Alberti and L.P. Krall, editors
© 1987 Elsevier Science Publishers, B.V.

20   Insulin secretion in vitro

GEOFFREY W.G. SHARP

In *The Diabetes Annual/2* the outline of the chapter on insulin secretion in vitro covered the cellular events involved in the rapid control of insulin release by physiological agents. The synthesis of insulin, long-term regulation and pharmacology of its release, e.g. the effects of the sulfonylureas, were not included. The articles reviewed this year cover similar ground to that delineated in the previous volume with the exception that drug effects are included in this Chapter where relevant to our understanding of the control of insulin secretion. Some of the sections in this Chapter are arbitrarily divided, e.g. Ca^{2+} handling is dealt with separately from membrane permeability. This is done in the belief that it makes the material easier to follow, provided one does not forget to reintegrate the sections subsequently!

Methodology

Several studies have appeared in which islet cells or pancreatic islets have been maintained under different conditions in tissue culture. Comparisons have been made between free-floating dissociated cells and monolayer cultures (1) and the characteristics of the cells in suspension documented (2). Comparison has also been made between cells grown on an extracellular matrix with those on plastic and the conclusion drawn that growth on an extracellular matrix enhanced attachment, proliferation and long-term maintenance (3). Following the report last year of RINm5F cells grown on microcarriers (4), dispersed islet cells have now been attached to microcarrier beads. After 72 hours in culture, A, B and D cells were well attached to the beads and responded to glucose stimulation with biphasic insulin secretion (5). The technique should be extremely useful for the study of homogenous populations of isolated and purified A, B and D cells. Long-term culture of pancreatic islet cells, both neonatal and adult, resulted in the occurrence of giant cells thought to contain insulin, which were used for patch clamping (6). While this may allow for easy patch clamping and the study of ion channels, the usefulness of these cells for the study of normal B cell functions can only be evaluated after their physiological characteristics become known. The topic of islet cell maintenance under tissue culture conditions was reviewed by Nielsen (7) and differences noted under the various conditions, times and species used. Once again, it is timely to point out that direct extrapolation from experiments on animal cells to the human situation must be made with caution.

Islet cells encapsulated in cellulose sulfate and maintained for up to 3 weeks in tissue culture were found to be unaffected by the encapsulation when tested for insulin content, secretion and biosynthesis in comparison with non-encapsulated controls (8).

The clonal pancreatic B-cell line obtained by SV40 transformation of hamster cells has attracted increased attention as a B-cell for experimental study. Under perifusion conditions the cells were stimulated by high glucose concentrations to release insulin in a concentration-dependent manner, although the response was neither biphasic nor sustained. The combination of glucose and 3-isobutyl-1-methylxanthine (IBMX) caused a large increase in the release rate and elicited a biphasic response. Depolarization of the B-cell membrane by KCl also stimulated release (9). These cells may well prove to be useful for mechanistic studies on the chain of events leading from glucose to exocytosis.

Finally, there are three unrelated methodological reports. Islets have been isolated from atrophied pancreas after short-term duct ligation and found to exhibit normal behavior with respect to insulin release (10). A homologous teleost insulin radioimmunoassay has been developed and used to study the effect of epinephrine on insulin secretion from isolated pancreatic tissue of the rainbow trout (11). The need for careful control of chemicals and reagents was emphasized by the finding that two commercial preparations of aprotinin contained high concentrations of somatostatin (12)!

B cell models

The C57BL/KsJ db/db mouse has been widely used as a model of diabetes and lean litter mates used as controls. The appropriateness of such controls and the possibility of a gene-dosage effect have been studied. Perifusion experiments were performed using islets isolated from diabetic (db/db), heterozygous (+/db), and normal (+/+) mice. In response to glucose the islets from the heterozygous mice had a two-fold greater release of insulin than that from diabetic mice, while the islets from the normal mice had a 5-fold greater increase. A biphasic release of insulin in response to glucose was only observed in the normal mice. However, all three sets of islets gave a biphasic response to d-glyceraldehyde while the islets from diabetic and heterozygous mice still had diminished responses. The results indicate a gene dosage effect upon the ability of the islets to release insulin in response to nutrient secretagogues (13).

Pancreatic islets from uremic rats were studied in comparison with control rats under perifusion conditions in support columns of Bio-Gel P-2 polyac-rylamide beads. Only the first phase of insulin release, which was diminished in islets from the uremic rats, was significantly different from the controls (14).

Streptozotocin-induced diabetes

The rat model of diabetes produced by the injection of submaximal concentra-tions of streptozotocin into neonates is extremely useful for the light it sheds on the development of diabetes in these animals, and the potential value of this knowledge to some forms of human diabetes. It is known that in this model of diabetes the pancreas is markedly less responsive to a glucose challenge. It has now been shown that the pancreas is similarly unresponsive to a reduction in the concentration of glucose (15). The animals were studied after the diabetes had developed in parallel with control animals. When the isolated perfused pan-creas was subjected to a decrease in glucose concentration, from 11.2 to 2.8 mM, a decrease in insulin release occurred in the pancreas of control, but not of the diabetic rats. However, pancreas from both groups behaved similarly to ex-posure to epinephrine or somatostatin. The decrease in glucose concentrations stimulated glucagon secretion in control rat pancreas but not the diabetic, whereas the stimulatory and inhibitory effects of epinephrine and somatostatin were comparable in both groups. These, and other data, demonstrate the selec-tivity of the defect in the diabetic animals. Both A and B cells are non-respon-sive to glucose but normally responsive to the other agents tested.

Further studies were performed to test the hypothesis that hyperglycemia plays a major role in the abnormal influence of glucose on arginine-stimulated insulin secretion (16). Four groups of animals were used: i.e. the diabetic and control groups and diabetic and control animals made hypoglycemic by the in-jection of insulin for 24 hours prior to the study of insulin and glucagon secre-tion. The perfused pancreas of both control groups, i.e. insulin-treated and un-treated, gave only a slight response to 10 mM arginine at 2.8 mM glucose but a larger one in the presence of 16.7 mM glucose. The response to arginine in the untreated diabetic animals at 2.8 mM glucose was abnormally high, but after 24 hours of insulin-induced hypoglycemia the response was the same as in the con-trol groups. Responsiveness to glucose was not restored by the hypoglycemia. The results of this study suggest that the abnormal response to arginine in the diabetic mice was induced by the hyperglycemia associated with the condition.

The consequence of prolonged hyperglycemia and its role in the develop-ment of diabetes was also examined by Unger and Grundy (17), who postulated that hyperglycemia diminishes the ability of A and B cells to respond to changed glucose concentrations, thus setting up a progressive cycle of deleterious conse-quences. It is stated that the restoration of normoglycemia can stop the cycle, prevent further deterioration and restore, even if only transiently, metabolic compensation both in IDDM and NIDDM.

Islet A and B cell function was tested in human volunteers whose plasma glucose levels were clamped for 12 hours at 5 or 11 mM glucose. Changed sensitivity of the A and B cells was observed in the subjects maintained hyperglycemic and the conclusion, from even a relatively short period of hyperglycemia, was that the abnormal A and B response seen in diabetes cannot be entirely due to intrinsic defects and that hyperglycemia is playing a role (18).

Two studies examined mechanisms underlying the diabetogenic effect of streptozotocin. In the first, a series of compounds were tested for protection against the effects of streptozotocin and alloxan on monolayer culture of rat pancreatic islets. Scavengers of hydroxyl radicals protected against alloxan, and inhibitors of poly(ADP-ribose)synthetase protected against streptozotocin (19). The second study investigated the effect of pancreatic islet blood flow on the diabetogenic effect of streptozotocin (20). While no association was apparent between the rate of islet blood flow and diabetogenicity, those animals with increased insulin secretory activity, following injections of glucose, phentolamine or yohimbine, did develop hyperglycemia several days later, indicating streptozotocin toxicity. Animals treated similarly but injected with saline, epinephrine or propranolol failed to develop diabetes.

Finally, with respect to streptozotocin, there is a study of the tumor-promoting ability of streptozotocin. As is now well known, the injection of streptozotocin with sufficient nicotinamide to block its diabetogenic effect results, after a long latent period, in the development of B-cell-rich islet cell tumors. The tumors respond to glucose but secrete a higher proportion of proinsulin to insulin than normal islets. Other differences include altered proportions of hormone content and the presence of some D-cell-like granulated cells of uncertain classification. The development of a B cell line from these glucose-responsive cells might provide a useful experimental model (21).

Membrane permeability and electrical activity

Since the original description of an ATP-sensitive K^+-selective channel which was proposed as the link between glucose metabolism and B cell membrane depolarization (22) and the direct demonstration of its closure in response to glucose (23) (see *The Diabetes Annual/2*) few new findings have been published. This is surprising and will, no doubt, be remedied soon. The ability of the patch-clamped K^+ channel to serve as a bioassay of the glucose-induced signal to close the channel is of great importance. Of equal importance, and wider applicability, is our ability to monitor exocytosis in single cells by capacitance measurements (24). The ATP sensitivity of the K^+ channel seems curious because the information we have at present suggests that the ATP levels in the B cell should keep the channel permanently closed. Furthermore, ATP would seem to be a most unlikely signal in view of the small range of concentration over which it can change. If ATP is the 'closing agent', it would seem possible that in the intact B cell an opening signal is dominant. The removal of this by glucose metabolism or a metabolite to permit ATP action would appear to be a more likely mechanism than a simple increase in ATP. Importantly, the techniques are now available for us to discover the link between glucose metabolism and membrane depolarization. The possibility that activation of protein kinase C could cause a decrease in K^+ channel activity already has experimental support in some cells, though this does not appear to be the case in B cells (25, 26). Furthermore, there is evidence that the sulfonylureas, which depolarize the B cell membrane, act by decreasing the activity of the K^+ channel (27).

The Ca^{2+}-activated K^+ channel has also been studied under patch clamp conditions and characterized in some detail (28). There is a complex relationship between the channel, membrane potential and the internal Ca^{2+} concentration, to which the channel is sensitive precisely over the presumed physiological range of Ca^{2+} concentration in the cells. It seems clear that this channel has a major role to play in the control of membrane potential during periods of cell activation. Both major K^+ channels were studied with respect to the actions of quinine and the tetraethylammonium ion with surprising conclusions (29). The widely held assumption that quinine blocks the Ca^{2+}- activated K^+ channel was dispelled. The finding follows logically from the observation that the Ca^{2+}-activated K^+ channel should be completely inactive, with no K^+ ion flow, under basal conditions (Ca^{2+} ca. 10^{-7} M) and normal membrane potential (28). Direct measurement of channel activity under patch clamp conditions showed that quinine blocks the Ca^{2+}-independent (ATP- and glucose-sensitive) K^+ channel, as had been reported by Cook and Hales (22), and tetraethylammonium affects the Ca^{2+}-activated channel. This requires the reinterpretation of previous data and conclusions from experiments using these two pharmacological agents.

Other studies of membrane K^+ channels and electrical activity have demonstrated that sparteine (30) and cesium (31) both decrease K^+ permeability, as judged using $^{86}Rb^+$ as a marker, and can produce depolarization. The actions of cesium were complex as, depending upon the conditions, both hyperpolarization and depolarization could be achieved.

The last paper in this section to deal with K^+ channels is one which relates to insulin secretion, electrical activity and cyclic AMP levels (32). Cyclic AMP is generally recognized as a potentiator of insulin release. Controversy exists as to whether it mobilizes intracellularly stored Ca^{2+}, and it has been described as having an effect upon Ca^{2+} entry via voltage-dependent channels by kinase-mediated phosphorylation of the channel (33). Eddlestone and colleagues observed that forskolin and IBMX both increased cyclic AMP levels in the islet and potentiated insulin release. Both agents potentiated the silent depolarization of the membrane in response to substimulatory glucose concentrations, whereas they increased the plateau phase with stimulatory glucose concentrations, much as would a further increase in the glucose concentration. The authors interpret their results as showing a phosphorylation reaction which changes the activity of the Ca^{2+}-sensitive K^+ channel. The increase in Ca^{2+} entry into the B cell that would result from these changes would then account for the cyclic-AMP-induced potentiation of insulin secretion (32). I would prefer to interpret these data rather differently and place the effect on the Ca^{2+}-insensitive K^+ channel, believing that it is the closure of this channel which is responsible for the silent depolarization phase. Further studies, including specific phosphorylation studies, are required to determine whether cyclic AMP changes the phosphorylation state of the K^+ channel, the voltage-dependent Ca^{2+} channel or both.

Phosphorylation must also be involved in the effects of the phorbol esters, which activate C-kinase, and which have been shown also to affect the electrical activity of the B cell (34). In this study TPA (12-O-tetradecanoyl-13-phorbol acetate) did not affect the membrane potential in the presence of 0-5.6 mM glucose but increased the active phase of oscillatory spike activity more than twofold. The data were interpreted to indicate that TPA increased the influx of Ca^{2+} via the voltage-dependent Ca^{2+} channels. The latter have been studied and characterized using the whole-cell voltage clamp technique and cultured neonatal rat pancreatic B cells (35).

Calcium handling by islet cells

After all the interest and excitement in the study of Ca^{2+} and its role in the control of exocytosis over the past several years, major new advances in our understanding in the last year have been few. Using the fluorescent indicator for Ca^{2+}, Quin-2, it was again shown in RINm5F cells that glyceraldehyde, carbamylcholine and alanine all raise Ca^{2+} levels and stimulate insulin release (36). An increase in Ca^{2+} in ob/ob mouse B cells in response to glucose was reported in *The Diabetes Annual/2* (37) and has also been independently confirmed in rat pancreatic islet cells (38). Under conditions of low extracellular Ca^{2+}, glucose caused a decrease in the cytosol Ca^{2+} concentration, presumably due to uptake into stores or increased protein binding (39). With the Ca^{2+}-sensitive electrode and isolated organelles from a rat insulinoma, the coordinate control of cytosolic Ca^{2+} has been demonstrated, while no role can be ascribed to the granules (40). Inositol 1,4,5-trisphosphate was shown to mobilize Ca^{2+} from the endoplasmic reticulum (41, 42). A gradual working out of the relative values of the different Ca^{2+} control systems for the various secretagogues will no doubt occur over the next few years. However, it already seems clear that extracellular Ca^{2+}, entering via the voltage-dependent channel, exerts the major influence in the stimulation of insulin secretion by glucose. The converse will be true for vagally stimulated release which must depend to a large extent on increased turnover of the phosphatidylinositol cycle.

Studies of the voltage-dependent channel have continued with various pharmacological antagonists and agonists:

Dihydropyridine derivatives with agonist properties potentiate glucose-stimulated insulin release and cause a left-shift in the glucose concentration-response relationship by increasing Ca^{2+} entry into the B cell (43-45). Verapamil, a Ca^{2+} antagonist, has the reverse, inhibitory affect on glucose-stimulated insulin secretion and was reported, as one would expect, to cause glucose intolerance in conscious, non-diabetic rats (46).

Studies with cobalt, thought by many to be a relatively specific blocking agent for the voltage-dependent Ca^{2+} channel, suggest an additional action on pancreatic islets which appeared to be on a distal step in stimulus-secretion coupling (47).

The role of extracellular Ca^{2+} in the control of B cell function was assessed by studying insulin release from RINm5F cells in media with different concentrations of $CaCl_2$ from 0.16 to 4.4 mM. No difference in the ability to release insulin was detected. Furthermore, the cells were resistant to low Ca^{2+} in that their calcium content did not decrease in the presence of low extracellular Ca^{2+} and D-600, the Ca^{2+} channel antagonist. However, when the cells were cultured with 4.4 mM Ca^{2+}, their calcium content increased and the insulin content decreased (48). In a study of the sensitivity of islet cells relative to extracellular Ca^{2+} content, the D cell was less sensitive to the regulatory effects of Ca^{2+} than the A and B cells. After treatment with EGTA (egtazic acid), reintroduction of Ca^{2+} stimulated insulin and glucagon secretion, this being maximal at 0.5 mM. In contrast, stimulation of somatostatin secretion was proportional to the Ca^{2+} concentration over the range of 0.5-6.5 mM (49).

Defective or missing voltage-dependent Ca^{2+} channels would appear to be the reason for the lack of responsiveness of a benign islet cell tumor and a transplantable rat insulinoma. After culturing the tumors in RPMI-1640 (11 mM glucose) for 3 days, no effects on $^{45}Ca^{2+}$ uptake or insulin release were detected in response to glucose alone or in combination with theophylline, glyceraldehyde, mannoheptulose, diazoxide, KCl, verapamil and D-600, and trifluoperazine (50). The most surprising result is the lack of effect of KCl. Consequently, paired studies with a positive control, such as stimulation of insulin release with a Ca^{2+} ionophore, would be useful before the conclusions can be fully accepted.

Studies on $^{45}Ca^{2+}$ efflux include one paper on the RINm5F cells which were attached to fibronectin-coated plastic beads. Evidence in accord with the existence of Ca^{2+}/Ca^{2+} and Ca^{2+}/Na^+ exchangers was obtained because $^{45}Ca^{2+}$

efflux was increased when the cells were changed from Ca^{2+}-deficient to Ca^{2+}-containing media, and because the removal of Na^+ from the media caused a decrease in $^{45}Ca^{2+}$ efflux. Definitive studies on Ca^{2+} handling systems in B cell plasma membranes remain to be performed. In media containing low concentrations of extracellular Ca^{2+} the efflux of $^{45}Ca^{2+}$ was decreased by glucose as it is in pancreatic islets. Depolarizing concentrations of KCl increased $^{45}Ca^{2+}$ efflux, an effect which was blocked by D-600, the Ca^{2+} channel antagonist. Thus, in these cells, voltage-dependent Ca^{2+} channels appear to be fully functional. Glucose was found to be a poor stimulator of $^{45}Ca^{2+}$ efflux, suggesting that one reason for the lack of glucose responsiveness in these cells was the inability of glucose to depolarize the membrane (4).

Glucose stimulation of intracellular buffering of calcium was further documented by experiments performed on pancreatic B cells (51). This effect of glucose is specific, in the sense that it cannot be mimicked by agents such as KCl or sulfonylureas.

While controversy still surrounds the possible role of calmodulin as a major participant in stimulus-secretion coupling, there is no doubt about its importance in the regulation of other specific cell functions and 'general housekeeping'. Studies on the localization of calmodulin-binding proteins have been carried out. As calmodulin mediates its actions directly on enzymes, or indirectly via enzymes affecting protein phosphorylation, one can anticipate a large number of calmodulin-binding proteins to be present in cells. Three major binding proteins were detected on secretion granules. The binding of ^{125}I-calmodulin was Ca^{2+}-dependent and inhibited by the calmodulin antagonists, trifluoperazine and calmidazolium. It was specific to the extent that binding was blocked by unlabeled calmodulin, whereas troponin C and parvalbumin were a 100- to a 1000-fold less effective (52). These studies should lead to a greater understanding of B cell function. However, as the evidence for a role of calmodulin in stimulus-secretion coupling is largely indirect and rigorously unconvincing, it remains to be seen whether this will help us to understand the control of insulin release.

Phosphoinositide metabolism

The involvement of phosphoinositides in stimulus-secretion coupling in the B cell is now obvious and the major outlines have been drawn. Acceleration of polyphosphoinositide turnover results in: (a) increased amounts of inositol 1,4,5-triphosphate (IP_3), which is able to mobilize Ca^{2+} from a store believed to be the endoplasmic reticulum; (b) increased amounts of arachidonic acid which (i) will result in increased activity in the cyclo-oxygenase, epoxygenase and lipoxygenase pathways, the latter being considered a stimulatory pathway with respect to insulin release and which (ii) is capable of mobilizing Ca^{2+} from intra-cellular stores (53); and (c) can increase the content of diacylglycerol which is an activator of protein kinase C.

By analogy with the effects of the phorbol esters the C-kinase pathway could also be involved in insulin secretion and it appears as though C-kinase activation increases the sensitivity of the insulin 'release machinery' to Ca^{2+} (54). Thus, polyphosphoinositide turnover, which is increased by glucose and by hormones such as acetylcholine, can activate pathways capable of stimulating insulin re-lease. The complications of this system appear to be considerable and its impor-tance is not understood. At this time one might conclude that the importance of polyphosphoinositide turnover for glucose-stimulated insulin secretion is rather slight. In contrast, the contribution of these pathways to acetylcholine-stimu-lated insulin secretion may be total. The next few years will see a detailed assess-ment of the pathways and their relative contributions under different conditions of B cell activation.

Two papers during the past year dealt with phospholipid methyltransferase activity (55, 56). Using *S*-adenosyl-L-methionine as the donor, phos-phatidylethanolamine was primarily methylated to mono- and dimethylphos-phatidylethanolamine and phosphatidylcholine. The V_{max} of methyltransferase was accelerated by an action of Ca^{2+} without an effect on the K_m. β-Adrenergic stimulation or high glucose in intact islets both stimulated the methylation (this, of course could be via indirect effects such as provision of more substrate or Ca^{2+}; nevertheless the effect is present). Neither cyclic AMP nor GMP stimu-lated the enzyme activity. Trifluoperazine, chlorpromazine and dibucaine did inhibit the enzyme. The methyltransferase inhibitor, 3-deaza-adenosine, inhi-bited both the enzyme and insulin release. Based on these data, and the pre-sence of the enzyme in the secretory granule fraction from islets, it seems possi-ble that the phospholipid methyltransferase activity in the B cell could play a role in the stimulation of insulin release by glucose and other agents.

Arachidonic acid metabolites

The roles of arachidonic acid metabolites in the control of insulin secretion have been the subject of much confusion and controversy. The reasons for this are obvious: incomplete knowledge of the pathways and products of arachidonic acid metabolism; no appreciation until recently that arachidonic acid itself could mobilize Ca^{2+} in islets; a reliance on presumptions of specificity for in-hibitors of arachidonic acid metabolism; the interpretation of whole animal or tissue studies despite the high probability of secondary effects and interactions; and the use of a diverse variety of species, preparations and experimental condi-tions. Nevertheless, some aspects of the role of these pathways in the control of insulin release by mechanisms within the B cell are now becoming clearer.

Arachidonic acid is produced by the action on phospholipids of phospholipase A_2, and of phospholipase C followed by diacylglycerol lipase. Both pathways are operative in B cells. Arachidonic acid is subsequently metabolized by the cyclo-oxygenase, lipoxygenase and epoxygenase enzymes, with the latter having received less attention than the former two. At the risk of making sweeping generalizations, opinion is focusing around an inhibitory 'tone' exerted by prostaglandins produced by cyclo-oxygenase and a stimulatory effect of some metabolite(s) of the lipoxygenase pathway. The evidence in favor of stimulation via the lipoxygenase pathway is far stronger than that for inhibition by prostaglandins. The five papers reviewed here all emphasize the potential importance of the lipoxygenase pathway for the stimulation of insulin secretion and raise the possibility of an obligatory role.

Arachidonic acid was found to be metabolized through the lipoxygenase pathway to 12-hydroxyeicosatetraenoic acid (12-HETE) and via the cyclo-oxygenase pathway to prostaglandin E_2, $F_{2\alpha}$ and prostacyclin by both dispersed endocrine-cell-rich pancreatic cells of neonatal rat and pancreatic islets (57). Exogenous arachidonic acid stimulated insulin release from monolayer cultures of pancreatic cells in a concentration- and time-dependent manner and was reversible on removal of the arachidonate. Indomethacin, a non-specific inhibitor of cyclo-oxygenase (which can also inhibit cyclic nucleotide phosphodiesterase), potentiated the response to arachidonic acid. However, the lipoxygenase inhibitors, BW-755c and eicosa-5,8,11,14-tetraynoic acid, blocked the effect of arachidonic acid. Glucose, ionophore A23187 and bradykinin all activate phospholipase and increase arachidonic acid production, and all increase insulin secretion. Insulin release stimulated by these three agents was inhibited by the lipoxygenase inhibitors. Exogenous 12-HETE in large amounts failed to stimulate insulin release, whereas 12-hydroxyperoxyeicosatetraenoic acid (12-HPETE) did. Furthermore, 5,6-epoxy-8,11,14-eicosatrienoic acid, a more stable analogue of leukotriene A_4, potentiated glucose-stimulated insulin release. The authors concluded that the metabolism of arachidonic acid provided a dual control of insulin secretion, with an inhibitory effect via cyclo-oxygenase and a stimulatory effect via the lipoxygenase (57).

As stated earlier, the evidence for the stimulatory effect of the lipoxygenase pathway seems much stronger than that for the inhibitory cyclo-oxygenase pathway. Certainly the fact that cyclo-oxygenase inhibitors were found to stimulate insulin secretion at a time when arachidonic acid was known to be converted to prostaglandins could have biased our interpretations towards an inhibitory role for prostaglandins. The shunt of arachidonic acid down the lipoxygenase pathway, when the cyclo-oxygenase pathway is blocked, provides an acceptable alternative explanation for the stimulation of insulin release. Furthermore, it has been shown that 12-HPETE, which stimulates insulin secretion, is converted by pancreatic islets to two hydroxy-epoxides, 8H-11,12-EPETE and 10H-11,12-EPETE, which were named hepoxilin A and B, respectively (58). Hepoxilin A was found to potentiate glucose-stimulated insulin secretion and could therefore be the stimulatory component (or one of the components) of the lipoxygenase pathway. This compound could account for the stimulation of insulin secretion seen with the cyclo-oxygenase inhibitors, arachidonic acid and 12-HPETE. As glucose also increases the amount of lipoxygenase products in pancreatic islets (59), hepoxilin could mediate some of the insulin secretion response to glucose.

The generalized importance of the lipoxygenase pathway in insulin secretion is suggested by the inhibitory effect of lipoxygenase inhibitors on insulin secretion stimulated by increased cyclic AMP levels (60). Nordihydroguaiaretic acid and 1-phenyl-3-pyrazolidinone inhibited the stimulation and potentiation of insulin secretion by forskolin, without affecting the rise in cyclic AMP levels, and by theophylline and dibutyryl cyclic AMP. The results lead to the conclusion that a lipoxygenase product may be an intermediary in the insulinotropic effect of cyclic AMP, or play a permissive role in insulin secretion or, as the conclusions are based on inhibitor studies, the inhibitors may have 'non-specific' inhibitory effects on secretion which are unrelated to the lipoxygenase pathway.

Effect of hormones on insulin secretion

A study of norepinephrine has characterized its concentration-response relationship with respect to inhibition of insulin secretion, its blockade by the α_2-adrenergic receptor blocker, yohimbine, but not by the α_1-blocker, prazosin (61). Norepinephrine blocked up to 50% of the increased $^{45}Ca^{2+}$ uptake stimulated by high glucose concentrations, thus confirming a previous report (62). The effect of norepinephrine on $^{45}Ca^{2+}$ uptake was not seen in the presence of dibutyryl cyclic AMP, which suggests that the effect on $^{45}Ca^{2+}$ uptake was due to a lowered cyclic AMP level in the islets. The inhibitory effect of norepinephrine on insulin secretion in the presence of raised cyclic AMP levels was also confirmed. The data support the idea of a distal site of action for α_2-adrenergic receptor agonists. Xylazine, a sedative extensively used in veterinary medicine, was characterized as a partial α_2-adrenergic receptor agonist, thus accounting for its 'side effects' on plasma insulin and blood glucose in animals sedated with the drug (63). Evidence that the inhibitory effect of dopamine on insulin secretion is via α_2-adrenergic receptors and not dopamine receptors was obtained by comparative studies on isolated rat pancreatic islets with analogs of dopamine, yohimbine and sulpiride (a dopamine receptor antagonist). An indirect effect of dopamine to inhibit insulin release via the adrenal medulla was observed (64).

There is, as yet, no rigorous evidence that islet B cells contain β-adrenergic receptors, although potentiation of insulin release by β-adrenergic receptor agonists has been observed. From studies with different concentrations of iso-prenaline, in the absence and presence of the α_2-blocker, rauwolscine, and of glucagon, it has been concluded that β-adrenergic receptor agonists exert their effects via the paracrine effect of stimulated glucagon secretion in the islet (65). Glucagon has also been implicated in the regulation of insulin secretion by arginine (66). In these studies, animals given glucagon antibodies released less insulin in response to arginine than did controls, whereas glucose-stimulated insulin secretion was unaffected. It would be useful to study the effect of β-adrenergic receptor agonists under similar glucagon-ineffective conditions, especially as binding of ^{3}H-dihydroalprenolol (a β-adrenergic receptor antagonist) to pancreatic islet cells has been reported (67). Confirmation that forskolin, a diterpene that stimulates adenylate cyclase and increases cell cyclic AMP levels, is a useful tool for the study of cyclic AMP effects (and therefore of glucagon and β-adrenergic receptor agents) was obtained during the year (68) with results on insulin secretion similar to those obtained in the initial report (69).

Binding sites for gastric inhibitory peptide (GIP) were reported in 1985 and claimed to represent 'the first analysis of functionally relevant GIP binding sites in an insulin-secreting cell' (70), despite the 1984 publication characterizing specific high-affinity binding sites for GIP in pancreatic B cells (71)! Both groups, using membranes from hamster B cell tumors, present evidence for two sets of binding sites for ^{125}I-labeled GIP, with those of high affinity being, presumably, the physiologically active receptors.

Two conflicting reports appeared with respect to thyroid state and insulin release. In one, hyperthyroidism was associated with decreased insulin secretion in response to glucose (72), while in the other it was reported to augment both phases of glucose-stimulated insulin release (73). In the latter, hypothyroidism caused by a low iodine diet and propylthiouracil decreased the second phase of release. Thyrotrophin-releasing hormone and its metabolite histidylproline di-ketopiperazine, both of which are putative neurotransmitters and present in pancreatic islets, were not found to have any effect upon insulin secretion.

Effects of drugs

In any particular year, one usually finds a variety of miscellaneous drugs being studied for their effect on insulin secretion. Motivation for such studies can be more varied than the types of drugs involved. Thus, a drug may be the 'specific inhibitor of the year', in which case the study must be done quickly because by next year it will be non-specific and the results unpublishable; sometimes an agent is trendy; occasionally, the drugs used allow us to gain insights into a mechanism or effect, and of course they are studied so that we can understand the action of the drug. So this year we have a range from a paper entitled 'Effects of some drugs on islet function in catfish' (74) to the 'Degranulation effect of ferric nitrilotriacetate on the pancreatic islet beta-cells' (75). Adriamycin, an antineoplastic agent, was found to affect multiple functions in pancreatic islets including insulin secretion, Ca^{2+} handling and glucose oxidation (76). Cyclizine was also studied for its toxicity (77). Phalloidin, known to stabilize F-actin, had no effect upon intact islets, but in islets made permeable by the technique of high-voltage discharge it increased insulin release. Thus the effect of this 'highly specific' drug suggests a role for F-actin in the regulation of insulin secretion (78). A possible explanation for the decreased insulin levels found in vitamin-B_6-deficient rats was proposed on the basis of studies with tryptophan and its metabolites on leucine-stimulated insulin secretion (79). Insulin secretion was inhibited by 3-hydroxykynurenine, 3-hydroxyanthranilic acid and *o*-aminophenol, whereas tryptophan, kynurenine and kynurenic, xanthurenic and anthranilic acids were without effect. Thus, selected metabolites (those with electron-donating aromatic amino and hydroxyl groups) may be responsible for diminished secretion in vitamin B_6 deficiency.

Enflurane has a marked inhibitory effect upon glucose-stimulated insulin release by an action which is not understood (80). At a concentration causing over 80% inhibition of release, in separate experiments, islet cyclic AMP levels and adenylate cyclase activity were both slightly decreased. These changes, as the authors point out, are unlikely to be the cause of such profound inhibition of insulin secretion.

Developmental and integrative studies

The maturation of stimulus-secretion coupling can be studied under different conditions by the use of islets from fetal rats kept in tissue culture (81). In order to evaluate the differential effects of age and the ambient glucose concentration, islets from 21.5-day fetuses were cultured in RPMI 1640 and 10% fetal calf serum with either 2.8 or 11.1 mM glucose. After 1 day of culture, a challenge with 16.7 mM glucose after basal perifusion in 2.8 mM glucose elicited only transient and small responses in insulin release and only minor 'phosphate flushes' regardless of the glucose concentration in the culture media. After 7 days in culture the effects were different. A high glucose challenge in both sets of islets caused an increase in islet oxygen consumption, phosphate flush, and ATP and GTP content. However, only the islets maintained in 11.1 mM glucose responded with an adult-like biphasic pattern of insulin secretion. The islets kept in 2.8 mM glucose responded with only a small first phase and a slight second phase. Thus, exposure to a high glucose concentration appears to be necessary to the development of some elements of stimulus-secretion coupling, though not all. It was stressed that while the 7-day (11.1 mM glucose) cultured islets responded to glucose with biphasic insulin release, the second phase could not be sustained. Thus, further development is required for the full, adult response. The importance of the study lies in the potential of the developing islet as an experimental model for the understanding of stimulus-secretion coupling.

Glucose is known to decrease the B cell membrane permeability to K^+ via an effect upon one type of K^+ channel, which is blocked by quinine and, of course, sensitive to glucose via a glucose metabolite or signal. The decreased K^+ permeability leads to depolarization, increased Ca^{2+} entry via the voltage-dependent Ca^{2+} channel and increased insulin secretion. K^+ permeability can be monitored by ^{86}Rb efflux and Ca^{2+} uptake with $^{45}Ca^{2+}$. Ammon et al (82) have shown that in fetal islets which do not secrete insulin in response to glucose, the islets show no decrease in ^{86}Rb efflux and no increase in $^{45}Ca^{2+}$ uptake. Both of these effects are consistently observed in mature, responding islets. It may be concluded that one missing element in the non-responding fetal islet is the inability of glucose to decrease plasma membrane K^+ permeability. Whether this is due to an inability of glucose metabolism to generate the signal to the channel or failure of the channel to receive the signal, or a combination of the two, remains to be determined.

In studies on the decline of glucose-stimulated insulin secretion observed with age, islets from 13-month-old rats had a 36% decrease in insulin release relative to islets from 2.5-month-old rats, and showed a blunted first phase. However, in response to stimulatory concentrations of glyceraldehyde, no age-related differences were observed. The authors conclude that the cause of the diminished response to glucose in older rats lies at a point in stimulus-secretion coupling prior to the metabolism of trioses (83).

The mechanisms underlying the synergy between glucose and cyclic AMP were studied under perifusion conditions and attempts made to differentiate between the effect of cyclic AMP to increase the sensitivity of the process of exocytosis to Ca^{2+}, and the effect of glucose to potentiate the action of Ca^{2+} by retaining it in the cell by reduced efflux. While the ability of cyclic AMP to potentiate insulin secretion is well recognized, the potentiating effect of glucose has not been clearly defined. In comparative studies, the potentiating effect of cyclic AMP was only 1.4 times greater than the potentiating effect of glucose (84). This potentiating effect of glucose, exerted via restrained Ca^{2+} efflux across the plasma membrane, provides an explanation for some, if not all, of the so-called permissive effects of glucose with respect to other secretagogues.

Conclusions

Studies on insulin secretion in vitro are leading steadily to a complete knowledge of stimulus-secretion coupling in the B cell. It is noteworthy that we have little knowledge of the signals generated by secretagogues prior to changes in Ca^{2+} handling by the B cell, nor do we know how Ca^{2+} causes granule membrane / plasma membrane fusion and exocytosis. Fortunately, recent advances in electrophysiology, allowing the study of single channels and membrane capacitance changes, provide the means for rapid advances over the next few years. Given a complete understanding of the control of insulin secretion, we may then unravel the B cell defects in some forms of diabetes.

References

1. Ohgawara H, Machiyama E, Mizuno Y et al (1985): A comparative study of insulin secretion from pancreatic islets maintained in free-floating and monolayer cultures. *J. Jpn. Diabetic Soc., 28,* 537.
2. Campbell IL (1985): Functional and metabolic characteristics of dissociated mouse pancreatic islet cells in suspension. *Aust. J. Exp. Biol. Med. Sci., 63,* 139.
3. Thivolet CH, Chatelain P, Nicoloso H et al (1985): Morphological and functional effects of extracellular matrix on pancreatic islet cell cultures. *Exp. Cell Res., 159,* 313.
4. Abrahamson H, Berggren P-O, Hellman B (1984): Mobilization of ^{45}Ca from insulin-producing RINm5F cells attached to microcarriers. *Am. J. Physiol., 10,* E719.
5. Hopcroft DW, Mason DR, Scott RS (1985): Adult rat pancreatic islet cells adherent to microcarrier beads: evaluation of function and morphology. *In Vitro, 21,* 485.
6. Mathers DA, Buchan AMJ, Brown JC et al (1985): Rat pancreatic islet cells in primary culture: occurrence of giant cells amenable to patch clamping. *Experientia, 41,* 116.
7. Nielsen JH (1985): Growth and function of the pancreatic beta cell in vitro: effects of glucose, hormones and serum factors on mouse, rat and human pancreatic islets in organ culture. *Acta Endocrinol., Suppl., 108,* 39.
8. Braun K, Besch W, Jahr H et al (1985): The encapsulation of pancreatic islets: investigation of insulin secretion and content in vitro. *Biomed. Biochim. Acta, 44,* 143.
9. Hill RS, Boyd III AE (1985): Perifusion of a clonal cell line of Simian virus 40-transformed beta cells: insulin secretory dynamics in response to glucose, 3-isobutyl-1-methylxanthine, and potassium. *Diabetes, 34,* 115.
10. Bodziony J, Schwille PO (1985): Islet isolation from atrophied pancreas after short-term duct ligature - evidence for normal in vitro release of insulin and somatostatin. *Horm. Metab. Res., 17,* 314.
11. Tilzey JF, Waights V, Holmes R (1985): The development of the homologous teleost insulin radioimmunoassay and its use in the study of adrenaline on insulin secretion from isolated pancreatic islet tissue of the rainbow trout, *Salmo gairdineri* (R.). *Comp. Biochem. Physiol. A, 81,* 821.
12. Baldissera FGA, Holst JJ (1984): On the contamination of commercially available aprotinins with pancreatic islet peptides. *Scand. J. Clin. Lab. Invest., 44,* 669.
13. Molina JM, Premdas FH, Klenck RE et al (1984): The dynamic insulin secretory response of isolated pancreatic islets of the diabetic mouse: evidence of a gene dosage effect on insulin secretion. *Diabetes, 33,* 1120.

14. Nakamura Y, Yoshida T, Kajiyama S et al (1985): Insulin release from column-perifused isolated islets of uremic rats. *Nephron, 40,* 467.
15. Leahy JL, Weir GC (1985): Unresponsiveness to glucose in a streptozotocin model of diabetes: inappropriate insulin and glucagon responses to a reduction of glucose concentration. *Diabetes, 34,* 653.
16. Leahy JL, Bonner-Weir S, Weir GC (1985): Abnormal insulin secretion in a streptozotocin model of diabetes: effects of insulin treatment. *Diabetes, 34,* 660.
17. Unger RH, Grundy S (1985): Hyperglycaemia as an inducer as well as a consequence of impaired islet cell function and insulin resistance: implications for the management of diabetes. *Diabetologia, 28,* 119.
18. Dimitriadis G, Cryer P, Gerich J (1985): Prolonged hyperglycaemia during infusion of glucose and somatostatin impairs pancreatic A- and B-cell responses to decrements in plasma glucose in normal man: evidence for induction of altered sensitivity to glucose. *Diabetologia, 28,* 63.
19. Wilson GL, Patton NJ, McCord JM et al (1984): Mechanisms of streptozotocin- and alloxan-induced damage in the rat B cells. *Diabetologia, 27,* 587.
20. Jansson L, Sandler S (1985): Pancreatic islet circulation in relation to the diabetogenic action of streptozotocin in the rat. *Endocrinology, 116,* 896.
21. Masiello P, Wollheim CB, Gori Z et al (1984): Streptozotocin-induced functioning islet cell tumor in the rat: high frequency of induction and biological properties of the tumor cells. *Toxicol. Pathol., 12,* 274.
22. Cook DL, Hales N (1984): Intracellular ATP directly blocks K^+ channels in pancreatic β-cells. *Nature (London), 311,* 271.
23. Ashcroft FM, Harrison DE, Ashcroft SJH (1984): Glucose induces closure of single potassium channels in isolated rat pancreatic beta-cells. *Nature (London), 312,* 446.
24. Fernandez JM, Neher E, Gomperts BD (1984): Capacitance measurements reveal stepwise fusion events in degranulating mast cells. *Nature (London), 312,* 453.
25. Malaisse WJ, Lebrun P, Merchuelz A et al (1983): Synergistic effect of a tumor-promoting phorbol ester and a hypoglycemic sulfonyl urea upon insulin release. *Endocrinology, 113,* 1870.
26. Pace CS, Goldsmith KT (1985): Action of a phorbol ester on β-cells: potentiation of stimulant-induced electrical activity. *Am. J. Physiol., 248,* C527.
27. Sturgess NC, Ashford MLJ, Cook DL, Hales CN (1985): The sulphonylurea receptor may be an ATP-sensitive potassium channel. *Lancet, 2,* 474.
28. Findlay I, Dunne MJ, Petersen OH (1985): High-conductance K^+ channel in pancreatic islet cells can be activated and inactivated by internal calcium. *J. Membr. Biol., 83,* 169.
29. Findlay I, Dunne MJ, Ullrich S et al (1985): Quinine inhibits Ca^{2+}-independent K^+ channels whereas tetraethylammonium inhibits Ca^{2+}-activated K^+ channels in insulin-secreting cells. *FEBS Lett., 195,* 4.
30. Paolisso G, Nenquin M, Schmeer W et al (1985): Sparteine increases insulin release by decreasing the K^+ permeability of the B-cell membrane. *Biochem. Pharmacol., 34,* 2355.
31. Paolisso G, Nenquin M, Meissner HP, Henguin JC (1985): The effects of cesium chloride on insulin release, ionic fluxes and membrane potential in pancreatic B-cells. *Biochim. Biophys. Acta, 844,* 200.
32. Eddlestone GT, Oldham SB, Lipson LG et al (1985): Electrical activity, cAMP concentration, and insulin release in mouse islets of Langerhans. *Am. J. Physiol., 17,* C145.
33. Henquin JC, Meissner HP (1984): The ionic, electrical, and secretory effects of endogenous cyclic adenosine monophosphate in mouse pancreatic β cells: studies with forskolin. *Endocrinology, 115,* 1125.
34. Pace CS (1984): Influence of a tumor-promoting phorbol ester on the electrical response of B-cells to glucose and glyburide. *Mol. Pharmacol., 26,* 267.

35. Satin LS, Cook DL (1985): Voltage-gated Ca^{2+} current in pancreatic B-cells. *Pflügers Arch. Eur. J. Physiol., 404*, 385.
36. Prentki M, Wollheim CB (1984): Cytosolic free Ca^{2+} in insulin secreting cells and its regulation by isolated organelles. *Experientia, 40*, 1052.
37. Rorsman P, Abrahmsson H, Gylfe E et al (1984): Dual effects of glucose on the cytosolic Ca^{2+} activity of mouse pancreatic β-cells. *FEBS Lett., 170*, 196.
38. Deleers M, Mahy M, Malaisse WJ (1985): Glucose increases cytosolic Ca^{2+} activity in pancreatic islet cells. *Biochem. Int., 10*, 97.
39. Hellman B, Hallgren R, Abrahamsson H et al (1985): The dual action of glucose on the cytosolic Ca^{2+} activity in pancreatic beta-cells: demonstration of an inhibitory effect of glucose on insulin release in the mouse and man. *Biomed. Biochim. Acta, 44*, 63.
40. Prentki M, Janjic D, Biden TJ et al (1984): Regulation of Ca^{2+} transport by isolated organelles of a rat insulinoma: studies with endoplasmic reticulum and secretory granules. *J. Biol. Chem., 259*, 10118.
41. Prentki M, Biden TJ, Janjic D et al (1984): Rapid mobilization of Ca^{2+} from rat insulinoma microsomes by inositol 1,4,5,-trisphosphate. *Nature (London), 309*, 562.
42. Biden TJ, Prentki M, Irvine RF et al (1984): Inositol 1,4,5-trisphosphate mobilizes intracellular Ca^{2+} from permeabilized insulin-secreting cells. *Biochem. J., 223*, 467.
43. Panten U, Zielmann S, Schrader M-T, Lenzen S (1985): The dihydropyridine derivative, Bay K 8644, enhances insulin secretion by isolated pancreatic islets. *Naunyn-Schmiedeberg's. Arch. Pharmacol., 328*, 351.
44. Malaisse WJ, Mathias PCF (1985): Stimulation of insulin release by an organic calcium agonist. *Diabetologia, 28*, 153.
45. Malaisse-Lagae F, Mathias PCF, Malaisse WJ (1984): Gating and blocking of calcium channels by dihydropyridines in the pancreatic B-cell. *Biochem. Biophys. Res. Commun., 123*, 1062.
46. Eng LA, Lee JC (1985): Verapamil induces glucose intolerance in conscious, nondiabetic rats. *Res. Commun. Chem. Pathol. Pharmacol., 48*, 157.
47. Wollheim CB, Janjic D (1984): Cobalt inhibition of insulin release: evidence for an action not related to Ca^{2+} uptake. *Am. J. Physiol., 15*, C57.
48. Hoftiezer V, Berggren P-O, Hellman B (1985): Effects of glucose deprivation and altered Ca^{2+} concentrations on clonal insulin-producing cells (RINm5F). *Biomed. Biochim. Acta, 44*, 77.
49. Grill V, Efendic S (1984): Stimulation by calcium and barium of somatostatin release: evidence for lower sensitivity of D- vis-à-vis B- and A-cells. *Acta Physiol. Scand., 122*, 401.
50. Flatt PR, Swanston-Flatt SK (1985): Role of calcium in defective insulin secretion from human and transplantable rat islet cell tumours. *Biomed. Biochim. Acta, 44*, 71.
51. Hellman B, Gylfe E (1984): Evidence for glucose stimulation of intracellular buffering of calcium in pancreatic beta-cell. *Q. J. Exp. Physiol., 69*, 867.
52. Watkins D, White BA (1985): Identification and characterization of calmodulin-binding proteins in islet secretion granules. *J. Biol. Chem., 260*, 5161.
53. Wolf BA, Turk J, Sherman WR, McDaniel ML (1986): Intracellular Ca^{2+} mobilization by arachidonic acid. *J. Biol. Chem., 261*, 3501.
54. Tamagawa T, Niki H, Niki A (1985): Insulin release independent of a rise in cytosolic free Ca^{2+} by forskolin and phorbol ester. *FEBS Lett., 183*, 430.
55. Laychock SG (1985): Phosphatidylethanolamine *N*-methylation and insulin release in isolated pancreatic islets of the rat. *Mol. Pharmacol., 27*, 66.
56. Kowluru A, Rana RS, MacDonald MJ (1985): Phospholipid methyltransferase activity in pancreatic islets: activation by calcium. *Arch.Biochem. Biophys., 242*, 72.
57. Metz S, VanRollins M, Strife R et al (1983): Lipoxygenase pathway in islet endocrine cells: oxidative metabolism of arachidonic acid promotes insulin release. *J. Clin. Invest., 71*, 1191.

58. Pace-Asciak CR, Martin JM (1984): Hepoxilin, a new family of insulin secretagogues formed by intact rat pancreatic islets. *Prostaglandins Leukotrienes Med., 16,* 173.
59. Metz SA (1985): Glucose increases the synthesis of lipoxygenase-mediated metabolites of arachidonic acid in intact rat islets. *Proc. Natl. Acad. Sci. USA, 82,* 198.
60. Yamamoto S, Nakadate T, Uzamaki H, Kato R (1985): Lipoxygenase inhibitors and cyclic AMP-mediated insulin secretion caused by forskolin, theophylline and dibutyryl cyclic AMP. *J. Pharmacol. Exp. Ther., 233,* 176.
61. Morgan NG, Montague W (1985): Studies on the mechanism of inhibition of glucose-stimulated insulin secretion by noradrenaline in rat islets of Langerhans. *Biochem. J., 226,* 571.
62. Wollheim CB, Kikuchi M, Renold AE, Sharp GWG (1977): Somatostatin- and epinephrine-induced modifications of $^{45}Ca^{++}$ fluxes and insulin release in rat pancreatic islets maintained in tissue culture. *J. Clin. Invest., 60,* 1165.
63. Abdel El-Motal SM, Sharp GWG (1985): Inhibition of glucose-induced insulin release by xylazine. *Endocrinology, 116,* 2337.
64. Arneric SP, Chow SA, Long JP, Fischer LJ (1984): Inhibition of insulin release from rat pancreatic islets by drugs that are analogues of dopamine. *Diabetes, 33,* 888.
65. Zielmann S, Schutte G, Lenzen S, Panten U (1985): Effects of isoprenaline and glucagon on insulin secretion from pancreatic islets. *Naunyn-Schmiedeberg's Arch. Pharmacol., 329,* 299.
66. Tan K, Atabani G, Marks V (1985): Divergent effect of glucagon antibodies on arginine and glucose-stimulated insulin secretion in the rat. *Diabetologia, 28,* 441.
67. Cherksey BD, Mendelsohn SA, Zadunaisky JA, Altszuler N (1985): Direct insertion and fluorescence studies of rhodamine-labeled beta-adrenergic receptors in cell membranes. *J. Membr. Biol., 84,* 105.
68. Hermansen K (1985): Forskolin, an activator of adenylate cyclase, stimulates pancreatic insulin, glucagon, and somatostatin release in the dog: studies in vitro. *Endocrinology, 116,* 2251.
69. Wiedenkeller DE, Sharp GWG (1983): Effects of forskolin on insulin release and cyclic AMP content in rat pancreatic islets. *Endocrinology, 113,* 2311.
70. Amiranoff B, Vauclin-Jacques N, Laburthe M (1985): Interaction of gastric inhibitory polypeptide (GIP) with the insulin-secreting pancreatic beta cell line, In III: characteristics of GIP binding sites. *Life Sci., 36,* 807.
71. Maletti M, Portha B, Carlquist M et al (1984): Evidence for and characterization of specific high affinity binding sites for the gastric inhibitory polypeptide in pancreatic beta-cells. *Endocrinology, 115,* 1324.
72. Varnum B, Davidson MB, Venkatesan N (1985): Insulin secretion and action in the hyperthyroid rat. *Horm. Metab. Res., 17,* 383.
73. Awouters P, Meissner HP, Henquin JC (1985): Thyrotropin-releasing hormone and insulin release: in vitro studies with islets of normal and dysthyroid mice. *Diabetes Res., 2,* 105.
74. Bhatt SD, Bora PS (1984): Effects of some drugs on islet function in catfish. *Indian J. Physiol. Pharmacol., 28,* 201.
75. Yamanoi Y, Awai M, Seno S (1984): Degranulation effect of ferric nitrilotriacetate (Fe^{3+}-NTA) on the pancreatic islet beta-cells: its acute toxic effect on glucose metabolism. *Acta Med. Okayama, 38,* 423.
76. Deleers M, Goormaghtigh E (1985): Adriamycin effects on insulin secretion, Ca^{2+} movements and glucose oxidation in pancreatic islet cells. *Pharmacol. Res. Commun., 17,* 227.
77. Hanai N (1984): Morphological and immunocytochemical study of rat pancreatic beta cell changes induced by cyclizine. *J. Appl. Toxicol., 4,* 308.
78. Stutchfield J, Howell SL (1984): The effect of phalloidin on insulin secretion from islets of Langerhans isolated from rat pancreas. *FEBS Lett., 175,* 393.

79. Rogers KS, Evangelista SJ (1985): 3-Hydroxykynurenine, 3-hydroxyanthranilic acid, and *o*-aminophenol inhibit leucine-stimulated insulin release from rat pancreatic islets. *Proc. Soc. Exp. Biol. Med., 178,* 275.

80. Ewart RBL, Rusy BF, Bradford MW (1985): Enflurane and adenosine 3',5'-cyclic monophosphate metabolism in pancreatic islets. *Anesth. Analg., 64,* 18.

81. Freinkel N, Lewis NJ, Johnson R et al (1984): Differential effects of age versus glycemic stimulation on the maturation of insulin stimulus-secretion coupling during culture of fetal rat islets. *Diabetes, 33,* 1028.

82. Ammon HPT, Fahmy A, Mark M et al (1985): Failure of glucose to affect [86]rubidium efflux and [45]calcium uptake of fetal rat pancreatic islets. *J. Physiol. (London), 358,* 365.

83. Molina JM, Premdas FH, Lipson LG (1985): Insulin release in aging: dynamic response of isolated islets of Langerhans of the rat to D-glucose and D-glyceraldehyde. *Endocrinology, 116,* 821.

84. Phang W, Domboski L, Krausz Y et al (1984): Mechanisms of synergism between glucose and cAMP on stimulation of insulin release. *Am. J. Physiol., 10,* E701.

The Diabetes Annual/3
K.G.M.M. Alberti and L.P. Krall, editors
© 1987 Elsevier Science Publishers, B.V.

21 C-Peptide and proinsulin

SVEND G. HARTLING, CHRISTIAN BINDER AND OLE K. FABER

C-Peptide

In vivo studies in laboratory animals and man most often use peripheral insulin concentrations as a reflection of B-cell secretory activity. This approach assumes that the peripheral insulin concentration changes in proportion to changes in its systemic delivery rate. There is considerable evidence, however, that the rate of insulin clearance may vary under different conditions. Furthermore, the liver extracts a large and variable proportion of the insulin delivered to it.

C-Peptide and insulin are both secreted from the B cell in equimolar concentrations, the hepatic extraction of C-peptide is negligible and its metabolic clearance rate is constant over a range of concentrations encountered under physiological conditions. It may therefore be argued that measurement of C-peptide in peripheral venous plasma gives a more direct reflection of B-cell secretory activity than measurements of insulin. Since it is possible, also in insulin-treated subjects, to determine B-cell secretion accurately using C-peptide measurements, these measurements have been widely used for the assessment of B-cell function.

In this review, we shall confine ourselves to aspects of the determination of C-peptide as a measure of B-cell function. For information about specific features of B-cell function under various physiological and pathophysiological conditions, the reader is referred to the other chapters in this and preceding *Annuals*.

Methodological aspects

C-Peptide is measured radioimmunologically. The inter-laboratory differences in ranges of normal values, discussed in *The Diabetes Annual/1,* still exist. These different values are due to differences in the antibodies and the labelled C-peptide preparations as well as to different standards used in the assays. In this context, it is important that the user of commercial assays be aware that the materials in these assay kits, especially the antibodies, may gradually be changed. This may introduce changes in the level of the C-peptide measured as well as in the cross-reactivity with human proinsulin and other aspects of the assay system. Thus, in the Novo C-peptide kit, the M1230 antibody has been changed to either K6 or M1221, both polyclonal antibodies. The change to M1221 (1), which has a higher cross-reactivity with proinsulin, induces a 5-8% increase in the normal fasting C-peptide level measured with the assay system (B. Tronier, personal communication).

Plasma C-peptide immunoreactivity is heterogeneous with different contributions to total C-peptide immunoreactivity from different components (2). Recently Oyama et al (3), using high-performance liquid chromatography (HPLC) and subsequent radioimmunoassay, have demonstrated heterogeneity of C-peptide immunoreactivity in urine. They found at least 4 different components. The major one, which accounts for over 50% of total reactivity, elutes in a position identical to that of a synthetic human C-peptide preparation. In their assay system, all components showed parallel serial dilution curves to the displacement curves of synthetic human C-peptide. However, one would like to see a similar parallelism in other assay systems with antibodies directed towards different antigenetic sites on the C-peptide molecule before finally accepting this similarity of the different components of C-peptide.

Measurements of B-cell function

With the availability of large quantities of synthetic C-peptide from different species including dog and man, new insights into the kinetics of C-peptide have become available. In the first direct study of the metabolic clearance rate of human C-peptide Faber and co-workers, using intravenous bolus injection of synthetic human C-peptide in normal volunteers, found an average metabolic clearance rate of 4.4 ml/kg/min (4). These findings have now been confirmed in elegant studies by Polonsky et al (5), who found the average metabolic clearance rate of C-peptide to be 4.0 ml/kg/min in normal subjects, after both intravenous bolus injection and constant rate infusion. Since the kinetics of C-peptide have been shown to be linear (4, 5), it is possible, under steady-state conditions, to calculate directly the C-peptide and consequently the insulin secretory rate from the plasma concentration of C-peptide and the metabolic clearance rate. The metabolic clearance rate varies between individuals with a coefficient of variation of about 8%. The determination of kinetic parameters of C-peptide in individual subjects should therefore increase the accuracy with which its secretion rate can be derived from peripheral plasma concentrations. This becomes even more important when the insulin secretion rate is calculated under non-steady-state conditions (6). When insulin secretion rate is calculated directly from the plasma concentration of C-peptide, an underestimate will appear during increasing peptide secretion rate whereas an overestimate of secretion rate will be found during decreasing peptide secretion rate (6). Consequently, more appropriate descriptions of C-peptide kinetics must be used. The most general impression of these kinetics is the equation describing the decay curve of plasma C-peptide levels from a single intravenous bolus injection of C-peptide (6). Using this equation, it is possible to calculate the rates of insulin secretion by B cells in a continuous fashion. The limit of error of such a calculation is in the order of 10%. No further information seems to be obtained in the two-compartment methods used by Eaton et al (7).

In combination, these studies have shown that it is possible, from measurements of peripheral venous C-peptide concentrations, under both steady-state and non-steady-state conditions, to calculate insulin secretion rates. However, this requires that C-peptide kinetics are studied after a single-bolus intravenous injection of C-peptide in each subject. Furthermore, it may be concluded that comparison of the rate of insulin secretion in the same subjects under two sets of physiological or pathophysiological conditions is possible from the direct measurement of plasma C-peptide concentration curves.

When larger populations are studied, the less stringent direct use of plasma C-peptide concentrations without individual knowledge of C-peptide kinetics is feasible. This also applies to the clinical use of C-peptide determinations under most circumstances.

Ten years ago we introduced the measurement of C-peptide 6 minutes after intravenous injection of 1 mg of glucagon as a convenient test for B-cell function in patients with insulin-dependent diabetes mellitus (IDDM) (8, 9). In recent years, the test has been increasingly used also in non-insulin-dependent diabetic (NIDDM) patients. We argued that the test was easy to perform, it was not time-consuming, the stimulus was reproducible, and discomfort during the test was limited. Furthermore, the test results correlated well with the C-peptide values found after the more time-consuming and less reproducible mixed-meal stimulus (10). In the following years, the glucagon/C-peptide test has become, at least in European countries, a routine test for several purposes. It is used as a test for insulin dependency: i.e., if a patient has an undetectable C-peptide concentration in plasma after glucagon stimulation, B-cell destruction is so extensive that exogenous insulin is needed to maintain life. At the other end of the spectrum, a C-peptide concentration that exceeds a certain level indicates that acceptable glycaemic control can be obtained without exogenous insulin, i.e. that the patient is non-insulin-requiring (11).

This concept has recently been substantiated by Koskinen et al (12), who studied 105 adult diabetic patients. Based on predefined clinical criteria, 56 patients were classified as requiring insulin therapy during a follow-up period of 6-18 months. They found that a glucagon-stimulated C-peptide level of 0.60 nmol/l (measured with antibody M1230) (1) predicted insulin requirement with a high sensitivity (95%) and a high specificity (96%). Measurement of fasting levels of C-peptide correctly predicted therapy in 70 of the patients (67%). Thus, the authors suggest that in the classification of diabetic patients, fasting C-peptide should be measured. If it is below 0.20 nmol/l, insulin treatment is necessary, whereas fasting levels exceeding 0.60 nmol/l indicate non-insulin-requirement. Subjects with values between these extremes are studied with a glucagon test, and insulin treatment is being instituted in those with stimulated C-peptide levels lower than 0.60 nmol/l. These findings are in strict accordance with previous findings by ourselves (11) and others (13). It should be emphasized that these specific C-peptide concentration levels are only relevant when samples are measured with M1230 antibody.

In other assay systems, other cut-off levels will apply. Thus, Matsuda et al (14), in a study of 68 diabetic patients with varying degrees of hyperglycaemia and insulin dependence, found that patients with a C-peptide level lower than 1 ng/ml (0.33 nmol/l) were insulin-dependent while many patients in the non-insulin-dependent group had C-peptide levels lower than 2.0 ng/ml (0.6 nmol/l). These findings are basically similar to those of Koskinen et al (12), although the actual levels discriminating between treatment groups are considerably lower, the most probable explanation being the different C-peptide assays used (Daiichi Radioisotope Laboratories, Tokyo).

Other factors that may influence discriminatory C-peptide levels are the stimulus used as well as the criteria for insulin treatment. Grant et al (15), in 34 insulin-treated diabetic patients, selected for evaluation of insulin requirement based on clinical criteria, found that a C-peptide level 2 hours after 50 g oral glucose of ≥ 0.10 nmol/l (Novo kit, antibody M1230) identified 75% of patients not requiring insulin and excluded all those who needed insulin. Although not specifically stated, they seem to define those who do not need insulin as patients whose glycaemic control did not deteriorate after cessation of insulin treatment. Thus, the group considered non-insulin-requiring after 3 months of evaluation had a high mean fasting plasma glucose concentration of 10.9 mmol/l with a range of 6-19 mmol/l. Consequently, most clinicians would not accept the majority of their patients not treated with insulin as non-insulin-requiring, a fact that probably explained the low discriminatory C-peptide level.

In our original studies, we were unable to demonstrate any effect of the prevailing blood glucose level on the C-peptide response to glucagon (8, 9). Such an effect was to be expected, however, from studies in normal subjects (16). Furthermore, Ward et al (17) have demonstrated a potentiation by glucose of non-glucose insulin secretagogues in both normal and diabetic subjects.

Recently, Rönnemaa studied the C-peptide response to repeated glucagon stimulation in 15 insulin-treated patients both in the fasting state and 1.5 hours after a breakfast meal (18). By chance, 4 patients had low blood glucose levels of 2.5-6.2 mmol/l during the fasting test and low glucagon stimulated C-peptide levels from undetectable to 0.32 nmol/l. When tested after the breakfast meal, blood glucose was 9.2-14.5 mmol/l and C-peptide levels 0.28-1.38 nmol/l. While some of the variation in C-peptide response may be a direct effect of a meal, as found in the other 11 subjects studied, it must also be concluded that low blood glucose levels will suppress the B-cell response to glucagon. Similar findings have been reported in a more extensive study, hitherto only published in abstract form (19).

It may be concluded that C-peptide determination in the fasting state and, with greater value in the stimulated state, is of considerable benefit in the selection of patients who need insulin to obtain acceptable glycaemic control. The conditions of testing as well as the C-peptide assay used determine the discriminatory C-peptide levels that should be employed. Caution should be observed to avoid testing after stimulation with non-glucose stimuli in subjects with low blood glucose concentrations, i.e. lower than 6-7 mmol/l. In clinical practice, this seems to be of minor importance since most of the patients studied with the glucagon C-peptide test are non-insulin-treated diabetics with unacceptable hyperglycaemia in whom clinicians want to know whether or not this is caused by loss of B-cell function.

Proinsulin

In *The Diabetes Annual/2* we raised the question of whether proinsulin is a hormone in its own right and not just a prohormone (precursor) for insulin. We defined a hormone as an organic compound synthesized in and secreted from specific cells. It exerts its action via specific receptors. The compound itself and/or its induced specific actions form part of an integrated system, which also controls synthesis and/or secretion of the compound.

Cells that synthesize and secrete proinsulin separately from those making insulin have still not been demonstrated. The question is therefore whether the secretion of proinsulin and insulin varies quantitatively in a systematic way, thus forming the basis for a differential proinsulin action. The synthesis of proinsulin (and thereby of insulin) depends on the amount of and the translational rate of preproinsulin mRNA. At low glucose concentrations (2-4 mmol/l) proinsulin synthesis comprises less than 5% of islet protein synthesis. At glucose concentrations above 15 mmol/l it increases to 20-30% (20). This response to glucose has been suggested to be dependent on an increased translational rate rather than on an increased mRNA level (21). Glucose will stimulate an increase in proinsulin mRNA, but only after long incubation in rat islet cultures. Recently, this has been questioned by Giddings et al (20) who found that an increased proinsulin mRNA level (increased transcription or reduced degradation) at high glucose (28 mmol/l) correlated with insulin biosynthesis, and that translational activity of RNA at both 2.8 and 28 mmol/l was decreased after 4 hours of incubation. It has also been shown in pancreatectomized rats that an increased cellular proinsulin mRNA concentration can compensate for a decreased B-cell mass (22). In rats subjected to 50% pancreatectomy, an increase in proinsulin mRNA nearly normalized glucose metabolism and serum insulin, while 90% pancreatectomy led to increased proinsulin mRNA at 1 and 3 weeks. However, at 14 weeks post-pancreatectomy a severely reduced level of proinsulin mRNA was present, leading to low serum insulin levels and hyperglycaemia.

The conversion of proinsulin to insulin in the normal B cell is so effective that only 3-5% of proinsulin escapes cleavage. Experimentally, the converting-enzyme system can be blocked or stimulated. Halban et al (23) have shown in rat islets that tris(hydroxymethyl)aminomethane (Tris) at 10 and 50 mmol/l inhibits proinsulin conversion in a dose-related manner. Also, Tris at 50 mmol/l inhibited the release of newly synthesized proinsulin/insulin while the release of 'old' stored insulin was not affected. In rats treatment with tolbutamide in pharmacological amounts increased the conversion rate of proinsulin to insulin so that the $t_{1/2}$ for the conversion of labelled proinsulin to insulin was reduced from 36 to 20 minutes, without affecting the rate of proinsulin synthesis (24).

Proinsulin secretion in man

Clinically, a family has been described in whom proinsulin accounted for approximately two-thirds of the insulin immunoreactivity due to a defective conversion process (25). The basic defect is probably located in or near the insulin gene (26). In two other families a genetically determined hyperproinsulinaemia was caused by a substitution of arginine with histidine at amino acid position 65, leading to incomplete conversion with the C-peptide attached to the A-chain (27-29).

Hyperproinsulinaemia is well described in patients with insulinoma in which proinsulin may be the only B-cell product found in increased concentration in the peripheral blood (30). In these patients exogenous hyperinsulinaemia during an euglycaemic clamp will not suppress proinsulin secretion (31). In normal and obese subjects, insulin levels of 600-700 pmol/l (90-100 mU/l) during euglycaemia clearly suppressed proinsulin secretion (31) just as insulin and C-peptide secretion were decreased (32-34). Hyperproinsulinaemia, on the other hand, seems to suppress C-peptide release (35). This mutual feedback inhibition speaks against a selective and specific integrated system controlling only proinsulin synthesis and/or secretion.

The mechanism of elevated insulin immunoreactivity found in liver cirrhosis is still under debate. Reduced liver extraction of insulin without increased B-cell secretion has been proposed (36). Increased proinsulin secretion explaining most of the increased insulin immunoreactivity has been demonstrated (37);

however, recently, normal proinsulin levels in liver cirrhosis were found while insulin and C-peptide levels were elevated (38). Probably, differences in assay techniques and certainly in the selection of patients explain these discrepancies.

In patients with cystic fibrosis having normal fasting blood glucose levels, proinsulin was found to be elevated in those with impaired glucose tolerance (39). This finding of elevated proinsulin in cystic fibrosis patients not suspected of having disturbed glucose metabolism at the time of the study has led to investigation of another diabetes-prone group, i.e. siblings of IDDM patients. Here, fasting proinsulin was elevated in one-third of these healthy siblings along with normal insulin values (40). In 10 non-diabetic identical twins of IDDM patients, a comparable result has been found (41). It seems as if proinsulin levels under certain pathophysiological conditions are elevated. This may be a controlled compensatory mechanism or it may only reflect a diseased B cell. In the former case, one could consider proinsulin as a backup hormone when insulin subsides; in the latter, proinsulin elevation could be an early indicator of altered B-cell function at a 'subclinical' stage of diabetes mellitus.

Measurement of proinsulin

The measurement of proinsulin in biological fluids is still a challenging problem. Previous methods using gel filtration (42, 43) or an 'insulin-specific protease' (44) have largely been discontinued. The gel filtration method is laborious and does not ensure complete separation of the immunoreactive components. The protease method is unreliable since degradation of insulin is incomplete and some proinsulin may also be degraded (45, 46).

During the past 10 years, several proinsulin immunoassays have been developed (47-55). Even though the standardisation of proinsulin is still not solved (56) and these assays use or have used different standards, the proinsulin levels (fasting or stimulated) in normal and NIDDM subjects are surprisingly comparable. Proinsulin cleavage to insulin and C-peptide may follow two pathways (Fig. 1). None of the assays published is proinsulin-specific since the intermediate conversion products of insulin cross-react to varying degrees. One assay seems to measure preferentially split 65-A1 and split 32-33 instead of intact proinsulin (57); another measures intact proinsulin and split 65-A1, but split 32-33 barely at all (49), while some assays measure both intact proinsulin and the main split forms (52, 51).

Proinsulin kinetics and metabolism

Whereas insulin is mainly metabolized in the liver, proinsulin metabolism occurs primarily extrahepatically. From studies where pharmacological amounts of proinsulin were infused, the fractional hepatic extraction of proinsulin

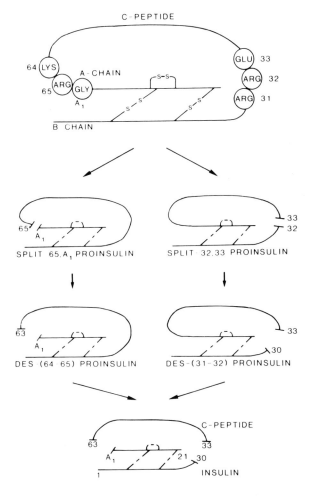

FIG. 1. *Scheme for the processing of human proinsulin to major conversion intermediates, and to C-peptide and insulin.*

appeared to be less than 5% under steady-state conditions at plasma proinsulin concentrations of 1.41-40 nmol/l. This is more than 100 times that of normal fasting levels (35, 58).

The metabolic clearance rate (MCR) determined from similar infusion studies varied from 1.6 to 3.49 ml/kg/min (35, 59-61), which is 10-30% that of insulin (59-61). So far, there are no data on the MCR of proinsulin at physiological plasma concentrations. Within the concentration range studied, the metabolic clearance process of proinsulin seems unsaturable. The differences in results obtained by various groups are not related to dosage or plasma concentration, but are most likely to be due to methodological problems.

Furthermore, proinsulin shows some peculiarities in its kinetics when administered intravenously. Adapting the recognized technique of infusing a priming dose over 10 min followed by a constant infusion where doses are calculated on estimates of MCR and the concentration level aimed at (62), the plasma proinsulin concentration does not follow the expected time course (59). Thus, there was no initial peak and the steady-state concentration was not achieved within the expected time. These results could indicate that the infused proinsulin is partly and rapidly cleared within the vascular compartment by a partly reversible process.

The lack of specificity of most proinsulin assays is another major methodological problem. The intermediate products of the conversion of proinsulin to insulin cross-react in almost all assays. Degradation of infused proinsulin within the vascular compartment and a release of intermediates back into the circulation from extravascular compartments will of course influence the data when non-specific assays are used.

By combining HPLC and an assay specific for proinsulin and its intermediate conversion products, Given et al (63) have elegantly demonstrated that the amount of circulating conversion intermediates comprised less than 1% of proinsulin immunoreactivity after intravenous infusion of supraphysiological amounts of proinsulin. The major conversion product was des-(31-32)proinsulin. By contrast, subcutaneous infusion of proinsulin resulted in the appearance of variable amounts of biologically active intermediates comprising up to 11% of total proinsulin immunoreactivity. Conversion to significant amounts of circulating insulin could not be demonstrated after either of the two routes of administration. The results indicate that proinsulin, when cleared from the circulation, is degraded into products other than insulin or known conversion intermediates of proinsulin. Furthermore, subcutaneous tissue contains enzyme systems capable of splitting proinsulin into biologically active components which become absorbed in significant amounts. These facts should be borne in mind when evaluating proinsulin for treatment of diabetes mellitus. One cannot deduce from the results achieved by intravenous infusion what will happen after subcutaneous administration.

From studies in vivo of the metabolism of non-homologous proinsulin in rats, the kidney seems to be a major site of degradation (58, 64). Although proinsulin and several of its conversion intermediates bind to the insulin receptor and become internalized (65, 66), it is not known whether the major degradation takes place via a receptor-binding mechanism.

Many more studies will be needed before we obtain a clear picture of the overall distribution and metabolism of proinsulin. The development of more sensitive and specific assays will be required before we can study the kinetics and metabolism of proinsulin within its physiological range of secretion. Until then we cannot judge whether proinsulin is a hormone in its own right or just an escaped precursor of insulin.

Biological activity of proinsulin

Infusion of porcine proinsulin in man had a stimulatory effect on uptake of glucose by muscle (67). It also appeared to be an effect of proinsulin *per se* and not dependent on its conversion to insulin (68).

In 1984 the first studies of the metabolic effect of biosynthetic human proinsulin in normal man was published by Revers et al (60) and in IDDM subjects by Bergenstal et al (59). By performing serial euglycaemic glucose-clamp studies using different infusion rates of biosynthetic human proinsulin, it was shown from dose-response curve analysis that proinsulin was 8% as potent as insulin in stimulating peripheral glucose uptake and 12% as potent in suppressing hepatic glucose production in normal man (60). However, the maximum effect upon the two processes was the same as for insulin. The plasma concentration of proinsulin required to maintain a normal fasting glucose level in IDDM subjects was 13.7 times higher than that of insulin and more than 100 times higher than fasting proinsulin levels in normal man (59).

After an overnight infusion of insulin aiming at normoglycaemia an infusion of either physiological amounts of proinsulin (8-21 pmol/kg/h) or saline was given. Similar responses of plasma glucose, 3-hydroxybutyrate and glycerol were observed in 4 IDDM patients (59). This indicates that a normal fasting proinsulin concentration does not protect against the development of ketoacidosis. At proinsulin concentrations of about 2.5 nmol/l there was suppression of hepatic glucose output as complete as that observed in the same study at a plasma insulin level of 0.26 nmol/l. At this level, proinsulin was only 70% as effective in stimulating glucose disposal. However, the activation of these two processes appeared to be slower during proinsulin than insulin infusion (60). When the hormone infusions were discontinued, stimulation of glucose disposal disappeared within 2-4 hours (fastest after insulin). The recovery of hepatic glucose output showed almost 1 hour's delay after proinsulin. A further 2½ hours later, it had regained only 50% of its initial value. This is in contrast to the recovery of hepatic glucose output after insulin which reached 50% within 1 hour after discontinuation (69). When infused together with insulin in doses sufficient to suppress hepatic glucose output, biosynthetic proinsulin and human insulin had additive and not synergistic effects on glucose disposal in normal man (70). Pretreatment with biosynthetic proinsulin did not enhance the combined action of insulin and proinsulin on glucose disposal (71).

The doses of proinsulin used have been extremely high when viewed in a physiological context. Therefore, a synergistic effect on hepatic glucose output and even on glucose disposal cannot be excluded at normal or slightly elevated physiological concentrations of the hormones.

Receptor binding in vitro

There is good evidence that proinsulin binds competitively to the insulin receptor (65, 66, 72, 73). Kinetic studies at 16°C showed a decreased affinity of biosynthetic human proinsulin in isolated adipocytes which was due to a much lower association constant with little difference in dissociation rate between ^{125}I-proinsulin and ^{125}I-insulin (66). In the same study, native insulin and proinsulin were capable of mutually displacing their radiolabelled ligands in a dose-dependent manner. The maximum effective proinsulin concentration was however, 10 times higher than that of insulin. The reduced affinity has also been demonstrated in human monocytes (74), in IM-9 lymphocytes and purified rat liver plasma membranes (65). The ratios of binding characteristics between human biosynthetic proinsulin and insulin vary among studies due mostly to varying constants of proinsulin binding. This can only partly be explained by differences in the assay conditions, although differences in the cell numbers studied may be of importance. Further confirmatory studies are awaited in which the radiolabelled as well as the native proinsulin used is chemically and biochemically characterized in detail.

It should however be borne in mind that conversion intermediates of proinsulin show higher binding as well as biological potency than proinsulin itself (65, 74). It is not known whether such intermediates are produced under certain assay conditions.

When bound to the receptor, biosynthetic human proinsulin becomes internalized even to a greater extent than the insulin-occupied receptors (66). There is some evidence that the intracellular degradation of proinsulin may be different and substantially slower than that of insulin (66).

Biological activity in vitro

The stimulation by biosynthetic human proinsulin of several hepatic metabolic processes has been studied in vitro using rat hepatocytes (75, 76) and perfused rat liver (75). A feature common to all dose-response curves of the effects of proinsulin and its intermediate conversion products, on ketogenic, gluconeogenic, and glycogenic enzymes, is that they parallel those of insulin but with a rightward shift. However, the maximal effects are similar for the two hormones (65, 76). Evaluated from the effects at half-maximal concentrations, insulin was 10-30 times more active than biosynthetic human proinsulin. The hormonal concentrations at this level were 2.5-5 and 30-100 nmol/l for insulin and proinsulin, respectively (65, 76).

In contrast to these findings, biosynthetic human proinsulin was found to be as potent as insulin in counteracting glucagon-stimulated glycolysis in the perfused rat liver (75). Studying 2-deoxyglucose transport (67, 73), lipolysis and lipogenesis (66, 74) in isolated rat adipocytes, the dose-response curves of proinsulin also parallel those of insulin with a rightward shift. However, the concentration needed for the half-maximal effect was higher than that observed for hepatocytes, but with the same order of magnitude of the potency ratio between proinsulin and insulin.

To determine whether the prolonged biological activity in vivo of human biosynthetic proinsulin was due to persistent hormone action at the cellular level, deactivation of 2-deoxyglucose transport into adipocytes was studied after stimulation and subsequent removal of insulin or biosynthetic human proinsulin. No difference in deactivation rate was found.

It should be borne in mind that, however interesting all these observations are, one should be cautious before extrapolating the results to man. Firstly, non-homologous proinsulin was used, and secondly, biologically significant effects could only be demonstrated at concentrations of proinsulin much higher than can be seen physiologically; and therapeutically massive doses of proinsulin would have to be given.

Therapeutic effects of biosynthetic human proinsulin

During steady-state infusion of either proinsulin or insulin, it was shown that a proinsulin concentration about 14 times higher is required to maintain euglycaemia in IDDM patients compared with insulin (59). When administered subcutaneously into a few subjects at a rate predicted to have 25% the biological activity of an initial insulin infusion, it was shown that proinsulin did not act synergistically but additively to insulin which was infused at 75% of the rate necessary to maintain euglycaemia (59).

It has been shown that subcutaneous injection into man of biosynthetic human proinsulin gives rise to a significant number of conversion intermediates in the circulation (63). Subcutaneous administration of proinsulin will therefore involve a complex pharmacokinetic situation. At present it is difficult to judge whether this is beneficial or not in the treatment of diabetes mellitus. The rationale for using biosynthetic human proinsulin at all therapeutically is the experimental evidence for its having a more prolonged effect than insulin on hepatic glucose output. At present, several clinical trials are under way to test the clinical usefulness of this compound.

So far, results have only been presented in abstract form. In one study, subcutaneous proinsulin (0.31 ± 0.02 U/kg) before dinner or at bedtime normalized fasting blood glucose and hepatic glucose output in NIDDM patients. This effect could not be achieved by injection of similar doses of NPH insulin (0.34 ± 0.02 U/kg) given at similar times (77). From another multicentre study, preliminary data surprisingly show that the mean dose of biosynthetic human proinsulin was only 60% that of insulin (78).

There are no indications that it is *unsafe* to evaluate further the therapeutic potential of proinsulin, but much more substantial data are needed before the efficacy and the side effects of such treatment can be reviewed.

References

1. Faber OK, Markussen J, Naithani VK, Binder C (1976): Systemic production of antisera to synthetic benzyloxycarbonyl C-peptide in human proinsulin. *Hoppe-Seylers Z. Physiol. Chem., 357*, 751.
2. Kuzuya H, Blix P, Horwitz DL et al (1977): Heterogeneity of C-peptide antibodies and of circulating C-peptide. *J. Clin. Endocrinol. Metab., 44*, 952.
3. Oyama H, Endoh M, Yoneda M et al (1985): New application of high-performance liquid chromatography for analysis of urinary C-peptide. *J. Chromatogr., 338*, 71.
4. Faber OK, Hagen C, Binder C et al (1978): Kinetics of human connecting peptide in normal and diabetic subjects. *J. Clin. Invest., 62*, 197.
5. Polonsky KS, Licinio-Paixao J, Given BD et al (1986): Use of biosynthetic human C-peptide in the measurement of insulin secretion rates in normal volunteers and type I diabetic patients. *J. Clin. Invest., 77*, 98.
6. Morishima R, Pye S, Polonsky K, Radziuk J (1986): The measurement and validation of the nonsteady-state rates of C-peptide appearance in the dog. *Diabetologia, 29*, 440.
7. Eaton RP, Allen RC, Schade DS et al (1980): Prehepatic insulin production in man: kinetic analysis using peripheral connecting peptide behavior. *J. Clin. Endocrinol. Metab., 51*, 520.
8. Faber OK, Binder C (1977): C-Peptide response to glucagon: a test for the residual B-cell function in diabetes mellitus. *Diabetes, 26*, 605.
9. Hendriksen C, Faber OK, Drejer J, Binder C (1977): Prevalence of preserved B-cell function in insulin dependent diabetes mellitus of long duration. *Diabetologia, 13*, 615.
10. Binder C, Faber OK (1978): Residual beta-cell function and its metabolic consequences. *Diabetes, 27*, 226.
11. Madsbad S, Krarup T, McNair P et al (1981): Practical clinical value of the C-peptide response to glucagon stimulation in the choice of treatment in diabetes mellitus. *Acta Med. Scand., 210*, 153.
12. Koskinen P, Viikari J, Irjala K et al (1985): C-Peptide determination in the choice of treatment in diabetes mellitus. *Scand. J. Clin. Invest., 45*, 589.
13. Hoekstra JBL, Van Rijn HJM, Thijssen JHH, Erkelens DW (1982): C-Peptide reactivity as a measure of insulin dependency in obese diabetic patients treated with insulin. *Diabetes Care, 5*, 585.
14. Matsuda A, Kamata I, Iwamoto Y et al (1985): A comparison of serum C-peptide response to intravenous glucagon, and urine C-peptide, as indexes of insulin dependence. *Diabetes Res. Clin. Pract., 1*, 161.
15. Grant PJ, Barlow E, Miles DW (1984): Plasma C-peptide levels identify insulin-treated diabetic patients suitable for oral hypoglycaemic therapy. *Diabetic Med., 1*, 284.
16. Oakley NW, Harrigan P, Kissebah AH et al (1972): Factors affecting insulin response to glucagon in man. *Metabolism, 21*, 1001.
17. Ward WK, Bolgiano DC, McKnight B et al (1984): Diminished B cell secretory capacity in patients with non insulin dependent diabetes mellitus. *J. Clin. Invest., 74*, 1318.
18. Rönnemaa T (1986): Practical aspects in performing the glucagon test in the measurement of C-peptide secretion in diabetic patients. *Scand. J. Clin. Lab. Invest., 46*, 345.

19. Krarup T, Madsbad S, Arnold-Larsen S et al (1986): Blood glucose dependency and reproducibility of the glucagon test. *Diabetologia, 29,* 560A.
20. Giddings SJ, Chirgwin JM, Permutt MA (1985): Glucose regulated insulin biosynthesis in isolated rat pancreatic islets is accompanied by changes in proinsulin mRNA. *Diabetes Res., 2,* 71.
21. Itoh N, Ohshima Y, Nose K, Okamoto H (1982): Glucose stimulates proinsulin synthesis in pancreatic islets without a concomitant increase in proinsulin mRNA synthesis. *Biochem. Int., 4,* 315.
22. Orland MJ, Chyn R, Permutt MA (1985): Modulation of proinsulin messenger RNA after partial pancreatectomy in rats. *J. Clin. Invest., 75,* 2047.
23. Halban PA, Amherdt M, Orci L, Renold AE (1986): Tris(hydroxymethyl)aminomethane inhibits the synthesis and processing of proinsulin in isolated rat pancreatic islets without affecting release of insulin stores. *Diabetes, 35,* 433.
24. Gold G, Pou J, Gishizky ML et al (1986): Effects of tolbutamide pretreatment on the rate of conversion of newly synthesized proinsulin to insulin and the compartmental characteristics of insulin storage in isolated rat islets. *Diabetes, 35,* 6.
25. Gruppuso PA, Gorden P, Kahn CR et al (1984): Familial hyperproinsulinemia due to a proposed defect in conversion of proinsulin to insulin. *N. Engl. J. Med., 311,* 629.
26. Elbein SC, Gruppuso P, Schwartz R et al (1985): Hyperproinsulinemia in a family with a proposed defect in conversion is linked to the insulin gene. *Diabetes, 34,* 821.
27. Robbins DC, Blix PM, Rubenstein AH et al (1981): A human proinsulin variant at arginine 65. *Nature (London), 291,* 679.
28. Shibasaki Y, Kawakami T, Kanazawa Y et al (1985): Posttranslational cleavage of proinsulin is blocked by a point mutation in familial hyperproinsulinemia. *J. Clin. Invest., 76,* 378.
29. Robbins DC, Shoelson SE, Rubenstein AH et al (1984): Familial hyperproinsulinemia: two cohorts secreting indistinguishable type II intermediates of proinsulin conversion. *J. Clin. Invest., 73,* 714.
30. Heding LG, Faber O, Kasperska-Czyzykowa T et al (1978): Radioimmunoassay of proinsulin and hyperproinsulinemic states. In: Baba S, Kaneko T, Yanaihara N (Eds), *Proinsulin, Insulin, C-peptide.* Excerpta Medica, Amsterdam.
31. Koivisto VA, Yki-Järvinen H, Hartling SG, Pelkonen R (1986): The effect of exogenous hyperinsulinemia on proinsulin secretion in normal man, obese subjects, and patients with insulinoma. *J. Clin. Endocrinol. Metab., 63,* 1117.
32. Yki-Järvinen H, Pelkonen R, Koivisto VA (1985): Failure to suppress C-peptide secretion by euglycaemic hyperinsulinaemia: a new diagnostic test for insulinoma? *Clin. Endocrinol., 23,* 461.
33. DeFronzo RA, Binder C, Wahren J et al (1981): Sensitivity of insulin secretion to feedback inhibition by hyperinsulinemia. *Acta Endocrinol., 98,* 81.
34. Elahi D, Nagulesparan M, Herchcopf RJ et al (1982): Feedback inhibition of insulin secretion by insulin: relation to the hyperinsulinemia of obesity. *N. Engl. J. Med., 306,* 1196.
35. Waldhäusl WK, Bratusch-Marrain P, Gasic S et al (1986): Inhibition by proinsulin of endogenous C-peptide release in healthy man. *Am. J. Physiol., 251,* E139.
36. Johnston DG, Alberti KGMM, Faber OK et al (1977): Hyperinsulinism of hepatic cirrhosis: diminished degradation or hypersecretion? *Lancet, 1,* 10.
37. Kasperska-Czyzykowa T, Heding LG, Czyzyk A (1983): Serum levels of true insulin, C-peptide and proinsulin in peripheral blood of patients with cirrhosis. *Diabetologia, 25,* 506.
38. Ballmann M, Hartmann H, Deacon CF et al (1986): Hypersecretion of proinsulin does not explain the hyperinsulinaemia of patients with liver cirrhosis. *Clin. Endocrinol., 25,* 351.

39. Garne S, Hartling SG, Binder C (1986): Exaggerated proinsulin response in cystic fibrosis with abnormal glucose tolerance. *Diabetologia, 29,* 539A.
40. Hartling SG, Lindgren F, Dahlquist G et al (1986): Proinsulin — a possible subclinical indicator for B-cell dysfunction. *Diabetologia, 29,* 547A.
41. Leslie RDG, Heaton DA, Millward BA et al (1986): Identical co-twins of type I (insulin-dependent) diabetic patients can show evidence of B-cell dysfunction which does not lead to diabetes. *Diabetologia, 29,* 564A.
42. Gorden P, Roth J (1969): Plasma insulin: fluctuations in the 'big' insulin component in man after glucose and other stimuli. *J. Clin. Invest., 48,* 2225.
43. Melani F, Rubenstein AH, Oyer PE, Steiner DF (1970): Identification of proinsulin and C-peptide in human serum by a specific immunoassay. *Proc. Natl Acad. Sci. USA, 67,* 148.
44. Kitabchi AE, Duckworth WC, Brush JS, Heinemann M (1971): Direct measurement of proinsulin in human plasma by the use of an insulin-degrading enzyme. *J. Clin. Invest., 50,* 1792.
45. Cresto JC, Lavine RL, Fink G, Recant L (1974): Plasma proinsulin: comparison of insulin specific protease and gel filtration assays. *Diabetes, 23,* 505.
46. Starr JI, Juhn DD, Rubenstein AH, Kitabchi AE (1975): Degradation of insulin in serum by insulin-specific protease. *J. Lab. Clin. Med., 86,* 631.
47. Heding LG (1977): Specific and direct radioimmunoassay for human proinsulin in serum. *Diabetologia, 13,* 467.
48. Rainbow SJ, Woodhead JS, Yue DK et al (1979): Measurement of human proinsulin by an indirect two-site immunoradiometric assay. *Diabetologia, 17,* 229.
49. Cohen RM, Nakabayashi T, Blix PM et al (1985): A radioimmunoassay for circulating human proinsulin. *Diabetes, 34,* 84.
50. Deacon CF, Conlon JM (1985): Measurement of circulating human proinsulin concentrations using a proinsulin-specific antiserum. *Diabetes, 34,* 491.
51. Hartling SG, Dinesen B, Kappelgård AM et al (1986): ELISA for human proinsulin. *Clin. Chim. Acta, 156,* 289.
52. Ward WK, Paquette TL, Frank BH, Porte Jr D (1986): A sensitive radioimmunoassay for human proinsulin, with sequential use of antisera to C-peptide and insulin. *Clin. Chem., 32,* 728.
53. Gray IP, Siddle K, Frank BH, Hales CN (1985): Use of monoclonal antibodies to human proinsulin in a specific two-site immunoradiometric assay. *Diabetes Res. Clin. Pract., Suppl. 1,* 204.
54. Cohen RM, Provow S, Nakabayashi T et al (1984): Site-specific radioimmunoassay in the evaluation of circulating proinsulin and its intermediates. *Clin. Res., 32,* 518A.
55. Hampton SM, Beyzavi K, Marks V (1985): Development and use of human specific proinsulin radioimmunoassay. *Diabetes Res. Clin. Pract., Suppl. 1,* 219.
56. Kruse V, Heding LG, Jørgensen KH et al (1984): Human proinsulin standards. *Diabetologia, 27,* 414.
57. Gray IP, Siddle K, Docherty K et al (1984): Proinsulin in human serum: problems in measurement and interpretation. *Clin. Endocrinol., 21,* 43.
58. Sodoyez JC, Sodoyez-Goffaux F, De Vos C, Frank BH (1986): Comparison of insulin and proinsulin binding to liver receptors: in vivo studies using 123-I-Tyr A14 labeled derivatives and external detection by scintillation scanning. *Diabetologia, 29,* 595A.
59. Bergenstal RM, Cohen RM, Lever E et al (1984): The metabolic effects of biosynthetic human proinsulin in individuals with type I diabetes. *J. Clin. Endocrinol. Metab., 58,* 973.
60. Revers RR, Henry R, Schmeiser L et al (1984): The effects of biosynthetic human proinsulin on carbohydrate metabolism. *Diabetes, 33,* 762.

61. Nauck M, Stöckmann F, Ebert R, Creutzfeldt W (1986): Pharmacokinetic properties of human biosynthetic proinsulin and insulin under euglycaemic clamp conditions in healthy subjects. *Diabetologia, 29*, 575A.
62. DeFronzo RA, Tobin JD, Andres R (1979): Glucose clamp technique: a method for quantifying insulin secretion and resistance. *Am. J. Physiol., 237*, E214.
63. Given BD, Cohen RM, Shoelson SE et al (1985): Biochemical and clinical implications of proinsulin conversion intermediates. *J. Clin. Invest., 76*, 1398.
64. Katz AI, Rubenstein AH (1973): Metabolism of proinsulin, insulin and C-peptide in the rat. *J. Clin. Invest., 52*, 1113.
65. Peavy DE, Brunner MR, Duckworth WC et al (1985): Receptor binding and biological potency of several split forms (conversion intermediates) of human proinsulin. *J. Biol. Chem., 260*, 13989.
66. Podlecki DA, Frank BH, Olefsky JM (1984): In vitro characterization of biosynthetic human proinsulin. *Diabetes, 33*, 111.
67. Fineberg SE, Merimee TJ (1970): Proinsulin: metabolic effects in the human forearm. *Science, 167*, 998.
68. Lazarus NR, Penhos JC, Tanese T et al (1970): Studies on the biological activity of porcine proinsulin. *J. Clin. Invest., 49*, 487.
69. Glauber HS, Revers RR, Henry R et al (1984): In vivo deactivation of proinsulin action on glucose disposal and hepatic glucose production in normal man. *Diabetes, 35*, 311.
70. Revers RR, Henry R, Schmeiser L et al (1984): Biosynthetic human insulin and proinsulin have additive but not synergistic effects on total body glucose disposal. *J. Clin. Endocrinol. Metab., 58*, 1094.
71. Glauber HS, Wallace P, Galloway J et al (1986): The effects of proinsulin pretreatment on the combined actions of insulin and proinsulin in normal man. *J. Clin. Endocrinol. Metab., 62*, 785.
72. Ciaraldi TP, Brady D, Olefsky JM (1986): Kinetics of biosynthetic human proinsulin action in isolated rat adipocytes. *Diabetes, 35*, 318.
73. Peavy DE, Abram JD, Frank BH, Duckworth WC (1984): In vitro activity of biosynthetic human proinsulin. *Diabetes, 33*, 1062.
74. Yu SS, Kitabchi AE (1973): Biological activity of proinsulin and related polypeptides in the fat tissue. *J. Biol. Chem., 248*, 3753.
75. Probst I, Hartmann H, Jungermann K, Creutzfeldt W (1985): Insulin-like action of proinsulin on rat liver carbohydrate metabolism in vitro. *Diabetes, 34*, 415.
76. Agius L, Chowdhury MH, Davis SN, Alberti KGMM (1986): Regulation of ketogenesis, gluconeogenesis, and glycogen synthesis by insulin and proinsulin in rat hepatocyte monolayer cultures. *Diabetes, 35*, 1286.
77. Henry RR, Glauber HS, Galloway JA, Olefsky JM (1986): Treatment of type 2 (non-insulin-dependent) diabetes mellitus with subcutaneous human proinsulin. *Diabetologia, 29*, 548A.
78. Galloway JA, Spradlin CT, Fineberg SE et al (1986): Human proinsulin (rDNA) in the treatment of diabetes mellitus in multicenter US trials. *Diabetologia, 29*, 609A.

The Diabetes Annual/3
K.G.M.M. Alberti and L.P. Krall, editors
© 1987 Elsevier Science Publishers, B.V.

22   Insulin action in vivo

OWEN P. McGUINNESS, KURT E. STEINER, NAJI N. ABUMRAD
AND ALAN D. CHERRINGTON

Introduction

In recent years there has been considerable increase in our knowledge of the physiology of insulin. Many advances have been made regarding its action in the contiol of carbohydrate, fat and protein metabolism. The purpose of this Chapter is to update our earlier review of insulin action in vivo in each of these areas with particular emphasis on recent findings and issues which are currently controversial. The role of insulin in regulating the disposal of a glucose load and its involvement in the determination of insulin sensitivity will be discussed first. Next, the role of insulin in the regulation in vivo of ketogenesis and lipolysis will be discussed, and lastly the role that the hormone is thought to play in regulating protein metabolism in vivo will be reviewed (see also Chapter 26).

Regulation of carbohydrate metabolism by insulin

Insulin and glucose disposal

Oral administration of glucose to man or dog results in the uptake of glucose by both peripheral and hepatic (or splanchnic) tissues (1-6). However, the relative roles of hyperinsulinemia, hyperglycemia and the route of glucose delivery in promoting these responses remain controversial.

Hyperinsulinemia and euglycemia   Insulin has long been known to stimulate glucose uptake by the peripheral tissues of the body. Small (20-30 μU/ml) increments in plasma insulin have been shown to increase glucose uptake by the forearm in euglycemic man (7, 8). Further studies have shown that when plasma insulin concentration was increased to pharmacological levels by intravenous infusion and euglycemia was maintained by glucose infusion, total body glucose uptake increased to a maximum of 10-12 mg/kg/min (Fig. 1). However, inhibition of hepatic glucose output was relatively more sensitive to insulin than

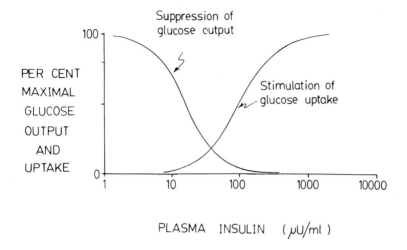

FIG. 1 *Normal dose-response characteristics of insulin on glucose output and glucose uptake in man using the euglycemia clamp technique (based on data from Refs 9-12). Arterial insulin concentrations are depicted.*

stimulation of glucose uptake by peripheral tissues (9-12), although it must be emphasized that the portal insulin level is 2-3 times the arterial insulin level.

Although suppression of glucose output by insulin in the postabsorptive animal is almost entirely due to inhibition of hepatic glycogenolysis, it cannot be concluded that gluconeogenesis is unresponsive to insulin (13-16). Indeed, the gluconeogenic process is already markedly inhibited after an overnight fast due to the potent effect of low levels of insulin. Basal insulin levels maintain the glycogenolytic process in a 50% inhibited state, so that selective insulin removal causes a rapid 2-fold increase in glucose production while gluconeogenesis is in a 75% inhibited state with selective insulin removal causing a 4-fold increase in gluconeogenesis (17). When the insulin concentration was raised 4-fold in portal and arterial blood, hepatic glycogenolysis was virtually completely suppressed (92%), as was hepatic gluconeogenesis (80%). This represented, however, an 84% reduction in the basal glycogenolytic rate but only a 20% reduction in the basal gluconeogenic rate. Much higher insulin levels were required to suppress gluconeogenesis totally, an important point since it shows that postprandial insulin excursions are not capable of turning off gluconeogenesis. This is important in view of the current hypothesis that much of the carbon deposited in hepatic glycogen is derived from precursors which traverse the gluconeogenic pathway.

It is also apparent that while pharmacological concentrations of insulin can inhibit hepatic glucose output, they cannot stimulate any significant uptake of glucose by the splanchnic bed. At insulin concentrations of 400-1000 μU/ml produced by intravenous insulin infusion during euglycemic conditions in man, splanchnic glucose uptake contributed a maximum of only 8% to total glucose metabolism (9, 10).

Intraportal infusion of insulin at 5.0 mU/kg/min into the conscious dog under euglycemic conditions caused a net hepatic glucose uptake of only 0.5 mg/kg/min (Frizzell et al, unpublished observation). At insulin levels as high as 2000 μU/ml in the conscious dog overall glucose uptake was 22.8 mg/kg/min while glucose uptake by the liver reached 2.2 mg/kg/min (McGuinness et al, unpublished observation). Insulin can thus activate the uptake response, but only at pharmacologic levels.

It is also clear that a decrease in glucagon brought about under euglycemic conditions cannot cause a net hepatic glucose uptake (18). Similarly, hyperglycemia in the presence of basal levels of insulin and glucagon cannot trigger any significant net hepatic glucose uptake (19). Thus, multiple signals must be present in order to trigger a marked nèt hepatic glucose uptake.

Hyperglycemia   If one combines hyperglycemia with an increase in the insulin/glucagon molar ratio, brought about either by raising the insulin or by lowering the glucagon concentration, a significant net hepatic glucose uptake can occur. Figure 2 shows data from an experiment in which overnight-fasted dogs underwent a 'pancreatic clamp' to fix the insulin and glucagon levels at basal values; they were then given glucose through a peripheral vein to create hyperglycemia (≃240 mg/100 ml; 13.3 mM and extra insulin to create simultaneous hyperinsulinemia (38 μU/ml in arterial blood and ≃102 μU/ml in portal blood). The combination of these two signals caused a significant net hepatic glucose uptake (2.8 mg/kg/min) (19).

When the same study was carried out, but the glucagon level was decreased instead of the insulin level being raised, a similar response was seen. In this case, the net hepatic glucose uptake averaged 1.8 mg/kg/min during the last hour of the infusion period (20). Thus, the combination of a change in the plasma level of the pancreatic hormones and an increase in blood glucose concentration can cause a net glucose uptake by the liver. Studies in man, where splanchnic rather than hepatic glucose balance can be measured, have suggested that only a slight hepatic glucose uptake occurs in response to a combined hormone and glucose signal (21).

A detailed examination of the interaction between increases in insulin, decreases in glucagon and hyperglycemia in vivo has not been carried out. It is of interest, however, to compare the net hepatic glucose uptake that occurred in response to glucose, insulin and glucagon levels apparent following oral glucose administration (22) with the net hepatic glucose uptake that occurred in a study in which similar hormone levels were created by intraportal insulin and

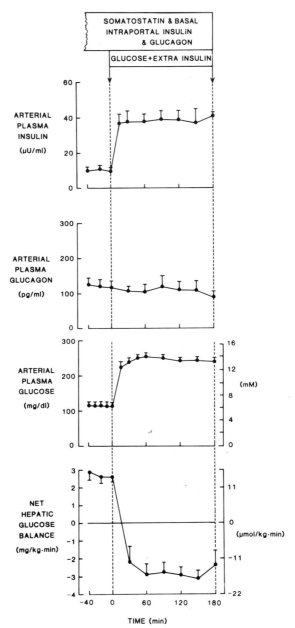

FIG. 2   *Effect of combined hyperinsulinemia and hyperglycemia on net hepatic glucose balance in the overnight-fasted conscious dog brought about in the presence of fixed basal glucagon levels. The glucagon level was fixed by peripheral infusion of somatostatin (0.8 μg/kg/min) and intraportal infusion of replacement amounts of glucagon (0.65 ng/kg/min). Hyperinsulinemia was brought about by the intraportal infusion of insulin (1 mU/kg/min). Hyperglycemia was established by peripheral glucose infusion. Net hepatic glucose balance was calculated using blood glucose values and hepatic blood flow. Data are expressed as means ± SEM and are redrawn from those in Ref. 19.*

glucagon infusion and similar glucose levels were created by peripheral glucose infusion (23). Hepatic glucose uptake was almost twice as great following oral glucose administration as after peripheral intravenous glucose infusion. Data from Ishida et al (24) and Barrett et al (25) also demonstrate a marked difference between the net hepatic glucose uptake seen after oral glucose feeding and that seen after peripheral intravenous glucose infusion. Perhaps the best studies in this regard were carried out by Barrett et al (25). In their studies insulin was given through a peripheral vein to achieve levels of 384 μU/ml in arterial (and presumably portal) blood and glucose was given through a peripheral vein so as to raise the glucose level in the blood entering the liver to 290 mg/100 ml. In response to the combined signals of hyperinsulinemia and hyperglycemia they observed a net hepatic glucose uptake of 2.8±0.4 mg/kg/min. When the authors gave glucose orally, it resulted in a peak glucose concentration of 203 mg/100 ml in the blood entering the liver and a coincident arterial insulin level of 93 μU/ml (portal level of approx. 270 μU/ml). Net hepatic glucose uptake was 4.2±1.0 mg/kg/min. Thus, even though the insulin and glucose levels were approximately 30% less with oral glucose administration, the latter resulted in a greater net hepatic glucose uptake than after peripheral intravenous glucose infusion. It would appear, therefore, that some factor related to the absorption of glucose or the delivery of glucose into the hepatic-portal system may play an important role in the response of the liver.

To determine whether the portal route of glucose entry was associated with greater hepatic glucose uptake than a peripheral intravenous route, insulin and glucagon levels (arterial and portal) in overnight-fasted dogs were fixed in basal values using the 'pancreatic clamp' (26, 27). Each experiment consisted of a control period and two 90-min glucose infusion periods. The latter were randomized, glucose being given through a peripheral vein or through several vessels draining into the hepatic portal vein. The infusion rate of glucose was adjusted so that the load of glucose reaching the liver (inflowing blood glucose concentration × blood flow) was the same during both periods (Fig. 3). Under this condition, hyperglycemia of peripheral intravenous origin suppressed net hepatic glucose production as expected but did not cause a net hepatic glucose uptake (Fig. 4). On the other hand, when glucose was given portally, uptake of glucose was observed, even though the glucose load, the insulin and glucagon levels, and the hepatic insulin extraction rate were no different from those present during peripheral glucose infusion (Fig. 4). Indeed, during portal glucose delivery one-third of the infused glucose was taken up by the liver and two-thirds by peripheral tissues, whereas none was taken up by the liver when the peripheral route was used for glucose infusion. Thus, even though insulin secretion did not occur, portal glucose delivery was able to bring about the same distribution of glucose between the liver and peripheral tissues as is normally observed after oral glucose administration.

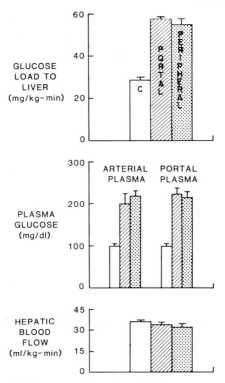

FIG. 3 *Glucose load to the liver, arterial and portal glucose concentrations, and hepatic blood flow during the control period (C) and during a portal (Po) and a peripheral (Pe) glucose infusion. Data are expressed as means ± SEM.*

Work by Ishida et al (24) and Barrett et al (25) in which glucose was infused intraportally supports the concept that the route of glucose administration would affect the distribution of a glucose load in the presence of an altered I/G molar ratio.

In a study similar to that described above the intraportal insulin infusion rate was increased 4-fold at the same time as hyperglycemia was induced (26). Once again the insulin levels in the artery were similar (34±7 and 36±4 μU/ml) regardless of the route of glucose delivery, as were the arterial glucagon levels (61±13 and 59±7 pg/ml), the loads of glucose reaching the liver (57±3 and 57±3 mg/kg/min), and the insulin extraction rates. Again, net hepatic glucose uptake was much greater (3.6±0.8 mg/kg/min) in the presence of portal glucose delivery than in the presence of peripheral glucose delivery (1.4±0.7 mg/kg/min).

The significance of portal versus peripheral glucose delivery has now been examined over a wide range of hepatic glucose loads (27). In the presence of

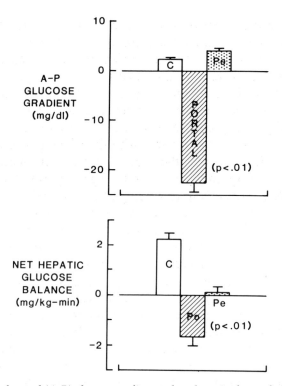

FIG. 4 *Arterial-portal (A-P) glucose gradient and net hepatic glucose balance during the control period (C) and during a portal (Po) and a peripheral (Pe) glucose infusion. Data are expressed as means ± SEM.*

moderate hyperinsulinemia (i.e. 4-fold basal) there is a linear relationship between net hepatic glucose uptake and the load of glucose reaching the liver regardless of the route of glucose administration. However, the relationship is significantly different when the glucose is delivered into the hepatic portal system. The threshold load required for net hepatic glucose uptake was much lower (24 mg/kg/min) when glucose was delivered portally than when it was delivered peripherally (40 mg/kg/min). Since the resting glucose load to the liver in an overnight-fasted dog is approximately 25 mg/kg/min, these data suggest that in the presence of the appropriate portal signal any hyperglycemic excursion will cause glucose uptake by the liver. The data also suggest, therefore, that portal glucose delivery might be particularly important in the case of small physiologic glucose loads.

The question thus arises as to what signal is generated by portal glucose infusion in order to trigger an enhanced response. Most obvious perhaps is the markedly negative arterial-portal (A-P) glucose gradient which exists during portal but not during peripheral glucose delivery. There was a significant correlation between the A-P glucose gradient and net hepatic glucose uptake in our studies in which the importance of the route of administration was assessed in the presence of basal insulin (26). A recent study in vitro has also suggested that the A-P glucose gradient may play a role in triggering a net hepatic glucose uptake (28). Regardless of the exact mechanism of the response, it is clear that it is not simply an increased portal glucose level which explains the difference. When net hepatic glucose uptake was correlated with the portal glucose load rather than the total glucose load reaching the liver, there was still a marked effect of the route of glucose delivery. In other words, for a given portal glucose load significantly more glucose was taken up when glucose entered the body via the hepatic portal system than when it entered via a peripheral vein.

In summary, insulin, glucose and glucagon play critical roles in regulating net hepatic glucose uptake. Modification of any of these variables alone, however, cannot trigger net hepatic glucose uptake. Modification of the I/G molar ratio (either by increasing insulin or decreasing glucagon) and the glucose level (bringing about hyperglycemia) can, on the other hand, cause a significant net glucose uptake. The amount of glucose taken up under that condition is proportional to the load of glucose reaching the liver. The fraction of the load that is extracted, however, depends on whether the glucose enters the body via the hepatic portal system. Three factors are critical to normal postprandial glucose tolerance: the I/G molar ratio, the load of glucose reaching the liver, and the route of glucose entry into the body. The relationship between these 3 variables needs to be clarified, the intracellular signals involved in mediating their responses need to be determined, and the fate of the glucose taken up by the liver needs to be ascertained.

Peripheral glucose utilization

In this section the roles that insulin and glucose play in disposing of the glucose load by peripheral tissues will be discussed.

Glucose-dependent glucose removal   Glucose uptake by the body decreases by 25% when insulin secretion is suppressed. This means that only 25% of basal glucose utilization is insulin-dependent (29, 30). The greater part of the insulin-independent glucose uptake supports brain glucose metabolism (31, 32). In the absence of changes in insulin concentration, glucose disposal increases as the plasma glucose concentration increases (33-35). Using the data of Baron et al (30) and Best et al (33), increasing the plasma glucose concentration by 100 mg/ 100 ml (5.5 mM) raises glucose removal by 40% independent of insulin. Although most tissues in the body require insulin to take up glucose in any significant amounts, in the absence of insulin their contribution to whole-body utilization must be small if the brain can account for nearly 90% of the glucose uptake. However, the contribution of non-neural tissues may increase as the glucose concentration increases.

The awareness that peripheral glucose uptake increases as glycemia increases has forced some investigators to normalize differences in basal glycemia in different situations by expressing results as a ratio of glucose utilization to glucose concentration (metabolic clearance rate: MCR). Using the MCR in this way produces a linear relationship between glucose uptake and glucose concentration and the correlation line if extrapolated passes through zero. This is inaccurate. Glucose MCR decreases as glycemia is increased (33, 34), although for small differences in glycemia the error is small. In the presence of near-basal insulin levels a rise in plasma glucose of 100 mg/100 ml (5.5 mM) decreases the clearance rate of glucose by 16% (33).

Insulin and glucose are synergistic in enhancing glucose disposal even with physiologic changes in insulin level. This increase in glucose disposal associated with an increase in insulin concentration occurs by changing the V_{max} rather than the K_m of glucose uptake (29). It is this synergism between insulin-dependent and glycemia-dependent glucose uptake that allows for rapid disposal of a glucose load.

Baron et al (30) looked at the rate of non-insulin-mediated glucose uptake in normal and diabetic individuals. When endogenous insulin secretion was suppressed by somatostatin, subjects with non-insulin-dependent diabetes mellitus (NIDDM) had higher rates of glucose utilization. However, they were also hyperglycemic relative to the normal group. When the glycemia was matched, the groups were not different. Hansen et al (36) examined the interaction between hyperglycemia and hyperinsulinemia in IDDM patients. Although these patients were insulin-resistant, glycemia-dependent glucose uptake was normal. At present the effectiveness of glucose in enhancing its own disposal seems to be normal in the elderly and IDDM (36-38). This may also be true for NIDDM, although more data are required. The contribution that hyperglycemia makes to enhancing glucose removal following a meal is substantial because of the large glycemic excursions, and any alteration in glycemia-dependent glucose uptake would exacerbate the hyperglycemic excursions in NIDDM subjects.

Estimation of insulin sensitivity

In a recent review Bergman et al (39) described methods for assessing insulin action in vivo. The method most frequently used is the euglycemic hyperinsulinemic clamp. A known insulin infusion rate is given with a concomitant exogenous glucose infusion to maintain euglycemia. When the insulin concentration and glucose infusion rate reach a steady state, the total rate of glucose utilization is equal to the responsiveness of the whole body to insulin at a given steady-state insulin concentration. The total rate of glucose utilization (the sum of endogenous glucose production and exogenous glucose infusion rate) is assessed by the rate of dilution of isotopically labeled glucose. It is critical in these studies that a relative steady state be achieved. To obtain a true steady state, one must maintain the clamp for at least 90 min and in some cases for 2 hours (40, 41). When whole-body glucose uptake at 90 min is compared to that at 3 hours, glucose uptake is underestimated by 17% during a 2 mU/kg/min insulin infusion (McGuinness et al, personal communication). If different doses of insulin are used, then a dose-response curve relating total glucose utilization to insulin concentration can be generated (42, 43). There have been some suggestions to modify the presentation of the data, which will not qualitatively change the results in most cases but would change them quantitatively. One suggestion by Donner et al (44) is to subtract the glucose utilization by insulin-independent tissues, thus magnifying the insulin insensitivity.

Another method for assessing insulin sensitivity is the 'minimal model' method for examining the intravenous glucose tolerance test (IVGTT), which has since been modified (39). This involves the determination of the time course of the plasma insulin and glucose values during an IVGTT. The method is easy to perform. One problem, however, is obtaining a large enough insulin secretory response in NIDDM subjects to determine the model parameters accurately. The method has since been modified by administering a bolus of tolbutamide to exaggerate the insulin response to the glucose load (45). The use of the modified IVGTT has another advantage in that it uses physiological insulin levels, but many assumptions are necessary, such as the linearity of insulin action and a minimal change in glucose effectiveness throughout the range of glucose and insulin concentrations seen in the IVGTT. A constant delay between an increase in insulin concentration and onset of action must also be assumed. However, this is not a problem in the clinical situation where a delay in insulin action should be treated as an *impairment* of insulin action because it leads to inefficient glucose removal. A comparison made in both dogs and normal human subjects of the sensitivity results obtained using the IVGTT and the euglycemic clamp indicates that there is a positive and relatively strong correlation between the two approaches (45). These approaches to assess peripheral insulin sensitivity cannot, however, be used easily to assess hepatic insulin sensitivity.

Two methods are available to assess hepatic insulin sensitivity, both of which use the euglycemic hyperinsulinemic clamp. Recently Cobelli et al (46) have developed a model which uses the IVGTT coupled with a bolus of labeled glucose to assess hepatic insulin sensitivity. The validity of this approach has not been tested. If the euglycemic clamp is used, a dose-response curve must be generated. Instead of measuring peripheral glucose utilization, the suppression of hepatic glucose production at a given insulin concentration is estimated. The direct method determines hepatic glucose production as the product of hepatic blood flow and the arterial-venous difference of glucose across the splanchnic bed (47). The indirect approach uses a primed tracer glucose infusion to assess total glucose turnover and the exogenous glucose infusion rate required to maintain euglycemia is then subtracted, the difference being the endogenous glucose production (43). The indirect method assumes that the glucose kinetics can be measured accurately since a very small number (hepatic glucose production) is obtained after subtracting two large numbers (glucose turnover and exogenous glucose infusion rate). When assessing glucose production during a euglycemic hyperinsulinemic clamp, many investigators obtain negative net hepatic glucose production when a one-compartment model of glucose kinetics is used. A negative net hepatic glucose production is theoretically impossible using the tracer method. Investigators have suggested that the one-compartment models that are commonly used should be replaced by multicompartmental models, which may give a more accurate estimate of glucose production (48). When the magnitude of the error in estimating hepatic glucose production was assessed directly by comparing the direct with the indirect method, glucose turnover was underestimated by 3-5%, resulting in an overestimation of the suppression of endogenous glucose production (97 *vs* 80%) (49). One suggestion is to mix the tracer with the glucose prior to infusing so that one error — the assumption of a rapidly mixing pool — is minimized (50). When the tracer is mixed with the glucose, the error is eliminated (49). Recent evidence indicates that the use of $[3-^3H]$glucose rather than $[6-^{14}C]$glucose may underestimate glucose turnover (51). Because of this error in estimating turnover, the indirect estimation of hepatic insulin sensitivity is difficult.

If one assumes that hepatic glucose balance can be measured accurately either directly or indirectly, another potential error arises. Insulin suppresses glucagon secretion. Liljenquist et al (52) showed that in man in the absence of a fall in glucagon the ability of insulin to suppress hepatic glucose production was impaired. In making an insulin dose-response curve to assess hepatic insulin sensitivity either glucagon secretion should be completely suppressed or glucagon should be infused to maintain constant basal glucagon levels. At present, this approach has not been used and the potential error has not been quantified.

Insulin sensitivity

Insulin sensitivity can vary considerably throughout the normal day. Using the euglycemic hyperinsulinemic clamp technique, insulin sensitivity was found to increase by nearly 45% 2 hours after receiving a 15 or 25 g glucose load (53). When the normal insulin response to the glucose load was mimicked in the absence of a glucose load, insulin sensitivity increased by 34%. This would suggest that normal fluctuations in insulin secretion have long-lasting effects on insulin action. The normal early-morning decrease in glucose clearance has complicated the life of IDDM subjects who manifest inappropriate hyperglycemia. This has been called the 'dawn phenomenon'. Increased growth hormone secretion and increased insulin clearance (54, 55) have been implicated. Campbell et al (55) prevented the normal morning increase in growth hormone using a somatostatin analog, which prevented the decrease in glucose clearance. Replacing growth hormone decreased glucose clearance to levels seen in the absence of somatostatin.

Insulin action can vary considerably during a lifetime because of dietary changes, puberty and aging. The consumption of a high-fat diet for 3 weeks, which was not accompanied by weight gain, decreased insulin action markedly (34%) in rats compared to animals fed a high-carbohydrate diet. At maximally effective insulin concentrations there was a 12% fall in glucose uptake (56). Puberty is associated with as much as a 50% decrease in insulin action (57). The average daily growth hormone levels were found to be higher at puberty than in prepubescent children and adults, which may help explain the resistance.

Glucose intolerance is also said to develop with age. Chen et al (38) attributed the intolerance to both a decrease in insulin action and an inappropriate insulin meal response as assessed by the minimal model approach. Fink et al (37) measured glucose disposal rates at different glucose concentrations in elderly subjects in the presence of hyperinsulinemia. Insulin-mediated glucose disposal was decreased by 30-35%. The K_m of the glucose transport system was unaltered, suggesting that the resistance is due to a decrease in the number of glucose transporters.

Several hormones antagonize insulin-mediated glucose uptake. A recent study by Lager et al (58) demonstrated that the inhibitory effect of epinephrine on glucose utilization was mediated mostly by the β_2-adrenergic receptor both at the periphery and in the liver. The antagonistic effect of glucagon on insulin action occurs at the liver; glucagon has no known peripheral effect on insulin action (52).

Insulin can also alter its own action. When Rizza et al (59) produced 40 hours of mild hyperinsulinemia in man, raising basal insulin levels from 15 to 35 μU/ml, they were able to demonstrate a small decrease in insulin action. Mild hyperinsulinemia produced by the intraportal infusion of insulin for 30 days decreased insulin action by 60% in the dog (60). This was not readily reversed after 30 days of discontinuation of the hyperinsulinemia. Decreases in insulin action associated with severe hyperinsulinemia have been correlated with both increases and decreases in insulin binding (61, 62). Other investigators have suggested that there is a post-binding defect (63). Chronic hypoinsulinemia can also lead to the development of insulin resistance. In the dog partial and total destruction of the pancreas by streptozotocin treatment leads to a progressive decrease in insulin action (64). Therefore, both chronic hyperinsulinemia and hypoinsulinemia can decrease insulin-mediated glucose uptake.

Hyperinsulinemia is seen in NIDDM, obesity and IDDM. The basal hyperinsulinemia of NIDDM and obesity is presumably compensation by the pancreas for peripheral insulin insensitivity. IDDM subjects are also hyperinsulinemic because insulin must be administered peripherally rather than intraportally. Normally portal insulin levels are at least 20 µU/ml higher than in the periphery. To obtain equivalent suppression of the liver by intravenous injection of insulin, hyperinsulinemia must be produced (65). Spangler (66) has attempted to reverse this situation in man by peripheral administration of insulin bound in lipid vesicles that are specifically taken up by the liver. In this way insulin can be delivered directly to the liver even when it is administered peripherally. Insulinoma patients are insulin-resistant compared to a normal population. However, resection of the insulinoma did not reverse the resistance (67). In populations which have a higher incidence of NIDDM, such as Mexican Americans, hyperinsulinemia is greater than what can be accounted for by adiposity (68). Reversal of the hyperinsulinemia by diazoxide increased insulin action in obese patients (69). Whether the hyperinsulinemia seen in diabetic patients can explain their insensitivity is unknown at present.

The insulin resistance seen in diabetes is common to both IDDM and NIDDM. Two weeks after diagnosis insulin action was 32% lower than normal. Except for the 'honeymoon' period in which insulin secretion returns to normal, the resistance is seen in all patients with varying degrees of control (70). Fat tissue removed from these patients is poorly responsive to insulin and shows decreased insulin binding. Examinations of the dose-response curve to insulin demonstrated a decrease in maximal insulin responsiveness (71). This was not readily reversed by intensive therapy (71, 72).

The insulin insensitivity of NIDDM subjects is variable (73). Glucose-intolerant patients have a normal maximal response to insulin but demonstrate a decrease in insulin sensitivity. The non-obese NIDDM subject not only is insulin-insensitive but also has a decreased maximal responsiveness, suggesting not only a receptor but also a post-receptor defect. This resistance is exaggerated if obesity is also present. The change in insulin action in vivo is manifest as a decrease in glucose transport in isolated adipocytes, and a decrease in glucose oxidation and storage in response to a meal. Liver membranes isolated from NIDDM patients demonstrated an increase in insulin binding (74). This is in contrast to the decrease in binding seen in obesity (75). In another study Caro et al (76) looked at liver biopsies obtained from obese NIDDM patients. Binding was similar when based on cell numbers, but decreased when based on surface area. Insulin receptor kinase activity was decreased in diabetic patients.

Hepatic handling of carbohydrate suggests that there is rapid futile cycling in the liver as assessed by comparing [3-^{3}H] and [2-^{3}H]glucose turnover (77). This futile cycling is consistent with a relative decrease in glycogen synthase or increase in glucose-6-phosphatase; no change in futile cycling was found in IDDM (78). Sacca et al (47) examined the role of splanchnic and peripheral tissues in the pathogenesis of impaired glucose tolerance. Hepatic uptake of an intravenous glucose load increased in the impaired glucose-tolerant group and peripheral glucose uptake was decreased by 37%. Hepatic glucose uptake increased because a greater glycemic excursion occurred in the impaired tolerance group. Pehling et al (79) examined the disposal of a meal-derived glucose load on carbohydrate disposition in IDDM. They concluded that the major problem was a lack of complete suppression of endogenous glucose production during the absorption of the meal. They showed further that 2 weeks of CSII therapy improved tolerance. The mechanism is uncertain because the insulin response to a meal was different in the two groups. Firth et al (78) examined the contribution of the peripheral and splanchnic tissues in disposing of a glucose load in NIDDM. They found that hepatic glucose production was equally suppressed. However, since basal glucose production was greater in the NIDDM subjects, the absolute rate of glucose production during the meal was higher than in the controls. The postprandial hyperglycemia of the diabetic patient is further exacerbated by the poor insulin response and the lack of an appropriate increase in glucose uptake.

Recently, intensive insulin therapy has been suggested as a means to improve glycemic control in poorly controlled diabetic patients. Not all studies support the idea that intensive insulin therapy is beneficial. Pedersen and Hjollund (80) looked at continuous subcutaneous insulin infusion (CSII) for 6 months in IDDM and found that it reduced the already depressed transport activity in fat cells, although insulin receptor number was not aggravated. Blackshear et al (81) showed that 2 years of intravenous insulin therapy using an implanted pump in 2 patients resulted in an improvement in glucose control, pancreatic insulin secretion, HbA$_1$, cholesterol and triglycerides. This was achieved, however, by producing a chronic hyperinsulinemia (basal insulin levels were more than doubled). These patients were severely insulin-resistant and this resistance did not improve after therapy. Therefore, although intensive therapy does improve glycemic control, it may have as yet unknown long-term consequences which may or may not be beneficial.

Indirect calorimetry and insulin action

The technique of indirect calorimetry uses the rates of whole body oxygen consumption and carbon dioxide production to assess the rates of glucose and lipid oxidation after correcting for nitrogen excretion. As long as lipogenesis and gluconeogenesis from amino acids are low, accurate estimations of substrate oxidation rates can be made (82). In the basal state, peripheral glucose utilization is approximately 2.2 mg/kg/min; approximately 60% of this is oxidized (1.2 mg/kg/min). In the absence of insulin, glucose oxidation decreases by 40%. When insulin levels are raised to 100 and 160 µU/ml during a euglycemic clamp, glucose oxidation increases to 2.3 and 2.9 mg/kg/min, respectively. At higher insulin levels, glucose oxidation can increase to 4 mg/kg/min (83).

The rest of the glucose utilized during the clamp is presumably stored as glycogen in both muscle and liver. The data of Defronzo et al (84) would suggest that over 85% of the glucose is taken up by muscle and the rest can be accounted for by the brain and other ncn-muscle tissue. Net splanchnic glucose uptake could account for a very minor part of the total glucose uptake (5%).

The increase in glucose oxidation in the presence of hyperinsulinemia may be due in part to the fall in non-esterified fatty acid (NEFA) levels and lipid oxidation (85) in addition to the direct effect of insulin on glucose oxidation. Prevention of the fall in NEFA in the presence of insulin inhibited glucose oxidation by 60%. Felber and Jequire (86) reported that there may be a rise in NEFA oxidation in the obese population at rest and during oral glucose tolerance test (OGTT). This was also seen in obese NIDDM subjects. Part of the decrease in glucose oxidation may be due to the rise in NEFA levels. Only 15% of the glucose disposal after OGTT is oxidized immediately (87). Therefore, oxidation is still a minor route for glucose disposal although in some situations glucose oxidation can be a significant route of glucose disposal (e.g. Graves' disease). During a euglycemic hyperinsulinemic clamp, glucose oxidation contributed nearly 74% of the total glucose utilized compared to 36% in euthyroid subjects (88).

Basal glucose oxidation in the diabetic patient tends to be lower than or the same as in the normal individual. This is mainly because most of the glucose is oxidized in the basal state by insulin-independent tissues. In addition, the hyperglycemia and the higher resting insulin levels in NIDDM may help to maintain the normal resting glucose oxidation. In looking at the response to a meal in severe NIDDM subjects there is only a small increment in glucose oxidation (68). This may be due in part to a poor insulin response to the meal. Although under hyperinsulinemic conditions diabetic patients tend to have lower glucose oxidation rates, the defect in glucose utilization is mostly at glucose storage level (89).

A normal person can dispose of 15% of glucose by oxidation in response to an oral glucose load (100 g). The NIDDM patient also disposes of approximately 15% of the total by oxidation. However, IDDM patients have shown a nearly 5% increase in glucose oxidation with little or no fall in NEFA oxidation (90, 91).

Regulation of fat metabolism by insulin

In addition to its crucial role in glucose metabolism, insulin is an important regulator of fat metabolism in vivo. The net overall changes in fat metabolism caused by insulin are the sum of its stimulatory action on lipogenesis and its inhibitory actions on lipolysis and ketogenesis. The nature of these actions makes it the major antagonist of glucagon, epinephrine, norepinephrine and cortisol, all of which can have lipolytic and ketogenic effects under certain circumstances. Not only do basal amounts of insulin potently restrain the lipolysis and ketogenesis which would normally occur in response to these counter-regulatory hormones, but increments in insulin can virtually abolish both processes.

Effects of selective hyperinsulinemia

Several studies have shown that both the release of non-esterified fatty acids (NEFA) from fat depots and their conversion to ketone bodies in the liver can be affected by relatively small increases in circulating insulin. Early studies by Zierler and Rabinowitz (92) in the human forearm showed that an increment of 38 μU/ml in insulin in the brachial artery was sufficient to inhibit completely NEFA release from the limb. A fall in NEFA level was also observed in overnight-fasted human subjects by Jackson et al (93) for a similar increment in insulin (40 μU/ml). In the latter studies selective hyperinsulinemia was induced by concomitant infusions of insulin, somatostatin (to inhibit endocrine pancreatic secretion of insulin and glucagon) and basal amounts of glucagon.

Massi-Benedetti et al (94) also observed potent antilipolytic and antiketogenic effects of increments in circulating insulin in normal overnight-fasted human subjects in studies which compared the metabolic effects of human and porcine insulins. When a human or porcine insulin was infused into a peripheral vein in successive increments creating plasma insulin levels of 30, 40 and 50 μU/ml, compared with basal levels of 9 μU/ml, the plasma glycerol level (a good indicator of lipolysis because it must be released from the fat cell following hydrolysis of triglyceride) fell by 50, 75 and 80%, respectively. The glucose level was prevented from falling by virtue of a coincident glucose infusion. Changes in NEFA were not reported, but 3-hydroxybutyrate levels were almost completely suppressed with each increment of insulin. Fernandez et al (95) examined in overnight-fasted human subjects during induction of and recovery from hypoglycemia caused by infusion of equivalent amounts of either human or porcine insulin and also found no difference between the two species.

Although a large portion of the antiketogenic effect of insulin is probably due to a decreased supply of NEFA reaching the liver, direct effects of insulin on hepatic ketogenesis have also been demonstrated in man. Gerber et al (96) studied the effects of selective hyperinsulinemia while maintaining plasma NEFA levels by the infusion of intralipid and heparin. Glucose was infused to preserve euglycemia and prevent counterregulatory hormone release. In the presence of basal unchanged NEFA levels, a 90 μU/ml increment in insulin caused a 66% fall in the hepatic production of ketone bodies, indicating a direct inhibitory effect of insulin on ketogenesis. It is interesting to note that the effect of insulin on NEFA levels is the same whether equivalent amounts of insulin are given as a constant infusion or in a series of pulses (97) since it has been hypothesized that normal secretion of the hormone is pulsatile in nature (98).

The antilipolytic and antiketogenic effects of increments in insulin (as little as 7 μU/ml) have also been studied in insulin-deprived diabetic subjects (99). Many years ago, Schade and Eaton (99) showed the effects of insulin on fat metabolism to be dose-dependent, with maximum inhibition at an increment of 100 μM/ml. Additional studies (100) indicate that the sensitivity of fat metabolism to regulation by insulin may be altered by IDDM. Trevisan et al (100), in recent studies using the euglycemic hyperinsulinemic clamp technique in normal subjects and patients with IDDM, found that for a given increment in insulin the decline in NEFA and glycerol was reduced in IDDM.

Effects of acute insulin deficiency

The effects of basal amounts of insulin on lipolysis and ketogenesis in vivo have been assessed by studying the effects of acute insulin deficiency. Wahren et al (101), using somatostatin to create insulin deficiency, examined changes in lipolysis and ketogenesis in both overnight- and 60 hour-fasted normal human subjects. In those fasted overnight both insulin and glucagon levels declined while NEFA levels rose 3-fold 1 hour after somatostatin infusion was begun. Changes in ketone body levels were not measured. In the 60-hour-fasted subjects, NEFA levels increased over 2-fold, but 3-hydroxybutyrate levels did not change. Measurements of splanchnic 3-hydroxybutyrate output, however, showed a 2-fold rise. Since the rise in splanchnic NEFA uptake could account for the rise in ketone production, it seems likely that in these studies ketogenic stimulation resulted entirely from increased delivery of NEFA to the liver rather than from any direct hepatic effects. In similar studies on the effects of acute insulin deficiency Metcalfe et al (102) observed a 3-fold increase in ketone body levels, but only about a 2-fold increase in NEFA levels. These changes accompanied a 50% fall in insulin and a 30-40% fall in glucagon. Contrary to the data of Wahren et al (101), the latter studies suggest that insulin deficiency can reveal a direct stimulatory effect on hepatic ketone body production. These conclusions are supported by studies on acute insulin deficiency in the dog. During selective insulin deficiency when basal glucagon levels were maintained, glycerol and NEFA levels rose by more than 20%, but ketone body production increased by 85% (103). These data indicate that lipolysis was minimally altered by insulin deficiency but that hepatic ketogenesis was significantly augmented. The studies in man summarized above provide a conservative estimate of the antilipolytic and antiketogenic potential of basal insulin since a fall in glucagon concentration, a ketogenic hormone in vivo (at least during insulin deficiency), was also observed during infusion of somatostatin.

The antilipolytic and antiketogenic role of basal insulin in IDDM subjects has also been assessed in vivo (104-108) by the withdrawal of exogenous insulin. Pickup et al (104) observed a progressive rise in 3-hydroxybutyrate levels as free insulin concentrations fell following insulin withdrawal from IDDM. After 9 hours 3-hydroxybutyrate levels had still not plateaued. In similar studies Keller et al (105) noted a rise in acetoacetate turnover with insulin withdrawal. These results were extended by Miles et al (106) in their studies on the effects of insulin deprivation in IDDM subjects. During a 10-hour observation period, insulin levels fell from 18 ± 4 to 7 ± 1 μU/ml, glucagon increased from 67 ± 6 to 259 ± 67 pg/ml, and ketone body levels increased 5-fold from 1.4 ± 0.4 to 7.2 ± 1.5 mmol/l. Both ketone body production (5.4 ± 1.4 to 18.3 ± 3.9 mmol/kg/min) and utilization (5.5 ± 1.1 to 14.7 ± 2.1 μmol/kg/min) increased in association with a 3-fold rise in fatty acid levels. Wahren et al (107) have also observed increases in NEFA levels and hepatic uptake of NEFA as well as ketone body levels after insulin withdrawal. Hepatic fractional extraction of NEFA was unchanged. A 3-fold increase in NEFA levels was accompanied by a 10-fold increase in ketone body production, indicating that basal levels of insulin have a direct inhibitory effect on hepatic ketogenesis as well as an indirect effect through restraint of lipolysis. The interpretation of these studies in diabetic patients, however, is complicated by the fact that glucagon levels rise during insulin withdrawal, and it is difficult to distinguish between those metabolic changes due solely to insulin deficiency and those due to the rise in glucagon. Indeed, Gerich et al (108) have shown that increases in NEFA, glycerol and ketone body levels are reduced when glucagon secretion is prevented by somatostatin infusion during insulin withdrawal in IDDM subjects. It is safe to conclude nonetheless that basal insulin restrains both lipolysis and ketogenesis in normal subjects and IDDM patients.

Effects of obesity and NIDDM

Obesity and NIDDM can also affect the regulation of fat metabolism by insulin. In the original studies by Bagdade et al (109) diabetic and non-diabetic subjects, both lean and obese, they found that obesity or NIDDM alone was not correlated with elevated NEFA or glycerol levels. A delayed decline in NEFA levels during an OGTT was also observed only in obese diabetic subjects, indicating impaired re-esterification. However, glycerol levels declined similarly in both diabetic and non-diabetic subjects, indicating that no impairment of the anti-lipolytic effect of insulin had taken place. Recent studies by Howard et al (110) support the conclusion that the superimposition of NIDDM on the obese state does not affect the inhibitory effect of insulin on lipolysis.

Howard and her associates studied the effects of an OGTT on NEFA and glycerol levels in obese diabetic and obese Pima Indians as well as obese Caucasians. They observed similar declines in NEFA for all 3 groups accompanied by parallel falls in the glycerol levels. These observations were surprising in light of the almost non-existent insulin response to the OGTT observed in the obese diabetic subjects compared to the obese control groups. It was concluded that NIDDM had not reduced the antilipolytic response to insulin, but if anything had actually enhanced it. This normal antilipolytic response occurred even though these subjects demonstrated an abnormal glucose tolerance test (indicative or peripheral insulin resistance with regard to glucose utilization and/or production). Golay et al (111) in studies on 3 groups of obese subjects (obese, obese with impaired glucose tolerance (IGT) and obese NIDDM), found elevated NEFA levels in obese NIDDM but not in the obese IGT group. The absolute and relative suppression of NEFA was reduced during an OGTT in the obese NIDDM group despite hyperinsulinemia, while in the obese IGT group no significant depression was noted. Either re-esterification and/or lipolysis could have been altered, but since glycerol levels were not reported the contribution of changes in either cannot be determined. The latter studies indicate that the degree of carbohydrate intolerance can play a significant role in the alteration of the response of fat metabolism to insulin.

Despite the observations of Bagdade et al (109), other studies have shown that obesity alone can cause abnormal regulation of NEFA levels even when insulin levels are elevated (112). Elevated levels of NEFA and insulin were observed throughout the day in obese as compared to non-obese subjects. However, the decline in NEFA in response to incremental changes in insulin was similar in both groups. Comparisons between obese and non-obese Pima Indians by Howard et al (113) showed a similar decline in NEFA levels in both groups for equivalent increments in insulin. However, in these studies obesity was not acompanied by elevated levels of NEFA following an overnight fast as had been observed by Golay et al (112). Thus, whether responses to basal insulin are altered by obesity is still unclear, but responses to increments in insulin are apparently unaffected by obesity.

In order to determine the effects of NIDDM alone on regulation of fat metabolism by insulin, Fraze et al (114) compared NEFA, insulin and glucose levels over the course of the day in lean subjects with varying degrees of NIDDM. Subjects with mild carbohydrate intolerance maintained NEFA levels similar to those of subjects with normal glucose tolerance, while subjects with more severe NIDDM had elevated NEFA levels even though their insulin levels were also elevated. The relative fall in NEFA after the midday meal was also significantly reduced compared to controls, showing an abnormal response of fat metabolism to the incremental change in insulin. These studies would indicate that NIDDM (depending on its severity) can alter regulation of fat metabolism by insulin independent of obesity.

Effects of hyperglucagonemia in the presence of basal insulin or insulin deficiency

Studies in overnight-fasted human subjects (115, 116) have shown that physiologic increments in glucagon (120-400 pg/ml) in the presence of basal insulin are unable to stimulate ketogenesis. However, during acute insulin deficiency similar increments in glucagon were ketogenic (116, 117). Earlier studies by Gerich et al (118) also showed that a physiologic increment in glucagon in insulin deprived diabetic subjects increased NEFA, glycerol and 3-hydroxybutyrate levels. Others (115), however, observed no lipolytic or ketogenic effects of similar increments in glucagon even during acute insulin deficiency in overnight-fasted normal human subjects. The above studies indicate that if physiologic increments of glucagon are to stimulate ketogenesis and/or lipolysis in vivo, a relative or absolute insulin deficiency is required. Whether the inhibitory effects of basal insulin on lipolysis and ketogenesis could be overcome by a larger physiologic increment in circulating glucagon has not been examined.

Effects of catecholamines in the presence of basal insulin or insulin deficiency

The ability of basal insulin to inhibit the lipolytic and ketogenic effects of increments in catecholamines in normal human subjects has recently been assessed (119-123). Acute insulin deficiency caused by concomitant somatostatin infusion greatly enhanced the increase in ketone body levels which accompanied epinephrine infusion. Weiss et al (122) and Keller et al (123) have shown that somatostatin-induced insulin deficiency in man enhances the ketogenic and lipolytic effects of epinephrine and norepinephrine, respectively. These studies probably underestimate the ketogenic and lipolytic enhancement of the catecholamines due to the relative glucagon deficiency caused by somatostatin infusion. The effects of norepinephrine and epinephrine on fat metabolism in IDDM subjects have also been investigated (124-127). Recent studies by Berk et al (128) in normal and IDDM subjects have shown that patients with IDDM have an enhanced ketogenic but not a lipolytic response to physiologic increments in epinephrine when compared to normal individuals. These data indicate that epinephrine and norepinephrine have a greater ability to augment ketogenesis in the absence of insulin in both normal and diabetic subjects and provide some measure of the ability of basal insulin to restrain the lipolytic and

BASAL INSULIN

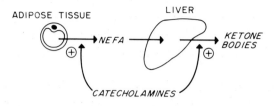

INSULIN DEFICIENCY

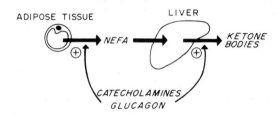

FIG. 5 *Effects of glucagon and catecholamines in the presence of basal insulin and insulin defi-ciency on lipolysis and ketogenesis in vivo. NEFA = non-esterified fatty acids.*

ketogenic effects of catecholamines.

The potent antilipolytic and antiketogenic effects of insulin in vivo are apparent from the studies cited in this review and are diagrammatically sum-marized in Figure 5. Under normal conditions the hormone acts as a potent re-straint on the lipolytic and ketogenic effects of basal glucagon and also of in-creases in glucagon, epinephrine and norepinephrine. Its absence can lead to large increases in both circulating NEFA and ketone bodies, particularly in situ-ations where glucagon and/or catecholamine levels may be increased.

Role of insulin in regulating protein metabolism in vivo

Insulin plays a major role in the maintenance of nitrogen balance in vivo, com-plementing its role as a regulator of carbohydrate and fat homeostasis. The effect of insulin is exerted in several tissues, the most important of which are the liver and the muscle. In vitro effects are reviewed in detail in Chapter 26. The most recently reported in vivo effects are outlined below.

Role of insulin in nitrogen accretion in normal human subjects

In keeping with the observations in vitro, supplementation of nutrients with in-sulin to non-diabetic patients was proposed as a method for enhancing nitrogen accretion. Woolfson et al (129) noted a reduction in urea nitrogen excretion in non-diabetic trauma patients fed parenterally. On the other hand, Fern et al (130) and Powell-Tuck et al (131, 132) noted an increase in urinary excretion of urea and ammonia nitrogen with insulin supplementation in a similar group of trauma patients.

The role that insulin plays in modulating nitrogen accumulation was examined for 4 hours after a beefsteak meal (5 g/kg) in 4 groups of healthy male volunteers fasted overnight. Balance data across the forearm (nmol/100 ml/min) for amino acids were estimated by arterio-venous difference measurements multiplied by blood flow determined using capacitance plethysmography (133). The first group (n=7) received the steak meal only. The second and third groups (n=6, each) had in addition a hyperinsulinemic-euglycemic clamp started 1 hour prior to beef ingestion and continued throughout the study. Beginning 35-48 hours before, the fourth group (n=7) received a graded infusion of 20% dextrose in water adjusted to achieve a glucose delivery of 5.5 mg/kg/min for 16-24 hours prior to beef ingestion and continued throughout the study. A fifth group (n=6) that did not receive a steak meal was studied for the same time period and acted as a saline control. The data are presented in Table 1.

TABLE 1 *The effect of acute (4 h) and prolonged (16-24 h) hyperinsulinemia on nitrogen accumulation across the human forearm in overnight-fasted male volunteers*

Parameter	Group I	Group II	Group III	Group IV	Group V
Peak insulin* (μU/ml)	61± 12	55± 9	95± 7	64± 12	8± 1
Peak plasma Leu**(μM)	243± 24	173±31	169± 27	148± 16	103± 12
Leucine uptake[+]	75± 17	71±15	66± 18	138± 34	−47± 19
Total AA uptake[++]	763±117	727±98	811±132	1127±291	−622±118

* V < I = II = IV < III (P<0.01).
** V < IV < II = III < I (P<0.01).
[+] V << I = II = III < IV (P<0.01).
[++] V << I = II = III < IV (P<0.01).
* and ** values correspond to peak insulin and plasma leucine levels, respectively achieved following steak meal ingestion.
[+] and [++] correspond to average uptake (or release) of leucine or total amino acids integrated over the whole 4 h period following meal ingestion.

The data indicate that acute physiologic (4-9-fold) elevations of plasma insulin (in Groups I-III) had no effect on nitrogen accumulation in human skeletal muscle. These data are consistent with those of Eriksson et al (134). On the other hand, more prolonged hyperinsulinemia (36-48 h) resulted in a significant increase in nitrogen accumulation. The mechanism behind this increase is not clear and may be related to a time-dependent induction of enzymes.

Selective acute insulin deficiency and amino acid metabolism in vivo

The effects of acute and prolonged physiologic changes in plasma insulin on leucine kinetics and protein turnover have been studied by us in both conscious dog and man using a constant infusion of isotopically labeled leucine (^{3}H or ^{14}C) to assess total body leucine kinetics (see also Chapter 26). Since leucine is an essential amino acid, in the absence of any exogenous dietary intake, changes in plasma specific activity of leucine at steady state can be used to estimate flux rates that represent overall traffic within the plasma pool.

The effect of selective insulin withdrawal, achieved by the simultaneous administration of peripheral somatostatin with intraportal replacement of basal glucagon on leucine kinetics in the conscious overnight-fasted dog has been studied (135). Insulin deficiency for 4 hours resulted in a nearly 50% increase in plasma leucine from basal values of 131 ± 9 to 187 ± 12 µmol/l. This was mainly a result of decreased outflow of leucine from the plasma compartment (clearance fell from basal values of 25 ± 3 to 15 ± 0.3 ml/mg/min by the end of 4 h) without a change in its rate of appearance (3.2 ± 0.2 µmol/kg/min). Similar studies carried out in overnight-fasted normal human subjects (136) showed that within 30 min of selective insulin withdrawal, brought about by peripheral infusion of somatostatin at 500 µg/h, plasma leucine rose progressively from basal values of 103 ± 4 µmol/l to a new plateau in 150 min which averaged 189 ± 6 µmol/l for the last 90 min of a 4-hour experimental period. This was due, as in the dog, to a net decrease in leucine outflow from the plasma compartment (clearance fell from basal values of 17 ± 1 to 10 ± 1 ml/mg/min). In addition, insulin withdrawal resulted in a nearly 60% increase in the rate of leucine oxidation from 0.27 ± 0.06 to 0.43 ± 0.07 µmol/kg/min. In man, as in the dog, leucine R_a did not change in response to insulin deficiency. All the changes in concentrations and clearance were reversible when insulin was supplemented to basal levels. The rate of leucine disappearance, as calculated by the isotopic method, represents the sum of the rate of leucine oxidation and a non-oxidative component which represents the amount of amino acid entering the intracellular pool. Therefore, these data indicate that the decrease in leucine outflow represented the minimum estimate by which protein synthesis was depressed. It is reasonable to conclude that acute insulin withdrawal had its major effect on protein synthesis without affecting protein breakdown.

Selective acute hyperinsulinemia and amino acid metabolism in vivo

Selective twice-basal hyperinsulinemia, brought about by the infusion of somatostatin peripherally and basal glucagon intraportally, resulted in a 35% decrease in plasma leucine, accompanied by a generalized hypo-aminoacidemia, (except for alanine, glycine and glutamine) most notably for the other two branched-chain amino acids, isoleucine and valine. This decrease in plasma leucine was primarily the result of decreased entry of leucine into the plasma compartment (R_a dropped from 3.08 ± 0.2 to 2.7 ± 0.1 µmol/kg/min in 4 h).

In these studies leucine kinetics were measured using ^{3}H-leucine label and hence leucine oxidation was not assessed. Recently, similar studies were performed in man (unpublished observations). A peripheral somatostatin infusion was accompanied by insulin (0.20 mU/kg/min) and glucagon (1.2 ng/kg/min) infusions; euglycemia was maintained with an exogenous infusion of glucose. The results from this study were identical to those obtained with the dog (135) except that the effect on plasma leucine (-16%) and leucine R_a (-120%) were less prominent. Leucine oxidation was not changed. Together, the data in man and the dog indicate that physiologic elevations of plasma insulin have their main effect on inhibiting protein breakdown, with little, if any, effect exerted on protein synthesis.

The effect of various doses of insulin on leucine kinetics in man has also been examined. The hyperinsulinemic-euglycemic clamp was used in conjunction with a primed continuous infusion of L-1-^{14}C-leucine infusion and measurement of the specific activities of plasma leucine and KIC and breath $^{14}CO_2$. Because of the known effects of insulin in lowering plasma amino acids, two studies were performed with each clamp, once when hypoleucinemia was allowed to develop, and the other when plasma leucine was maintained near basal levels by an exogenous infusion of leucine (hyperinsulinemic-euglycemic-euleucinemic clamp). The latter study was made feasible with the development of a rapid HPLC method for the measurement of plasma leucine concentration in less than 5 min from the time of blood sampling. Blood and breath samples were obtained for a 60-min basal period and a 3-hour experimental period. Insulin was then administered at 0.6, 2.5 or 5.0 mU/kg/min to each of the groups (n=10) studied. Table 2 shows the mean leucine concentrations (µmol/l), and the percent change from basal values in the rates of appearance of endogenous leucine in the plasma compartment and its oxidation.

It is clear that insulin, in pharmacologic doses, exerts its primary effect on suppressing endogenous R_a which, in the absence of a dietary source, represents an estimate of proteolysis. In order to obviate the criticism that the associated hypoaminoacidemia could limit the availability of amino acids for protein synthesis the study was repeated in 3 normal volunteers using peripheral in-

TABLE 2 *The effect of graded insulin infusions on leucine kinetics in overnight-fasted normal male volunteers*

Type of infusion	Percent change in leucine*		Rate of oxidation
	Leu concentration	Endogenous R_a	
Saline	− 4.2	0	+ 8.3
Insulin (mU/kg/min)			
0.6 (− Leu)	− 12.1[a]	− 9.1[a]	− 1.3
(+ Leu)	+ 5.6	− 8.8[a]	+ 70.5[a,b]
2.5 (− Leu)	− 30.9[a]	− 21.2[a]	− 2.4
(+ Leu)	+ 3.2	− 23.8	+ 72.7[a,b]
5.0 (− Leu)	− 42.9	− 30.0[a]	− 3.8
(+ Leu)	+ 2.1	− 33.1[a]	+ 60.0[a,b]

*Values are expressed as average of percent change from basal during the last 30 min of the 3 h experimental period. Basal plasma leucine (112 ± 8 µmol/l), endogenous R_a (1.56 ± 0.1 µmol/kg/min) and rate of oxidation (0.23 ± 0.06 µmol/kg/min) did not differ among the groups. Two groups were studied for each insulin dose, once with exogenous leucine infused (+ Leu) and the other when hypoleucinemia was allowed to develop during the insulin infusion (− Leu). The values in the table represent the mean ± SEM.
[a]Significance from basal, $P<0.01$.
[b]Significance from corresponding (− Leu) value, $P<0.01$.
[b]V < IV < II = III < I ($P<0.01$).

fusion of a commercially available L-amino acid mixture. The results were identical to those shown in Table 2. It is therefore safe to conclude that insulin exerts its primary effect on inhibiting proteolysis, with minimal, if any, effect on leucine incorporation into protein. Furthermore, it is quite apparent that insulin suppression of proteolysis is not complete, indicating the presence of an insulin-sensitive (dose-dependent) and another insulin-insensitive portion of proteolysis.

The effect of insulin on the rate of leucine oxidation in vivo is not well understood. Several studies in vitro and in vivo have indicated that both absolute insulin deficiency in normal man (136) or IDDM patients (137) and relative insulin deficiency as in fasting (138) are associated with enhanced leucine oxidation. These conditions are reversed with insulin supplementation (138, 139). On the other hand, the role of hyperinsulinemia on leucine oxidation is not well understood. Based on a study in normal volunteers, similar to that described above with the (-Leu) group, Tessari et al (140) concluded that hyperinsulinemia had no effect on leucine oxidation. It is clear, however, from the present data that in the presence of euleucinemia insulin exerted a marked stimulatory effect on leucine oxidation. Furthermore, this effect was observed at the lowest dose of insulin used (0.3 mU/kg/min; data not shown). The mechanism and exact site of action of insulin are not clear from our study and further studies are required.

Fasting and amino acid metabolism

Fasting is another condition where low insulin concentrations are presumed to play the major role in regulating protein turnover. It has been suggested that low insulin levels associated with starvation allow for the orderly transfer of amino acids from skeletal muscle to the liver where they are either deaminated, converted to glucose, urea or fat, or are completely oxidized. As a result the essential (E) amino acids, particularly the branched-chain amino acids and their corresponding ketoacids, are markedly elevated, while the non-essential (N) amino acids decline, resulting in higher E/N ratios.

Recent observations in our laboratory (141, 142), however, do not totally support this hypothesis. Since the plasma insulin level in the dog fasted for 24 or 48 hours does not change significantly while leucine R_a increases in the absence of a change in leucine clearance, the changes seen with early fasting (24 and 48 h) obviously can occur independently of changes in plasma insulin levels. Only when fasting is prolonged beyond 2 days do the changes resemble those seen with insulin deficiency (141). Fasting resulted in a rise in plasma leucine from 116 ± 8 to 147 ± 8 µmol/l ($P<0.05$). Its rate of appearance also increased (30%, $P<0.05$) from 3.3 ± 0.2 to 4.4 ± 0.3 µmol/kg/min, while clearance rate remained unchanged. Acute insulin deficiency, induced by somatostatin and replacement glucagon infusion in 48-hour-fasted dogs caused a 45% increase in leucine levels ($P<0.05$). Leucine R_a rose from 4.3 ± 0.3 to 5.0 ± 0.3 µmol/kg/min ($P<0.05$) while the metabolic clearance rate fell by 20% in the 48-hour group. In summary, it appears that early (up to 4 d) fasting in dog and man (unpublished observations) is associated with changes in both rates of protein synthesis and degradation which are not solely related to changes in insulin levels. This complexity in insulin interaction has also been emphasized by the observations of Garlick et al (143) that infusion of insulin to overnight-fasted rats to achieve levels comparable to those seen with feeding failed to raise the rates of protein synthesis in gastrocnemius muscle to levels seen postprandially. All these data suggest that the response of protein synthesis of both fasting and feeding is complex and involves more than the effects of changing insulin concentrations alone.

Chronic insulin deficiency

The effect of chronic insulin deficiency on protein and amino acid turnover in vivo is not well characterized. Diabetes is characterized by a generalized increase in the rates of oxidation in most of the essential amino acids (144-146). Older studies in rats rendered diabetic with streptozotocin (147) have shown that diabetes is also characterized by a generalized decrease in protein synthesis in various tissues. Studies in man have been less revealing. It is well established that diabetic patients with ketoacidosis have marked protein wasting, and this has been attributed to enhanced gluconeogenesis and amino acid release from skeletal muscle (148-150). Robert et al (139) found that poorly controlled IDDM patients have increased plasma leucine and increased leucine oxidation. They attributed the increased flux to enhanced proteolysis. Proper control of glycemia, however, reverted leucine kinetic parameters to within the limits of normal non-diabetic controls. These results were consistent with those obtained by Umpleby et al (151), who also found that proper strict control of blood glucose levels in IDDM patients resulted in near normalization of leucine flux, oxidation rate and plasma leucine levels. In addition, Tessari et al (140) showed that IDDM patients also manifest resistance to insulin in their amino acid (leucine) metabolism, similar to that found with glucose. These investigators noted that a progressive increase in circulating insulin resulted in a progressive decrease in both leucine and KIC fluxes in both IDDM subjects and normal volunteers, with the rates in the former, however, remaining higher at each insulin dose tested.

We recently assessed leucine kinetics in 9 depancreatectomized dogs (6 months — 3.5 years duration) using similar isotopic techniques to those described above. This animal model has the advantage of being similar to human IDDM (i.e. lack of insulin associated with high circulating glucagon). Leucine kinetics were measured after 48 hours of insulin withdrawal and a 24-hour fast. Following 2 days of insulin withdrawal the rate of leucine appearance in the plasma compartment was at least 65% higher than that seen in the normal postabsorptive dog, suggesting enhanced protein degradation. Thirty minutes after restoration of basal circulating insulin levels by intraportal insulin infusion, plasma leucine levels began to revert to normal as a result of both a decrease in its rate of appearance and an increase in its rate of clearance. Although rates of leucine oxidation were not measured, it is reasonable to assume that the effects observed relate to changes in the rates of synthesis and breakdown of protein. Although it is difficult from these studies to identify the tissues involved in this response, these studies are supportive of studies in vitro which have shown enhanced protein breakdown in skeletal muscle obtained from rats rendered diabetic with streptozotocin (152).

References

1. Felig P, Wahren J, Hendler R (1975): Influence of oral glucose ingestion on splanchnic glucose and gluconeogenic substrate metabolism in man. *Diabetes, 24,* 468.
2. DeFronzo RA, Ferrannini E, Hendler R et al (1978): Influence of hyperinsulinemia, hyperglycemia, and the route of glucose administration on splanchnic glucose exchange. *Proc. Natl. Acad. Sci. USA, 75,* 5173.
3. Bergman RN, Beir JR, Hourigan PM (1982): Intraportal glucose infusion matched to oral glucose absorption — Lack of evidence for 'gut' factor: involvement in hepatic glucose storage. *Diabetes, 31,* 27.
4. Abumrad NN, Cherrington AD, Williams PE et al (1982): Glucose absorption and disposition in the conscious dog. *Am. J. Physiol., 242,* E398.
5. Katz LD, Glickman MG, Rapoport S et al (1983): Splanchnic and peripheral disposal of oral glucose in man. *Diabetes, 32,* 675.
6. Ishida T, Chap Z, Chou J et al (1983): Differential effects of oral, peripheral intravenous, and intraportal glucose on hepatic glucose uptake and insulin and glucagon extraction in conscious dogs. *J. Clin. Invest., 72,* 590.
7. Zierler KL, Rabinowitz D (1963): Roles of insulin and growth hormone, based on studies of forearm metabolism in man. *Medicine, 42,* 385.
8. Pozefsky T, Felig P, Tobin JD et al (1969): Amino acid balance across tissues of the forearm in post-absorptive man: effects of insulin at two dose levels. *J. Clin. Invest., 48,* 2273.
9. DeFronzo RA, Jacot E, Jequier E et al (1981): The effect of insulin on the disposal of intravenous glucose: results from indirect calorimetry and hepatic and femoral vein venous catheterization. *Diabetes, 30,* 1000.
10. DeFronzo RA, Ferrannini E, Hendler R et al (1983): Regulation of splanchnic and peripheral glucose uptake by insulin and hyperglycemia in man. *Diabetes, 32,* 35.
11. Kolterman OG, Insel J, Saekow M, Olefsky JM (1980): Mechanisms of insulin resistance in human obesity: evidence for receptor and postreceptor defects. *J. Clin. Invest., 65,* 1272.
12. Rizza RA, Mandarino LJ, Gerich JE (1981): Dose-response characteristics for effects of insulin on production and utilization of glucose in man. *Am. J. Physiol., 240,* E630.
13. Chiasson JL, Liljenquist JE, Finger FE (1976): Differential sensitivity of glycogenolysis and gluconeogenesis to insulin infusions in dogs. *Diabetes, 25,* 283.
14. Chiasson JL, Atkinson RL, Cherrington AD (1979): Insulin regulation of gluconeogenesis from alanine in man. *Metabolism, 29,* 810.
15. Cherrington AD (1981): Gluconeogenesis: its regulation by insulin and glucagon. In: Brownlee M (Ed.), *Diabetes Mellitus,* p. 49. Garland Press, New York.
16. Steiner KE, Williams PE, Lacy WW, Cherrington AD (1981): Effects of the insulin/glucagon molar ratio on glucose production in the dog. *Fed. Proc., 40,* 3481.
17. Cherrington AD, Lacy WW, Chiasson JL (1978): Effect of glucagon on glucose production during insulin deficiency in the dog. *J. Clin. Invest., 62,* 664.
18. Cherrington AD, Liljenquist JE, Shulman GI et al (1979): The importance of hypoglycemia induced glucose production during selective glucagon deficiency. *Am. J. Physiol., 236,* E263.
19. Cherrington AD, Stevenson RW, Steiner KE et al (1987): Insulin, glucagon and glucose as regulators of hepatic glucose uptake and production in vivo. In: DeFronzo R (Ed.), *Diabetes/Metabolism Reviews,* p. 307. Wiley, New York.
20. Shulman GI, Liljenquist JE, Williams PE et al (1978): Glucose disposal during insulinopenia in somatostatin-treated dogs: the roles of glucose and glucagon. *J. Clin. Invest., 62,* 487.

21. DeFronzo RA, Ferrannini E, Hendler R et al (1978): Influence of hyperinsulinemia, hyperglycemia, and the route of glucose administration on splanchnic glucose exchange. *Proc. Natl. Acad. Sci. USA, 15,* 5173.
22. Abumrad NN, Cherrington AD, Williams PE et al (1982): Glucose absorption and disposition in the conscious dog. *Am. J. Physiol., 242,* E398.
23. Cherrington AD, Williams PE, Abou Mourad N et al (1982): Insulin as a mediator of hepatic glucose uptake in the conscious dog. *Am. J. Physiol., 5,* E97.
24. Ishida T, Chap Z, Chou J et al (1983): Differential effects of oral, peripheral intravenous, and intraportal glucose on hepatic glucose uptake and insulin and glucagon extraction in conscious dogs. *J. Clin. Invest., 72,* 590.
25. Barrett EJ, Ferrannini E, Gusberg R et al (1985): Hepatic and extrahepatic splanchnic glucose metabolism in the postabsorptive and glucose fed dog. *Metabolism, 34,* 410.
26. Adkins BA, Meyers SR, Hendrick GK et al (1985): Interaction between insulin and the route of intravenous glucose delivery in the regulation of net hepatic glucose uptake in the conscious dog. *Diabetes Res. Clin. Pract., Suppl. 1,* 10.
27. Myers SR, Biggers DW, Cherrington AD (1986): Dependence of net hepatic uptake (NHGU) on the hepatic glucose load is enhanced by portal glucose delivery. *Diabetes, 35, Suppl. 1,* 85a.
28. Gardemann A, Strulik H, Jungermann K (1986): A portal-arterial glucose concentration gradient as a signal for insulin-dependent net glucose uptake in perfused rat liver. *FEBS Lett., 202,* 255.
29. Gottesman I, Mandarino LI, Gerich J (1983): Estimation and kinetic analysis of insulin independent glucose uptake in human subjects. *Am. J. Physiol., 244,* E632.
30. Baron AD, Kolterman OG, Bell J et al (1985): Rates of non-insulin-mediated glucose uptake are elevated in type II diabetic subjects. *J. Clin. Invest., 76,* 1782.
31. Huang S, Phelps ME, Hoffman EJ et al (1980): Non-invasive determination of local cerebral metabolic rate of glucose in man. *Am. J. Physiol., 238,* E69.
32. Growden WA, Bratton TS, Houston MC et al (1971): Brain glucose metabolism in the intact mouse. *Am. J. Physiol., 221,* 1738.
33. Best JD, Taborsky Jr GJ, Halter JB, Porte Jr D (1981): Glucose disposal is not proportional to plasma glucose level in man. *Diabetes, 30,* 847.
34. Verdonk C, Rizza R, Gerich J (1981): Effects of plasma glucose concentration on glucose utilization and clearance in normal man. *Diabetes, 30,* 535.
35. Defronzo RA, Ferrannini E, Hendler R et al (1978): The influence of hyperinsulinemia, hyperglycemia and the route of glucose administration on splanchnic glucose exchange. *Proc. Natl. Acad. Sci. USA, 75,* 5173.
36. Hansen IL, Cryer PE, Rizza RA (1985): Comparison of insulin-mediated and glucose-mediated glucose disposal in patients with insulin-dependent diabetes mellitus and in non-diabetic subjects. *Diabetes, 34,* 751.
37. Fink RI, Wallace P, Olefsky JM (1986): Effects of aging on glucose-mediated glucose disposal and glucose transport. *J. Clin. Invest., 77,* 2034.
38. Chen M, Bergman RN, Pacini G, Porte D (1985): Pathogenesis of age-related glucose intolerance in man: insulin resistance and decreased B-cell function. *J. Clin. Endocrinol. Metab., 60,* 13.
39. Bergman RN, Finegood DT, Ader M (1985): Assessment of insulin sensitivity in vivo. *Endocr. Rev., 6,* 45.
40. Doberne L, Greenfield MS, Schultz B, Reaven GM (1981): Enhanced glucose utilization during prolonged glucose clamp studies. *Diabetes, 30,* 829.
41. Liu G, Chen YDI, Hollenbeck CB et al (1984): Insulin-stimulated glucose disposal increases with time in patients with non-insulin dependent diabetes mellitus. *Diabetes, 33,* 643.

42. Proietto J, Harewood M, Aitken P et al (1982): Validation of a practical in vivo insulin dose response curve in man. *Metabolism, 31,* 354.
43. Rizza RA, Mandanio LH, Gerich JE (1981): Dose-response characteristics for effects of insulin on production and utilization of glucose in man. *Am. J. Physiol., 240,* E630.
44. Donner CC, Fraze E, Chen YDI, Reven GM (1985): Quantitation of insulin-stimulated glucose disposal in patients with non-insulin dependent diabetes mellitus. *Diabetes, 34,* 831.
45. Beard JC, Bergman RN, Ward WK, Porte Jr D (1986): The insulin sensitivity index in non-diabetic man: correlation between clamp derived and IVGTT-derived values. *Diabetes, 35,* 362.
46. Cobelli C, Pacine G, Toffolo G, Sacca L (1986): Estimation of insulin sensitivity and glucose clearance from minimal model: new insights from labeled IVGTT. *Am. J. Physiol., 250,* E591.
47. Sacca L, Orfino G, Petrone A, Vigorito C (1984): Differential roles of splanchnic and peripheral tissues in the pathogenesis of impaired glucose tolerance. *J. Clin. Invest., 73,* 1683.
48. Ferrannini E, Smith KD, Cobelli C et al (1985): Effect of insulin on the distribution and disposition of glucose in man. *J. Clin. Invest., 76,* 357.
49. McGuinness O, Ivy R, Mari A et al (1987): The error in estimating endogenous glucose production using 3-^{3}H glucose during the euglycemic hyperinsulinemic clamp. *Diabetes, 36,* in press.
50. Finegood DT, Vranic M (1986): Inadequacy of 1-compartmental constant pool fraction model for calculating endogenous glucose production from euglycemic glucose clamps. *Diabetes, 35, Suppl. 1,* 14A.
51. Bell PM, Firth RG, Rizza RA (1986): Assessment of insulin action in insulin-dependent diabetes mellitus using [6-^{14}C]glucose, [3-^{3}H]glucose, and [2-^{3}H]glucose. *J. Clin. Invest., 78,* 1479.
52. Liljenquist JE, Bloomgarden ET, Cherrington AD et al (1979): Possible mechanism by which somatostatin-induced glucagon suppression improved glucose tolerance during insulinopenia in man. *Diabetologia, 17,* 139.
53. Kingston WJ, Livingston JN, Moxley III RT (1986): Enhancement of insulin action after oral glucose ingestion. *J. Clin. Invest., 77,* 1153.
54. Dox SM, White NH, Sjor DA, Santiago JW (1985): Insulin clearance contributes to the variability of nocturnal insulin requirements in insulin-dependent diabetes mellitus. *Diabetes, 34,* 1260.
55. Campbell PJ, Molli GB, Cryer PE, Gerich JE (1985): Pathogenesis of the dawn phenomenon in patients with insulin-dependent diabetes mellitus. *N. Engl. J. Med., 312,* 1473.
56. Kraegen SW, James DE, Storlien LH et al (1986): In vivo insulin resistance in individual peripheral tissues of a high fat rat assessment by euglycemic clamp plus deoxyglucose administration. *Diabetologia, 29,* 192.
57. Amiel SA, Sherwin RS, Simonson DC et al (1986): Impaired insulin action in puberty. *N. Engl. J. Med., 315,* 216.
58. Lager I, Attvall S, Eriksson BM et al (1986): Studies on the insulin-antagonistic effect of catecholamines in normal man. *Diabetologia, 29,* 409.
59. Rizza RA, Mandarino LJ, Genest J et al (1985): Production of insulin resistance by hyper-insulinemia in man. *Diabetologia, 28,* 70.
60. McGuinness QP, Friedman AH (1986): Insulin sensitivity can be reduced by a mild hyper-secretion of insulin. *Diabetes, 35, Suppl. 1,* 54A.
61. Mandarino L, Baker B, Rizza R et al (1984): Infusion of insulin impairs human adipocyte glucose metabolism in vitro without decreasing insulin receptor binding. *Diabetologia, 27,* 358.

62. Wardzala LJ, Hirshman M, Potcher E et al (1985): Regulation of glucose utilization in adipose cells and muscle after long term experimental hyperinsulinemia in rats. *J. Clin. Invest., 76,* 460.

63. Garvey WT, Olefsky JM, Marshall S (1986): Insulin induces progressive insulin resistance in cultured rat adipocytes: sequential effects at a receptor and multiple post-receptor sites. *Diabetes, 35,* 258.

64. Bevilacqua S, Barrett EJ, Smith D et al (1985): Hepatic and peripheral insulin resistance following streptozotocin-induced insulin deficiency in the dog. *Metabolism, 34,* 817.

65. Eaton EP, Allen RC, Schade DS, Standefer JC (1980): Normal insulin secretion: the goal of artificial insulin delivery systems. *Diabetes Care, 3,* 270.

66. Spangler RS (1985): Selective insulinization of liver in conscious diabetic dogs. *Am. J. Physiol., 249,* E152.

67. Nankervis A, Prosetto J, Aitken P, Alford F (1985): Hyperinsulinemia and insulin insensitivity in subjects with insulinoma. *Diabetologia, 28,* 427.

68. Haffner SM, Stein MP, Hazuda HP et al (1986): Hyperinsulinemia in a population at high risk for non-insulin dependent diabetes mellitus. *N. Engl. J. Med., 315,* 220.

69. Ratzman KP, Ruhnke R, Kohnert KD (1983): Effect of pharmacological suppression of insulin secretion on tissue sensitivity to insulin in subjects with moderate obesity. *Int. J. Obesity, 7,* 453.

70. Jarvisen H, Koivisto VA (1986): Natural course of insulin resistance in type I diabetes. *N. Engl. J. Med., 315,* 224.

71. Del Prato S, Nosadini R, Tiengo A et al (1983): Insulin-mediated glucose disposal in type I diabetes: evidence for insulin resistance. *J. Clin. Endocrinol. Metab., 57,* 904.

72. Nankervis A, Prosetto J, Aitken P, Alford P (1984): Impaired insulin action in newly diagnosed type I (insulin-dependent) diabetes mellitus. *Diabetologia, 27,* 497.

73. Kolterman OG, Gray RS, Friffin J et al (1981): Receptor and post-receptor defects contribute to the insulin resistance in non-insulin-dependent diabetes mellitus. *J. Clin. Invest., 68,* 957.

74. Arner P, Einarsson K, Ewerth S, Livingston J (1986): Studies of the human liver insulin receptor in non-insulin-dependent diabetes mellitus. *J. Clin. Invest., 77,* 1716.

75. Arner P, Einarsson K, Backman L et al (1983): Studies of liver insulin receptors in non-obese and obese human subjects. *J. Clin. Invest., 72,* 1729.

76. Caro JF, Ittoop O, Pories NJ et al (1986): Studies on the mechanism of insulin resistance in the liver from humans with non-insulin-dependent diabetes. *J. Clin. Invest., 78,* 249.

77. Effendic S, Wajngot A, Vranic M (1985): Increased activity of the glucose cycle in the liver: early characteristic of type 2 diabetes. *Proc. Natl Acad. Sci. USA, 82,* 2965.

78. Firth RG, Bell PM, Marsh HM et al (1986): Postprandial hyperglycemia in patients with non-insulin-dependent diabetes mellitus. *J. Clin. Invest., 77,* 1525.

79. Pehling G, Tessani P, Gerich JE et al (1984): Abnormal meal carbohydrate disposition in insulin dependent diabetes: relation contribution of endogenous glucose production and initial splanchnic uptake and effect of intensive insulin therapy. *J. Clin. Invest., 74,* 985.

80. Pedersen O, Hjollund E (1982): Insulin receptor binding to fat and blood cells and insulin action in fat cells from insulin dependent diabetics. *Diabetes, 31,* 706.

81. Blackshear PJ, Shulman GI, Roussell AM et al (1986): Metabolic response to three years of continuous basal rate intravenous insulin infusion in type II diabetic patients. *J. Clin. Endocrinol. Metab., 61,* 753.

82. Frayn KN (1983): Calculation of substrate oxidation rates in vivo from gaseous exchange. *Am. J. Physiol., 55,* 628.

83. Thiebaud D, Jacot E, Defronzo RA et al (1982): The effect of graded doses of insulin on total glucose uptake, glucose oxidation and glucose storage in man. *Diabetes, 31,* 1957.

84. Defronzo RA, Jacot E, Jequire E et al (1981): The effect of insulin on the disposal of intra-venous glucose: results from indirect calorimetry and hepatic and femoral venous catheterization. *Diabetes, 30,* 1000.

85. Thiebaud D, Defronzo RA, Jacot E et al (1982): Effect of long chain triglyceride infusion on glucose metabolism in man. *Metabolism, 31,* 1128.

86. Felber JHP, Jequire E (1985): Differential influence of obesity and type II diabetes on oxidative and non-oxidative glucose metabolism. *Diabetes, 34, Suppl. 1,* 21A.

87. Lillioja S, Mott DM, Zawadzki JK et al (1986): Glucose storage is a major determinant of in vivo 'insulin resistance' in subjects with normal glucose tolerance. *J. Clin. Endocrinol. Metab., 62,* 922.

88. Randin JP, Tappy L, Scazziga B et al (1986): Insulin sensitivity and exogenous insulin clearance in Graves' disease. *Diabetes, 35,* 178.

89. Bogardus C, Lillioja S, Howard BU et al (1984): Relationships between insulin secretion, insulin action and fasting plasma glucose concentration in non-diabetic and non-insulin-dependent diabetic subjects. *J. Clin. Invest., 74,* 1238.

90. Felber JP, Meyer HU, Curchad B et al (1981): Glucose storage and oxidation in degrees of human obesity measured by continuous indirect colorimetry. *Diabetologia, 20,* 39.

91. Felber JP, Magnenat G, Casthelaz M et al (1977): Carbohydrate and lipid oxidation in normal and diabetic subjects. *Diabetes, 26,* 693.

92. Zierler KL, Rabinowitz D (1964): Effect of very small concentrations of insulin on forearm metabolism: persistence of its action on potassium and free fatty acids without its effect on glucose. *J. Clin. Invest., 43,* 950.

93. Jackson RA, Hamling JB, Blis PM et al (1986): The influence of graded hyperglycemia with and without physiological hyperinsulinemia on forearm glucose uptake and other metabolic responses in man. *J. Clin. Endocrinol. Metab., 63,* 594.

94. Massi-Benedetti M, Burrin JM, Capaldo B, Alberti KGMM (1981): A comparative study of the activity of biosynthetic human insulin and pork insulin using the glucose clamp technique in normal subjects. *Diabetes Care, 4,* 163.

95. Fernandez RP, Casaneuva FF, Devesa J, Cabezas-Cerrato J (1985): Metabolic and hormonal parameters after insulin-induced hypoglycemia in man: comparison between biosynthetic human insulin and purified pork insulin. *Horm. Metab. Res., 17,* 351.

96. Gerber PPG, Keller U, Stauffacher W (1983): Direct effect of insulin on liver ketogenic capacity in man. *Diabetologia, 25,* 156.

97. Paolisso G, Scheen AJ, Verdin EM et al (1986): Insulin oscillations *per se* do not affect glucose turnover parameters in normal man. *J. Clin. Endocrinol. Metab., 63,* 520.

98. Lang DA, Matthews DR, Peto J, Turner RC (1979): Cyclic oscillations of basal plasma glucose and insulin concentrations in human beings. *N. Engl. J. Med., 301,* 1023.

99. Schade DS, Eaton RP (1977): Dose response to insulin in man: differential effects on glucose and ketone body regulation. *J. Clin. Endocrinol. Metab., 44,* 1038.

100. Trevisan R, Nosadini R, Avogaro A et al (1986): Type I diabetes is characterized by insulin resistance not only with regard to glucose, but also to lipid and amino acid metabolism. *J. Clin. Endocrinol. Metab., 62,* 1155.

101. Wahren JH, Effendic S, Lift R et al (1977): Influence of somatostatin on splanchnic glucose metabolism in post-absorptive and 60-hour fasted humans. *J. Clin. Invest., 59,* 299.

102. Metcalfe P, Johnston DG, Nosadini et al (1981): Metabolic effects of acute and prolonged growth hormone excess in normal and insulin deficient man. *Diabetologia, 20,* 123.

103. Keller U, Chiasson JL, Liljenquist JE et al (1977): The role of insulin, glucagon and free fatty acids in the regulation of ketogenesis in dogs. *Diabetes, 26,* 1040.

104. Pickup JC, Viberti GC, Billous RW et al (1982): Safety of continuous subcutaneous insulin infusion: metabolic deterioration and glycemic autoregulation after deliberate cessation of infusion. *Diabetologia, 22,* 175.

105. Keller U, Sonnenberg GE, Berger W (1980): Ketone body turnover rates in insulin dependent diabetics following short term withdrawal of a continuous sub-cutaneous infusion of insulin. *Eur. J. Clin. Invest., 10*, 18.
106. Miles JM, Rizza RA, Harmond MW, Gerich JE (1980): Effects of acute insulin deficiency on glucose and ketone body turnover in man. *Diabetes, 29*, 926.
107. Wahren J, Sato Y, Ostmann J et al (1984): Turnover and splanchnic metabolism of free fatty acids and ketones in insulin dependent diabetics at rest and in response to exercise. *J. Clin. Invest., 73*, 1367.
108. Gerich JE, Lorenzi M, Bier DM et al (1976): Effects of physiologic levels of glucagon and growth hormone on human carbohydrate and lipid metabolism. *J. Clin. Invest., 57*, 875.
109. Bagdade JD, Porte D, Bierman EL (1969): The interaction of diabetes and obesity on the regulation of fat mobilization in man. *Diabetes, 18*, 759.
110. Howard BV, Savage PJ, Nagulesparan M et al (1979): Evidence for marked sensitivity to the antilipolytic action of insulin in obese maturity-onset diabetics. *Metabolism, 28*, 744.
111. Golay A, Chen YDI, Reaven GM (1986): Effect of differences in glucose tolerance on insulin's ability to regulate carbohydrate and free fatty acid metabolism in obese individuals. *J. Clin. Endocrinol. Metab., 62*, 1081.
112. Golay A, Swislocki ALM, Chen YDI et al (1986): Effect of obesity on ambient plasma glucose, free fatty acid, insulin, growth hormone, and glucagon concentrations. *J. Clin. Endocrinol. Metab., 63*, 481.
113. Howard BV, Klimes I, Vasquez B et al (1984): The antilipolytic action of insulin in obese subjects with resistance to its glucoregulatory action. *J. Clin. Endocrinol. Metab., 58*, 544.
114. Fraze E, Conner CC, Swislocki ALM et al (1985): Ambient plasma free fatty acid concentrations in insulin-dependent diabetes mellitus: evidence for insulin resistance. *J. Clin. Endocrinol. Metab., 61*, 807.
115. Sonnenberg GE, Stauffacher W, Keller U (1982): Failure of glucagon to stimulate ketone body production during acute insulin deficiency on insulin replacement in man. *Diabetologia, 23*, 94.
116. Miles JM, Haymond MW, Nissen SL, Gerich JE (1983): Effects of free fatty acid availability, glucagon excess, and insulin deficiency on ketone body production in postabsorptive man. *J. Clin. Invest., 71*, 1554.
117. Keller U, Shulman GI (1979): Effect of glucagon on hepatic fatty acid oxidation and ketogenesis in conscious dogs. *Am. J. Physiol., 237*, E121.
118. Gerich JE, Lorenzi M, Bier DM et al (1976): Effects of physiologic levels of glucagon and growth hormone on human carbohydrate and lipid metabolism. *J. Clin. Invest., 57*, 875.
119. Chideckel EW, Goodner CJ, Koerker DJ et al (1977): Role of glucagon in mediating metabolic effects of epinephrine. *Am. J. Physiol., 232*, E464.
120. Johnston DG, Alberti KGMM (1982): Hormonal control of ketone body metabolism in the normal and diabetic state. *Clin. Endocrinol. Metab., 11*, 329.
121. Pernet A, Walker M, Gill GV (1980): Ketogenic effect of catecholamines in normal man. *Diabetologia, 19*, 306.
122. Weiss M, Keller U, Stauffacher W (1984): Effect of epinephrine and somatostatin induced insulin deficiency on ketone body kinetics and lipolysis in man. *Diabetes, 33*, 738.
123. Keller U, Gerber PPOG, Stauffacher W (1984): Stimulatory effect of norepinephrine on ketogenesis in normal and insulin deficient humans. *Am. J. Physiol., 247*, E732.
124. Willms B, Bottcher M, Walters V et al (1969): Relationships between fat and ketone body metabolism in obese and nonobese diabetics and nondiabetics during norepinephrine infusion. *Diabetologia, 5*, 88.
125. Schade D, Eaton RP (1977): The regulation of plasma ketone body concentration by counterregulatory hormones in man. *Diabetes, 26*, 989.

126. Baker L, Kaye R, Haque N (1969): Metabolic homeostasis in juvenile diabetes mellitus. *Diabetes, 18,* 421.
127. Schade DS, Eaton RP (1979): The regulation of plasma ketone body concentration by counter-regulatory hormones in man. *Diabetes, 28,* 5.
128. Berk MA, Clutter WE, Skor D et al (1985): Enhanced glycemic responsiveness to epinephrine in insulin-dependent diabetes mellitus is the result of the inability to secrete insulin. *J. Clin. Invest., 75,* 1842.
129. Woolfson AMJ, Heatley RV, Allisson SP (1979): Insulin to inhibit protein catabolism. *N. Engl. J. Med., 300,* 14.
130. Fern EB, Garlick PJ, McNurlan MA, Waterlow JC (1981): The excretion of isotope in urea and ammonia for estimating protein turnover in man with ^{14}N-glycine. *Clin. Sci., 61,* 217.
131. Powell-Tuck J, Fern EB, Garlick PJ, Waterlow JC (1984): The effect of surgical trauma and insulin on whole body protein turnover in parenterally fed undernourished patients. *Hum. Nutr. Clin. Nutr., 38C,* 11.
132. Powell-Tuck J, Glynn MJ (1985): The effect of insulin infusion on whole body protein metabolism in patients with gastrointestinal disease fed parenterally. *Hum. Nutr. Clin. Nutr., 39C,* 181.
133. Abumrad NN, Wise KL, Rabin D, Lacy WW (1982): The disposal of an intravenously administered amino acid load across the human forearm. *Metabolism, 31,* 463.
134. Eriksson LS, Hagenfeldt L, Felig P, Wahren J (1983): Leucine uptake by splanchnic and leg tissues in man: relative independence of insulin levels. *Clin. Sci., 65,* 491.
135. Abumrad NN, Jefferson LS, Rannels SR et al (1982): The role of insulin in the regulation of leucine kinetics in the conscious dog. *J. Clin. Invest., 70,* 1031.
136. Powell CS, Abumrad NN (1982): Effect of basal insulin levels on leucine metabolism in normal man. *Surg. Forum, XVIII,* 91.
137. Robert JJ, Beaufrère B, Koziet J et al (1985): Whole body *de novo* amino acid synthesis in type I (insulin-dependent) diabetes studies with stable isotope-labelled leucine, alanine and glycine. *Diabetes, 34,* 67.
138. Rennie MJ, Edwards HT, Halliday D et al (1982): Muscle protein synthesis measured by stable isotope techniques in man: the effects of feeding and fasting. *Clin. Sci., 63,* 519.
139. Robert JJ, Bier DM, Zhao XH et al (1982): Glucose and insulin effects on *de novo* amino acid synthesis in young men: studies with stable isotope labelled alanine, glycine, leucine and lysine. *Metabolism, 31,* 1210.
140. Tessari P, Nosadine R, Trevisan R et al (1986): Defective suppression by insulin of leucine-carbon appearance and oxidation in type 1, insulin dependent diabetes mellitus. *J. Clin. Invest., 77,* 1977.
141. Abumrad NN, Williams PE, Wise KL et al (1981): The effect of starvation on leucine kinetics in the conscious dog. In: Walser M, Williams JR (Ed.), *Metabolism and Clinical Implications of Branched Chain Amino and Ketoacids,* p. 355. Elsevier/North-Holland, New York.
142. Hoxworth B, Radosevich P, Buckspan R et al (1985): Insulin's effect on leucine turnover changes during early fasting in the conscious dog. *Diabetes, 34,* 295.
143. Garlick PJ, Fern M, Preedy VR (1983): The effect of insulin infusion and food intake on muscle protein synthesis in post-absorptive rats. *Biochem. J., 210,* 669.
144. Paul HS, Adibi SA (1978): Leucine oxidation in diabetes and starvation: effects of ketone bodies on branched chain amino acid oxidation in vitro. *Metabolism, 27,* 185.
145. May ME, Mancussi VJ, Aftring RP, Buse MG (1980): Effects of diabetes on oxidative de-carboxylation of branched chain keto acids. *Am. J. Physiol., 239,* E215.
146. Hutson SM, Zapalowski C, Cree TC, Harper AE (1980): Regulation of leucine and ketoisocaproate acid metabolism in skeletal muscle: effects of starvation and insulin. *J. Biol. Chem., 255,* 2418.

147. Manchester KL (1974): Effect of insulin and denervation on the activity of ribosomes of rat diaphragm muscle. *Biochemistry, 13,* 3062.
148. Huszar G, Koioisto V, Davis E, Felig PP (1982): Urinary 3-methylhistidine excretion in juvenile onset diabetes: evidence of increased protein catabolism in the absence of ketoacidosis. *Metabolism, 31,* 188.
149. Marchesini G, Forlani G, Zoli M et al (1982): Muscle protein breakdown in uncontrolled diabetes as assessed by urinary 3-methylhistidine excretion. *Diabetologia, 23,* 456.
150. Saunders J, Boroujerdi MA, Brown PM et al (1982): Isotope turnover studies in uncontrolled diabetes and the effects of insulin in metabolic acidosis. In: *Ciba Foundation Symposium 81,* p. 273. Pitman, London.
151. Umpleby AM, Boroujerdi MA, Brown PM et al (1986): The effect of metabolic control on leucine metabolism in type 1 (insulin dependent) diabetic patients. *Diabetologia, 29,* 131.
152. Pain VM, Alberse EC, Garlick PJ (1983): Protein metabolism in skeletal muscle, diaphragm and heart of diabetic rats. *Am. J. Physiol., 245,* E604.

The Diabetes Annual/3
K.G.M.M. Alberti and L.P. Krall, editors
© 1987 Elsevier Science Publishers, B.V.

23   Insulin action: mechanisms involved in the rapid effects of insulin on carbohydrate metabolism*

J.M. TAVARÉ AND R.M. DENTON

Introduction

Substantial progress has been made in the understanding of some of the actions of insulin in recent years. The primary aim of this Chapter is to review some of the advances made in unravelling the means whereby the hormone has rapid and profound effects on the metabolism of carbohydrate in its major target tissues: liver, muscle and adipose tissue.

The major acute effects of insulin on carbohydrate metabolism are summarized in Table 1. Their combined effect is to increase the net uptake of glucose from blood and to enhance its conversion to glycogen and triacylglycerol. These changes in metabolism can be largely explained in terms of the activation of glucose transport across the plasma membrane of fat and muscle cells together with the dephosphorylation of a number of key intracellular enzymes.

In this Chapter, we will summarize first the recent progress in our understanding of the action of insulin on glucose transport and in particular the extent to which it may be explained by the translocation of glucose transporters to the plasma membrane from an intracellular location. In fact, it has recently become evident that insulin also causes the translocation of a number of other proteins into and out of the plasma membrane.

We then consider the means whereby insulin may stimulate the dephosphorylation of intracellular proteins with particular emphasis on glycogen synthase and pyruvate dehydrogenase. The action of insulin on these two enzymes is of special interest because dephosphorylation and activation of these enzymes is most easily observed under basal conditions (in the absence of other hormones) when there are typically no detectable changes in cAMP levels and

*Studies from the authors' laboratory were supported by grants from the Medical Research Council (U.K.), the British Diabetic Association and the Waite Salmon Bequest.

TABLE 1   *Principal effects of insulin on carbohydrate metabolism*

Process	Effect	Tissue	Mechanisms involved
Glucose transport	increase	F, M	translocation of glucose transporters
Glycogen synthesis	increase	L, F, M	dephosphorylation of glycogen synthase
Glycogen breakdown	decrease*	L, F, M	dephosphorylation of phosphorylase kinase and hence phosphorylase
Glycolysis	increase*	L ⎫	dephosphorylation of pyruvate kinase
Gluconeogenesis	decrease*	L ⎬	and fructose-2, 6-bisphosphate kinase
Pyruvate → acetyl- CoA	increase	(L), F	dephosphorylation of pyruvate dehydrogenase

*These effects are not usually apparent unless tissue cAMP levels are increased by the presence of another hormone.
The changes listed under mechanisms involved are not necessarily complete. F = white and brown adipose tissue; M = muscle; L = liver. For further details including specific references see Ref. 2.

dephosphorylation occurs at sites which are probably not phosphorylated by cAMP-dependent protein kinase. In contrast, the dephosphorylation of the other proteins can be explained, at least in part, by a decrease in activity of cAMP-dependent protein kinase. Such effects of insulin are usually only evident when cell cAMP concentrations are first elevated by other hormones such as glucagon or β-adrenergic receptor agonists. Nevertheless, the mechanisms whereby insulin lowers intracellular cAMP are of considerable relevance to an understanding of insulin actions in general and on carbohydrate metabolism in particular and so this topic is also discussed.

Many aspects of insulin action are not included here, but are covered in a number of recent reviews (1-4) and by two books on the topic (5, 6).

Glucose transport

The entry of glucose into most mammalian cells is mediated by an integral membrane transport protein through a facilitated diffusion mechanism. In only two mammalian tissues, however, is glucose uptake acutely regulated by insulin, namely muscle and adipose tissue. Since adipose tissue has been more amenable to a detailed study of the mechanism by which insulin stimulates glucose uptake, much of the remainder of this section will be devoted to this tissue.

The elegant independent studies of Kono and Cushman and their respective co-workers have revealed that the binding of insulin to its receptor results in the rapid translocation of glucose transporter proteins from an apparently intracellular membrane location to the plasma membrane (7, 8). Early studies involved the use of either the binding of cytochalasin B (a specific inhibitor of glucose transport) (9) to glucose transporters in subcellular membrane fractions (7) or the reconstitution of glucose transport activity derived from similar subcellular membrane fractions into artificial liposomes (8). This has been substantiated more recently by the use of photochemical cross-linking of glucose transporters with [^{3}H]cytochalasin B (10, 11) and the use of western blotting with specific antisera raised against the glucose transporter (12, 13). The use of such antisera has also allowed the isolation and sequencing of the gene coding for a human glucose transporter (14). This information has revealed that this glucose transporter is a Mr 55,000 protein consisting of 12 putative transmembrane domains which probably form a hydrophilic channel through which glucose can be transported.

In unstimulated fat cells, it appears that approximately 10% of the total cellular complement of glucose transporters reside in the plasma membrane. Addition of insulin to cells increases this number 5- to 8-fold with a concomitant decrease in the number of glucose transporters associated with the intracellular membrane compartment (15, 16). This translocation event is energy-dependent and protein-synthesis-independent, and occurs with a half-time of 2-3 min (17, 18) (Table 2). The translocation hypothesis explains the general observation that under most conditions insulin increases the maximal rate of glucose transport into fat cells without having a major effect on the K_m (19-21). However, a translocation event of this scale does not appear to account fully for the overall increase in glucose transport into fat cells promoted by insulin which can be up to 40-fold, for the changes in K_m which have been reported to occur under certain conditions (22), or for the apparent changes in specific activity of plasma-

TABLE 2   *Effects of insulin on the distribution of fat-cell membrane proteins*

Class*	Protein	Time course of response (min)		ED$_{50}$ for insulin (nM)	References
		Half-time	Steady state		
I	Insulin receptor	2-3	5-10	3	33, 87, 88
II	Glucose transporter	2-3	10	0.1	17, 18, 89
	IGF-II receptor	1	10	0.1	29, 30
	Transferrin receptor**	<2	2	1	31
	Mr-90,000 protein***	0.5	2	0.07	90

* Class I and Class II represent those proteins which move out of the plasma membrane to an intracellular membrane fraction in response to insulin and vice versa, respectively.
** The data involved measurements of binding to intact cells and not subcellular membrane fractions (31).
*** The identity of the subcellular membrane fraction to which this protein moved was not specified.
The table indicates the approximate time courses and half-maximal responses to insulin of the listed proteins (see text for more details).

membrane-associated transporters in cells exposed to catecholamines and adenosine (23). Very recently, it has been reported that treatment of fat cells with the protein synthesis inhibitor cycloheximide greatly diminishes translocation without having an effect on the extent of insulin stimulated glucose transport (23a). Perhaps insulin also causes a change in the inherent activity of the individual transporters when they are located within the plasma membrane, e.g. through changes in phosphorylation or association with other proteins such as GTP-binding proteins. Phorbol esters mimic the effects of insulin on translocation of glucose transporters to the plasma membrane of Swiss 3T3-L1 cells (24). This could occur through the phosphorylation of the glucose transporter by protein kinase C which is the major receptor for phorbol esters (25). Indeed, Witters et al (26) have shown that the erythrocyte glucose transporter is a substrate for purified protein kinase C and that the glucose transporter is phosphorylated upon addition of phorbol esters to intact erythrocytes. It remains to be seen whether this phosphorylation event affects the intrinsic activity or membrane location of the glucose transporter. At present, however, the evidence suggests that the fat cell glucose transporter itself is not phosphorylated in response to insulin (2, 24a) although changes in phosphorylation of associated proteins remains a possibility.

Much still remains to be learnt about the precise mechanism by which insulin stimulates glucose transport. The effect of insulin on the translocation of glucose transport has also been demonstrated in rat heart and diaphragm muscle (27, 28). Insulin also promotes the translocation of IGF-II receptors and transferrin receptors to the plasma membrane from an intracellular membrane compartment with very similar characteristics to that which contains the insulin-sensitive pool of glucose transporters (29-32). Furthermore, the time course and extent of the translocations of glucose transporters, IGF-II receptors and transferrin receptors are all very similar (Table 2).

In contrast, insulin promotes the translocation of insulin receptors from the plasma membrane to an 'endocytic' subcellular membrane compartment with broadly similar characteristics to those described above. The half-maximal response of this internalization follows the binding of insulin to its receptor (33). However, the response to insulin of the translocation of glucose transporters and IGF-II receptors is shifted one order of magnitude to the left of insulin binding (Table 2), suggesting that the mechanisms involved differ. There are also huge differences in the numbers involved. It can be calculated that the binding of insulin to no more than 2000 receptors per cell is sufficient to cause the translocation of more than one million glucose transporters.

The next few years should reveal much more about the relationships between all these translocation events in both spatial and mechanistic terms and should also establish the extent to which changes in specific protein phosphorylation are involved.

Glycogen synthase

Insulin activates rabbit muscle glycogen synthase through stimulating its dephosphorylation on 3 specific serine residues termed 'Sites 3a,b,c' (34, 35) and it is in this tissue that the enzyme has been most extensively studied. Insulin has also been shown to activate glycogen synthase through an apparently similar dephosphorylation mechanism in both rat adipocytes (36) and rat diaphragm muscle (37).

Studies on glycogen synthase phosphorylation have been considerably hampered by the fact that it can be phosphorylated on 7 serines by at least 7 distinct protein kinases (for review see Ref. 38) and that, in the resting state, the enzyme contains approximately 3 moles of phosphate per mole of enzyme shared between the 7 phosphorylation sites (35, 39). Only through the analysis of the extent of phosphorylation of each individual site has it become clear that insulin promotes the dephosphorylation of Sites 3a,b,c found near the C-terminus of the polypeptide chain. Sheorain et al (35) and Lawrence et al (37) have also suggested that insulin promotes the additional dephosphorylation of a further site known as 'Site 2'.

In contrast, agents which promote increases in cAMP concentrations, such as adrenaline and glucagon, inhibit glycogen synthase activity through increasing the phosphorylation state of Sites 1a, 1b, 2 and 3a,b,c (39, 40) with no effect on Site 5. Parker et al (39) believe that it is the level of phosphorylation of Sites 3a,b,c that is the major influence on the activity of glycogen synthase. Increased phosphorylation of Sites 1a, 1b and 2 is most likely the result of phosphorylation by cAMP-dependent protein kinase while the increased phosphorylation of Sites 3a,b,c may be largely due to phosphorylation of inhibitor-1. This protein inhibits phosphatase-1 but only when phosphorylated by cAMP-dependent protein kinase (41).

Sites 3a,b,c are phosphorylated by a cAMP- and Ca^{2+}-independent protein kinase known as GSK-3 (42) and dephosphorylated by both phosphatase-1 and -2A (43). Cohen has argued, therefore, that at least in rabbit muscle insulin could act through inhibition of GSK-3, activation of either protein phosphatase-1 or -2A, or a combination of these events. However, protein kinases other than GSK-3 can phosphorylate these sites including cAMP-dependent protein kinase (44-46). In rabbit muscle these other kinases may not be able to phosphorylate these sites at a sufficient rate to be important, but this may not be true in other tissues (47). There are currently no reports of any changes, with insulin, in the activities of GSK-3 or protein phosphatase-1 or -2A which survive cell breakage and conventional assay techniques, so it may be difficult to identify which of these enzymes are important in bringing about the observed dephosphorylation of Sites 3a,b,c.

Insulin may act, in part, by activation of protein phosphatase-1. Foulkes et al

(48) demonstrated that insulin was capable of decreasing inhibitor-1 activity (and by inference, phosphorylation state) in the presence of raised levels of β-catecholamines (and hence raised cAMP levels). This could be due to the ability of insulin to oppose β-catecholamine-induced increases in cAMP. Insulin might, therefore, stimulate dephosphorylation of Sites 3a,b,c by preventing inhibitor-1 phosphorylation and hence enhancing protein phosphatase-1 activity; however, such a mechanism does not appear to operate under basal conditions (34, 49) where the levels of cAMP and the extent of inhibitor-1 phosphorylation are both very low (42).

Larner and colleagues have suggested that insulin promotes the release of low-molecular-weight mediators which might be responsible for the dephosphorylation of glycogen synthase by both inhibiting cAMP-dependent kinase activity and stimulating phosphatase activity (50). Similar substances may be involved in the regulation of pyruvate dehydrogenase, phosphodiesterase and other intracellular effects of insulin and are discussed further in the following sections. The Larner group have recently concluded that up to 4 separate mediators are probably involved in the regulation of the different targets of insulin action and that they are acidic peptides or peptide conjugates with molecular weights in the range 2000-5000 (51). However, purification and characterization of these mediators have been very incomplete.

Recently, Tung et al (52) have shown that spermine (a highly basic polyamine) promotes the dephosphorylation of Sites 3a,b,c by purified protein phosphatase-2A while affecting the dephosphorylation of other sites on glycogen synthase to a much smaller extent. Tung et al (52) concluded, therefore, that insulin might act by increasing the cellular concentration of spermine. Separate studies have shown that spermine also has an insulin-like effect in the pyruvate dehydrogenase system and thus further consideration of the possible role of spermine in insulin action is given in the next section.

Pyruvate dehydrogenase

Once pyruvate is converted to acetyl-coenzyme A (acetyl-CoA) by this exclusively intramitochondrial enzyme complex, there is no means in mammals whereby the acetyl-CoA can be used for the resynthesis of glucose. The enzyme must, by inference, be under exact control and, in particular, during starvation the enzyme must be greatly inhibited to conserve the restricted reserves of carbohydrate. Regulation of the enzyme is achieved in part by end-product inhibition by acetyl-CoA and NADH and in part by reversible phosphorylation. The phosphorylated form of the enzyme is essentially inactive (53, 54).

Exposure to insulin of tissues such as adipose tissue, liver and mammary gland where the complex plays an essentially biosynthetic role (since much of the acetyl-CoA formed is used for the synthesis of fatty acids) results in the rapid activation of pyruvate dehydrogenase (for reviews, see Refs 54-56). Such short-term effects are not found in muscle where pyruvate dehydrogenase has an essentially catabolic role as acetyl-CoA formed is mainly oxidized via the citrate cycle to CO_2. Most studies have been concerned with the means whereby insulin causes a 2- to 3-fold increase in activity in rat epididymal fat cells. The increase in activity has been shown directly to be the result of dephosphorylation (57) and persists during the preparation and subsequent incubation of intact mitochondria (58) and this property has greatly facilitated investigations into the mechanism involved. In particular, it has allowed good evidence to be obtained that the effect of insulin is brought about by the activation of pyruvate dehydrogenase phosphatase rather than inhibition of the kinase (57-59). However, no changes in phosphatase activity are detectable in extracts of mitochondria from insulin-treated tissue (58, 59). This suggests that insulin may cause a change in the concentration of some effector of the phosphatase within mitochondria that then dissociates from the phosphatase during the preparation of extracts.

The activity of the phosphatase is known to be regulated by Ca^{2+}, Mg^{2+} and possibly changes in the $NADH/NAD^+$ ratio, but there is now considerable evidence that insulin does not alter the activity of the phosphatase through changes in these particular regulators (58-60). Thus, the effect of insulin is still apparent within mitochondria made permeable to Mg^{2+} or Ca^{2+} by incubation with A23187 or to all substances up to a molecular weight of 1000-2000 by treatment with toluene (59, 60). In both instances the major change is an increase in the sensitivity of pyruvate dehydrogenase phosphatase to Mg^{2+}. As first demonstrated by Damuni et al (61), spermine has a similar effect on purified preparations of pyruvate dehydrogenase phosphatase. Thus, the intriguing situation has arisen that spermine can be linked with the actions of insulin, not only on dephosphorylation of glycogen synthase, but also on that of pyruvate dehydrogenase. However, it is most unlikely that insulin acts by the simple means of increasing the concentration of spermine in the appropriate cell compartments since the cell content of spermine would appear to be too high to have a conventional second-messenger role and insulin appears to have little or no short-term effect on the amount of spermine in cells (62).

The simplest explanation of these observations on pyruvate dehydrogenase would appear to be that insulin causes a change in the concentration of a spermine-like compound in mitochondria. The persistence of the activation in toluene-permeabilized mitochondria suggests that the compound is not small and/ or water-soluble. An attractive explanation would be that insulin may lead to some change in the interactions between the pyruvate dehydrogenase system and the inner mitochondrial membrane (60).

However, such an explanation is not easily reconciled with the proposal of

Jarett and Seals (63) that the activation of pyruvate dehydrogenase by insulin involves a low-molecular-weight mediator apparently similar to that proposed by Larner to be involved in the activation of glycogen synthase (for reviews, see Refs 64 and 65). This putative mediator was first proposed following the demonstration that addition of insulin to fat-cell plasma membranes resulted in formation of a low-molecular-weight factor which was capable of increasing pyruvate dehydrogenase activity when added to fat-cell mitochondria (63, 66). The mediator appears to act by stimulating the phosphatase (67), although characterization has been difficult. One reason for this may be the assay systems used which would appear to be far from optimal (2). Nevertheless, the putative mediator appears to have a molecular weight of 1000-3000, to be acid- and heat-stable and to have a net negative charge at pH 7.0 (65). Spermine, of course, has a net positive charge at this pH.

Insulin and regulation of cAMP concentrations

As emphasised in the Introduction, a number of the actions of insulin on carbohydrate metabolism are undoubtedly brought about via decreases in cellular cAMP levels — at least in liver and adipose tissue previously exposed to a hormone which increases cAMP levels. The effect of insulin probably involves a combination of the activation of phosphodiesterase activity and inhibition of adenyl cyclase. The former may be quantitatively more important since decreases are rather less evident when phosphodiesterase activity is blocked by methylxanthines (68).

Direct inhibitory effects of insulin on adenyl cyclase activity in plasma membranes can be observed, but rather precise conditions are necessary and the effects are quite small (69-71). In a recent study, Heyworth and Houslay (70) found inhibition of adenyl cyclase activity in rat liver plasma membranes only in the presence of glucagon, Mg^{2+} and, most interestingly, an adequate concentration of GTP.

Activation of a phosphodiesterase activity with a low K_m for cAMP has been observed by many groups in both fat and liver cells (e.g. Refs 72 and 73). What is rather mystifying is that conditions which result in high levels of cAMP in liver and fat cells also lead to persistent activation of phosphodiesterase activity (68, 74). Thus, under the very conditions in which insulin causes the greatest diminution in cAMP concentrations there may be little or no persistent effect of insulin on particulate phosphodiesterase activity.

In liver, two distinct membrane-bound phosphodiesterases have been found to be activated by insulin. One is associated with the plasma membrane, the other with intracellular 'dense vesicles'. However, neither appears to play an essential role in lowering cAMP as decreases can be observed on addition of insulin to liver cells exposed to glucagon under conditions where no persistent changes in these enzymes occur (4, 75). However, the liver plasma membrane enzyme shows a number of fascinating properties. Activation can be demonstrated on addition of insulin to liver plasma membrane preparations and this appears to involve phosphorylation of the enzyme; moreover, guanine nucleotides also activate the enzyme and under appropriate conditions may potentiate the effect of insulin (4, 68, 76). Houslay (4) has concluded that a guanine-nucleotide-binding protein may be involved in the action of insulin on adenyl cyclase and phosphodiesterase and that this protein may be distinct from the well-characterized G_s and G_i. Direct evidence for such a nucleotide-binding protein is lacking, but recently insulin has been reported to inhibit the cholera-toxin-induced ADP-ribosylation of a protein of Mr 25,000 in liver plasma membranes. This protein could represent an α-subunit of a nucleotide-binding protein closely associated with the insulin receptor (77).

The low K_m particulate enzyme from adipose tissue has been reported to be activated by plasma-membrane-derived, low-molecular-weight mediators apparently similar to those suggested to be involved in the activation of glycogen synthase and pyruvate dehydrogenase (65, 78). Recently Saltiel and colleagues (79, 80) have obtained evidence that the mediators (or 'modulators' as they are called by these workers) may be a complex of glycosylated inositol-phosphates derived from novel plasma-membrane-associated, inositol-containing glycolipids by the action of a specific insulin-activated phospholipase C. Their hypothesis is outlined in Figure 1.

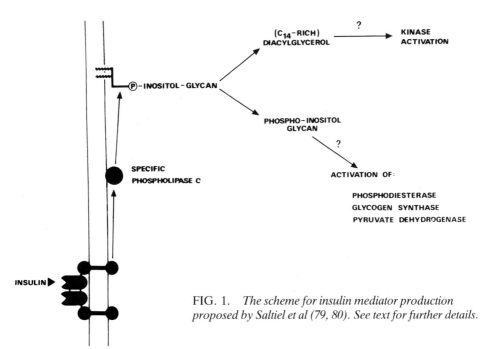

FIG. 1.   *The scheme for insulin mediator production proposed by Saltiel et al (79, 80). See text for further details.*

Evidence for the hypothesis has been obtained with isolated liver plasma membranes which have been shown to release two apparently related activators of particulate phosphodiesterase activity from fat cells on addition of insulin or a phosphatidyl-inositol-specific phospholipase C derived from *Staphylococcus aureus*. The chemical properties of the released activators and precursor are compatible with the hypothetical structure given in Figure 1. The molecular weight appears to be about 1500 (79). Furthermore, in intact cultured myocyte BC$_3$H1 cells, addition of insulin seems to increase the concentration of apparently identical inositol- and glucosamine-containing substances while decreasing the concentration of the precursor which appears to be rich in myristic acid. Much further work is required before this interesting hypothesis is established. For example, it is not clear how such low-molecular-weight mediators could alter the activity of the phosphodiesterase in such a way that the activation persists during cell extraction and partial purification. It has been suggested that the mediator may result in dephosphorylation, but there is no direct evidence that the phosphodiesterase involved is regulated by this means. Further comments on this hypothesis are made in the following concluding section.

Some general conclusions

The effects of insulin on carbohydrate metabolism can be explained largely in terms of the activation of glucose transport together with the dephosphorylation of several key intracellular enzymes which are substrates for cAMP-dependent protein kinase (e.g. pyruvate kinase and phosphorylase kinase). Under appropriate conditions, the ability of insulin to decrease cAMP levels (especially in liver and fat tissue) can partly explain the latter. However, the effects of insulin on dephosphorylation of pyruvate dehydrogenase and glycogen synthase can occur quite independently of changes in cAMP and probably involve activation of the appropriate phosphatases through rather different mechanisms. One possibility is that these involve some polybasic compound as the effects of insulin can be mimicked rather strikingly in vitro by spermine. Alternatively, these phosphatases may be activated by one or more of a group of low-molecular-weight acidic mediators. The structures of these putative mediators have not been established. However, the possibility must be considered that they are related to the glycosylated inositol phosphates proposed by Saltiel and colleagues to be involved in activation of phosphodiesterase by insulin. In the case of pyruvate dehydrogenase these mediators would have to cross the inner mitochondrial membrane through a carrier-mediated mechanism or bind to a specific mitochondrial membrane receptor which then mediates pyruvate dehydrogenase phosphatase activation. Perhaps the latter mechanism is most likely due to the observations that the effects of insulin persist in permeabilized mitochondria from which molecules of molecular weight of about 1500 would be readily lost.

Nevertheless, the hypothesis of Saltiel has a number of real attractions as it could explain the large degree of amplification involved in insulin action. The binding of insulin to less than 5000 receptors is sufficient to alter the activity of many millions of enzyme or transporter molecules in each cell (2, 81).

Insulin also stimulates serine phosphorylation of several intracellular proteins such as acetyl CoA carboxylase, ATP citrate lyase and the insulin receptor itself, most likely through the activation of specific protein serine kinases (see Refs 2 and 81). The hypothesis of Saltiel proposes that the activation of phospholipase C not only causes the formation of the glycosylated inositol phosphate (which may activate protein phosphatases), but also the formation of an unusual diacylglycerol which is rich in myristoyl groups. This unusual diacylglycerol might activate a protein serine kinase related to protein kinase C which results directly or indirectly in the increased phosphorylation of many intracellular proteins. It seems unlikely that insulin acts through protein kinase C itself as increased phosphorylations can occur in cells apparently depleted of the kinase (82, 83). Such a unifying hypothesis is outlined in Figure 1.

The insulin receptor contains an intrinsic insulin-stimulated protein tyrosine kinase activity capable of phosphorylating the insulin receptor itself (for review, see Ref. 84). At the time of writing, the role of this activity in the mechanism of insulin action is a mystery. The only known physiological function is autophosphorylation and further activation of the kinase (85, 86), a process which might also increase the interaction of the insulin receptor with other membrane proteins involved in insulin action such as the proposed specific phospholipase C, GTP-binding proteins or protein serine kinases. However, the formation of the modulators proposed by Saltiel appears to occur on addition of insulin to plasma membranes in the absence of added ATP, Mg^{2+} or GTP, suggesting that the activation of the phospholipase C does not involve a tyrosine or serine kinase activity or a GTP binding protein.

References

1. Czech MP (1985): The nature and regulation of the insulin receptor: structure and function. *Ann. Rev. Physiol., 47,* 357.
2. Denton RM (1986): Early events in insulin actions. *Adv. Cyclic Nucleot. Prot. Phos. Res., 20,* 289.
3. Kahn CR (1985): The molecular mechanism of insulin action. *Ann. Rev. Med., 36,* 429.
4. Houslay MD (1985): The insulin receptor and signal generation at the plasma membrane. In Cohen P, Houslay MD (Eds), *Molecular Mechanisms of Transmembrane Signalling. Molecular Aspects of Cellular Regulation, Vol. 4,* pp. 279-333. Elsevier Biomedical Press, Amsterdam.

5. Czech MP (Ed.) (1985): *Molecular Basis of Insulin Action.* Plenum Press, New York-London.
6. Belfrage P, Donnér J, Strålfors P (Eds) (1986): *Mechanisms of Insulin Action.* Elsevier, Amsterdam.
7. Cushman SW, Wardzala LJ (1980): Potential mechanism of insulin action on glucose transport in the isolated rat adipose cell: apparent translocation of intracellular transport systems to the plasma membrane. *J. Biol. Chem., 255,* 4758.
8. Susuki K, Kono T (1980): Evidence that insulin causes translocation of glucose transport activity to the plasma membrane from an intracellular storage site. *Proc. Natl Acad. Sci. USA, 77,* 2542.
9. Lin S, Spudich JA (1974): Biochemical studies on the mode of action of cytochalasin B. *J. Biol. Chem., 249,* 5778.
10. Shanahan MF, Olson SA, Weber MJ et al (1982): Photolabelling of glucose sensitive cytochalasin B binding proteins in erythrocyte, fibroblast and adipocyte membranes. *Biochem. Biophys. Res. Commun., 107,* 38.
11. Oka Y, Czech MP (1984): Photoaffinity labelling of insulin-sensitivity hexose transporters in intact rat adipocytes: direct evidence that latent transporters become exposed to the extracellular space in response to insulin. *J. Biol. Chem., 259,* 8125.
12. Lienhard GE, Kim HH, Ransome KJ et al (1982): Immunological identification of an insulin-responsive glucose transporter. *Biochem. Biophys. Res. Commun., 105,* 1150.
13. Wheeler TJ, Simpson IA, Sogin DC et al (1982): Detection of the rat adipose cell glucose transporter with antibody against the human red cell glucose transporter. *Biochem. Biophys. Res. Commun., 105,* 89.
14. Mueckler M, Caruso C, Baldwin SA et al (1985): Sequence and structure of a human glucose transporter. *Science, 229,* 941.
15. Simpson IA, Yver DR, Hissin PJ et al (1983): Insulin-stimulated translocation of glucose transporters in the isolated rat adipose cell: characterisation of subcellular fractions. *Biochim. Biophys. Acta, 763,* 393.
16. Kono T, Robinson FW, Blevins TL et al (1982): Evidence that translocation of the glucose transport activity is the major mechanism of insulin action on glucose transport in fat cells. *J. Biol. Chem., 257,* 10942.
17. Kono T (1985): Insulin-dependent apparent translocation of glucose transport activity. In: Czech MP (Ed.), *Molecular Basis of Insulin Action,* Ch. 24, pp. 423-431. Plenum Press, New York.
18. Simpson IA, Cushman SW (1985): Hexose transport regulation by insulin in the isolated rat adipose cell. In: Czech MP (Ed.), *Molecular Basis of Insulin Action,* Ch. 23, pp. 399-422. Plenum Press, New York.
19. Vinten J, Gliemann J, Østerlind K (1976): Exchange of 3-*O*-methylglucose in isolated fat cells: concentration dependence and effect of insulin. *J. Biol. Chem., 251,* 794.
20. Czech MP (1980): Insulin action and the regulation of hexose transport. *Diabetes, 29,* 399.
21. Gliemann J, Rees WD (1983): The insulin-sensitive hexose transport system in adipocytes. *Curr. Top. Membranes Transp., 18,* 337.
22. Whitesell RR, Abumrad NA (1985): Increased affinity predominates in insulin stimulation of glucose transport in the adipocyte. *J. Biol. Chem., 260,* 2894.
23. Joost HG, Weber TM, Cushman SW et al (1986): Insulin stimulated glucose transport in rat adipose cells. *J. Biol. Chem., 261,* 10033.
23a. Baly DL, Horuk R (1987): Dissociation of insulin-stimulated glucose transport from the translocation of glucose carriers in rat adipose cells. *J. Biol. Chem., 262,* 21.
24. Kitigawa K, Nishino H, Iwashima A (1985): Tumor promoter-stimulated translocation of glucose transport system in mouse embryo fibroblast Swiss 3T3 cell. *Biochem. Biophys. Res. Commun., 128,* 1303.

24a. Gibbs EM, Allard WJ, Lierhard GE (1986): The glucose transporter in 3T3-L1 adipocytes is phosphorylated in response to phorbol ester but not in response to insulin. *J. Biol. Chem.*, *261*, 16597.

25. Nishizuka Y (1984): The role of protein kinase C in cell surface signal transduction and tumour promotion. *Nature (London)*, *308*, 693.

26. Witters LA, Vater CA, Lienhard GE (1985): Phosphorylation of the glucose transporter in vitro and in vivo by protein kinase C. *Nature (London)*, *316*, 777.

27. Wardzala LJ, Jeanrenaud B (1983): Identification of the D-glucose-inhibitable cytochalasin B binding site as the glucose transporter in rat diaphragm plasma and microsomal membranes. *Biochim. Biophys. Acta*, *730*, 49.

28. Watanabe T, Smith MM, Robinson FW et al (1984): Insulin action on glucose transport in cardiac muscle. *J. Biol. Chem.*, *259*, 13117.

29. Oka Y, Mottola C, Oppenheimer CL et al (1984): Insulin activates the appearance of insulin-like growth-factor II receptors on the adipocyte cell surface. *Proc. Natl Acad. Sci. USA*, *81*, 4028.

30. Wardzala LJ, Simpson IA, Rechler MM et al (1984): Potential mechanism of the stimulatory action of insulin on insulin-like growth factor II binding to the isolated rat adipose cell: apparent redistribution of receptors cycling between a large intracellular pool and the plasma membrane. *J. Biol. Chem.*, *259*, 8378.

31. Corvera S, Czech MP (1985): Mechanism of insulin action on membrane protein recycling: a selective decrease in the phosphorylation state of insulin-like growth factor II receptors in the cell surface membrane. *Proc. Natl Acad. Sci. USA*, *82*, 7314.

32. Davis RJ, Corvera S, Czech MP (1986): Insulin stimulates cellular iron uptake and causes the redistribution of intracellular transferrin receptors to the plasma membrane. *J. Biol. Chem.*, *261*, 8708.

33. Sonne O, Simpson IA (1984): Internalisation of insulin and its receptor in the isolated rat adipose cell: time-course and insulin concentration dependency. *Biochim. Biophys. Acta*, *804*, 404.

34. Parker PJ, Caudwell FB, Cohen P (1983): Glycogen synthase from rabbit skeletal muscle: effect of insulin on the state of phosphorylation of the seven phosphoserine residues in vivo. *Eur. J. Biochem.*, *130*, 227.

35. Sheorain VS, Juhl H, Bass M et al (1984): Effects of epinephrine, diabetes, and insulin on rabbit skeletal muscle glycogen synthase: phosphorylation site occupancies *J. Biol. Chem.*, *259*, 7024.

36. Lawrence JC, James C (1984): Activation of glycogen synthase by insulin in rat adipocytes: evidence of hormonal stimulation of multisite dephosphorylation by glucose transport-dependent and -independent pathways. *J. Biol. Chem.*, *259*, 7975.

37. Lawrence Jr JC, Hiken JF, Depaoli-Roach AA et al (1983): Hormonal control of glycogen synthase in rat hemidiaphragms. *J. Biol. Chem.*, *258*, 10710.

38. Cohen P (1987): Role of multisite phosphorylation in the hormonal control of glycogen synthase from mammalian muscle. In: Krebs EG, Boyer PD (Eds), *The Enzymes, Vol. 18*. In press.

39. Parker PJ, Caudwell FB, Cohen P (1982): Glycogen synthase from rabbit skeletal muscle: state of phosphorylation of the seven phosphoserine residues in vivo in the presence and absence of adrenaline. *Eur. J. Biochem.*, *124*, 47.

40. Soderling TR, Sheorain VS (1985): Skeletal muscle glycogen synthase: hormonal regulation. In: Czech MP (Ed.), *Molecular Basis of Insulin Action*, Ch. 14, pp. 235-245. Plenum Press, New York.

41. Cohen P (1978): The role of cAMP-dependent protein kinase in the regulation of glycogen metabolism in mammalian skeletal muscle. *Curr. Top. Cell. Regul.*, *14*, 117.

42. Cohen P, Parker PJ, Woodgett JR (1984): The molecular mechanism by which insulin activates glycogen synthase in mammalian skeletal muscle. In: Czech MP (Ed.), *Molecular Basis of Insulin Action,* Ch. 13, pp. 213-233. Plenum Press, New York.
43. Ingrebritsen TS, Cohen P (1983): The protein phosphatases involved in cellular regulation. I. Classification and substrate specificities. *Eur. J. Biochem., 132,* 255.
44. Sheorain VS, Corbin JD, Soderling TR (1985): Phosphorylation of sites 3 and 4 in rabbit skeletal muscle glycogen synthase by cAMP-dependent protein kinase. *J. Biol. Chem., 260,*1567.
45. Sheorain VS, Ramakrishna S, Benjamin WB et al (1985): Phosphorylation of sites 3 and 2 in rabbit skeletal muscle glycogen synthase by a multifunctional protein kinase. *J. Biol. Chem., 260,* 12287.
46. Ahmad Z, Camici M, Depaoli-Roach AA et al (1984): Glycogen synthase kinase: classification of a rabbit liver casein and glycogen synthase kinase (casein kinase-1) as a distinct enzyme. *J. Biol. Chem., 259,* 3420.
47. Lawrence Jr JL, James C, Hiken JF (1986): Control of glycogen synthase by insulin and iso-proterenol in rat adipocytes: changes in the distribution of phosphate in the synthase sub-unit in response to insulin and β-adrenergic receptor activation. *J. Biol. Chem., 261,* 669.
48. Foulkes JG, Cohen P, Strada SJ et al (1982): Antagonistic effects of insulin and β-adrenergic agonists on the activity of protein phosphatase inhibitor-1 in skeletal muscle of the perfused rat hemicorpus. *J. Biol. Chem., 257,* 12493.
49. Kahtra BS, Chiasson JL, Shikama H et al (1980): Effect of epinephrine and insulin on the phosphorylation of phosphorylase phosphatase inhibitor 1 in perfused rat skeletal muscle. *FEBS Lett., 114,* 253.
50. Larner J, Lawrence JC, Walkenbach RJ et al (1978): Insulin control of glycogen synthesis. *Adv. Cyclic. Nucleot. Res., 9,* 425.
51. Cheng K, Thompson M, Schwartz C et al (1985): Multiple intracellular peptide mediators of insulin action. In: Czech MP (Ed.), *Molecular Basis of Insulin Action,* Ch. 10, pp. 171-182. Plenum Press, New York.
52. Tung HYL, Pelech S, Fisher MJ et al (1985): The protein phosphatases involved in cellular regulation: influence of polyamines on the activities of protein phosphatase-1 and protein phosphatase-2A. *Eur. J. Biochem., 149,* 305.
53. Denton RM, Halestrap AP (1979): Regulation of pyruvate metabolism in mammalian tissues. *Essays Biochem., 15,* 37.
54. Wieland OH (1983): The mammalian pyruvate dehydrogenase complex: structure and regulation. *Rev. Physiol. Biochem. Pharmacol., 96,* 123.
55. Denton RM, Hughes WA (1978): Mini-review: pyruvate dehydrogenase and the hormonal regulation of fat synthesis in mammalian tissues. *Int. J. Biochem., 9,* 545.
56. Denton RM, Thomas AP, Tavaré JM et al (1985): Mechanisms involved in the stimulation of fatty acid synthesis by insulin. In: Belfrage P, Donnér J, Strålfors P (Eds), *Mechanisms of Insulin Action,* Ch. 20, pp. 283-304. Elsevier, Amsterdam.
57. Hughes WA, Denton RM (1976): Incorporation of ^{32}P into pyruvate dehydrogenase phosphate in mitochondria from control and insulin-treated adipose tissue. *Nature (London), 264,* 471.
58. Denton RM, McCormack JG, Marshall SE (1984): Persistence of the effect of insulin on pyruvate dehydrogenase activity in rat white and brown adipose tissue during the preparation and subsequent incubation of mitochondria. *Biochem. J., 217,* 441.
59. Thomas AP, Diggle TA, Denton RM (1986): Sensitivity of pyruvate dehydrogenase phosphate phosphatase to magnesium ions: similar effects of spermine and insulin. *Biochem. J., 238,* 83.

60. Thomas AP, Denton RM (1986): Use of toluene-permeabilised mitochondria to study the regulation of adipose tissue pyruvate dehydrogenase in situ: further evidence that insulin acts through stimulation of pyruvate dehydrogenase phosphate phosphatase. *Biochem. J.*, *238*, 93.

61. Damuni Z, Humphreys JS, Reed LJ (1984): Stimulation of pyruvate dehydrogenase phosphatase activity by polyamines. *Biochem. Biophys. Res. Commun.*, *124*, 95.

62. Grillo MA (1985): Metabolism and function of polyamines. *Int. J. Biochem.*, *17*, 943.

63. Jarett L, Seals JR (1979): Pyruvate dehydrogenase activation in adipocyte mitochondria by an insulin generated mediator from muscle. *Science*, *206*, 1407.

64. Jarett L, Kiechle FJ (1984): Intracellular mediators of insulin action. *Vitam. Horm.*, *41*, 51.

65. Jarett L, Kiechle FL, Macaulay SL et al (1985): Intracellular mediators of insulin action. In: Czech MP (Ed.), *Molecular Basis of Insulin Action*, Ch. 11, pp. 183-198. Plenum Press, New York.

66. Seals JR, Czech MP (1981): Characterisation of a pyruvate dehydrogenase activator released by adipocyte plasma membrane in response to insulin. *J. Biol. Chem.*, *256*, 2894.

67. Macaulay SL, Jarett L (1985): Insulin mediator causes dephosphorylation of the alpha-subunit of PDH by stimulating phosphatase activity. *Arch. Biochem. Biophys.*, *237*, 142.

68. Heyworth CM, Wallace AV, Houslay MD (1983): Insulin and glucagon regulate the activation of two distinct membrane-bound cAMP phosphodiesterases in hepatocytes. *Biochem. J.*, *214*, 99.

69. Hepp DK, Renner R (1972): Insulin action on the adenyl cyclase system: antagonism to activation by lipolytic hormones. *FEBS Lett.*, *20*, 191.

70. Heyworth CM, Houslay MD (1983): Insulin exerts actions through a distinct species of guanine nucleotide regulatory protein: inhibition of adenylate cyclase. *Biochem. J.*, *214*, 547.

71. Lambert B, Jacquemin C (1979): Inhibition by insulin of the adrenaline-stimulated adenylate cyclase in rat adipose tissue. *FEBS Lett.*, *105*, 19.

72. Kono T, Robinson FW, Sarver JA (1975): Insulin-sensitive phosphodiesterase: its localization, hormonal stimulation and oxidative stabilization. *J. Biol. Chem.*, *250*, 7826.

73. Loten EG, Sneyd JGT (1970): An effect of insulin on adipose tissue adenosine- 3′ 5′-cyclic monophosphate phosphodiesterase. *Biochem. J.*, *120*, 187.

74. Makino H, Kono T (1980): Characterization of insulin-sensitive phosphodiesterase in fat cells. II. Comparison of enzyme activities stimulated by insulin and by isoproterenol. *J. Biol. Chem.*, *255*, 7850.

75. Heyworth CM, Rawal S, Houslay MD (1983): Guanine nucleotides can activate the insulin stimulated phosphodiesterase in liver plasma membranes. *FEBS Lett.*, *154*, 87.

76. Marchmont RJ, Houslay MD (1980): Insulin controls the cAMP-dependent phosphorylation of integral and peripheral proteins associated with the rat liver plasma membrane. *FEBS Lett.*, *118*, 18.

77. Heyworth CM, Whetton AD, Wong S et al (1985): Insulin inhibits the cholera toxin catalysed ribosylation of a Mr-25,000 protein in rat liver plasma membranes. *Biochem. J.*, *228*, 593.

78. Kiechle FL, Jarett L (1981): The effect of an insulin sensitive chemical mediator from rat adipocytes on low K_m and high K_m cAMP phosphodiesterase. *FEBS Lett.*, *133*, 279.

79. Saltiel AR, Cuatrecasas P (1986): Insulin stimulates the generation from hepatic plasma membranes of modulators derived from an inositol glycolipid. *Proc. Natl Acad. Sci. USA*, *83*, 5793.

80. Satliel AR, Fox JA, Sherline P et al (1986): Insulin stimulated hydrolysis of a novel glycolipid generates modulators of cAMP phosphodiesterase. *Science*, *223*, 967.

81. Denton RM, Brownsey RW, Belsham GJ (1981): A partial view of the mechanism of insulin action. *Diabetologia*, *21*, 347.

82. Blackshear PJ, Witters LA, Girard PR et al (1985): Growth factor-stimulated protein phosphorylation in 3T3-L1 cells: evidence for protein kinase C-dependent and -independent pathways. *J. Biol. Chem., 260,* 13304.

83. Blackshear PJ (1986): Protein phosphorylation in cultured cells: interactions among insulin, growth factors and phorbol esters. In: Belfrage P, Donnér J, Strålfors J (Eds), *Mechanisms of Insulin Action,* Ch. 15, pp 211-227, Elsevier, Amsterdam.

84. Kahn CR, White MF, Grigorescu F et al (1985): The insulin receptor protein kinase. In: Czech MP (Ed.), *Molecular Basis of Insulin Action,* Ch. 4, pp, 67-94. Plenum Press, New York.

85. Rosen OM, Herrera R, Olowe Y et al (1983): Phosphorylation activates the insulin receptor tyrosine protein kinase. *Proc. Natl Acad. Sci. USA 80,* 3237.

86. Yu K-T, Czech MP (1984): Tyrosine phosphorylation of the insulin receptor β-subunit activates the receptor associated tyrosine kinase activity. *J. Biol. Chem., 259,* 5277.

87. Marshall S (1985): Kinetics of insulin receptor internalisation and recycling in adipocytes. *J. Biol. Chem., 260,* 4136.

88. Cushman SW, Simpson IA, Smith U (1986): Insulin-induced integral membrane protein translocations and their counter-regulation by lipolytic and antilipolytic hormones. In: Belfrage P, Donnér J, Strålfors P (Eds), *Mechanisms of Insulin Action,* Ch. 14, pp. 181-210. Elsevier, Amsterdam.

89. Karnieli E, Zarnowski MJ, Hissin PJ et al (1981): Insulin-stimulated translocation of glucose transport systems in the isolated rat adipose cell. *J. Biol. Chem., 256,* 4772.

90. Schoenle EJ, Adams LD, Sammons DW (1984): Insulin-induced rapid decrease of a major protein in fat cell plasma membranes. *J. Biol. Chem., 259,* 12112.

The Diabetes Annual/3
K.G.M.M. Alberti and L.P. Krall, editors
© 1987 Elsevier Science Publishers, B.V.

24   The insulin receptor: an update*

SETHU REDDY AND GEORGE L. KING

Introduction

The insulin receptor is a transmembranous glycoprotein composed of two disulfide-linked α- and β-subunits, having a total approximate weight of 350,000 (1). In this review, we will detail the structure and function of the insulin receptor, provide an update of the insulin receptor genetic studies, and relate progress in studies of autophosphorylation of the receptor and substrate phosphorylation. The relationship of the tyrosine kinase activity of the insulin receptor to insulin action and diabetes will also be discussed.

Structure

The insulin receptor is synthesized as a single polypeptide precursor which undergoes proteolytic cleavage and glycosylation (2). The precursors of the α- and β-subunits contain *N*-linked carbohydrate chains, which are capped by terminal sialic acids prior to maturation. There appears to be some *O*-linked glycosylation, as well, on the β-subunit (3). The mature α- and β-units have molecular weights of 135,000 and 95,000, respectively.

The receptor is a heterotetramer with disulfide-linked α- and β-subunits. The α-subunit is essentially an extracellular component involved in insulin binding, while the β-subunit contains a transmembranous portion and an intracellular domain which acts as a tyrosine kinase upon insulin stimulation. The receptor undergoes autophosphorylation and also has the ability to phosphorylate other substrates (4, 5).

Although each receptor could theoretically bind two insulin molecules, Pang and Shafer have shown that the affinity for a second molecule of insulin is almost 100 times less than that for the first (6).

---
*This work was supported by grants DK-36433 and EY-05110 (G.L.K.) from the National Institutes of Health, and by a Diabetes Canada Research Scholarship (S.R.).

Internalization

Once bound, the insulin/insulin receptor complex does not remain static. There is rapid internalization of the complex as well as subsequent recycling of the receptor back to the membrane (7). Normally, approximately 10% of the receptor pool is located intracellularly and this increases to a steady state of 30% after 6 min of hormone stimulation (8).

Carpentier et al (9) studying monocytes have shown that the insulin receptor complex is present initially in clear vesicles and later associates with lysosomes. It can then be recycled through clear vesicles.

King et al (10, 11) have studied intracellular processing of ^{125}I-insulin in vascular endothelial cells and have shown receptor-mediated transcytosis of insulin.

Hachiya et al (12) have also studied intracellular processing of ^{125}I-insulin and ^{125}I-labeled insulin-like growth factor II (^{125}I-IGF-II) in these cells and have shown that the internalized hormones can be processed via two pathways (Fig. 1): (a) a lysosomal-degradative pathway or (b) intact transport across the cells. The transcytosis appears to be unidirectional (12). Interestingly, unlike adipocytes, a minority of internalized insulin enters the degradative pathway.

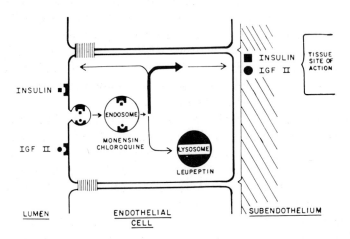

FIG. 1. *Schematic diagram of insulin and IGF-II processing by vascular endothelial cells. There is predominant transport of intact hormone across the cell to the tissue site of action. The hormones may also enter the recycling or degradative pathways after being internalized. Proposed sites of action for inhibitors of cellular processing are also shown. Reproduced from Hachiya et al (12) by courtesy of the Editors of Diabetes.*

Insulin receptor gene

Two groups have now cloned the cDNA (Fig. 2) of the insulin receptor which has clarified the structure of the insulin receptor and has given scientists a major tool for further elucidation of insulin receptor function. The insulin receptor has been shown (1) to have areas of homology with the IGF-I receptor such as the cross-linking domain in the α-subunit, the transmembrane area, the ATP binding site and a region similar to oncogene proteins (V-*vos*, V-*erb* and V-*src* family) (13, 14).

From the cDNA structure the amino acid sequence of the receptor can be deduced. The α-subunit consists of many hydrophilic amino acids, which suggests that it is an entirely extracellular protein. The β-subunit consists of 4 domains: an extracellular domain, a 23-amino-acid hydrophobic, α-helical transmembranous domain, an intracellular ATP binding site, and finally a domain containing possible sites of tyrosine autophosphorylation. This fourth domain contains 7 possible sites, the most likely of which are at positions 960, 1150 and 1316 or 1322. The 1150 site is similar to the major phosphorylation site of the product of V-*src*.

Ullrich et al (15) have recently determined the structure of the human insulin-like growth factor I (IGF-I) receptor from cloned cDNA. As expected, the structure is very similar to that of the insulin receptor (Fig. 2). Despite such a high degree of homology, some differences do exist and these areas may point to sites of hormone specificity. Thus, there is lower homology (48%) in the extracellular cysteine-rich domains, which is where hormone binding is likely to occur. Although there is 84% homology with the insulin receptor kinase domain, there appear to be 3 areas of difference in the amino acid sequence following positions 986, 1072 and 1208. Such areas may modify phosphorylation sites and confer receptor functional specificity.

The insulin receptor gene has been localized to human chromosome 19. The genes for complement component C3 and of the LDL receptor are also on this chromosome. The gene for myotonic dystrophy has also been mapped by linkage analysis to the short arm of chromosome 19. Interestingly, these patients have been reported to have insulin resistance (16), which raises the possibility of an abnormal insuiin receptor gene.

With the availability of insulin receptor cDNA, quantitative and qualitative studies are being performed on the insulin receptor gene and mRNAs. Since the entire sequence of the insulin receptor gene is not known, restriction-fragment length polymorphisms (RFLPs) have been studied, using labeled cDNA probes to hybridize with digested DNA from various cells. As a note of caution, there appear to be racial differences in RFLP patterns. Thus far, two studies have not found an association of any RFLP with non-insulin-dependent diabetes mellitus (NIDDM) (17, 18). However, Trembath et al (19) from the

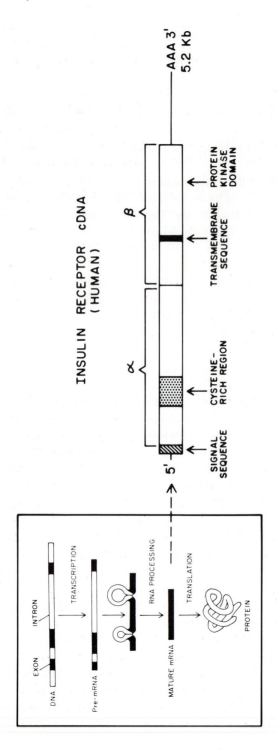

FIG. 2.   Schematic diagram of insulin receptor precursor cDNA. The actual insulin receptor gene has a series of exons and introns, with only exons being expressed in the mature mRNA. The cDNA, a copy of the mature mRNA, is a single chain of nucleotides coding for both the α- and β-subunits. Important coding sites are shown. The protein undergoes further processing and glycosylation (not shown). Reproduced by courtesy of Muller-Wieland and Kriauciunas.

United Kingdom have some preliminary data showing a higher frequency of two fragments (4.2 and 3.7 Kb) in NIDDM patients. It may be possible, in the future, to identify a subset of the NIDDM population with insulin receptor gene abnormalities.

The phenomenon of multiple species of mRNAs for the insulin receptor with varying length (2.9-8.2 Kb) has been observed. The significance of these is not clear, although, in at least 3T3-LI cells, the 6.5 and 6.2 Kb mRNAs seem most important (14). Since the smallest mRNAs are not capable of coding for the insulin proreceptor, it is possible that they are coding for the subunits. Their exact physiology remains to be elucidated.

Rutter et al (20) have been able to transfect Chinese hamster ovary (CHO) cells with human insulin receptor cDNA; these cells normally express little insulin receptor (20). The transfected cells produced human insulin receptor, and displayed insulin-stimulated autophosphorylation of the β-subunit and insulin-mediated 2-deoxyglucose uptake.

These techniques are currently being used to study genetic syndromes of insulin resistance and should shed further light on the pathophysiology of insulin receptor gene transcription and mRNA translation.

Phosphorylation

Since the recent discovery of the ability of the insulin receptor to phosphorylate itself upon insulin binding and the subsequent finding of its ability to be a tyrosine kinase, these functions have been thought to play a major role in insulin action. This has therefore been studied intensively in cell membrane preparations and intact cells. The kinase activity of the subunit is dependent upon ATP as a donor of phosphate and on Mn^{2+} as a necessary co-factor. Once phosphorylated, the insulin receptor becomes insulin-independent with respect to its tyrosine kinase activity. The initial rate of autophosphorylation is independent of receptor concentration and thus suggests that this is an intra- rather than an inter-molecular mechanism (21). In an in-vitro system, autophosphorylation is rapid with a $t_{1/2}$ of about 30 seconds; this is compatible with the rapid actions of insulin. Only tyrosine phosphorylation is seen in the in-vitro system, whereas in intact cells the receptor also undergoes serine and threonine phosphorylation. Studying well-differentiated hepatoma cells, White et al (22) showed differences in patterns of tyrosine phosphorylation between in-vitro and in-vivo systems. The non-tyrosine phosphorylation of the β-subunit must be due to another kinase and there is some suggestion that this affects receptor function (23). Findings by several groups that phorbol esters, activators of protein kinase C, produced serine phosphorylation of this receptor, suggest that this kinase is a likely candidate. Phorbol esters decrease tyrosine phosphorylation of the β-subunit. It is therefore hypothesized that the level of serine phosphorylation of the insulin receptor modifies the receptor tyrosine kinase activity (24, 25).

Other factors which have been shown to modify tyrosine kinase activity under experimental conditions are the presence of sialic acids on the receptor and the monomeric (α,β) versus dimeric (α_2,β_2) structure of the receptor. Fujita-Yamaguchi et al (26) have found that tyrosine kinase activity is enhanced by the removal of sialic acids and is higher in the monomeric form.

The insulin receptor, once autophosphorylated, has been shown to phosphorylate many proteins in an in-vitro system. These include ribosomal protein S6, ATP citrate lyase, calmodulin, several glycolytic enzymes, histone H2b, angiotensin II, cytoskeletal proteins such as tubulin, and microtubule-associated proteins and casein (5, 27). Endogenous substrates, however, have been more difficult to identify. Rees-Jones and Taylor (28, 29) recently described a liver-specific glycoprotein of $M_r = 120,000$ which was phosphorylated by the insulin receptor.

Sadoul et al (30) have described a 110 Kd protein substrate, in brown adipose tissue and lymphocytes. White et al (31) have reported a protein of $M_r = 185,000$ which is phosphorylated rapidly by the insulin receptor, in intact rat hepatoma cells (Fig. 3). An anti-phosphotyrosine antibody was used to detect

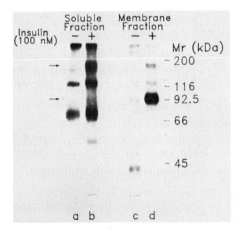

FIG. 3. *Fao rat hepatoma cells were labeled with ^{32}P-orthophosphate and incubated with and without 100 nM insulin for 1 min. The cells were then frozen, thawed and centrifuged. The soluble fraction (supernatant) containing cytosolic proteins (lanes a, b) was immunoprecipitated by phosphotyrosine antibody. The pellet (membrane proteins) was solubilized in 1% Triton X-100; after ultracentrifugation, the solubilized membranes were immunoprecipitated with the phosphotyrosine antibody. The 185 Kd protein appears to be a cytosolic protein while the phosphorylated 95 Kd β-subunit of the insulin receptor is present in the membrane fraction, as expected. Weaker stimulation of phosphorylation of a 120 Kd protein and a 70 Kd protein is also seen (lanes a, b). Reproduced by courtesy of White et al.*

this intriguing substrate. The exact role of any of these phosphorylated substrates in insulin action has still to be defined.

Whether the tyrosine kinase activity is of physiological importance is still debated, but some recent evidence favors an important role for autophosphorylation as well as substrate phosphorylation. Herrera et al (32) demonstrated that an antibody directed against a region surrounding tyrosine-960 inhibited autophosphorylation and exogenous substrate phosphorylation; Morgan et al (33) also showed that a monoclonal antibody which inhibited phosphorylation inhibited the growth response of cells to insulin. Ellis et al (34) were able to generate transfected CHO cells which have the 2 tyrosines in the V-*src* homologous region substituted by phenylalanine (34). No kinase activity of the insulin receptor was seen and a parallel decrease in insulin-stimulated 2-deoxyglucose uptake was observed. Kohanski et al (35) performed kinetic studies of β-subunit phosphorylation and changes in glucose transport rate which supported the plausibility of β-subunit phosphorylation as an intermediate step to increased glucose transport. Thus, although the insulin receptor tyrosine kinase does not interact with the glucose transporter protein directly, it may well play an important intermediary role (36).

Decreased tyrosine kinase activity of the insulin receptor, relative to insulin binding, has been described in skeletal muscle from insulin-resistant mice, in 2 patients with Type A syndrome of insulin resistance, in hepatocytes from streptozotocin-induced diabetic rats and in some patients with leprechaunism (submitted for publication) (37-39). Burant et al (40, 41) have recently demonstrated a similar defect in denervated skeletal muscle; they have also shown altered electrophoretic mobility of the insulin receptor β-subunit of skeletal muscle isolated from diabetic rats. A tyrosine kinase defect was also evident in this tissue. Recent studies of insulin action in hepatocytes from diabetic patients also suggest a post-binding defect (42).

Other groups have looked at generation of plasma membrane low-molecular-weight mediators by insulin-stimulated cells. Adipocytes, skeletal myocytes and hepatocytes have been studied most extensively; one of the mediators appears to be a phospholipid (43). How this approach relates to insulin receptor phosphorylation and is significant in pathological states of insulin action remains to be seen.

Conclusions

Many recent advances have been made in our understanding of the insulin receptor, but the exact mechanism of insulin action remains elusive. Certainly, from the many actions of insulin, several mechanisms may be playing a role. The future looks exciting in this quest.

Acknowledgment

The authors wish to thank Ms Frances Sarly and Ms Terri-Lyn Bellman for their excellent secretarial assistance in the preparation of this manuscript.

References

1. Jacobs S, Cuatrecasas P (1981): Insulin receptor: structure and function. *Endocr. Rev., 2,* 25.
2. Ronnett GV, Knutson VP, Kohanski et al (1984): Role of glycosylation in the processing of newly translated insulin proreceptor in 3T3-L1 adipocytes. *J. Biol. Chem., 259,* 4566.
3. Herzberg VL, Grigorescu F, Edge AB et al (1985): Characterization of insulin receptor carbohydrate by comparison of chemical and enzymatic deglycosylation. *Biochem. Biophys. Res. Commun., 129,* 789.
4. Kasuga M, Karlsson FA, Kahn CR (1982): Insulin stimulates the phosphorylation of the 95,000 subunit of its own receptor. *Science, 215,* 185.
5. Stadtmauer LA, Rosen OM (1983): Phosphorylation of exogenous substrates by the insulin receptor-associated protein kinase, *J. Biol. Chem., 258,* 6082.
6. Pang DT, Shafer JA (1984): Evidence that insulin receptor from human placenta has a high affinity for only one molecule of insulin. *J. Biol. Chem., 259,* 8589.
7. Marshall S, Heidenreich KA, Horikoshi H (1985): Stoichiometric translocation of adipocyte insulin receptor from the cell-surface to the cell-interior. *J. Biol. Chem., 259,* 15003.
8. Marschall S (1985): Kinetics of insulin receptor internalization and recycling in adipocytes. *J. Biol. Chem., 260,* 4136.
9. Carpentier JL, Dayer JM, Long U et al (1984): Down regulation and recycling of insulin receptor: effect of monensin on 1M-9 lymphocytes and U937 monocyte-like cells. *J. Biol. Chem., 259,* 14190.
10. Jialal I, King GL, Buchwald S et al (1984): Processing of insulin by bovine endothelial cells in culture: internalization without degradation. *Diabetes, 33,* 794.
11. King GL, Johnson SM (1985): Receptor-mediated transport of insulin across endothelial cells. *Science, 227,* 1583.
12. Hachiya HL, Carpentier JL, King GL (1986): Comparative studies on insulin-like growth factor II and insulin processing by vascular endothelial cells. *Diabetes, 35,*1065.
13. Ebina Y, Ellis L, Jarnagin M et al (1985): The human insulin receptor cDNA: the structure basis for hormone-activated transmembrane signalling. *Cell, 40,* 747.
14. Ullrich A, Bell JR, Chen EY et al (1985): Human insulin receptor and its relationship to the tyrosine kinase family of oncogenes. *Nature (London), 313,* 756.
15. Ullrich A, Grey A, Tam AW et al (1986): Insulin-like growth factor 1 receptor primary structure: comparison with insulin receptor suggests structural determinants that define functional specificity. *EMBO J., 5,* 2503.
16. Shaw DJ, Meredith AC, Break JD et al (1986): Linkage relationship of the insulin receptor gene with the complement component 3, LDL receptor, apolipoprotein C2 and myotonic dystrophy loci on chromosome 19. *Hum. Genet., 74,* 267.
17. Elbein SC, Corsetti L, Ullrich A, Permutt MA (1986): Multiple restriction fragment length polymorphisms at the insulin receptor locus: a highly informative marker for linkage analysis. *Proc. Natl Acad. Sci. USA, 83,* 5223.
18. Takeda J, Seino Y, Yoshimasa Y et al (1986): Restriction fragment length polymorphisms (RFLP) of the human insulin receptor gene: its possible usefulness as a genetic marker (in Japanese). *Diabetologia, 29,* 667.

19. Trembath RC, O'Connor G, Galton DJ (1986): An insulin receptor gene polymorphism and Type 2 (non-insulin-dependent) diabetes mellitus (Abstract). *Diabetologia, 28,* 601A.
20. Ebina Y, Ederly M, Ellis DN et al (1985): Expression of a functional human insulin receptor from a cloned cDNA in Chinese hamster ovary cells. *Proc. Natl Acad. Sci. USA, 82,* 8014.
21. Rosen OM, Herrera R, Olowe Y et al (1983): Phosphorylation activates the insulin receptor tyrosine protein kinase. *Proc. Natl Acad. Sci. USA, 80,* 3237.
22. White MF, Takayama S, Kahn CR (1984): Differences in the sites of phosphorylation of the insulin receptor in vivo and in vitro. *J. Biol. Chem., 260,* 9470.
23. Yu KT, Czeh M (1984): Tyrosine phosphorylation of the insulin receptor β-subunit activates the receptor-associated kinase activity. *J. Biol. Chem., 259,* 5277.
24. Takayama S, White MF, Lauris V, Kahn CR (1984): Phorbol esters modulate insulin receptor phosphorylation and insulin action in cultured hepatoma cells. *Proc. Natl Acad. Sci. USA, 81,* 7797.
25. Haring HO, White MF, Kahn CR et al (1985): Interaction of the insulin receptor with serine/threonine kinase in vitro. *J. Cell. Biochem., 28,* 171.
26. Fujita-Yamaguchi Y, Sato Y, Kathuria S (1985): Removal of sialic acids from the purified insulin receptor results in enhanced insulin binding and kinase activities. *Biochem. Biophys. Res. Commun., 129,* 739.
27. Kadowaki T, Fujita-Yamaguchi Y, Nishita E et al (1985): Phosphorylation of tubules and microtubule-associated proteins by the purified insulin receptor kinase. *J. Biol. Chem., 260,* 4016.
28. Rees-Jones RW, Taylor SI (1985): An endogenous substrate for the insulin receptor-associated tyrosine kinase. *J. Biol. Chem., 260,* 4461.
29. Accili D, Perrotti N, Rees-Jones R, Taylor SI (1986): Tissue distribution and subcellular localization of an endogenous substrate (pp. 120) for the insulin receptor associated tyrosine kinase. *Endocrinology, 119,* 1274.
30. Sadoul JL, Peyron JF, Ballotti R (1985): Identification of a cellular 110,000-Da protein for the insulin receptor kinase. *Biochem. J., 227,* 887.
31. White MF, Maron R, Kahn CR (1985): Insulin rapidly stimulates tyrosine phosphorylation of a $M_r = 185,000$ protein in intact cells. *Nature (London), 318,* 183.
32. Herrera R, Petruzelli L, Thorner N et al (1985): An antipeptide antibody that specifically inhibits insulin receptor autophosphorylation and protein kinase activity. *Proc. Natl Acad. Sci. USA, 82,* 7899.
33. Morgan DO, Ho L, Korn LJ, Roth RA (1980): Insulin action is blocked by a monoclonal antibody that inhibits the insulin receptor kinase. *Proc. Natl Acad. Sci. USA, 83,* 328.
34. Ellis L, Clauser E, Morgan DO et al (1986): Replacement of insulin receptor tyrosine 1162 and 1163 compromises insulin stimulated kinase activity and uptake of 2-deoxyglucose. *Cell, 45,* 721.
35. Kohanski R, Frost SC, Lane MD (1986): Insulin dependent phosphorylation of the insulin receptor-protein kinase and activation of glucose transport in 3T3-L1 adipocyte. *J. Biol. Chem., 261,* 12272.
36. Gibbs EM, Allard WJ, Lienhard GE (1986): The glucose transporter in 3T3-L1 adipocytes is phosphorylated in response to phorbol ester but not in response to insulin. *J. Biol. Chem., 261,* 16597.
37. Grunberger F, Flier JS, Gorden P (1984): Defect in phosphorylation of insulin receptors in cells from an insulin resistant patient with normal insulin binding. *Science, 223,* 932.
38. Grigorescu F, Flier JS, Kahn CR (1984): Defect in insulin receptor phosphorylation in erythrocyte and fibroblasts associated with severe insulin resistance. *J. Biol. Chem., 259,* 15003.

39. Okamoto M, White MF, Maron R, Kahn CR (1986): Autophosphorylation and kinase activity of insulin receptor in diabetic rats. *Am. J. Physiol., 251,* E542.
40. Burant CF, Treutelaar MK, Buse MG (1986): In vitro and in vivo activation of the insulin receptor kinase in control and denervated skeletal muscle. *J. Biol. Chem., 201,* 2985.
41. Burant CF, Treutelaar MK, Buse MG (1986): Diabetes induced functional and structured changes in insulin receptor from rat skeletal muscle. *J. Clin. Invest., 77,* 260.
42. Arner P, Einarsson K, Ewerth S, Livingston J (1986): Studies of the human liver insulin receptor in non-insulin-dependent diabetes mellitus. *J. Clin. Invest., 77,* 1716.
43. Kiechle FL, Jarrett L (1985): The molecular basis of insulin action: membrane associated reactions and intracellular mediators. In: Hollenberg MD (Ed.), *Insulin, Its Receptor and Diabetes,* p. 181. Dekker, New York.

The Diabetes Annual/3
K.G.M.M. Alberti and L.P. Krall, editors
© 1987 Elsevier Science Publishers, B.V.

25 Plasma lipids and lipoproteins in diabetes mellitus

M.F. LAKER

Introduction

Since lipids and lipoproteins were last reviewed in this series, 3 reviews considering this or related topics have appeared. These have focussed on metabolic aspects of diabetic hyperlipidaemia (1), the relationship of lipoproteins to atherosclerosis in diabetes (2), and diabetic vascular disease (3).

A large number of research papers have also been published and a comprehensive review of these would result in a disjointed presentation. Only selected aspects of the subject will therefore be considered. The following have been included: (a) lipoprotein abnormalities; (b) glycaemic control and blood lipids; (c) management of diabetic hyperlipidaemia; and (d) metabolism of lipoproteins in diabetes.

Lipoprotein abnormalities

Lipoprotein abnormalities in diabetes

A large cross-sectional study of 3300 Italian patients with diabetes has been undertaken to investigate the prevalence of hyperlipidaemia (4). The study included patients with IDDM and NIDDM. Overall, 5% of diabetic patients had Type IIA hyperlipidaemia as defined by the Fredrickson classification, 2% had Type IIB and 17% had Type IV hyperlipidaemia. The prevalence of macrovascular disease was 30% in hyperlipidaemic diabetic patients compared with 4.2% in diabetics with normal lipid levels. In hyperlipidaemic female diabetic subjects the prevalence of macrovascular disease was 43% compared to 16% in male patients, while 5.1% of normolipidaemic females had macrovascular disease compared to 2.9% of males. Smaller subgroups of matched patients with IDDM and NIDDM were investigated further. In 15 patients with IDDM there were positive correlations between concentrations of triglycerides, very-low-density lipoprotein (VLDL) and glycated haemoglobin, while in 15 patients with NIDDM glycated haemoglobin concentrations were not correlated with those of triglycerides or VLDL. In the latter group, however, there were positive correlations between concentrations of triglycerides, VLDL and body mass index.

A higher prevalence of hyperlipidaemia has been found in 23 patients with NIDDM who were not well controlled by diet or sulphonylurea treatment (5). Only 6 patients had normal lipid levels and the most common abnormalities — increased low-density lipoprotein (LDL) and increased VLDL concentrations — were found in 13 patients (56%). There was no significant relationship between insulin secretion, glycated haemoglobin, hepatic triglyceride lipase, lipoprotein lipase and lipids, although there was an increase in body weight in those patients with increased LDL and VLDL.

Lipoprotein abnormalities in IDDM have been studied by comparing findings in 51 male patients aged 35-70 years and 81 healthy control subjects (6). The mean glycated haemoglobin concentration was 9.1% in the diabetic patients. Mean total serum triglyceride concentrations were higher and total and LDL cholesterol concentrations were lower in IDDM although not significantly so. In contrast to an earlier study (7), apolipoprotein B (apo-B) concentrations were significantly lower in IDDM, a finding confirmed for male patients (8), although in the latter study similar concentrations of apo-B were found in female patients and control subjects. However, total cholesterol concentrations were higher in white female patients than in the corresponding controls (8). Winocour et al (6) calculated LDL-cholesterol/apo-B ratios and found that these were significantly elevated in IDDM, indicating that there was a substantially increased amount of cholesterol complexed with apo-B in LDL from these patients. These findings indicate that less dense particles were present. Since LDL concentrations were derived from the Freidwald calculation (9) intermediate-density lipoproteins (IDL) were included in the LDL fraction and the results were consistent with increased IDL particles accumulating in IDDM. The authors point out that the lipoprotein pattern is similar to that seen in Type III dyslipoproteinaemia in which accelerated peripheral vascular and coronary atherosclerosis both occur. The latter condition occurs in the presence of apo-E2 homozygosity, although it has also been described in patients with the E2/E3 phenotype and the E3/E3 phenotype (10). It was hypothesised that impaired binding of chylomicron remnants and IDL to hepatic receptors, which occurs in Type III dyslipoproteinaemia, also occurred in IDDM. Such findings might be expected if there were an increase in the E2 phenotype in IDDM, or if there were an increase in apo-CIII production, since this apolipoprotein blocks apo-E binding to hepatic receptors. It was also possible that insulin deficiency might affect the expression of the hepatic receptor or post-receptor events to produce these changes (6).

High-density lipoprotein (HDL) cholesterol is low in poorly controlled

IDDM, although it may be normal or raised in well-controlled IDDM and normal or low in NIDDM [see corresponding chapters in *The Diabetes Annual/1* (p. 463) and *2* (p.267)]. In the study by Winocour et al (6) HDL and HDL$_2$ cholesterol concentrations did not differ significantly from control values in IDDM and control subjects although HDL$_3$ cholesterol concentrations were higher in IDDM, as were the ratios of HDL cholesterol to LDL cholesterol and HDL cholesterol to total cholesterol. Higher HDL$_3$ cholesterol concentrations in diabetic boys and girls compared to those in their non-diabetic siblings have also been reported (11).

Using different criteria for the selection of patients, Laasko et al (12) have studied total HDL and HDL subfraction cholesterol concentration in diabetes. Serum lipids and lipoproteins were measured in 124 non-diabetic controls and in 170 patients (90 females and 80 males aged 45-64 years, mean glycated haemoglobin concentrations 10.4-11.3%) who were treated with insulin. In addition, the plasma C-peptide response to intravenous glucagon was investigated to classify patients according to their capacity for endogenous insulin secretion. Those with no C-peptide response (IDDM) had higher HDL and HDL$_2$ cholesterol concentrations than controls and HDL$_3$ cholesterol concentrations were lower in female but not male patients in this group. Patients with a high C-peptide response (NIDDM) had lower levels of HDL and HDL$_2$ cholesterol concentrations than the appropriate controls. Although not determined in this study, when the major apolipoproteins of HDL (apo-AI and AII) have been measured in NIDDM they have been low (7, 8, 13). Laasko et al (12) concluded that the elevated HDL and HDL$_2$ cholesterol concentrations in IDDM were not explained by the treatment but were associated with the type of diabetes. It is not clear to what extent differences in techniques used for lipoprotein subfractionation, the population studied or the degree of glycaemic control may have contributed to the contrasting findings of total HDL and HDL subfraction concentration in the studies by Winocour et al (6) and Laasko et al (12).

The above results were obtained from middle-aged patients. Plasma lipoprotein concentrations and lipoprotein lipase activities have been evaluated in young diabetic patients with and without episodes of ketonuria (14). Both ketotic and non-ketotic patients showed an impaired insulin and C-peptide responses to a glucose load in comparison with normal subjects. Ketotic patients had low HDL cholesterol and increased total and VLDL triglyceride and VLDL cholesterol concentrations with reduced lipoprotein lipase activity compared to control and non-ketotic NIDDM values.

Less marked changes in lipoproteins and lipolytic enzymes have been described in patients after pancreatectomy than occur in diabetes (15). Ten patients treated for chronic pancreatitis or carcinoma of the pancreas were studied after total pancreatectomy and compared with IDDM and controls matched for age, sex and weight. Insulin requirements in the pancreatectomised patients were less than in IDDM to achieve the same degree of glycaemic control. Concentrations of total, VLDL and HDL triglycerides were higher than in IDDM or in controls whereas total and LDL cholesterol concentrations were lower. HDL_2 cholesterol concentrations were similar in all 3 groups although HDL_2 triglyceride concentrations were higher after pancreatectomy. HDL_3 cholesterol concentrations were lower and HDL_3 triglyceride concentrations were higher in pancreatectomised patients. There were no significant differences in lipoprotein concentrations between IDDM and controls. Post-heparin lipoprotein lipase and hepatic triglyceride lipase activities were normal in all 3 groups, suggesting that the increased triglyceride concentrations were due to increased synthesis. It is not clear to what extent insulin, glucagon and exocrine deficiency may have affected the findings. It was suggested that exocrine deficiency, by inducing fat malabsorption, might be responsible for the lower LDL levels found after pancreatectomy.

Lipid and lipoprotein status has been studied in 85 Indian patients with non-insulin-dependent diabetes of the young (NIDDY) (16). The levels of glycaemic control were poorer than in the studies described above (mean glycated haemoglobin 13%). Serum total cholesterol, LDL cholesterol and apo-AI were similar to control values, although serum triglyceride and apo-B concentrations were higher in female patients. HDL cholesterol concentrations were lower in both male and female NIDDY patients. Serum triglycerides were significantly correlated with glycated haemoglobin and apo-B levels and negatively correlated with HDL cholesterol concentrations. These findings are similar to those found in a recent study of newly diagnosed adult patients with NIDDM (17).

Three studies have investigated the relationship between risk factors including lipoproteins and macrovascular disease in diabetes, two examining NIDDM (18, 19) and the other a mixed diabetic population (20). Total and LDL cholesterol had no significant association with definite myocardial infarction (18, 19) or cardiovascular disease (20). Lower HDL concentrations were noted in patients with vascular disease in all the studies, although in one (18) this finding was restricted to women. HDL subfraction analysis showed lower HDL_2 but similar HDL_3 cholesterol concentrations in post-myocardial-infarction NIDDM patients compared with those without vascular disease, although from the study design it was unclear whether the findings were predictive or a consequence of myocardial infarction. It is however of interest that HDL_2 has a stronger negative correlation with cardiovascular disease than total HDL or HDL_3 in non-diabetic patients (21).

Lipoproteins and 'potential abnormalities of glucose tolerance'

Results have recently been reported from two longitudinal studies which provide data on lipoproteins and potential abnormalities of glucose tolerance. In the Bogalusa Heart Study the relationship of lipoprotein concentrations and other cardiovascular risk factors to carbohydrate intolerance in children and a parental history of diabetes mellitus and cardiovascular disease has been examined (22-25). The design of the Framingham Study has also allowed the prevalence of hyperlipidaemia in subjects who later developed glucose intolerance to be studied (26).

The Bogalusa Heart Study is a long-term epidemiological investigation of cardiovascular risk factors in children from birth to 26 years of age living in Bogalusa, Louisiana. An initial cross-sectional survey of this population was undertaken in 1974, followed by 4 further cross-sectional surveys by 1982. The fourth survey collected data on 3312 children, 80% of the eligible population being included. Lipoprotein fraction concentrations, determined by electrophoresis, were related to measures of carbohydrate intolerance. Children with the highest β- and pre-β-lipoprotein concentrations were more obese and had greater serum insulin and glucose responses to an oral glucose load than their peers with lower lipid levels. Those with the lowest β and pre-β-lipoproteins had the lowest measures of obesity and carbohydrate tolerance (22). Fasting insulin levels were positively related to measures of obesity, blood pressure, serum triglycerides, pre-β- and β-cholesterol and negatively related to α-lipoprotein cholesterol concentrations. Fasting blood sugar was positively related to measures of obesity, blood pressure, serum triglycerides, pre-β-cholesterol and obesity (23). A parental history of diabetes was associated with the highest levels of total and LDL cholesterol, and triglycerides, particularly in those children whose lipid concentrations did not show regression to the mean (24, 25). The Framingham Study shows that elevated triglycerides and VLDL and reduced HDL are associated with obesity and precede the onset of diabetes (26).

Ganda et al (27) have examined plasma lipoproteins in the offspring of patients with NIDDM. Age- and weight-adjusted analyses of covariance were performed for glucose and insulin responses. Lipid concentrations in those offspring with normal glucose tolerance or in male offspring with abnormal glucose tolerance did not differ from control values; however, in female offspring with abnormal glucose tolerance, total and LDL cholesterol and total triglyceride were significantly elevated and HDL concentrations were lower than those in controls. It was concluded that significant sex differences in lipid metabolism occurred in the early stages of diabetes.

Eto et al (28) investigated lipoproteins and apolipoproteins in male subjects with impaired glucose tolerance and compared them with controls and NIDDM patients well matched for age and blood pressure. They showed that in NIDDM increased serum triglycerides, total and LDL cholesterol, apo-CII and apo-B concentrations were present with decreased HDL cholesterol concentrations. Apolipoprotein concentrations were similar to controls in subjects with impaired glucose tolerance, although triglycerides and LDL cholesterol and LDL/HDL cholesterol concentrations were greater than in controls. The relationship between the insulin response to intravenous glucose and plasma lipoproteins has been investigated in men with normal glucose tolerance by Capaldo et al (29). The insulin response was significantly correlated with VLDL triglyceride, VLDL cholesterol and VLDL + LDL/HDL cholesterol.

Glycaemic control and blood lipids

Diet

Conventional calorie-reduced diets are of limited effectiveness in treating obesity and thus very-low-calorie diets have been investigated to maximise particularly initial weight loss. Such diets have also been investigated in diabetes. Under closely supervised metabolic ward conditions, severe calorie restriction which allowed 200 kcal/d (30) or 300 kcal/d (31) have been shown to reduce significantly the serum cholesterol and triglyceride concentrations with no adverse medical effects. In one of these studies, caloric intake was gradually increased from severe restriction to amounts allowed in a conventional diabetic diet and although triglycerides and cholesterol increased with increasing calorie intake they were still significantly lower than values before the supplemented fast was commenced (30). Oral hypoglycaemic agents were withdrawn before these investigations were undertaken. The effect of more modest calorie restriction has been examined and whether this was more effective if combined with sulphonylurea treatment (32). Diets consisted of 1500 kcal/d less than the calculated requirements to maintain body weight, and two groups were studied (diet alone and diet plus glipizide). Cholesterol and triglycerides fell significantly in both groups, by similar amounts. Cholesterol fell by approximately 0.80 mmol/l and triglycerides by approximately 0.90 mmol/l. HDL cholesterol did not alter in either group.

The relationship between the composition of the diet and blood lipids in patients with IDDM has been explored in several studies. The influence of several dietary constituents has been examined by using the statistical technique of multiple regression analysis (33). A high consumption of polyunsaturated fats had a favourable influence on serum triglycerides while alcohol had an unfavourable influence. A high intake of vegetable protein and polyunsaturated fats was associated with lower serum cholesterol concentrations. Dietary fibre appeared to have an unfavourable influence on HDL cholesterol.

The question of whether sucrose affects blood lipids in diabetes has been examined in two recent studies (34, 35). In one, 45 g complex carbohydrate was replaced by 45 g sucrose in patients with IDDM and NIDDM: no significant difference in glycaemic control or blood lipids was noted (34). Differing results were obtained in the other study (35). Increasing sucrose from 1% to 16% of the caloric intake caused a significant elevation in total and VLDL triglyceride, and total and VLDL cholesterol concentrations. The increment in the sucrose content of the diet was greater in this study and the diet had a higher fat and lower fibre content. Increasing the simple sugar content of the diet in experimental animals while maintaining the amount of cereal fibre in the diet led to an increase in serum triglycerides, but this effect was negated if cereal fibre was replaced by leguminous fibre (36). Thus, the type of fibre may have an influence on the effect of simple sugars on serum lipids, at least in experimental animals.

Several further investigations of the effect of dietary fibre on lipids have been undertaken, either by simple additions to the diet, or increasing fibre while reducing the fat content. Reduction of fat from 45% of the caloric intake to 20% while increasing the polyunsaturated /saturated fat ratio and increasing the fibre content from 28 to 50 g/d over a 6-week period resulted in a 25% fall in total cholesterol due mainly to a fall in the LDL cholesterol concentration (37). The patients studied all had IDDM. Triglyceride concentrations initially rose on the experimental diet, although they appeared to return to control values in the last 2 weeks of the study.

Short-term investigation of the effects of fibre supplements have shown that some types of fibre lower serum cholesterol but have little effect on triglycerides (cf. *The Diabetes Annual/2*, p. 267). Longer-term studies have now been reported that demonstrate that the cholesterol-lowering action of guar gum is maintained over several months (38, 39). Some investigations have shown a hypocholesterolaemic effect with lower amounts of guar than previously described (40, 41), in one case with as low as 5 g guar per day incorporated into bread rolls (41). However, caloric intake was not constant in this study and it was suggested that self-imposed dietary restriction resulted from greater satiety while taking guar. Not all studies describe a lowering of serum cholesterol, however, no significant changes in blood cholesterol being noted by Jones et al (42) using guar granules, 10 g daily, for 2 months. Glycaemic control was however improved. Feeding 4-6 granola bars to which were added 6.6 g guar gum each day to a small group of obese patients with NIDDM resulted in a decrease in LDL cholesterol in male subjects but not in females after 6 months (43). Xanthan gum which, unlike guar, is resistant to bacterial breakdown in the colon, has been shown to have a hypocholesterolaemic effect, at least in short-term studies (44).

Other fibres which have been examined include wheat bran and cellulose. Total cholesterol fell with both, although the calculated LDL cholesterol concentration did not decrease with the addition of fibre supplements. Unlike some other fibres, adding 30 g cellulose per day to the diet also reduced serum triglycerides (45). A high cereal intake when combined with a high-carbohydrate, low-fat diet led to a decrease in LDL cholesterol in compliers (46); fibre supplements from vegetable sources have been shown to be well tolerated with the hypocholesterolaemic effect maintained over long periods (47). In contrast to a previous study (48), apple bran, while not affecting total cholesterol, was found to reduce LDL cholesterol while increasing HDL cholesterol concentrations (49). Increasing physical exercise, either by itself or when combined with dietary modification, did not improve blood lipids in IDDM or NIDDM (50-52).

A possible alternative to ingesting viscous fibre is to impair the intestinal digestion of simple carbohydrates with a non-digestible enzyme inhibitor. The α-glucosidase inhibitor, acarbose, inhibits the activities of α-amylase, sucrase and maltase. Its long-term effects have been investigated in a group of NIDDM patients, poorly controlled with diet and drugs (53). Treatment, which was undertaken for 1 year, resulted in an improvement in glycaemic control. Total cholesterol concentrations fell initially but were not significantly different from baseline after 20 weeks. There was an unexpected fall in cholesterol 6 weeks after treatment had stopped. HDL cholesterol initially rose, although this change was not maintained. Triglycerides were unaltered. Thus, there was no evidence for any sustained beneficial effect of acarbose on blood lipids.

Diets in experimental animals

The effects of safflower and marine fish oil have been investigated in rats (54). The animals were placed on a standard or oil-supplemented diet for 10 days and then rendered diabetic: blood metabolites and lipids were then followed. Total triglyceride concentrations were initially lower in the oil-fed groups but rose significantly after the administration of streptozotocin. They were unaltered in animals fed on standard chow. Cholesterol concentrations were also raised in oil-fed animals. It was considered that this was more likely to be due to defective clearance of lipoproteins, although lipolytic enzyme activities were not measured. The authors conclude that there should be caution in recommending fish-oil diets to diabetic patients, at least until further studies are undertaken.

The addition of vitamin E to the diet of diabetic rats limited the increase in blood triglycerides that otherwise occurred (55). Higher activities of hepatic triglyceride and lipoprotein lipase activities were noted in vitamin-E-treated animals and it was hypothesised that this effect was mediated by the vitamin protecting membrane-bound lipases against peroxidative damage.

Diabetic rats become hyperphagic when fed diets low in fat but reduce their caloric intake when fat is added to the diet (56). The possibility that this was due either to a response to the utilization of fat fuels or to reduced loss of urinary glucose with fat feeding was investigated. Animals were fed a fixed ration of food in which either fat or carbohydrate were reduced in equal caloric amounts, with substitution by cellulose. The animals did not increase feeding with prior reduction in carbohydrates but did so if fat was reduced. The more fat that was consumed during rationing, the greater the increase in blood triglycerides and ketone bodies when the animals were allowed to eat *ad libitum* and the less they then ate. Since the animals increased food intake with prior reduction of fat intake, but not carbohydrate, increased intake after the reduction appeared to be specific to fat.

Drug therapy of IDDM

A study of children and adolescents with IDDM has been reported in which the patients were divided into 3 groups according to their glycated haemoglobin concentrations: less than 9%, 9-11% and greater than 11% (57). In female adolescents with poor control, triglyceride and apo-B concentrations were raised while HDL cholesterol and phospholipids and the ratio of HDL/non-HDL cholesterol was reduced. Results were similar in male patients except that there were no reductions in HDL cholesterol or phospholipids. Glycated haemoglobin was directly correlated with triglyceride, total cholesterol, phospholipid and apo-B concentrations and inversely with HDL cholesterol, HDL phospholipid and HDL/non-HDL cholesterol. In well-controlled children, lipid concentrations are very similar to those in control subjects, although a small but significant increase in VLDL-cholesterol has been noted (58). Using multivariate analysis, serum glucose, glycated haemoglobin, glycated serum proteins and insulin dose were found to be significantly related to several serum lipid variables (triglyceride, VLDL and HDL cholesterol, apo-AI, apo-AII and apo-B) even in the absence of marked dyslipoproteinaemia. It was calculated that 40% of the variation in total cholesterol, HDL cholesterol and apo-AII might be explained by the combined effects of serum glucose, glycated haemoglobin, glycated serum proteins and insulin dose.

HDL composition may fluctuate rapidly during treatment of diabetic ketoacidosis with continuous low-dose intravenous infusion of insulin (59). In this study, 13 patients were investigated, 6 with IDDM of whom 3 presented for the first time with ketoacidosis. Seven patients were treated with oral hypoglycaemic agents but became ketotic during episodes of stress. Those with unequivocal IDDM had low HDL cholesterol concentrations on admission, although HDL cholesterol almost doubled within 24 hours of treatment. These findings were almost entirely due to changes in HDL_2 cholesterol concentrations. Those patients who had been treated with oral hypoglycaemic agents presented with near-normal HDL cholesterol concentrations, although these fell during the first 24 hours of treatment.

Insulin has also been shown to have acute effects on serum triglycerides and cholesterol in normolipidaemic patients with NIDDM who were investigated using the glucose clamp technique (60). Triglycerides decreased by 15% and cholesterol by 8%. The rate of decrease of cholesterol, but not of triglyceride, was correlated with the glucose infusion rate.

Intensification of insulin treatment, either by increasing the frequency of injections to 4-5 per day or by giving continuous infusion, has been reported to produce varying effects on lipoproteins, including reducing VLDL cholesterol (61), increasing HDL cholesterol and apo-A (62), and decreasing apo-B concentrations (8). Low HDL cholesterol concentrations in NIDDM may not increase when hyperglycaemia is controlled by insulin (63). In one study of two patients continuous intravenous infusion of insulin was without effect on serum cholesterol over 3 years, although triglycerides were reduced (64), while in another, continuous insulin infusion produced no change in triglycerides but reduced total cholesterol by a small amount, while increasing HDL/LDL cholesterol (65).

Biosynthetic human insulin produces no greater changes in lipoproteins in diabetes than does porcine insulin (66).

Oral hypoglycaemic drugs

The effect of sulphonylurea therapy on lipids and HDL composition has been investigated in a group of obese Pima Indians who were treated with tolazamide for 1 month (67). Diet did not change and weight remained constant. Therapy produced a significant fall in total and LDL cholesterol, and total and VLDL triglycerides, even though the patients were normolipidaemic at the start of treatment. HDL cholesterol and phospholipids, and apo-AI concentrations were unchanged although there was a change in HDL composition, increased HDL_2 cholesterol concentrations being noted, with a greater molar ratio of HDL_2 cholesterol/apo-AI. In hyperlipidaemic patients with NIDDM glyburide reduced VLDL cholesterol in Type IV hyperlipidaemia while HDL increased in patients with mixed hyperlipidaemia (68). The drug produced increased HDL cholesterol concentrations in some patients although the changes were not significant. Gliclazide reduces triglycerides in NIDDM although probably not independently of its hypoglycaemic effect (69).

Differing effects of combined insulin/sulphonylurea treatment have been reported. No changes in lipoproteins occurred when glyburide was combined with insulin therapy in NIDDM (70) while the addition of chlorpropamide to insulin treatment in IDDM lowered total, LDL and HDL_3 cholesterol concentrations without altering the HDL/LDL cholesterol ratio (71). When directly compared, no difference in lipoprotein levels was found in patients treated with insulin or sulphonylureas (72). Patients with NIDDM have low HDL cholesterol concentrations irrespective of the mode of treatment (73).

Management of diabetic hyperlipidaemia

The principles of the management of diabetic hyperlipidaemia have been outlined by Chait (74). The objectives of treatment are to try to slow the appearance and progression of atherosclerotic complications and to prevent the development of chylomicron-induced pancreatitis. Both the NIH (75) and the European Atherosclerosis Group (to be published) consider that a goal for serum cholesterol below 6.5 mmol/l is both desirable and achievable, although this figure will not be accepted by all. The guidelines outlined by Chait (74) for treating hypercholesterolaemia in diabetes were (74):

a. Where modest increases in cholesterol occur which result from increased HDL cholesterol, no action should be taken.
b. Where hypercholesterolaemia occurs because of increased LDL cholesterol, dietary management should be initially undertaken. Obese patients should be treated with a calorie-reduced diet, the amount of saturated dietary fat should be reduced and glycaemic control should be improved.
c. If elevated cholesterol with increased LDL cholesterol persists or is due to a familial cause, it should be treated with drugs. A bile-acid-sequestering agent is probably the most appropriate first-line drug, although such treatment may lead to increased serum triglycerides. Nicotinic acid, fibrate drugs and probucol may have a role, as may hydroxymethylglutaryl coenzyme A (HMG-CoA) reductase inhibitors, when they become more widely available (76).

Chait's approach to the treatment of diabetic hypertriglyceridaemia may be considered controversial by many. He does not recommend treating hypertriglyceridaemia to reduce the risks of atherosclerosis but only to prevent pancreatitis and he considers pancreatitis unlikely below 22 mmol/l triglyceride. For the management of diabetes in these circumstances oral hypoglycaemic agents, particularly sulphonylureas, are preferred to insulin as insulin may increase VLDL production. Fibrate drugs are agents of choice if hypertriglyceridaemia persists.

Beta-blocking drugs and diuretics

Beta-blockers and diuretics, particularly thiazides, cause disturbances in lipoprotein metabolism; diabetic patients, particularly those with NIDDM, are more likely to be treated with these drugs than their non-diabetic peers (18). Antihypertensive agents thought unlikely to worsen lipid risk factors in diabetes include prazosin (77), calcium antagonists (78), hydralazine (79) and reserpine (80). The beta-blocker, celiprolol, has been shown to raise triglycerides in diabetes (81).

Lipoprotein metabolism

The intestine and lipid metabolism in diabetes

The intestine is an insulin-insensitive organ that can synthesise triglycerides from endogenous substrates during times of fasting (82). The possibility that increased triglyceride synthesis from endogenous substrates occurs in diabetic rats has been investigated (83). Fatty acid esterification and the activities of acyl-CoA synthetase and acyl-CoA monoglyceride acyltransferase were the same in diabetic and control rats when expressed per milligram of protein. However, these activities were increased when expressed per centimetre of gut length because of marked intestinal hypertrophy. In animals with mesenteric lymphatic fistulae there was a twofold increase in triglyceride synthesis in fasting diabetic rats, VLDL production being increased. There were no differences in response to lipid infusion by diabetic and control animals. The rate of incorporation of exogenous triglyceride into chylomicrons was reduced in diabetic rats.

The small intestine appears more permeable to cholesterol in diabetic rats than in controls (84) and intestinal cholesterol synthesis is also increased (85). This may occur in all sections of the small intestine, although limiting the intake of food reduces cholesterol synthesis (86).

Chylomicron metabolism and lipolytic enzymes

There appear to be diabetes-induced changes in chylomicron composition which result in a reduced rate of catabolism of these lipoproteins. When chylomicrons from diabetic rats were injected into normal recipients, they were found to be removed more slowly than chylomicrons from non-diabetic animals (87). Chylomicrons and chylomicron remnants from diabetic animals were depleted in apo-E, and the apo-AI content was also reduced. Pre-incubation of these chylomicrons with normal rat HDL resulted in more rapid catabolism. The relative contribution of these changes and reduced lipoprotein lipase activity to impaired catabolism of triglyceride-rich particles in diabetes is unclear. Although it is well established that lipoprotein lipase activity is reduced in diabetes, it is unclear whether hepatic triglyceride lipase is insulin-sensitive (88-90).

Apolipoprotein E metabolism

The possibility that some of the lipoprotein abnormalities in IDDM may be explained by an unusual pattern of apo-E isoforms in diabetes has been referred to above (6) and reduced apo-E content of chylomicrons has been reported in diabetes (87). Others have noted reduced total serum apo-E (91) and reduced VLDL and HDL apo-E (92) in experimental diabetes. In addition to affecting the catabolism of triglyceride-rich particles, apo-E deficiency may reduce the hepatic uptake of cholesterol from HDL (93). Studies in man have shown that the E2/E3 phenotype occurs more frequently in diabetic patients than in control populations (94, 95) and the ratio returns towards a normal frequency with insulin treatment (95). These changes are thought to be due to increased sialation of apo-E in diabetes.

Glucosylation and lipoprotein metabolism

Lipoproteins may be modified by glucosylation and greater degrees of glucosylation of LDL apo-B have been reported in diabetic subjects than in controls, 2-5% of lysine residues on LDL apo-B being modified in IDDM compared with less than 2% in non-diabetic subjects (96, 97). In vitro metabolism of glycated apo-B has been studied by exposing LDL to very high glucose concentrations in the presence of sodium cyanoborohydride and radioactively labelling modified LDL. When this LDL was incubated with cultured fibroblasts, internalisation and catabolism via apo-B-specific receptors was reduced while catabolism receptor-independent pathways was unaffected (97, 98). If a greater proportion of LDL is catabolised by receptor-independent pathways the risk of atherosclerosis developing is thought to be greater (99). Using lipoproteins chemically modified by the above procedure, LDL catabolism may be impaired to an extent similar to that seen in heterozygous familial hypercholesterolaemia (100).

While there is little disagreement that chemically modified glycated LDL may be catabolised more slowly than normal LDL, it is unclear if native glycated LDL from diabetics is subject to altered metabolism. One group (101) have reported that LDL which was naturally glucosylated to an extent similar to that seen in diabetes was metabolised more slowly than normal LDL by receptor-mediated pathways, while others were unable to show such impairment (102). The reasons for these differences are not immediately apparent, but both depended on glucosylation in vitro for the preparation of test material.

Most experimental work on glucosylation of apoproteins has examined apo-B and LDL metabolism. However, apo-AI, AII, B, CI and E have all been shown to be glycosylated in hyperglycaemic diabetic subjects (103). The functional significance of these findings has yet to be investigated.

Glucosylation could also affect lipoprotein metabolism by other mechanisms, such as modifying receptors or by affecting molecules which in turn may affect lipoprotein metabolism. This latter possibility has received some attention in relation to advanced-glucosylation end-products (AGE). AGE are produced by further reactions and rearrangements to Amadori products in stable molecules such as collagen and nucleic acids. They are brown fluorescent chromophores which can cause additional cross-linkages to occur between proteins (104). Collagen has been demonstrated to form AGE in vitro and such collagen covalently binds LDL (105). If such a phenomenon occurred in vivo, it could cause increased trapping of LDL particles within arterial walls and lead to excessive fibrous plaque formation.

Cellular uptake and metabolism of lipids and lipoproteins

One of the most consistent findings in studies of lipoproteins in diabetes is that VLDL of abnormal composition are found or IDL particles accumulate. Kraemer et al (106) have investigated the uptake of VLDL from NIDDM patients by mouse peritoneal macrophages. Diabetic VLDL had a greater cholesterol and triglyceride content than VLDL from normal subjects and although VLDL from both sources were taken up by the macrophages there was greater accumulation of diabetic VLDL. Murine macrophages contain high-affinity VLDL receptors and thus these findings cannot be directly extrapolated to human macrophages.

The effect of insulin deficiency on cholesterol metabolism in mouse macrophages has been investigated (107). Thioglycolate-elicited macrophages from insulin-deficient animals showed increased activity of HMG-CoA reductase, the rate-limiting enzyme of cholesterol biosynthesis. Treatment with insulin returned HMG-CoA reductase activities to normal and the activities of this enzyme were normal in mice with diet-induced hyperlipidaemia. Cell-surface receptors for VLDL uptake were reduced in diabetic animals while insulin treatment increased their number. The net effect of these changes was that intracellular cholesterol synthesis was increased in diabetic animals.

The uptake of LDL from diabetic and non-diabetic hypertriglyceridaemic sources has been investigated in cultured human skin fibroblasts (108). Binding of LDL from diabetic and non-diabetic hypertriglyceridaemic patients was significantly decreased compared with diabetic and non-diabetic normolipidaemic controls; LDL from diabetic and non-diabetic hypertriglyceridaemic patients caused less inhibition of LDL receptor activity and intracellular sterol synthesis than LDL from healthy subjects. The ability to suppress LDL receptor activity was inversely related to the ratio of triglyceride to protein in LDL. Thus, although LDL from hypertriglyceridaemic diabetic subjects was less efficient at down-regulating LDL receptor activity and intracellular sterol synthesis than normal LDL, this appeared to be due to factors associated with hypertriglyceridaemia rather than diabetes.

The effect of diabetic lipoprotein-deficient serum (LPDS) on LDL uptake and degradation by fibroblasts has been investigated (109). Binding, internalization and degradation of LDL from normal or diabetic subjects was significantly reduced when LPDS from poorly controlled diabetic subjects was present. Such LPDS had higher non-esterified fatty acid, lecithin, apo-A, and immunoreactive insulin contents and the addition of palmitic and oleic acids to pooled normal LPDS reduced degradation of LDL. Thus, reduced internalization and degradation of LDL in diabetes may be due to factors other than lipoprotein composition.

Conclusions

Since this topic was last reviewed in this series (*The Diabetes Annual/ 2*, p. 267) approximately 100 papers describing research into lipids and lipoproteins in diabetes have appeared. These have confirmed that hyperlipidaemia is more common in diabetic than in non-diabetic subjects, with higher triglycerides being the most common abnormality. HDL cholesterol is low in poorly controlled IDDM but rises with effective treatment while HDL cholesterol is often low in NIDDM. Abnormalities of HDL subfractions have been described, although findings have differed. There is increasing evidence that the composition of lipoproteins is altered in diabetes, both lipid and apolipoproteins being affected. The metabolic consequences of these findings have yet to be established.

References

1. Gibbons GF (1986): Hyperlipidaemia of diabetes. *Clin. Sci., 71*, 477.
2. Schonfield G (1985): Diabetes, lipoproteins and atherosclerosis. *Metabolism, 34, Suppl. l*, 45.
3. Feingold KR, Siperstein MD (1986): Diabetic vascular disease. *Adv. Intern. Med., 31*, 309.
4. Solerte SB, Carnevale Schiana GP, Adamo S et al (1985): Lipid and lipoprotein changes in diabetes mellitus in relation to metabolic control and vascular degenerative complications. *Med. Biol. Environ., 13*, 755.
5. Hayashi K, Matsumoto H, Ito K et al (1984): The change of serum lipoproteins observed in non-insulin dependent diabetic patients and a study of its mechanism. *Hiroshima J. Med. Sci., 33*, 619.
6. Winocour PH, Durrington PN, Ishola M et al (1986): Lipoprotein abnormalities in insulin dependent diabetes mellitus. *Lancet, 1*, 1176.
7. Schernthauer G, Kostner GM, Dieplinger H et al (1983): Apoproteins (A-I, A-II, B), Lp(a) lipoprotein and lecithin: cholesterol acyl transferase activity in diabetes. *Atherosclerosis, 49*, 277.
8. Gonen B, White N, Schofield G et al (1985): Plasma levels of apolipoprotein B in patients with diabetes mellitus: the effect of glycaemic control. *Metabolism, 34*, 675.
9. Freidwald WT, Levy RI, Fredrickson DS (1972): Estimation of serum low density lipoprotein cholesterol concentration without the use of preparative ultracentrifugation. *Clin. Chem., 18*, 499.

10. Havel RJ, Kotite L, Kane JP et al (1983): Atypical familial dyslipoproteinaemia associated with apolipoprotein phenotype E3/E3. *J. Clin. Invest., 72*, 379.
11. Cruikshanks KJ, Orchard TJ, Becker DJ (1985): The cardiovascular risk profile of adolescents with insulin-independent diabetes mellitus. *Diabetes Care, 8*, 118.
12. Laasko M, Voultilainen E, Sarland S et al (1985): Inverse relationship of serum HDL and HDL$_2$ cholesterol to C-peptide level in middle-aged insulin treated diabetics. *Metabolism, 34*, 715.
13. Martin BC, Pometta D, Grab B et al (1984): Relations entre le cholestérol HDL et la glycémie à jeûn dans une population normale et un groupe de diabétiques. *Schweiz. Med. Wochenschr., 114*, 1834.
14. Rubba P, Capaldo B, Falanga A et al (1985): Plasma lipoproteins and lipoprotein lipase in young diabetics with and without ketonuria. *J. Endocrinol. Invest., 8*, 433.
15. Kiviluoto T, Schroder T, Karonen S-L et al (1985): Glycaemic control and serum lipoproteins after total pancreatectomy. *Ann. Clin. Res., 17*, 110.
16. Jialal I, Deppe W, Joubert SM (1985): Lipid and lipoprotein aberrations in Indian patients with non-insulin dependent diabetes in the young. *South Afr. Med. J., 67*, 1001.
17. Uusitupa M, Siitonen O, Pyorala K et al (1985): The relationship of cardiovascular risk factors to the prevalence of coronary heart disease in newly diagnosed type 2 (non-insulin dependent) diabetes. *Diabetologia, 28*, 653.
18. Uusitupa M, Siitonen O, Voutilainen E et al (1986): Serum lipids and lipoproteins in newly diagnosed non-insulin dependent (type II) diabetic patients, with special reference to factors influencing HDL-cholesterol and triglyceride levels. *Diabetes Care, 9*, 17.
19. Laasko M, Voutilainen E, Pyolara K et al (1985): Association of low HDL and HDL$_2$ cholesterol with coronary heart disease in non-insulin dependent diabetes. *Arteriosclerosis, 5*, 653.
20. Maserai JRL, Kiiveri HT, Stanton K (1986): Risk factors for cardiovascular disease in a diabetic population. *Pathology, 18*, 89.
21. Miller NE, Hammett F, Saltissi S et al (1981): Relation of angiographically defined coronary artery disease to plasma lipoprotein subfractions and apoproteins. *Br. Med. J., 282*, 1741.
22. Radhakrishnamurthy B, Srinivasan SR, Webber LS et al (1985): Relationship of carbohydrate intolerance to serum lipoprotein profiles in children: The Bogalusa Heart Study. *Metabolism, 34*, 850.
23. Burke GL, Webber LS, Srinivasan SR et al (1986): Fasting plasma glucose and insulin levels and their relationship to cardiovascular risk factors in children: Bogalusa Heart Study. *Metabolism, 35*, 441.
24. Shear CL, Webber LS, Freedman DS et al (1985): The relationship between parental history of vascular disease and cardiovascular disease risk factors in children: The Bogalusa Heart Study. *Am. J. Epidemiol., 122*, 762.
25. Freedman DS, Shear CL, Srinivasan SR et al (1985): Tracking of serum lipids and lipoproteins in children over an 8-year period: The Bogalusa Heart Study. *Prev. Med., 14*, 203.
26. Kannel WB (1985): Lipids, diabetes, and coronary heart disease: insights from the Framingham Study. *Am. Heart J., 110*, 1100.
27. Ganda OP, Soeldner JS, Gleason RE (1985): Alterations in plasma lipids in the presence of mild glucose intolerance in the offspring of two type II diabetic parents. *Diabetes Care, 8*, 254.
28. Eto M, Watanabe K, Sekiguchi M et al (1985): Plasma lipids, lipoproteins and apoproteins in subjects with impaired glucose tolerance. *J. Jpn. Diabetic Soc., 28*, 1049.
29. Capaldo B, Rivellese A, Santoro D et al (1985): Relationship between insulin response to intravenous glucose and plasma lipoprotein in healthy man. *Artery, 13*, 108.

30. Vessby V, Selinns I, Lithell H (1985): Serum lipoprotein and lipoprotein lipase in over-weight type II diabetics during and after supplemental fasting. *Arteriosclerosis, 5,* 93.
31. Henry RR, Wiest-Kent TA, Scheaffer L et al (1986): Metabolic consequences of very-low-calorie diet therapy in obese non-insulin-dependent diabetic and non-diabetic subjects. *Diabetes, 35,* 155.
32. Liu GC, Couston AM, Lardinois LK et al (1985): Moderate weight loss and sulfonylurea treatment of non-insulin-dependent diabetes mellitus. *Arch. Intern. Med., 145,* 665.
33. Van der Beek EJ, Wedel M, Van de Zedde A et al (1984): The relationship of diet, body composition, physical activity and the quality of metabolic control to blood lipid levels in type-1-diabetic men. *Int. J. Sports Med., 5, Suppl.,* 59.
34. Peterson DB, Lambert J, Gerring S et al (1986): Sucrose in the diet of diabetic patients — just another carbohydrate? *Diabetologia, 29,* 216.
35. Coulston AM, Hollenbeck CB, Donner CC et al (1985): Metabolic effects of added dietary sucrose in individuals with non-insulin dependent diabetes mellitus (NIDDM). *Metabolism, 34,* 962.
36. Calle-Pascual AL, Marenco G, Asis MJ et al (1986): Effects of different proportions of carbohydrates, polysaccharides/monosaccharides and different fibers on the metabolic control in diabetic rats. *Metabolism, 35,*919.
37. Hollenbeck CB, Connor WE, Riddle MC et al (1985): The effect of a high-carbohydrate low-fat cholesterol restricted diet on plasma lipid, lipoprotein and apoprotein concentrations in insulin-dependent (type I) diabetes mellitus. *Metabolism, 34,* 559.
38. Vaaler S, Hanssen KF, Dahl-Jorgensen K (1986): Diabetic control is improved by guar gum and wheat bran supplementation. *Diabetic Med., 3,* 230.
39. Uusitupa M, Tuomilehto J, Karttunen P et al (1984): Long term effects of guar gum on metabolic control, serum cholesterol and blood pressure levels in type 2 (non-insulin-dependent) diabetic patients with high blood pressure. *Ann. Clin. Res., 16, Suppl. 43,* 126.
40. Tagliaferro V, Cassader M, Bozzo C et al (1985): Moderate guar-gum addition to usual diet improves peripheral sensitivity to insulin and lipaemic profile in NIDDM. *Diabète Métab., 11,* 380.
41. McNaughton JP, Morrison DD, Huhner LJ et al (1985): Changes in total serum cholesterol levels of diabetic fed five grams guar gum daily. *Nutr. Rep. Int., 3,* 505.
42. Jones DB, Slaughter P, Lonsley S et al (1985): Low-dose guar improves diabetic control. *J. R. Soc. Med., 78,* 546.
43. McIvor ME, Cummings CC, Van Duyn MA et al (1986): Long-term effects of guar gum on blood lipids. *Atherosclerosis, 60,* 7.
44. Osilesi O, Trout DL, Glover EE et al (1985): Use of xanthan gum in dietary management of diabetes mellitus. *Am. J. Clin. Nutr., 42,* 597.
45. Harold MR, Reeves RD, Bolze MS et al (1985): Effect of dietary fiber in insulin-dependent diabetics: insulin requirements and serum lipids. *J. Am. Diet. Assoc., 85,* 1455.
46. Pacy PJ, Dodson PM, Fletcher RF (1986): Effect of a high carbohydrate, low sodium and low fat diet in type 2 diabetics with moderate hypertension. *Int. J. Obesity, 10,* 43.
47. Story L, Anderson JW, Chen W-JL et al (1985): Adherence to high-carbohydrate, high-fiber diets: long-term studies in non-obese diabetic man. *J. Am. Diet., Assoc., 85,* 1105.
48. Mahalko JR, Sandstead HH, Johnson LK et al (1984): Effect of consuming fiber from corn bran, soy husks or apple powder on glucose tolerance and plasma lipids in Type II diabetes. *Am. J. Clin. Nutr., 39,* 25.
49. Onumi T, Tsutsui M, Kudo M et al (1984): Clinical studies on apple fiber for diabetic patients — influence of the fiber on lipoprotein metabolism and glucose tolerance. *J. Jpn. Diabetic Soc., 27,* 759.

50. Kaplan RM, Wilson DK, Hartwell SL et al (1985): Prospective evaluation of HDL cholesterol changes after diet and physical conditioning programmes for patients with type II diabetes mellitus. *Diabetes Care, 8,* 343.
51. Wallberg-Henrickson H, Gunnarsson R, Rossner S et al (1986): Long-term physical training in female type 1 (insulin-dependent) diabetic patients: absence of significant effect on glycaemic control and lipoprotein levels. *Diabetologia, 29,* 53.
52. Lithell H, Krotkiewski M, Kiens B et al (1985): Non-response of muscle capillary density and lipoprotein-lipase activity to regular training in diabetic patients. *Diabetes Res., 2,* 17.
53. Uttenthal LO, Ukponmwan OO, Wood SM et al (1986): Long-term effects of intestinal alpha-glucosidase inhibition on postprandial glucose, pancreatic and gut hormone responses and fasting serum lipids in diabetics on sulphonylureas. *Diabetic Med., 3,* 155.
54. Illman RJ, Trimble RP, Storer GB et al (1986): Time-course of changes in plasma lipids in diabetic rats fed diets high in fish or safflower oils. *Atherosclerosis, 59,* 313.
55. Pritchard KA, Patel ST, Karpen CW et al (1986): Triglyceride-lowering effect of dietary vitamin E in streptozotocin induced diabetic rats: increased lipoprotein lipase activity in livers of diabetic rats fed high dietary vitamin E. *Diabetes, 35,* 278.
56. Friedman MI, Ramirez I, Edens MK et al (1985): Food intake in diabetic rats: isolation of primary metabolic effects of fat feeding. *Am. J. Physiol., 249,* R44.
57. Jos J, Thevenin M, Dumont G et al (1985): Effet du contrôle métabolique sur les lipides et lipoprotéines plasmatiques dans le diabète insulino-dépendant de l'enfant et de l'adolescent. *Diabète Métab., 11,* 174.
58. Stroble W, Widhalm K, Schoher E et al (1985): Apolipoproteins and lipoproteins in children with type 1 diabetes: relation to glycosylated serum proteins and HbA$_1$. *Acta Paediatr. Scand., 74,* 966.
59. Joven J, Rubies-Prat J, De la Figuera M et al (1985): High density lipoprotein changes during treatment of diabetic ketoacidosis. *Diabète Métab., 11,* 102.
60. Morita S, Nakata K, Tanaka T et al (1985): The acute effects of insulin on plasma triglyceride and cholesterol observed with the glucose clamp technique. *J. Jpn. Diabetic. Soc., 28,* 845.
61. Goldberg RB, Reeves MJ, Seigler DE et al (1985): Lack of a persistent reduction in serum lipid and apoprotein levels in insulin-dependent diabetic patients receiving intensified insulin treatment. *Acta Diabetol. Lat., 22,* 93.
62. Wilson DP, Fesmire JD, Endres RK et al (1985): Increased levels of HDL-cholesterol and apolipoprotein A-1 after intensified insulin therapy for diabetes. *South. Med. J., 78,* 636.
63. Hollenbeck CB, Chen Y-DI, Greenfield MS et al (1986): Reduced plasma high density lipoprotein-cholesterol concentrations need not increase when hyperglycaemia is controlled with insulin in non insulin-dependent diabetes mellitus. *J. Clin. Endocrinol. Metab., 62,* 605.
64. Blackshear PJ, Shulman GI, Koussell AM et al (1985): Metabolic response to three years of continuous, basal rate intravenous insulin infusion in type II diabetic patients. *J. Clin. Endocrinol. Metab., 61,* 753.
65. Chute EP, Barbosa JJ, Rupp WM et al (1985): Reduction of plasma cholesterol and LDL-cholesterol by continuous intravenous insulin infusion. *Surgery, 98,* 655.
66. Marchetti P, Benzi L, Cerri M et al (1986): Biosynthetic human insulin does not modify circulating lipid and apolipoprotein concentrations in type 1 diabetic patients. *Acta Diabetol. Lat., 23,* 63.
67. Howard BL, Xiaoren P, Harper I et al (1985): Effect of sulfonylurea therapy on plasma lipids and high-density lipoprotein composition in non-insulin-dependent diabetes mellitus. *Am. J. Med., 79, Suppl. 3B,* 78.

68. Hughes TA, Kramer JO, Segrest JP (1985): Effects of glyburide therapy on lipoproteins in non-insulin-dependent diabetes mellitus. *Am. J. Med., 79, Suppl. 3B,* 86.
69. Delargy M, McGovern M, Johnson A et al (1985): Gliclazide: the effects on lipids in type II diabetes. *Ir. J. Med. Sci., 154,* 102.
70. Falko JM, Osei K (1985): Combination of insulin/ glyburide therapy in type II diabetes mellitus. *Am. J. Med., 79, Suppl. 3B,* 92.
71. Seviour PW, Teal TK, Richmond W et al (1986): Chlorpropamide lowers serum and lipoprotein cholesterol in insulin-dependent diabetics. *Diabetic Med., 3,* 152.
72. Kasim SE, LeBoeuf RC, Rockett MJ et al (1986): The effects of oral agents or insulin-treatment on the plasma lipoproteins and the plasma lipoproteins lipase activator in diabetic patients. *Horm. Metab. Res., 18,* 190.
73. Laasko M, Voutilainen E, Sarland H et al (1985): Serum lipids and lipoproteins in middle-aged non-insulin-dependent diabetes. *Atherosclerosis, 56,* 271.
74. Chait A (1985): Hyperlipidaemia: forestalling complications in older diabetics. *Geriatrics, 40,* 71.
75. Consensus Conference (1985): Lowering blood cholesterol to prevent heart disease. *J. Am. Med. Assoc., 253,* 2080.
76. Yoshino G, Kazumi T, Uenogamia R et al (1986): Probucol versus eptastatin in hyper-cholesterolaemic diabetics. *Lancet, 2,* 740.
77. Weinberger MH (1986): Antihypertensive therapy and lipids. *Am. J. Med., 80, Suppl. 2A,* 64.
78. Trost BN, Weidmann P, Beretta-Piccoli C (1985): Antihypertensive treatment in diabetic patients. *Hypertension, 7, Suppl. II,* II-102.
79. Rodriguez B, Goyal RK, McNeill JH (1986): Effects of hydralazine on streptozotocin-induced diabetic rats: prevention of hyperlipidaemia and improvement in cardiac function. *J. Pharmacol. Exp. Ther., 237,* 292.
80. Vargase S, Devi KS (1985): Effects of serpasil on lipids, lipoprotein lipase and lipogenic enzymes in alloxan diabetic rats. *J. Biosci., 9,* 53.
81. Janka HU, Petschke H, Mehrert H (1985): The effects of beta-blocker therapy with celiprolol on metabolism in diabetics treated with insulin. *Med. Klin., 80,* 764.
82. Shiau Y-F, Holtzapple PG (1980): Effect of insulin on in vitro intestinal fatty acid esterification in the rat. *Am. J. Physiol., 238,* E364.
83. Popper DA, Shiau Y-F, Reed M (1985): Role of small intestine in pathogenesis of hyper-lipidaemia in diabetic rats. *Am. J. Physiol., 249,* G161.
84. Hotke C, McIntyre T, Thompson ABR (1985): Jejunal uptake of sugars, cholesterol, fatty acids, and fatty alcohols in vivo in diabetic rats. *Can. J. Physiol. Pharmacol., 63,* 1356.
85. Feingold KR, Wiley MH, MacRae G et al (1982): The effect of diabetes mellitus on sterol synthesis in the diabetic rat. *Diabetes, 31,* 388.
86. Feingold KR, Moser AH (1984): Localization of cholesterol synthesis in the small intestine of diabetic rats. *Am. J. Physiol., 247,* G494.
87. Levy E, Shefrir E, Ziv E et al (1985): Composition, removal and metabolic fate of chylomicrons derived from diabetic rats. *Biochim. Biophys. Acta, 834,* 376.
88. Nomora T, Hagino Y, Gotoh M et al (1984): The effects of streptozotocin diabetes on tissue specific lipase activities in the rat. *Lipids, 19,* 594.
89. Murase T, Inoue S (1985): Hepatic triglyceride lipase is not an insulin-dependent enzyme in rats. *Metabolism, 34,* 531.
90. Mueller DL, Sandek CB, Applebaum-Bowden D (1985): Hepatic triglyceride lipase in diabetic dogs. *Metabolism, 34,* 251.
91. Yamada N, Murase T, Iwamoto Y et al (1984): Reciprocal changes of plasma Apo A1 and E levels in streptozotocin-induced diabetic rats. *Horm. Metab. Res., 16,* 85.

92. O'Looney P, Irwin D, Briscoe P et al (1985): Lipoprotein composition as a component in the lipoprotein clearance defect in experimental diabetes. *J. Biol. Chem., 260*, 428.
93. Wilson DE, Chan I-F, Elstall M et al (1986): Apolipoprotein E-containing lipoproteins and lipoprotein remnants in experimental canine diabetes. *Diabetes, 35*, 933.
94. Sano R, Abe R, Oikawa S-I et al (1985): Apo E-2/E-3 ratio of very low density lipoprotein in diabetes mellitus. *Tohoku J. Exp. Med., 146*, 131.
95. Takegoshi T, Haba T, Takeshita H et al (1985): Analysis of lipoprotein pattern and VLDL apo C and E isoform of diabetic patients. *J. Jpn. Diabetic Soc., 28*, 721.
96. Schleicher E, Deufel T, Wieland OH (1981): Non-enzymatic glycosylation of human serum lipoproteins. *FEBS Lett., 129*, 1.
97. Witztum JL, Mahoney EM, Branks MJ et al (1982): Non enzymatic glucosylation of low-density lipoprotein alters its biologic activity. *Diabetes, 31*, 283.
98. Gonen B, Baenziger J, Schonfield G et al (1981): Nonenzymatic glycosylation of low density lipoprotein in vivo. *Diabetes, 30*, 875.
99. Ross R (1986): The pathogenesis of atherosclerosis — an update. *N. Engl. J. Med., 314*, 488.
100. Kesaniemi YA, Witztum JL, Steinbrecher UP (1983): Receptor-mediated catabolism of low density lipoprotein in man. *J. Clin. Invest., 71*, 950.
101. Steinbrecher UP, Witztum JL (1984): Glucosylation of low-density lipoproteins to an extent comparable to that seen in diabetes slows their catabolism. *Diabetes, 33*, 130.
102. Schleicher E, Olgemoller B, Schon J et al (1985): Limited non-enzymatic glucosylation of low-density lipoprotein does not alter its catabolism in tissue culture. *Biochim. Biophys. Acta, 846*, 226.
103. Curtiss LK, Witztum JL, (1985): Plasma apolipoproteins AI, AII, B, CI and E are glucosylated in hyperglycaemic diabetic subjects. *Diabetes, 34*, 452.
104. Cerami A, Vlassara H, Brownlee M (1985): Protein glycosylation and the pathogenesis of atherosclerosis. *Metabolism, 34, Suppl. 1*, 37.
105. Brownlee M, Vlassara H, Cerami A (1985): Non enzymatic glucosylation products on collagen covalently trap low-density lipoprotein. *Diabetes, 34*, 938.
106. Kraemer FB, Chan Y-DI, Lopez RD et al (1985): Effects on non-insulin-dependent diabetes mellitus on the uptake of very low density lipoproteins by thioglycolate-elicited mouse peritoneal macrophages. *J. Clin. Endocrinol. Metab., 61*, 335.
107. Kraemer FB (1986): Insulin deficiency alters cellular cholesterol metabolism in murine macrophages. *Diabetes, 35*, 764.
108. Hiramatsu K, Bierman EL, Chait A (1985): Metabolism of low-density lipoprotein from patients with diabetic hypertriglyceridaemia by cultured human stem fibroblasts. *Diabetes, 34*, 8.
109. Lopes-Virella MF, Sherer G, Wohltmann H et al (1985): Diabetic lipoprotein deficient serum: its effect in low density lipoprotein (LDL) uptake and degradation by fibroblasts. *Metabolism, 35*, 1079.

The Diabetes Annual/3
K.G.M.M. Alberti and L.P. Krall, editors
© 1987 Elsevier Science Publishers, B.V.

26   In vitro and in vivo effects of insulin on protein metabolism*

TERESA J. NELSON AND MOREY W. HAYMOND

Introduction

The protein anabolic effects of insulin were first recognized as the ability of insulin to reverse the nitrogen losses associated with uncontrolled diabetes mellitus (1). The mechanism(s) by which this protein anabolic effect is mediated has been the subject of a large number of investigations both in vitro and in vivo; both increased rates of protein synthesis and decreased rates of protein degradation have been reported. Although detailed, well-controlled studies have shed substantial light on the biochemical and molecular effects of insulin in a variety of body tissues in a number of species, the precise role which insulin plays in the physiological (or pathophysiological) regulation of amino acid and protein metabolism in specific tissues, among specific organs and, most pertinently, in man, remains to be clearly established. The present Chapter attempts to review some of the in vitro and in vivo data and identify areas of uncertainty which will require further exploration.

Studies involving the regulation of amino acid and/or protein metabolism are complex because of the presence of multiple amino acid pools, intracellular regulation of proteolysis and protein synthesis involving a variety of proteins and peptide molecules, as well as the effects of other substrates and hormones on amino acid and protein metabolism of the tissue(s) under investigation. Due to the complexity of these multiple factors, a given experimental model (or condition) cannot control all of the variables and every experimental strategy or probe has limitations. As a result, it is imperative that the experimental condition and the assumption(s) (whether stated or implied) of the model employed, whether in vitro or in vivo, be carefully and thoughtfully examined.

In vitro studies involving cell suspensions, incubated tissues or perfused organs have the distinct advantage that the milieu to which these tissues are exposed can be precisely defined and controlled. As a result, the effect of a single variable can be carefully examined. Whether the results of such experiments

*Supported by US Public Health Service, NIH AM 26989 and MAYO Clinic and Foundation.

can be extrapolated to the same tissue in vivo or to whole-body amino acid or protein metabolism must be confirmed. In addition, with the exception of cell cultures, the viability of the tissues or cells under examination in any in vitro investigation must be carefully examined. In vitro tissues have limited viability. Protein synthesis is highly energy-dependent, and therefore the relative rates of proteolysis and protein synthesis in any given tissue preparation may provide an indication of the tissue's viability. In many in vitro studies in which both of these processes have been evaluated, rates of proteolysis greatly exceed rates of protein synthesis, a condition which most likely does not exist in vivo (Table 1). The specific experimental conditions (e.g. temperature, type and concentrations of available substrates, utilization of collagenase) to which the tissue is exposed will affect the results obtained from such experiments. In addition, maintenance of passive stretch on incubated muscle has recently been reported to ameliorate the high rates of protein degradation observed in vitro (4).

TABLE 1   *Rates of tyrosine incorporation and release from incubated rat muscle: in vitro indicators of protein synthesis and proteolysis*

Muscle	Tyrosine incorporation into protein	Tyrosine release	Ref no.
Diaphragm (nmol of Tyr/h per mg of muscle)	0.15 ± 0.01	0.29 ± 0.02	2
Soleus (µmol of Tyr/g of protein per 3 h)	1.33 ± 0.10	4.29 ± 0.25	3
Extensor digitorum longus (µmol of Tyr/g of protein per 3 h)	0.69 ± 0.04	2.54 ± 0.10	3

Primary cell cultures provide a more viable system for the study of protein metabolism since they can be maintained viable for periods of days as opposed to hours for tissues incubated in vitro (5). Tissues that replicate in vitro are generally transformed or malignant cells whose protein and amino acid metabolism may not be normally regulated (6). Therefore, the results derived from the study of these tissues must be interpreted with caution. Despite these problems, the information obtained from such studies has been invaluable in exploring the cellular mechanisms involved in the regulation of both amino acid and protein metabolism.

In vivo studies of amino acid and protein metabolism should be superior to those of in vitro experiments because they are usually carried out under normal physiologic conditions. However, such studies are considerably more complex than in vitro experiments since it is nearly impossible to define and control all the experimental parameters. As a result, it may be difficult to compare experimental results between studies because of differences in species, strategies or experimental models employed.

Due to ethical considerations, human studies are generally limited to the sampling of plasma, breath, and/or waste products and the use of isotopically labeled compounds. In the absence of direct tissue or whole-body analysis, all indicators of tissue and/or whole-body protein metabolism are derived by indirect means. Thus, the plasma space is not in total equilibrium with the amino acid pool(s) where protein synthesis, proteolysis, or amino acid catabolism occur and therefore change in plasma amino acid concentrations or specific activities may not directly reflect changes in the intracellular metabolism of amino acids and protein. In addition, well-defined subject populations and experimental design may not completely control for the metabolic variables encountered in studies in vivo. Definition of the circulating substrate and hormone concentrations is imperative but generally limited to their peripheral circulating plasma concentrations and the breadth of analytical capacity of the investigating laboratory. Therefore, the influence of insulin on amino acid and protein metabolism can only be reviewed when the reader is aware of the constraints of both in vitro and in vivo models of amino acid and protein metabolism.

In vitro effects of insulin on amino acid and protein metabolism

On a cellular level, the total protein content at steady state is determined by a balance between the rates of protein synthesis and protein degradation (7). The rate of protein synthesis is determined by the availability of intracellular amino acids as well as the rate of each step involved in the process of protein synthesis. The availability of intracellular amino acids for protein synthesis is influenced by the rate of cellular uptake of amino acids, amino acid oxidation and the cytoplasmic appearance of amino acids from intracellular proteolysis. The rate of protein degradation is determined by the proteolytic enzymes present and factors which regulate their activities.

Protein synthesis

Whether intracellular amino acids are derived from the extracellular space (via transport) or from proteolysis within the cell, they enter a complex process ultimately resulting in the synthesis of protein. This protein synthetic process involves cellular uptake, formation of tRNA amino acyl complexes, mRNA, ribosomes, initiation of peptide chain formation, elongation of the peptide chain, as well as posttranslational modifications (8). The influence of insulin on each of these processes may vary with the tissue and the in vitro experimental conditions.

Cellular uptake of amino acids was the first component of protein metabolism on which the effect of insulin was studied in vitro. Studies of isolated rat diaphragm cultured with radiolabeled α-aminoisobutyrate (AIB), a non-metabolizable synthetic amino acid, demonstrated an increased intracellular uptake of AIB in the presence of insulin (9), suggesting that insulin might enhance amino acid uptake and thus protein synthesis. The enhancement of AIB uptake by insulin has also been demonstrated in hepatocytes (10). However, in these studies, the concentration of insulin required in vitro to demonstrate this effect on AIB uptake was between 100 and 13,000 μU/ml, the latter clearly outside the physiologic range (5). Furthermore, it remains doubtful that the influence of insulin on protein metabolism can result from increased amino acid uptake *per se* since insulin does not increase the transport of all essential amino acids, which would be required for a stimulatory effect on protein synthesis to occur by this mechanism alone (11-13). It has indeed become apparent that there are several specific amino acid transport systems on the cell membrane which may have differing responses to insulin (12). As a result, one may conclude that although amino acid availability can be rate-limiting for protein synthesis, the stimulatory effect of insulin on protein synthesis is not a result of an insulin-mediated effect on amino acid transport.

Insulin could also have an effect on the interaction of tRNAs with amino acids. In studies using embryonic chick heart and skeletal muscle cell cultures (14) and isolated rat epitrochlearis muscle (15), insulin enhanced the protein synthetic rate calculated by measuring the rate of incorporation of [3H]leucine into protein and the specific activity of tRNA-bound leucine. As opposed to the rapid effect of insulin on glucose metabolism in skeletal muscle, a lag period of more than 15 minutes was required before an insulin dose-dependent increase in protein synthesis became apparent (15). However, insulin had no influence on the specific activity of the tRNA-bound leucine (14, 15). These studies suggest that the effect on protein synthesis involves processes beyond the charging of tRNAs with amino acids. Both of these studies calculate protein synthesis based on the assumption that total tissue tRNA-specific activity represents a single intracellular pool from which protein synthesis occurs. Although this is logical, little information is available to validate this assumption (16).

The utilization of charged tRNA—amino acid complexes for the synthesis of protein requires the presence of mRNA. In vivo studies measuring the relative amount of [3H]leucine incorporated into hepatic total protein and albumin in alloxan-induced (17) and spontaneous diabetic rats (18) demonstrated a decrease in albumin synthesis relative to total protein synthesis when compared to controls. This decrease was accompanied by a specific reduction in albumin mRNA. The changes in albumin synthetic rates and albumin mRNA content occurred over a 3-day course after the induction of diabetes and normalized within 3 days of insulin therapy (19). Concomitant liver perfusion studies permitted measurement of the rate of protein synthesis based on the rate of incorporation of [^{3}H]leucine into total liver proteins and albumin. In these liver perfusion studies, livers from insulin-deficient diabetic rats had significantly lower rates of protein synthesis which was most marked with regard to albumin (17). In these animals, the rate of albumin synthesis in vitro was normal following in vivo insulin replacement. Perfusion studies which employed insulin replacement in the perfusate required more than an hour of perfusion before a change in the protein synthetic rate was demonstrated. In addition, no change in the half-life of albumin mRNA, ribosomal half-transit-time for total protein and albumin and the average sizes of total and albumin-synthesizing polysomes was observed in the insulin-deficient animals. However, there was a decrease in the number of albumin-synthesizing polysomes (19) and total cellular RNA (18). This suggests that protein synthesis in liver is decreased in the absence of insulin because of: (a) decreased total RNA, of which 80% is ribosomal (20), required for the actual process of protein synthesis; and (b) decreased amounts of specific mRNAs required for the production of a given protein such as albumin.

In the normal (21) and diabetic rat hemicorpus, insulin-deficient perfusion media (20) decreased total muscle RNA. In more recent studies, the production of several mRNA species in diabetic rat hearts are influenced (both increased and decreased) by insulin. The actual identification of the protein products of these mRNAs remains to be established (22, 23). However, this suggests that in cardiac muscle, as in liver, insulin may influence protein synthesis by altering the production of specific mRNAs.

The formation of ribosomes requires the presence of a peptide chain initiation factor(s). Using an isolated perfused rat heart model, impaired peptide chain initiation and protein synthesis were corrected by the addition of insulin to the perfusate (24). This has also been shown in rat skeletal muscle but requires more than 1 hour of insulin deficiency (24). The actual mechanism by which this occurs appears to be the result of the presence of an inhibitor of peptide chain initiation which is produced in response to insulin deficiency (25). This inhibitor is either present in an amount which does not interfere with peptide chain initiation or absent altogether in insulin-replete rat muscle (25). Thus, in rat liver and cardiac muscle, the rate of production of mRNA is influenced by insulin. In rat skeletal muscle, the effect of insulin on protein synthesis appears to be mediated, at least in part, via the activity of peptide-chain initiation factor. The specific effect of insulin on actin and myosin mRNA remains to be clarified.

The ability of insulin to stimulate protein synthesis may be tissue-dependent. Thus, the ability of insulin to stimulate protein synthesis is dependent in part on muscle fiber composition (red *vs* white) (26), whereas in other tissues such as rat lung, insulin may have little or no effect on protein synthesis (27).

Therefore, the effect of insulin on protein synthesis varies both in degree and mode of action between various tissue types, but does not appear to be related to enhanced amino acid uptake or charging of tRNA complexes. The tissue specificity of the effect of insulin on protein synthesis appears to be related to differences in rates of mRNA production and peptide chain initiation. Any effects of insulin on amino acid uptake may be secondary to stimulation of protein synthesis, i.e. enhanced protein synthesis which leads to decreased intracellular concentrations of free amino acids and a secondary increase in uptake of extracellular amino acids.

Proteolysis

In recent studies, rates of protein degradation have also been demonstrated to be influenced by insulin. These studies largely involve the use of rat liver perfusion systems and isotope dilution methods. In the absence of insulin in the perfused rat liver, negative nitrogen balance occurs as a result of release of free amino acids rather than the secretion of proteins. When insulin is added, this loss of free amino acids is decreased (28). In the presence of cycloheximide, a protein synthetic inhibitor, the net loss of free amino acids is increased, presumably due to the inhibition of reincorporation of amino acids released from proteolysis (28). However, in the presence of both insulin and cycloheximide, the net loss of free amino acids is reduced, suggesting that insulin decreases proteolysis within the liver. This hypothesis is further strengthened by the observation that insulin: (a) decreased the rate of catabolism of the enzyme, 5-adenosyl methionine decarboxylase, as estimated by changes in its activity in perfused heart (29); (b) decreased the release of [^{3}H]leucine from prelabeled hepatocytes (30); (c) increased the specific activity of [^{14}C]phenylalanine added to rat heart perfusate (29); and (d) decreased the release of free amino acids from the perfused rat hindquarter (31). Taken together, these data provide strong evidence that a major effect of insulin in vitro is to decrease proteolysis and that this effect is probably not tissue-specific.

The mechanism(s) by which insulin alters proteolysis at a cellular level is not well understood. In liver, lysosomes are the predominant site of proteolysis (30, 32). In muscle, cytosolic enzymes are responsible for myofibrillar proteolysis, a process which is probably not sensitive to insulin (4, 33). As in liver, muscle lysosomes appear to be insulin-sensitive and are responsible for the degradation of non-myofibrillar protein (33). The role that cytosolic enzymes play in the catabolism of non-myofibrillar protein in skeletal muscle and whether this process (if it occurs) is affected by insulin remains to be determined. However, these studies suggest that less than 25% of the proteolytic activity of muscle under these study conditions can be inhibited by pharmacologic amounts of insulin and is restricted to non-myofibrillar proteins (33). The investigation of muscle is further complicated by the fact that the proteins in the myofibrillar unit may not turn over at the same rate, suggesting selective protein degradation of some components and re-utilization of others (34).

Increased lysosomal size within hepatocytes has been reported in association with increased proteolysis. In liver perfusion studies, insulin decreases the number of enlarged lysosomes (35). Both biochemical and electron-microscopic evidence from experiments with hepatocyte monolayer suspensions suggests that insulin prevents autophagy (30). The decrease in proteolytic activity with ischemia or anoxia in the perfused heart suggests that proteolysis, as is known for protein synthesis, is at least in part an energy-requiring process (29), an observation in agreement with previous studies in *Escherichia coli* (36).

In summary, the preponderance of in vitro evidence suggests that an important role of insulin is the suppression of proteolysis. This insulin effect may be mediated via the regulation of lysosomes, and appears to be tissue-independent. However, the breakdown of myofibrillar protein, a major constituent of body protein, may not be sensitive to insulin. In addition, it remains to be determined whether insulin has a direct effect on protein catabolic enzymes or if its action is mediated indirectly by altering substrate availability for energy production since insulin affects the mobilization, transport and metabolism of a variety of nutrients.

In vivo studies

Although insulin affects the metabolism of both protein and amino acids in specific tissues, extrapolating these findings to whole-body protein metabolism is more difficult. It has been long recognized that, in diabetics, insulin deficiency leads to negative nitrogen balance and muscle wasting and that insulin replacement results in positive nitrogen balance (1) and a presumed normalization of amino acid and protein metabolism. Nitrogen balance studies require multiple accurate collections of urine and stool and knowledge of the dietary intake. The difference between nitrogen intake and losses provides an indication of net nitrogen balance. Changes in net nitrogen balance could be the result of changes in protein catabolism and/or anabolism. Thus, nitrogen balance studies can provide little insight into the mechanism(s) by which these changes occur. In contrast, isotope dilution methods employing ^{15}N-labeled non-essential amino acids or labeled essential amino acids may provide information about the mechanism(s) but may not be quantitative.

Nutritional (and presumably hormonal) factors regulate plasma amino acid concentrations (37). Fasting in obese individuals (38) or insulin withdrawal in diabetics (39) results in an increase in the plasma concentration of most amino acids, whereas refeeding or glucose infusion in normal volunteers (37) or insulin administration in diabetics (37, 39) decreases their plasma concentrations. In recent studies, an insulin dose-dependent decrease in the plasma concentrations of most amino acids (except glycine and alanine) has been observed in normal subjects (40-42).

To determine the role that skeletal muscle may play in insulin regulation of the plasma amino acid concentration, arterio-venous differences across the forearm have been carried out (43). Intra-arterial infusion of insulin increased the arterio-venous difference of most amino acids, demonstrating decreased release and/or increased uptake. Although the local insulin concentrations were very high, the local infusion of insulin did not affect the arterial circulating plasma concentrations of the amino acids and, in addition, had little systemic effect on glucose and free fatty acid concentrations. In normal volunteers with normal plasma amino acid concentrations, net amino acid release was observed from the splanchnic bed and leg (44) whereas paradoxically in insulin-withdrawn diabetics with high plasma amino acid concentrations, net uptake at both sites occurred (44). This raises questions about the source and mechanism of the high amino acid concentrations in poorly controlled diabetic patients and about the information and conclusions which can be drawn from organ balance studies.

The interpretation of amino acid data derived from organ balance studies is not straightforward due to the complexity of the metabolism of individual amino acids. Thus, the branched-chain amino acids (leucine, isoleucine and valine) can be taken up by tissues, incorporated into protein, or transaminated to their respective α-keto acids and either released or oxidized locally, making interpretation difficult, if not impossible. In contrast, phenylalanine, which is not metabolized by muscle, may provide a more appropriate measure of directions of change across muscle but cannot be used for splanchnic balance studies because of the hepatic metabolism of this essential amino acid (45). Inclusion of a labeled amino acid permits the calculation of a minimum rate of amino acid uptake and release, but due to differences in the intra- and extracellular specific activity of the infused amino acid tracer (see discussion below), organ rates of proteolysis and protein synthesis derived from such data can only be considered semiquantitative. Therefore, the exact interpretation of the effects of insulin on forearm amino acid metabolism requires further study.

Use of ^{15}N-labeled non-essential amino acids (primarily [^{15}N]glycine) has been widely applied to the study of whole-body protein metabolism. This method, as initially described by Picou and Taylor-Roberts (46), utilizes an infusion or oral administration of trace and measurement of the enrichment of ^{15}N in urinary urea (and as subsequently modified, urinary NH_3 as well) (47). To obtain steady-state enrichment in the end-products, a prolonged duration (24-36 h) of isotope administration is required (47). This analytical probe is advantageous in that total protein metabolism can be examined and the results are less dependent on the metabolism of any single amino acid (and any subsequent extrapolation to whole-body protein). This technique has been extremely useful for estimating whole-body rates of proteolysis and protein synthesis when comparing one nutritional state with another. However, the time required to achieve a new steady state constitutes the major drawback when attempting to discern the acute effects of a given hormone or substrate on amino acid and protein metabolism. In addition, recycling of trace (as discussed below) could result in a significant underestimation of the rate of protein turnover. As a result, recent studies have been carried out using a labeled infusion of an essential amino acid.

The most widely utilized essential amino acid trace for in vivo isotope dilution studies has been leucine which has been employed to investigate in vitro protein metabolism for many years (48). Intracellular leucine can be incorporated directly into cellular proteins or can be metabolized. The initial step in the catabolism of leucine is the reversible transamination to its α-ketoacid, α-ketoisocaproate (KIC). KIC can be re-aminated back to leucine, transported out of the cell, or undergo irreversible decarboxylation of its 1-carbon via branched-chain α-ketoacid dehydrogenase. This latter process results in the release of CO_2 and the production of isovaleryl coenzyme A (49). Thus, labeled leucine for in vivo studies is advantageous because the intra- and extracellular concentrations of the free amino acid pools are similar (50, 51) and the decarboxylation of the leucine carbon skeleton is a measure of the irreversible catabolism of this essential amino acid when the 1-^{14}C label is used.

Golden and Waterlow (47) originally described the use of labeled leucine in human studies. The dilution of the infused trace in the plasma space provides an estimate of the entry of unlabeled leucine (or rate of appearance, Ra). Under steady-state conditions, the rate of entry and removal of leucine are presumed to be equal and represent the flux (Q) of leucine through the metabolic pool being sampled. As a result, leucine entry can be from the diet (I, intake) and endogenous protein breakdown (B) and removal via oxidation (O) and protein synthesis (S). Thus,

$$Ra = Q = I + B = O + S$$

Since most studies have been carried out in the post-absorptive overnight fasted condition, the intake (I) is zero. Therefore,

$$Q = B = O + S$$

Using a constant infusion of [1-^{14}C]leucine and traditional isotope dilution methods, leucine flux (Q, μmol/min) is calculated by dividing the infusion rate of [1-^{14}C]leucine (dpm/min) by the plasma leucine-specific activity (dpm/μmol). Leucine oxidation is calculated by dividing the rate of expired $^{14}CO_2$ (dpm/min) by the plasma leucine specific activity and by 0.8 to correct for CO_2 fixation (52). Using the above equation, the rate of leucine entering protein can be estimamated by subtracting the rate of leucine oxidation from the rate of leucine flux (7).

Results obtained from studies employing an infusion of labeled leucine must also be interpreted with care and extrapolations to whole-body protein metabolism only considered in the light of the limitations of the isotope dilution model employed. At least 4 assumptions can be identified which must be considered in evaluating the accuracy and quantitative nature of leucine turnover and oxidation data (16): (a) the labeled and unlabeled leucine are metabolized identically (i.e. no isotope effect); (b) the label is distributed in a single metabolic pool; (c) release of label incorporated into body protein does not occur over the course of study (no recycling of label); and (d) the plasma specific activity (or enrichment) of the tracer accurately reflects that of the intracellular space.

The absence of an isotope effect in studies in vivo remains a basic assumption upon which all isotope dilution models are based. However, such effects have been clearly identified for a number of species of hydrogen-labeled glucose tracers (53-55). Different per cent recoveries of $^{13}CO_2$ and $^{14}CO_2$ have been reported during infusion of labeled bicarbonate (56). In addition, the peak rate of expiration of $^{13}CO_2$ has been reported to be later than that of $^{14}CO_2$ following simultaneous injection of the respective carbon-labeled leucine tracers (57), although the total fraction of expired label was similar over a 4-hour period of breath collection. Therefore, isotope effects may exist with tracers of leucine. This would not preclude their use in obtaining new and useful information but would prevent precise quantitative measurements.

The assumption that whole-body leucine exists in a single metabolic pool is clearly naive and a contrivance of the steady-state isotope dilution model used. When the decay data from a bolus infusion of a leucine tracer is plotted on a semilogarithmic scale, a curvilinear plot results. Using curve stripping techniques or more sophisticated data analysis programs at least 3 compartments can be identified (58). Interpretation of bolus kinetic data requires steady-state conditions throughout the sampling period and therefore does not permit the assessment of an acute metabolic effect during an experimental perturbation. It is for this reason that we have preferred to use the constant isotope infusion technique which will minimize pool differences under 'plateau' or pseudo-steady-state conditions. For a discussion of the advantages and disadvantages of bolus *versus* constant infusions of trace, the reader is referred to several reviews (16, 59, 60).

During infusion of leucine (and presumably any amino acid tracer), label is incorporated into body proteins which are being synthesized over the course of the experiment. For proteins with long biologic half-lives in relation to the duration of the study, the loss of trace is functionally irreversible. However, for proteins and peptides with short biologic half-lives, the leucine tracer may be incorporated into and subsequently released via proteolysis back into the free amino acid pool over the course of the experiment (recycling of tracer). Using a constant infusion of leucine trace and the isotope dilution calculations described above, the rate of entry of tracer into the vascular space will be greater than the measured exogenous infusion rate of isotope. Thus, assuming that the specific activity (or enrichment) of the plasma leucine can be accurately measured, the calculated rate of appearance of leucine will be underestimated.

In recent studies from our (61, 62) and other (63) laboratories, recycling of infused tracer has appeared to be a significant problem. Up to 30% of the tracer entering the plasma space following a 24-hour infusion of label would appear to be derived from such a process (61). Isotope recycling most likely begins within minutes of the initiation of an infusion of a leucine tracer and a portion of the time required to achieve a 'steady state' may involve the recycling of tracer out of these short-half-lived proteins. Use of bolus infusion of isotope may minimize this problem but will not eliminate it. This does not mean that meaningful data cannot be derived from in vivo isotope dilution techniques employing labeled amino acids — however, the calculated rate of appearance of the amino acid into the vascular space will be underestimated, as will any other estimates derived from this value. Therefore, these studies must be carefully designed to include appropriate control experiments, values derived from such studies must be considered to be semiquantitative, and conclusions drawn only after the impact of isotope recycling on the results is carefully considered.

An additional factor that may lead to an underestimation of leucine kinetics is the use of the plasma leucine specific activity (or enrichment) during infusion of labeled leucine (a primary pool model) (64). Since the isotope is delivered into the intravascular space and leucine derived from proteolysis enters the intracellular space, equilibration of the label between the intra- and extracellular leucine compartments is likely to be incomplete. However, leucine (together with the other branched-chain amino acids) is unique in that the first step in its catabolism involves reversible transamination to KIC, a substrate which can be measured in plasma. Matthews et al (65) and Rennie et al (66) originally proposed using the plasma enrichment of $[^{13}C]$KIC during infusion of $[1\text{-}^{13}C]$leucine as the precursor of leucine oxidation since KIC is the immediate substrate for the irreversible decarboxylation of the leucine carbon skeleton. We have extended this concept by using the plasma specific activity (or enrichment) of the transaminated product of the leucine carbon trace to estimate the specific activity of intracellular leucine (reciprocal pool model) (64). In rats, the intracellular leucine specific activity in liver and muscle during labeled leucine infusion was nearly identical to the plasma KIC specific activity (67). Additional work will be required to provide further validation for the use of the transaminated product of an infused leucine tracer as an indicator of the intracellular leucine specific activity. Plasma leucine specific activity during the infusion of labeled leucine may provide valid estimates of direction of change in the rate of appearance of endogenous leucine and oxidation in the postabsorptive state; however, this may not be the case when unlabeled leucine is administered orally or intravenously and estimates of appearance rate of endogenous leucine are calculated.

Only a limited number of studies have been carried out in diabetic human subjects using infusions of labeled leucine. In hyperglycemic diabetic patients withdrawn from insulin for 14-18 hours and fasted overnight, the rate of appearance of leucine into the plasma space and the rate of leucine oxidation were increased when compared to normal subjects or normoglycemic, insulin-infused diabetic subjects (68, 69). These data are consistent with an increased rate of whole-body proteolysis in the insulin-deficient state (Table 2). Since the in-

TABLE 2 *Effect of insulin withdrawal on leucine metabolism in diabetic human subjects*

	Rate of appearance	Oxidation $(\mu mol \cdot kg^{-1} \cdot h^{-1})$	Nonoxidative rate of disappearance
Nair et al (68)			
Normal subjects	85 ± 9	15 ± 3	70 ± 9
Insulin-withdrawn diabetic subjects	$116 \pm 7*$	$30 \pm 5*$	$87 \pm 13*$
Robert et al (69)			
Insulin-infused diabetic subjects	88 ± 4	19 ± 3	69 ± 1
Insulin-withdrawn diabetic subjects	$108 \pm 7*$	$35 \pm 9*$	73 ± 3

* < 0.05 compared with normal or insulin-infused diabetic subjects.

crease in leucine oxidation was not proportional to the increase in appearance rate of leucine, the calculated rate of leucine entering protein (non-oxidative rate of leucine disappearance) was not decreased, but rather increased (although the increase was significant in only one of the two studies). Although the results of these two studies (68, 69) are in close agreement, it is difficult to conclude that the changes in leucine metabolism were the result of insulin insufficiency *per se* since the circulating plasma concentrations of other hormones and substrates were not the same in the control and insulin-withdrawn subjects.

To evaluate the effects of acute insulin withdrawal on leucine metabolism, Abumrad et al (70) used the pancreatic clamp dog model of Cherrington. In these studies, an acute decrease in the plasma insulin concentration resulted in an increase in the plasma leucine concentration but no change in the rate of entry of unlabeled leucine. These results suggest that acute withdrawal of insulin below a certain basal concentration may have no effect on proteolysis but affect leucine removal (or clearance). We (71) and others (72) have obtained similar results during acute insulin withdrawal in diabetic human subjects and during somatostatin infusion in normal human subjects. However, several factors must be considered in the interpretation of these studies. A major difference between these studies and those of Nair et al (68) and Robert et al (69) is the duration of isotope infusion: 3-4 hours for those of Nair and Robert *versus* 7-10 hours for our study (71) and those of Abumrad (70, 72). Increased recycling of label with the longer isotope infusion might give rise to decreased estimates of leucine flux. Whether isotope recycling contributes to the differences between the studies of Abumrad and co-workers and those of Robert and Nair cannot be clearly ascertained. However, it should be pointed out that in the Abumrad studies (70), no increase in the net balance of leucine or KIC was observed across a number of tissue beds during acute insulin deficiency. However, when Tsalikian repeated the acute insulin withdrawal studies originally carried out in our laboratory but employing two 4-hour infusions of leucine trace (one during insulin infusion and one 4 hours after insulin withdrawal), a clear and significant increase in leucine flux was observed within 6 hours of discontinuation of the insulin (73). Therefore, during studies employing prolonged infusion of leucine tracer, recycling of trace must be considered when the plasma concentration of leucine increases in the absence of a change in entry of unlabeled leucine (62).

Insulin infusion not only leads to a decrease in the plasma concentration of leucine and other amino acids but to a decrease in the rate of appearance of unlabeled leucine. Recent studies by Fukagawa et al (74) and Tessari et al (41, 42) have demonstrated a dose-response relationship between the rate of appearance of unlabeled leucine and the plasma concentration of insulin employing the euglycemic clamp technique. Similar results were observed in both studies despite the fact that a sequential infusion of insulin was used in one (41, 42) and individual clamp studies were carried out on separate days in the other (74). Thus, despite potential problems of isotope recycling and the use of a primary pool model (plasma enrichment or specific activity of leucine), these data provide strong evidence that insulin decreases whole-body proteolysis. It is of interest to note that in both of these studies the absolute suppression of the rate of appearance of leucine was only 30%. If a reciprocal pool model (plasma enrichment or specific activity of KIC) was used as an indicator of the intracellular enrichment or specific activity of leucine, the suppression of the rate of appearance of leucine is closer to 20% despite unphysiologically high plasma concentrations of insulin. If extrapolations of these data to whole-body protein metabolism can be made, 70% or more of the proteolytic activity in man is unresponsive to acute and pharmacologic increases in the plasma insulin concentration. An additional factor that must be considered in these studies in whether the increasing rates of glucose infusion (and utilization) which are required to maintain euglycemia during exogenous insulin infusion affect leucine metabolism.

In similar studies carried out in diabetic subjects, a dose-response relationship between insulin and leucine was also observed, but the relative suppression of the rate of leucine entry was smaller than that observed in the normal subjects, suggesting insulin resistance (41). However, the diabetic patients had received a peripheral infusion of insulin prior to the clamp studies to achieve basal euglycemia (41). Whether this antecedent insulin infusion and the basal peripheral hyperinsulinemia observed resulted in partial suppression of the leucine plasma concentration and rate of appearance of leucine cannot be ascertained from these studies. If the ability of insulin to suppress proteolysis is limited, as appears to be the case, then the defective suppression of the rate of appearance of leucine ('insulin resistance') when expressed as percent of basal reported in these diabetic patients may be in part an artefact of the experimental design employed. It should, however, be pointed out that, throughout the study, leucine flux in the diabetic subjects was higher than that of the normal subjects.

In neither of the studies discussed above (41, 74) did insulin increase estimates of leucine entering protein. Such conclusions are not in keeping with the large body of in vitro data alluded to above. Once again, the experimental design of these studies must be carefully examined before one can conclude that insulin does not stimulate protein synthesis. In the companion studies reported from the insulin clamp data, Fukagawa et al (40) demonstrated that during insulin infusion the plasma concentrations of many amino acids decreased. Of particular note is that the plasma concentration of isoleucine decreased to almost zero at the higher rates of insulin infusion. Deficiency of a single essential amino acid could result in substrate limitation for the synthesis of any protein containing isoleucine. Thus, protein synthesis would be limited to the amout of isoleucine derived from endogenous protein degradation.

Substrate limitation is an important key factor which must be considered in experiments dealing with insulin effects on whole-body protein metabolism. The importance of availability of all amino acids is exemplified by recent studies carried out in our laboratory (75). In these studies, dogs were fed 3 separate isocaloric test meals: one containing fat and carbohydrate alone, one containing all the amino acids except the branched-chain amino acids, and a diet complete in fat, carbohydrate and all amino acids. Following ingestion of the fat and carbohydrate alone or in combination with all of the amino acids except the branched-chain amino acids, the plasma concentrations of leucine and KIC and the flux of leucine decreased, as did the estimates of leucine oxidation. Therefore, although leucine balance improved from the postabsorptive state, it remained negative throughout the meal study. Following ingestion of the complete amino acid diet, leucine flux remained constant and the rate of leucine oxidation increased. However, the endogenous rate of leucine appearance, calculated by subtracting the dietary contribution from the total leucine rate of appearance, decreased and the estimated rate of leucine entry into protein remained constant or increased slightly. As a result, during ingestion of the complete diet, these animals moved from a negative leucine balance in the postabsorptive state to a significantly positive leucine balance during meal absorption. Of greater importance to this discussion is the fact that these differences in the estimated rate of leucine entering protein occurred at similar plasma insulin concentrations.

Both Castellino and Luzi (76) and Tessari (77) have carried out studies combining euglycemic clamps at different plasma insulin concentrations with varying infusions of mixed amino acids to examine the effects of amino acid and insulin availability on leucine kinetic estimates of whole-body proteolysis and protein synthesis. When amino acid concentrations are maintained constant or increased during insulin infusion, the calculated rate of endogenous leucine Ra (total leucine flux minus the exogenous rate of leucine infused) decreased whereas the non-oxidative rate of leucine disappearance either remained constant or increased. However, when amino acids alone were infused with basal insulin (76) similar findings were observed. These data collectively emphasize the importance of amino acid availability for protein synthesis during experiments assessing the effects of insulin (or other hormones or substrates) on whole-body estimates of leucine (and protein) metabolism. However, studies employing infusions of unlabeled leucine (with or without the other amino acids) assume that the circulating plasma specific activity and/or enrichment of the infused isotope is identical to that of intracellular leucine, the site of protein synthesis and protein degradation. This most probably is not the case, and the rates of total leucine flux and oxidation will be underestimated. Therefore, when the known exogenous infusion of leucine is subtracted from the total leucine flux, the suppression of the rate of appearance of endogenous leucine will be overestimated. As a result, significant errors in quantitation of the effects of insulin on protein metabolism could occur which might lead to erroneous conclusions.

Conclusions

Although extensively studied, the precise role that insulin plays in the regulation of organ and whole-body amino acid and protein metabolism remains to be clarified. The present discussion attempts to outline various recent lines of evidence from both in vitro and in vivo studies to elucidate the role of insulin in the metabolism of some amino acids and protein. The preponderance of data provides evidence that a major role of insulin is to suppress proteolysis, but it is clear from both in vivo and in vitro studies that the majority of protein break-down is not responsive to insulin alone. The role insulin plays in stimulating pro-tein synthesis in less clear and may be model-dependent. Resolution of the ap-parent conflicting studies both in vivo and in vitro will require a better under-standing of the validity of the assumptions implicit in any given experiment. Ex-perimental models must be utilized in both in vitro and in vivo studies and al-though valid data can be accumulated, the interpretation of these data and the conclusions drawn from such models must be carefully examined. The role of insulin in the regulation of amino acid and protein metabolism in any given organ and the interrelationship of various body tissues in both the fasted and fed state continues to be a fertile and important area for future research.

References

1. Atchley DW, Loeb RF, Richardson DW et al (1933): On diabetic acidosis: a detailed study of electrolyte balances following the withdrawal and reestablishment of insulin therapy. *J. Clin. Invest., 12*, 297.
2. Fulks RM, Li JB, Goldberg AL (1975): Effects of insulin, glucose and amino acids on protein turnover in rat diaphragm. *J. Biol. Chem., 250*, 290.
3. Frayn KN, Maycock PF (1979): Regulation of protein metabolism by a physiological concentration of insulin in mouse soleus and extensor digitorum longus muscle: effects of starvation and scald injury. *Biochem. J., 184*, 323.
4. Furuno K, Goldberg AL (1986): The activation of protein degradation in muscle by Ca^{2+} or muscle injury does not involve a lysosomal mechanism. *Biochem. J., 237*, 859.
5. Kletzien RF, Pariza MW, Becker JE et al (1976): Induction of amino acid transport in primary cultures of adult rat liver parenchymal cells by insulin. *J. Biol. Chem., 241*, 3014.
6. Gunn JM, Clark MG, Knowles SE et al (1977): Reduced rates of proteolysis in transformed cells. *Nature (London), 266*, 58.
7. Waterlow JC, Garlick PJ, Millward DJ (1978): General principles of the measurement of whole body protein turnover. In: Waterlow JC, Garlick PJ, Millward DJ (Eds), *Protein Turnover in Mammalian Tissues and in the Whole Body*, Ch. 6, pp. 225-250. North-Holland, New York.
8. Waterlow JC, Garlick PJ, Millward DJ (1978): Protein synthesis and its regulation. In: Waterlow JC, Garlick PJ, Millward DJ, (Eds), *Protein Turnover in Mammalian Tissues and in the Whole Body*, Ch. 6, pp. 15-54. North-Holland, New York.
9. Kipnis DM, Noall MW (1958): Stimulation of amino acid transport by insulin in the isolated rat diaphragm. *Biochim. Biophys. Acta, 28*, 226.
10. Kilberg MS, Neuhaus OW (1977): Hormonal regulation of hepatic amino acid transport. *J. Supramol. Struct., 6*, 191.
11. Mohri T, Kitagawa H, Riggs TR (1974): Action of insulin on amino acid uptake by the immature rat uterus in vitro. *Biochim. Biophys. Acta, 363*, 249.
12. Barber EF, Handlogten ME, Vida TA et al (1982): Neutral amino acid transport in hepato-cytes isolated from streptozotocin-induced diabetic rats. *J. Biol. Chem., 257*, 14960.

13. Manchester KL (1970): The control by insulin of amino acid accumulation in muscle. *Biochem. J., 117*, 457.
14. Airhart J, Arnold HA, Stirewalt WS et al (1982): Insulin stimulation of protein synthesis in cultured skeletal and cardiac muscle cells. *Am. J. Physiol., 243*, C81.
15. Stirewalt WS, Low RB (1983): Effects of insulin in vitro on protein turnover in rat epitrochlearis muscle. *Biochem. J., 210*, 323.
16. Zak R, Martin AF, Blough R (1979): Assessment of protein turnover by use of radioisotopic tracers. *Physiol. Rev., 59*, 407.
17. Peavy DE, Taylor JM, Jefferson LS (1978): Correlation of albumin production rates and albumin mRNA levels in livers of normal, diabetic and insulin-treated diabetic rats. *Proc. Natl Acad. Sci. USA, 75*, 5879.
18. Jefferson LS, Liao WSL, Peavy DE et al (1983): Diabetes-induced alterations in liver protein synthesis: changes in the relative abundance of mRNAs for albumin and other plasma proteins. *J. Biol. Chem., 258*, 1369.
19. Peavy DE, Taylor JM, Jefferson LS (1985): Time course of changes in albumin synthesis and mRNA in diabetic and insulin treated diabetic rats. *Am. J. Physiol., 248*, E656.
20. Flaim KE, Copenhaver ME, Jefferson LS (1980): Effects of diabetes on protein synthesis in fast- and slow-twitch rat skeletal muscle. *Am. J. Physiol., 239*, E88.
21. Jefferson LS, Li JB, Rannels SR (1977): Regulation by insulin of amino acid release and protein turnover in the perfused rat hemicorpus. *J. Biol. Chem., 252*, 1476.
22. Barrieux A, Neeley WE, Dillmann WH (1985): Diabetes-induced alterations in the translational activity of specific mRNAS isolated from rat hearts. *Circ. Res., 57*, 296.
23. Shanker R, Neeley WE, Dillmann WH (1986): Rapid effects of insulin on in vitro translational activity of specific mRNA in diabetic rat heart. *Am. J. Physiol., 250*, E558.
24. Jefferson LS (1980): Role of insulin in the regulation of protein synthesis. *Diabetes, 29*, 487.
25. Buse MG, Cheema IR, Owens M et al (1984): Muscle protein synthesis: regulation of a translational inhibitor. *Am. J. Physiol., 246*, E510.
26. Monier S, Cam AL, Marchand-Brustel YL (1983): Insulin and insulin-like growth Factor I: effects on protein synthesis in isolated muscles from lean and goldthioglucose-obese mice. *Diabetes, 32*, 392.
27. Besterman JM, Watkins CA, Rannels DE (1983): Regulation of protein synthesis in lung by amino acids and insulin. *Am. J. Physiol., 245*, E508.
28. Mortimore GE, Mondon CE (1970): Inhibition by insulin of valine turnover in liver. *J. Biol. Chem., 245*, 2375.
29. Chua B, Kao R, Rannels DE et al (1978): Hormonal and metabolic control of proteolysis. *Biochem. Soc. Symp., 43*, 1.
30. Hopgood MF, Ballard FJ (1980): Regulation of protein breakdown in hepatocyte monolayers. *Ciba Found. Symp. 75*, 205.
31. Davis EJ, Less SHC (1985): Amino acid metabolism by perfused rat hindquarter: effects of insulin, leucine and 2-chloro-4-methylvalerate. *Biochem. J., 229*, 19.
32. Ward WF, Cox JR, Mortimore GE (1977): Lysosomal sequestration of intracellular protein as a regulatory step in hepatic proteolysis. *J. Biol. Chem., 252*, 6955.
33. Lowell BB, Ruderman HB, Goodman MN (1986): Evidence that lysosomes are not involved in the degradation of myofibrillar proteins in rat skeletal muscle. *Biochem. J., 234*, 237.
34. Low RB, Goldberg AL (1973): Nonuniform rates of turnover of myofibrillar protein in rat diaphragm. *J. Cell Biol., 56*, 590.
35. Neely AN, Cox JR, Fortney JA et al (1977): Alterations of lysosomal size and density during rat liver perfusion: suppression by insulin and amino acids. *J. Biol. Chem., 252*, 6948.

36. Murakami K, Voellmy R, Goldberg AL (1979): Protein degradation is stimulated by ATP in extracts of *Escherichia coli. J. Biol. Chem.*, *254*, 8194.
37. Adibi SA, Morse EL, Amin PM (1975): Role of insulin and glucose in the induction of hypoaminoacidemia in man: studies in normal, juvenile diabetic, and insulinoma patients. *J. Lab. Clin. Med.*, *86*, 395.
38. Cahill GF, Herrera MG, Morgan AP et al (1966): Hormone-fuel interrelationship during fasting. *J. Clin. Invest.*, *45*, 1751.
39. Carlsten A, Hallgren B, Jagenburg R et al (1966): Amino acids and free fatty acids in plasma in diabetics. I. The effect of insulin on the arterial levels. *Acta Med. Scand.*, *179*, 361.
40. Fukagawa NK, Minaker KL, Young VR et al (1986): Insulin dose-dependent reductions in plasma amino acids in man. *Am. J. Physiol.*, *250*, E13.
41. Tessari P, Nosadini R, Trevisan R et al (1986): Defective suppression by insulin of leucine-carbon appearance and oxidation in type I, insulin-dependent diabetes mellitus: evidence for insulin resistance involving glucose and amino acid metabolism. *J. Clin. Invest.*, *77*, 1797.
42. Tessari P, Trevisan R, Inchiostro S et al (1986): Dose-response curves of effects of insulin on leucine kinetics in humans. *Am. J. Physiol.*, *251*, E334.
43. Pozefsky T, Felig P, Tobin JD et al (1969): Amino acid balance across tissues of the forearm in postabsorptive man: effects of insulin at two dose levels. *J. Clin. Invest.*, *48*, 2273.
44. Wahren J, Felig P, Cerasi E et al (1972): Splanchnic and peripheral glucose and amino acid metabolism in diabetes mellitus. *J. Clin. Invest.*, *51*, 1870.
45. Tourian A, Sidbury JB (1983): Phenylketonuria and hyperphenylalaninemia. In: Stanbury JB, Wyngaarden JB, Fredrickson DS et al (Eds), *The Metabolic Basis of Inherited Disease*, Ch. 12, p. 271. McGraw-Hill, New York.
46. Picou D, Taylor-Roberts T (1969): The measurement of total protein synthesis and catabolism and nitrogen turnover in infants in different nutritional states and receiving different amounts of dietary protein. *Clin. Sci.*, *36*, 283.
47. Golden MNH, Waterlow JC (1977): Total protein synthesis in elderly people: a comparison of results with [^{15}N]glycine and [^{14}C]leucine. *Clin. Sci. Mol. Med.*, *53*, 277.
48. Schoenheimer R, Ratner S, Rittenberg D (1939): Studies in protein metabolism. X. The metabolic activity of body proteins investigated with 1($-$)-leucine containing two isotopes. *J. Biol. Chem.*, *130*, 703.
49. Harper AE, Miller RH, Block KP (1984): Branched chain amino acid metabolism. *Annu. Rev. Nutr.*, *4*, 409.
50. Bergstrom J, Furst P, Noree L-O et al (1974): Intracellular free amino acid concentration in human muscle tissue. *J. Appl. Physiol.*, *36*, 693.
51. Rennie MJ, Mathews DE, Bier DM et al (1980): Enrichment of muscle free amino acids during infusion of [1-^{13}C], [α-^{15}N]leucine. (Abstract). *Eur. J. Clin. Invest.*, *10*, Suppl. 31.
52. Allsop JR, Wolfe RR, Burke JF (1978): Tracer priming the bicarbonate pool. *J. Appl. Physiol.*, *45*, 137.
53. Rose IA (1961): The use of kinetic isotope effects in the study of metabolic control. I. Degradation of glucose-1-D by the hexose monophosphate pathway. *J. Biol. Chem.*, *236*, 603.
54. Gatley SJ, Wess MM, Govoni PL et al (1986): Deuterioglucose: alteration of biodistribution by an isotope effect. *J. Nucl. Med.*, *27*, 388.
55. Bielmann JF, O'Connell EL, Rose IA (1969): Secondary isotope effects in reactions catalyzed by yeast and muscle aldolase. *J. Am. Chem. Soc.*, *91*, 6484.
56. Irving CS, Wong WW, Shulman RJ et al (1983): [^{13}C]Bicarbonate kinetics in humans: intra- vs. interindividual variations. *Am. J. Physiol.*, *245*, R190.
57. Schwenk WF, Haymond MW (1986): Further evidence in man for rapid transamination of leucine and its alpha-keto acid. *Clin. Res.*, *34*, 906A.

58. Umpleby AM, Boroujerdi MA, Brown PM et al (1986): The effect of metabolic control on leucine metabolism in type I (insulin-dependent) diabetic patients. *Diabetologia, 29,* 131.

59. Shipley RA, Clark RE (1972): Mean transit time, mass, volume and constant infusion of tracer. In: Shipley RA, Clark RE (Eds), *Tracer Methods for In Vivo Kinetics and Applications,* Chs 7 and 9, pp. 111-127, 145-162. Academic Press, New York.

60. Waterlow JC, Garlick PJ, Millward OJ (1978): Total protein turnover from measurements on plasma and on the whole body. In: Waterlow JC, Garlick PJ, Millward OJ (Eds), *Protein Turnover in Mammalian Tissues and the Whole Body,* Ch. 8. pp. 303-308. North-Holland, New York.

61. Schwenk WF, Tsalikian E, Beaufrere B et al (1985): Recycling of an amino acid label with prolonged isotope infusion: implications for kinetic studies. *Am. J. Physiol. 248,* E482.

62. Tsalikian E, Howard C, Gerich JE et al (1984): Increased leucine flux in short-term fasted human subjects: evidence for increased proteolysis. *Am. J. Physiol., 247,* E323.

63. Abumrad NN, McRae JR, Lacy WW (1984): Inadequacy of leucine isotopic methods for measurements of whole body protein turnover in vivo. *Clin. Res., 32,* 387A.

64. Schwenk WF, Beaufrere B, Haymond MW (1985): Use of reciprocal pool specific activities to model leucine metabolism in humans. *Am. J. Physiol., 249,* E646.

65. Matthews DE, Schwarz HP, Yang RD et al (1983): Relationship of plasma leucine and α-ketoisocaproate during L-[1-^{13}C]leucine infusion in man: a method for measuring human intracellular leucine tracer enrichment. *Metabolism, 31,* 1105.

66. Rennie MJ, Edwards RHT, Halliday D et al (1982): Muscle protein synthesis by stable isotope techniques in man: the effects of feeding and fasting. *Clin. Sci., 63,* 519.

67. Vazquez JA, Paul HS, Adibi SA (1986): Relation between plasma and tissue parameters of leucine metabolism in fed and starved rats. *Am. J. Physiol., 250,* E615.

68. Nair KS, Garrow JS, Ford C et al (1983): Effect of poor diabetic control and obesity on whole body protein metabolism in man. *Diabetologia, 25,* 400.

69. Robert JJ, Beaufrere B, Koziet J et al (1985): Whole body de novo amino acid synthesis in type I (insulin dependent) diabetes studied with stable isotope-labeled leucine, alanine and glycine. *Diabetes, 34,* 67.

70. Abumrad NN, Jefferson LS, Rannels SR et al (1982): Role of insulin in the regulation of leucine kinetics in the conscious dog. *J. Clin. Invest., 70,* 1031.

71. Tsalikian E, Haymond MW (1986): Unpublished data.

72. Powell CS, Abumrad NN (1982): Effect of blood insulin levels on leucine metabolism in normal man. *Surg. Forum, 33,* 91.

73. Tsalikian E (1985): Acute insulin withdrawal in insulin dependent diabetes mellitus does not increase alanine de novo synthesis to provide a precursor for gluconeogenesis. *Diabetes, 34, Suppl. 1,* 22A.

74. Fukagawa NK, Minaker KL, Rowe JW et al (1985): Insulin mediated reduction of whole body protein breakdown: dose-response effects on leucine metabolism in postabsorptive man. *J. Clin. Invest., 76,* 2306.

75. Nissen S, Haymond MW (1986): Changes in leucine kinetics during meal absorption: effects of dietary leucine availability. *Am. J. Physiol., 250,* E695.

76. Castellino P, Luzi L (1985): Effect of insulin and amino acid concentration on leucine kinetics in man. *Diabetes, 34, Suppl. I,* 74A.

77. Tessari P (1986): Personal communication.

. Krall, editors
blishers, B.V.

Diabetic ketoacidosis

S.M. MARSHALL AND K.G.M.M. ALBERTI

Introduction

Diabetic ketoacidosis (DKA) remains a significant cause of morbidity and mortality in diabetes mellitus. Many comprehensive review articles have been published in the last few years (1-16). The purpose of this Chapter is not to reduplicate their efforts but to highlight those areas which remain controversial and to summarize and comment upon new information which has appeared in the last 2-3 years. Incidence and precipitating factors well be discussed first, followed by new observations on biochemical changes in both man and experimental animals. The final section discusses treatment concentrating on the main modalities: fluid, insulin, electrolytes, bicarbonate and associated measures.

Incidence

General

Good studies of true incidence remain few and far between, primarily because most studies have been hospital- rather than community-based. Incidence remains important, however, as it provides one yardstick of effectiveness of community control programmes for diabetes.

Comparison of studies estimating the incidence of DKA remains difficult because of lack of a uniform definition of DKA. The Rhode Island diabetic acidosis project was primarily designed to provide an epidemiological description of DKA (carefully defined) in a well-demarcated population (17). Exhaustive measures were undertaken to ensure that all cases were included. DKA accounted for 152 out of 9663 diabetic admissions (1.6%). New diabetic patients accounted for 20% of DKA cases. The annual incidence rate was 14/ 100,000 total population or 46/10,000 diabetic subjects. The rates for females were 1.5 times that of males. Age-specific rates were highest in those less than 15 years old.

Another useful study, from Denmark, used slightly different criteria for

498

defining ketoacidosis, but again the study population was well defined and the ascertainment rate probably very high (18). The incidence of DKA rose steadily from 2.5/100,000 total population/year in 1960-1964 to 8.5/100,000/year in 1975-1979, comparable to the Rhode Island study. Patients in the lowest social class and those residing in urban areas were at highest risk. After excluding changes in clinical practise, increasing incidence of diabetes, increasing population and increasing incidence of precipitating factors, the authors concluded that some exogenous factor or lack of education accounted for the rising incidence. This is contrary to present 'belief' that the increasing focus on education and improved technical methods of insulin therapy must be causing a fall in the incidence of DKA. It will be of interest to see the Danish figures for the post-1979 period.

A recent review in the invaluable compilation of data by the National Diabetes Data Group of the United States has quoted an annual incidence of DKA of 3-8 episodes/1000 diabetic patients with episodes occurring at onset of diabetes in 20-30% of newly diagnosed diabetic patients (19).

An American study concluded that DKA (not defined) accounted for 5.4% of all emergency-room attendances by diabetic patients (20). Hospital admission from the emergency room was 4 times commoner in diabetic than in non-diabetic attenders and most of the admissions were due to DKA. A similar study from New Zealand suggested that 8% of all hospital admissions in diabetic subjects were due to DKA (undefined) (21).

During continuous subcutaneous insulin infusion

With the more widespread use of continuous subcutaneous insulin infusion (CSII) under routine clinical conditions rather than strictly controlled research studies, have come reports suggesting that the incidence of DKA is higher on CSII than on injection therapy. Peden et al (22) reported an incidence rate of 1 episode/53 patient-months (29 episodes in 1880 patient-months). No control group on injection therapy was provided for comparison, but the authors felt that the rate on CSII was higher. Comment was also made, without data, that the incidence fell with increasing experience and more attention to detailed patient education.

Another large study, from the Mason Clinic in Seattle, of 161 patients with 2978 patient-months' experience of CSII reported an incidence of 1 episode of DKA per 78 patient-months (23). The same patients had an incidence rate of 1/425 patient-months on prior injection therapy ($P < 0.03$), and a carefully matched group of patients on injection therapy a rate of 1/495 patient-months, both significantly lower than the rate on CSII. Sixty-two percent of the episodes of DKA occurred within the first 5 months of initiation of CSII. In a more recent prospective study the same authors have shown a decrease in the DKA rate on CSII to 1 episode per 130 patient-months (24). At another centre, reduction in the rate of DKA from 1 episode per 86 patient-months in the first year of the centre's experience to 1/200 patient-months in the second and 1/150 in the third year (25). The decrease was attributed to more aggressive recommendations to the patient in the management of hyperglycaemia.

A U.K. centre with vast experience of CSII as a research tool has shown equal rates of DKA on injection therapy and after 6 months' use of CSII (26). All episodes of DKA occurred within 7 months of patients initiating pump therapy. There was an improvement in the incidence from 1/2 patient-months during 1978 (with only small numbers) to 1/475 in 1983. Similarly, in their report of mortality during CSII, Teutsch et al (27) showed that deaths from DKA occurred during the first few months of treatment. The feasibility phase of the Diabetes Control and Complications Trial has shown no difference in DKA rates between those using CSII and those using intensified conventional therapy (28). However, in a small randomised trial of CSII versus intensified injection therapy in children, there were 6 episodes of DKA on CSII and none on injection therapy (29).

Overall the main causes of DKA during CSII were intercurrent illness (23) and pump malfunction with inadequate monitoring (25). Improved pumps should diminish the latter.

It seems probable that the incidence of DKA on CSII is higher than on injection therapy during the physician's and patients' early experience. However, awareness by the physician and particularly effective patient education can reduce the rates to similar levels. The nature of the patients in whom CSII is used may also be significant. These are often patients with unstable diabetic control, where self-monitoring may not be optimal, and the lack of a subcutaneous depot of insulin may predispose to DKA.

Precipitating factors

The classical precipitating factors of infection and other intercurrent illness remain common, albeit with different frequencies in different studies, varying from 53% (17), 47% (18) to 27% (30). Faich and colleagues noted that the incidence of non-compliance as a precipitating factor of DKA increased from 19% in those patients with single episodes to 43% in those with multiple episodes (17). The importance of psychological and social problems in patients with recurrent episodes of DKA has been emphasised (31). Such problems are particularly important in childhood and adolescence. In a study of 15 adolescents with recurrent DKA, Orr and colleagues found psychological problems, depression and family difficulties to be common (32). In a larger retrospective study of children and adolescents with multiple episodes of DKA, overt manipulation was found in only a few (33). Most had behavioural and personality problems with families showing unresolved conflict and dysfunction. Such difficulties were not always easily identified.

A comparison of 45 adult patients with repeated episodes of DKA and 42 with single episodes showed that the repeat group had had less full-time education, were more likely to be single, had a higher incidence of neurosis, were more likely to use hospital rather than general practitioner as source of primary care and attended a general medical clinic rather than a specialist diabetic clinic (34).

Any of the above causes can obviously precipitate DKA whilst using CSII, but in addition, failure of insulin delivery — such as pump malfunction, battery failure, empty insulin reservoir, leakage, blockage or disconnection of insulin catheter — is also important. The incidence of such mishaps causing DKA has been reported as 42% (22), 11% (25) and 8% (23). Infection at the catheter insertion site may also precipitate DKA (22, 23, 35).

Unusual causes of DKA include Fournier's gangrene, either spontaneous (36) or following scrotal insulin injection as a remedy for impotence (37), and infusion of the β_2-sympathomimetic agent, ritodrine, to prevent premature labour (38). A recent case-report of recurrent DKA precipitated by increased fat consumption and stress in a patient with acquired total lipodystrophy has challenged the view that ketoacidosis does not occur in this condition (39). Anaphylaxis and immunological resistance to pork and beef insulins has also been reported as precipitating and complicating the treatment of DKA (40).

Biochemical changes

Glucose metabolism

For recent reviews, the reader is referred to References 1, 14, 15 and 41.

There are many older studies in insulin-dependent diabetic man and animals which have charted the time course of biochemical changes on withdrawal of insulin therapy. It is worth stressing that in the clinical situation the presence of precipitating factors with their accompanying surge of counterregulatory hormone secretion will inevitably modify this time course. The counterregulatory hormones themselves may also modify the biochemical response.

In man the study by Miles et al (42) has shown very clearly the effects of insulin withdrawal on glucose metabolism. They confirmed that plasma glucose increases rapidly, reaching a plateau of around 16 mmol/l after 2-4 hours. This was accounted for by a rapid increase in glucose production which, after 4 hours, gradually returned to normal. After an initial slight increase in glucose utilization, it also fell, rates of production and utilization becoming equal, and thus maintaining stable hyperglycaemia.

Our understanding of carbohydrate metabolism in diabetes has been increased by the discovery of the key regulator of glucose metabolism, fructose 2,6-bisphosphate. Fructose 2,6-bisphosphate activates phosphofructokinase-1 by preventing inhibition by ATP and enhancing stimulation by AMP and fructose 1,6-bisphosphate (43). Fructose 2,6-bisphosphate also inhibits fructose bisphosphatase, blocking conversion of fructose 1,6-bisphosphate to fructose 6-phosphate. Thus, with low levels of fructose 2,6-bisphosphate, flux through phosphofructokinase-1 to pyruvate is decreased and from pyruvate to glucose-6-phosphate increased. Fructose 2,6-bisphosphate is synthesized from fructose 6-phosphate by phosphofructokinase-2 and dephosphorylated by fructose 2,6-bisphosphatase. Phosphofructokinase-2 and fructose 2,6-bisphosphatase appear to be one and the same molecule, phosphorylation of the kinase by a protein kinase under the control of cAMP converting the enzyme to the phosphatase form (44, 45).

In DKA relatively high levels of glucagon stimulate protein kinases, resulting in phosphorylation of phosphofructokinase-2 and a decrease in the level of fructose 2,6-bisphosphate, thus increasing flux from pyruvate to glucose-6-phosphate (46). Glucagon also stimulates hepatic glycogenolysis (47). The end-result is a vast increase in hepatic glucose output.

Levels of hepatic fructose 2,6-bisphosphate and phosphofructokinase-2 have been compared in ketotic and non-ketotic hyperglycaemic streptozotocin-diabetic mice (48). The groups had equivalent blood glucose levels, but fructose 2,6-bisphosphate and phosphofructokinase-2 levels were decreased only in the ketotic group, reaching levels seen in starved non-diabetic mice. Values in the ketotic group returned to normal after 24 hours of insulin therapy, whilst in starved animals levels were normalised within 30 minutes of glucose feeding. The authors concluded that ketosis and not hyperglycaemia is related to the depressed levels of fructose 2,6-bisphosphate and speculated that the falling levels and consequent slower rate of glycolysis produced the trigger to switch hepatic fatty acid metabolism towards oxidation and ketone body formation.

The situation is obviously more complex in human DKA, although glucagon levels are always increased early in the course of the disorder. In one clinical study of 26 patients with hyperglycaemia and variable ketosis, multiple regression analysis demonstrated that blood glucose correlated strongly with increased glucagon levels but not with ketone body levels, the latter correlating with increased non-esterified fatty acid levels, falling C-peptide levels and increased body mass index (49). Thus, ketone bodies seem less important than glucagon in determining the degree of hyperglycaemia.

Ketone bodies

A comprehensive review of ketone body metabolism can be found in Reference 50. Relative insulin deficiency leads to peripheral adipocyte lipolysis with a rapid rise in plasma non-esterified fatty acid (NEFA) levels. Lipolysis may be enhanced by concomitant rises in glucagon, growth hormone, adrenaline and noradrenaline in DKA. In the liver, the fatty acids are oxidised rather than re-esterified, producing the ketone bodies, 3-hydroxybutyrate and acetoacetate. Insulin withdrawal studies have demonstrated a continuous rise in plasma ketone body levels for 10 hours after insulin withdrawal (41, 42). Although both ketone body production and utilization increased, production always exceeded utilization, resulting in a net increase in plasma ketone body levels. Plasma glucagon levels also increased progressively and there was a significant correlation between maximal plasma glucagon level and rate of ketone body production. It is interesting to note, however, that once DKA is established, there is no correlation between plasma glucagon and blood ketone body levels (49).

Key determinants of ketogenesis are the amount of fatty acid reaching the liver and the pathway followed by those fatty acids once in the hepatocyte.

In the hepatic cytosol, fatty acids are condensed with coenzyme A. Transfer of the resulting acyl-coenzyme A into the mitochondrion is by the carnitine shuttle, acyl-coenzyme A condensing with carnitine under the influence of carnitine acyltransferase I (CAT-I). Once across the mitochondrial membrane, acyl-coenzyme A is released by carnitine acyltransferase II (CAT-II). CAT-I is inhibited by malonyl-coenzyme A. In diabetic ketoacidosis, the switch from hepatic re-esterification of free fatty acids to oxidation is achieved by a relative excess of glucagon. Glucagon increases levels of carnitine by an unknown mechanism, hence favouring formation of fatty acylcarnitine and enhancing fatty acid flux into oxidation (51). Excess glucagon also causes a decrease in levels of malonyl-coenzyme A, resulting in a further increase in fatty acid movement into mitochondria through stimulation of CAT-I (52). Fatty acids themselves are powerful inhibitors of malonyl-coenzyme A formation and the relative roles of fatty acid and glucagon are unclear (53). It is thought that after oxidation has been primed by glucagon, increased levels of the substrate (fatty acid) drive the oxidation process even faster. Control of fatty acid oxidation may also be exerted by changing sensitivity of CAT-I to inhibition by malonyl-coenzyme A. In fasting normal (54) and ketotic, streptozotocin-diabetic rats (55), the sensitivity of CAT-I to malonyl-coenzyme A appears to decrease.

In ketotic and ketoacidotic diabetic children, free carnitine levels are decreased as opposed to the increase that might be expected, but acylcarnitine levels are increased (56). Insulin therapy returns the levels to normal. This study, however, also demonstrated an inverse correlation between ketone body and free carnitine levels but not between ketone bodies and acylcarnitine or between free carnitine and acylcarnitine, suggesting that the fall in free carnitine levels was not due solely to acylation.

The dogma that ketone bodies can only be synthesized in the liver is no longer tenable. Thus, one study showed that approximately 16% of ketone bodies may be synthesized outside the liver in ketotic diabetic rats, presumably in the kidney (57). Isotope studies suggest that the ketone bodies are secreted from the kidneys into the circulation and not directly excreted.

Debate continues on the existence of a specific deficit in ketone body clearance in DKA. Isotope studies have confirmed that ketosis in uncontrolled diabetes is associated with increased rates of ketogenesis and decreased clearance rates. One study demonstrated increased synthesis of 3-hydroxybutyrate and decreased clearance, the clearance of 3-hydroxybutyrate falling more than that of acetoacetate. Similar results were obtained in uncontrolled diabetes, in obesity and in obese subjects after 1-2 weeks' starvation (58, 59). Another tracer study in obese, non-starved subjects and ketoacidotic diabetes revealed normal acetoacetate clearance in both groups and decreased 3-hydroxybutyrate clearance only in the diabetic group (60). The different results may be due to different kinetic modelling.

Acetone

Acetone is formed by spontaneous, non-enzymatic decarboxylation of acetoacetate. Enzymatic test for ketone bodies do not measure acetone whilst acetone reacts much less avidly than acetoacetate in the nitroprusside test, so that acetone has largely been ignored. A recent study using a bolus tracer technique has demonstrated widely variable rates of production of acetone in DKA (61). Plasma acetone concentration was generally related to but higher than acetoacetate concentration and accounted for approximately 52% of the estimated acetoacetate production rate. Urine excretion of acetone was constant at around 7% of the production rate. As plasma acetone levels rose, so did the amount of the production rate which could be accounted for by excretion in the breath, and the percent undergoing in vivo metabolism fell. Radioactivity from the tracer was found in plasma acetone, glucose, lipids and proteins but not in acetoacetate, 3-hydroxybutyrate or NEFA. Acetone is a substrate for gluconeogenesis in starved rats (62) and in human subjects in diabetic ketoacidosis (63). Acetol and 1,2-propanediol, possible metabolites of acetone, were also found in plasma of ketoacidotic patients at concentrations of up to 0.5 mmol/l (63).

Lipids

A careful study of the acute effects of insulin deficiency on lipoprotein metabolism has been performed in 14 insulin-dependent diabetic patients with ketoacidosis treated by standard means (64). Initial plasma triglyceride levels were grossly elevated (6.48 mmol/l) falling to 2.35 mmol/l after 24 hours therapy, accompanied by a marked fall in very-low-density lipoproteins (VLDL) and chylomicrons. Cholesterol levels were relatively normal and remained unchanged. Levels of intermediate-density lipoprotein (IDL), high-density lipoprotein (HDL) and LDL-cholesterol were initially low. HDL cholesterol rose with therapy whilst IDL and LDL cholesterol did not change. The ratio of apoprotein A-I to cholesterol in HDL fell significantly with therapy. Mean apoprotein A-I levels fell from normal initially but subsequently increased again. The authors concluded that insulin may decrease secretion or increase catabolism of apoprotein A-I.

A further report has confirmed initial very high levels of plasma triglycerides falling rapidly with therapy for DKA (65). Serum cholesterol levels remained unchanged as did apoprotein A. Total phospholipids, HDL phospholipids and apoprotein B fell after 24 hours therapy.

In a newly presenting Type I diabetic patient with ketoacidosis and acute pancreatitis, extreme lipid abnormalities were associated with profound coma (66). Correction of the acidosis did not produce clinical improvement, so plasma exchange was undertaken. Coma regressed during the exchange. Triglyceride levels fell from 148 to 40 mmol/l and cholesterol from 46 to 8 mmol/l.

Acid-base balance

Recent reviews of acid-base disturbance in DKA can be found in References 1, 3, 4, 6, 15, 16, 67, 68 and 69. The classical biochemical picture is of a metabolic acidosis with an increased anion gap due to ketoacids. However, a recent large study, partly retrospective, demonstrated that a broad spectrum of acid-base disturbances existed at presentation of DKA, from a classical metabolic acidosis with increased anion gap to a hyperchloraemic acidosis with normal anion gap (70).

Those patients with hyperchloraemic acidosis had normal renal function whilst those with classical metabolic acidosis had evidence of prerenal failure. The authors suggested that the first group had been able to maintain salt and water intake, preventing prerenal failure and thus allowing the excretion of ketone bodies balanced by sodium as the cation. This leads to relative retention of chloride. Infusion of saline may increase the excretion of ketone salts and lead to a treatment-induced hyperchloraemic acidosis. In this study most patients, treated in a standard manner, developed hyperchloraemic acidosis 4-8 hours after initiation of therapy. The authors found a slower rate of recovery in those patients presenting with hyperchloraemic acidosis and suggested that administration of bicarbonate may be appropriate. By contrast, when there is severe volume depletion, ketone bodies are retained and there is less hyperchloraemia. A further recent report has emphasised that DKA may be accompanied by a normal anion gap (71).

If there is doubt about the diagnosis, the urine anion gap may be helpful (72). Two cases of DKA with metabolic alkalosis secondary to diuretics (73) and copious vomiting (74) have also been recorded recently.

Blood changes

Coagulation

Thromboembolic disease is a not infrequent complication of DKA. In a prospective trial of 11 patients in DKA, Paton demonstrated, after correction for dehydration, elevation of clotting Factors VIII-C and VIII-R:Ag and depression of antithrombin III levels (75). Seven of the 11 subjects also had significant quantities of fibrin degradation products. It was concluded that controlled trials of anticoagulants and anti-platelet agents were warranted. However, a further study provided evidence of increased platelet activity in vivo as judged by elevated serum levels of β-thromboglobulin but decreased aggregation in vitro when exposed to ADP and prostacyclin (76), confirming an earlier study reported in a brief letter (77). There was a significant correlation between blood glucose levels and platelet sensitivity. This evidence suggests that anti-platelet agents may be harmful in DKA. Nonetheless, the use of anticoagulants seems warranted.

Prostaglandins

Increased levels of prostaglandin E_2 (PGE_2) and its major metabolite, 13,14-dihydro-15-keto-PGE_2 (PGE_m), and thromboxane B_2 have been found in streptozotocin-diabetic rats (78), in insulin-dependent diabetic subjects during insulin withdrawal (79) and in ketoacidosis (80). Levels fell towards normal with insulin therapy. In ketoacidosis, prostaglandin levels correlated with plasma NEFA levels initially and during therapy, arousing speculation that the increased plasma levels of prostaglandin signified adipocyte overproduction in a local counterregulatory effort to inhibit lipolysis. In rats, the cyclo-oxygenase inhibitors, meclofenamic acid and indomethacin, significantly decreased the elevated levels of PGE_2 and PGE_m whilst the α-adrenoceptor blocker, phentolamine, had an effect only on the levels of thromboxane B_2. The β-adrenoceptor blocker, propranolol, had no effect on prostaglandin levels but did lower levels of blood glucose, NEFA and ketone bodies (81). The place of cyclo-oxygenase inhibitors in the routine therapy of DKA has not been evaluated.

Macrocytosis

Red blood cell volume is elevated in DKA when measured by Coulter counter but not when calculated from haematocrit, and macrocytosis is not seen on blood films (82). In one patient, Coulter-measured MCV fell as plasma osmolality fell with therapy for DKA. The authors postulated that red blood cells become hypertonic in the hyperglycaemic, dehydrated plasma of DKA. On exposure to the hypotonic fluid in the Coulter counter, the cells swell, giving an erroneously high count.

A more detailed study confirmed the above findings and went on to show in vitro that true red cell swelling resulted from decreased sodium concentration and was not related to varying glucose concentrations (83). Similar volume changes were documented in a diabetic patient parallel to daily variations in blood glucose.

Diagnosis

The mainstay of diagnosis remains a thorough history and examination coupled with bedside measurement of blood and urine glucose and ketones.

Laboratory analysis of blood glucose, urea, electrolytes, ketones and pH confirms the diagnosis. The development of a sensitive paper-strip test for 3-hydroxybutyrate, detecting levels as low as 0.1 mmol/l, may prove useful (84). The nitroprusside-based tests for the detection of ketones do not react with 3-hydroxybutyrate. Thus, in cases of DKA where there is a high ratio of 3-hydro-xybutyrate to acetoacetate, diagnosis may be difficult. It has been suggested that if a few drops of hydrogen peroxide were added to urine initially negative for ketones, conversion to a positive test would confirm the presence of 3-hydroxybutyrate (85). However, the detection level for urinary 3-hydroxybuty-rate was 50 mmol/l and for serum 100 mmol/l, making the modified test clearly worthless (86).

Treatment

Insulin

The use of low-dose insulin regimes, either intravenous or intramuscular, now seems generally accepted (1, 3-6, 9, 10, 16, 87, 88) in adults and in children (89-92). Low-dose intermittent intramuscular therapy appears particularly suitable when resources are minimal (8, 93, 94). Debate continues on the relative fre-quencies of hypoglycaemia and hypokalaemia with low- and high-dose insulin therapy.

Perhaps not surprisingly, recombinant insulin has been shown to be just as effective in the treatment of DKA in a low-dose regime as highly purified porcine insulin (95).

Insulin resistance

Marked insulin resistance is present in virtually all diabetic patients in ketoacidosis. In a study comparing the effect of low-dose insulin infusion on diabetic subjects admitted in DKA and normal controls made hyperglycaemic by infusion of somatostatin and glucose, the fractional glucose turnover and the half-time of the fall in plasma glucose during insulin treatment were both reduced 10-fold (96). In ketoacidotic patients, a history of prior exposure to insulin was associated with a more rapid decline in blood glucose concentration.

Specific ^{125}I-insulin binding to erythrocytes were found to be significantly higher at presentation of DKA than after 24 hours and 5 days, values after treatment being similar to those of a control group (97). The affinity constant was significantly higher in DKA, indicating increased receptor affinity rather than receptor member. Insulin binding correlated inversely with arterial pH. The relevance of this to insulin action in insulin-sensitive tissues is uncertain. Indeed, by contrast, in cultured adipocytes, acute lowering of pH produced a decrease in insulin binding due to a decrease in the rate of association with a concomitant decrease in insulin sensitivity but no change in insulin responsiveness (98). After culture at pH 6.9 for 24 hours, insulin binding and sensitivity were normal, but the insulin response was substantially impaired. These post-receptor changes could be reversed by further culture for 48 hours at pH 7.4. Exposure to ketoacids had little effect on insulin effectiveness. The authors concluded that insulin resistance in DKA is due to low-pH-induced insulin receptor binding and post-binding alterations.

Despite these experimental findings it is worth commenting that clinically important insulin resistance is rare in DKA. When it occurs, it is more likely due to inadequate rehydration than profound insensitivity of tissues *per se* to insulin.

Fluids

The water loss in severe DKA may be as much as 100 ml/kg with a sodium deficit of 7-10 mmol/kg. Most authors recommend replacement with 'isotonic' 0.154 mol/l (0.9%) saline, switching to 0.077 mol/l (0.45%) if hypernatraemia develops, although some mistakenly prefer 0.077 mol/l saline throughout (see below). Blood or colloid should be infused if hypotension does not improve rapidly. Simple rehydration, by improving renal excretion, may lower blood glucose concentrations significantly, without affecting the acidosis (99-101). Indeed, West and colleagues have shown that in the first phase of therapy in hyperosmolar coma at least as much glucose is lost in the urine as metabolised (102) whilst haemodilution due to rehydration can account for a 23% fall in blood glucose. Rehydration, with sodium bicarbonate infusion (if pH<7.2), also reduces the level of the counterregulatory hormones adrenaline, noradrenaline, glucagon and cortisol, and also of lactate, aldosterone and renin (100).

Electrolyte

Potassium

Serum potassium levels may be low, normal or high on presentation in DKA although the majority are normal or at the upper end of the normal range. This occurs despite a vast total body potassium deficit of 3-12 mmol/kg body weight (103, 104). Conventional wisdom suggests that loss of intracellular potassium in DKA is due to: (a) insulin deficiency *per se* — insulin normally stimulates (Na^+ + K^+) -ATPase promoting potassium entry into cells (105); (b) acidaemia with exchange of potassium for hydrogen ions entering cells; and (c) intracellular volume depletion. Much of the potassium displaced from cells will be lost in urine although rapid onset of severe DKA will result in hyperkalaemia. Overall, hyperkalaemia (K > 6.0 mmol/l) has been reported in one-fifth to one-third of cases of DKA (106, 107) with a particularly high incidence in CSII failures (108). Studies in which CSII has been discontinued have shown conflicting results with Knight et al (108) showing small changes, but Pickup (109) showed a more significant increase in plasma K^+ over a 9-hour period.

Recently the role of the metabolic acidosis in causing the hyperkalaemia has been questioned (110). Thus, although infusion of mineral acids into experimental animals causes potassium displacement from cells (111), the infusion of organic acids such as 3-hydroxybutyric acid or lactic acid does not cause hyperkalaemia (112). Similarly, acute lactic acidosis may not be associated with hyperkalaemia (113) while blood pH does not always correlate with serum K^+ in DKA (113) although other studies report a correlation (114).

One suggestion has been that organic acid anions diffuse into cells readily so that extrusion of K^+ is not required to maintain ionic balance (114). On the other hand, if there is excessive organic anion loss in the urine, then H^+/K^+ exchange would still be expected. The unknown fraction in the equation is generally renal function. Thus, in experimental animals there will be substantial urine K^+ loss as the animals will not be dehydrated. In severe dehydration there will be prerenal impairment of renal function and K^+ will accumulate in the extracellular fluid, although some have contested as to how important this is in determining serum K^+ concentration (114).

Adrogue et al (114) have carried out a careful analysis of factors influencing plasma potassium in 132 admissions for severe DKA in Houston. They found highly significant positive correlations of plasma K^+ with plasma glucose, osmolality, BUN and anion gap, and negative correlations with pH and TCO_2. Multiple linear regression showed that only 3 variables — glucose, pH and anion gap — had truly independent effects. They report that the equation:

$$K^+_p = 25.4 - 3.02pH + 0.001G + 0.028AG$$

best describes the relationship. It is worth noting that the correlation coefficient was only 0.52, so that at best 27% of the K^+ can be explained on this basis. They conclude that endogenous ketoacidaemia and hyperglycaemia are the main determinants of an elevated plasma K^+ and both of these are secondary to insulin deficiency. Prerenal azotaemia contributes by preventing loss of K^+ in the urine.

Two further factors should be considered when seeking mechanisms for the loss of intracellular K^+. Thus, hyperglycaemia *per se* causes hyperkalaemia in IDDM patients (115, 116) and will be important in DKA. The mechanism of this is uncertain, although it could be an osmotic effect. Second, glucagon can also cause hyperkalaemia (117) and glucagon levels are greatly elevated in DKA.

Once treatment of DKA has commenced, then plasma potassium levels will always fall due to intracellular and extracellular volume repletion, to loss of K^+ in urine, to reversal of the acidaemia and to direct action of insulin on K^+ transport into cells. Nonetheless, opinion varies as to when potassium replacement should commence: immediately (2, 5, 10); when serum potassium values are known (7, 12, 14, 15); or when urine output is established (4, 6, 18).

A recent study showed significant hyperkalaemia ($K^+ > 6.0$ mmol/l) in 1.4% of all hospital admissions, of which 0.03% were in DKA. Of these 12 patients, 8 had a serum potassium level > 6.5 mmol/l. Four of these had hyperkalaemia on admission, but in the others it developed during treatment of DKA, due to a combination of renal impairment and excessive intravenous replacement (118). Two deaths have been reported in patients on maintenance haemodialysis who in addition became hyperglycaemic but not ketotic (119). In streptozotocin-diabetic rats with normal renal function, renal potassium handling is normal despite decreased levels of renin and aldosterone (120, 121). In far the majority of patients, hypokalaemia is a greater threat to survival than hyperkalaemia and cautious early replacement (20-30 mmol/h), when insulin infusion is started, seems warranted. Thereafter the rate of potassium replacement should be adjusted in the light of serum levels, electrocardiograph monitoring and urine output. It has been suggested that potassium be infused as the phosphate salt since there is commonly a total body deficit of phosphate in DKA (13); however, the extent of the phosphate deficit is much less than that of potassium, and separate replacement is wiser.

Phosphate

There is significant total body phosphate loss during the development of DKA, although plasma levels tend to be normal on presentation. However, as has been known for many years, severe hypophosphataemia occurs commonly during the treatment of DKA. It is still debated whether phosphate replacement is necessary or desirable, although it has been suggested that the low levels prevent the recovery of red cell 2,3-diphosphoglycerate levels (122). This could impair oxygen delivery to the tissues.

A randomised study of replacement with one single dose of 15 mmol sodium PO_4 at 4 hours or 3 doses of 15 mmol PO_4 at 2, 6 and 10 hours, or no replacement has been performed (123). The group given 3 doses had significantly higher serum phosphate levels at all times within the first 24 hours whilst the group given only one dose had higher levels only at 8 hours. However, there was no difference in the rates of clinical or biochemical recovery between the 3 groups and no patient became clinically hypophosphataemic. Serum calcium levels fell in all 3 groups, whilst Mg^{2+} levels remained stable.

A second study compared KCl replacement alone to potassium phosphate alone (8.5 mmol/h) for 24 hour (124). Unfortunately, initial serum phosphate and magnesium levels were higher in the group given phosphate, and remained so throughout the 24 hours, falling to control level as soon as the phosphate infusion was stopped. Both groups developed biochemical hypocalcaemia, although the serum calcium level was significantly lower in the phosphate-treated group at the 24th hour only. There was no difference in 2,3-diphosphoglycerate levels or oxygen dissociation throughout the study.

In a study in children with DKA given intravenous potassium replacement as phosphate or chloride, serum phosphate and ionised calcium levels were unchanged, but phosphate excretion was higher in those given phosphate (125). Intravenous bicarbonate therapy appeared to produce a further fall in serum phosphate levels.

Thus, although biochemical hypophosphataemia is common during therapy of DKA, replacement does not appear to speed clinical or biochemical recovery and is probably unnecessary. However, 2 cases of acute haemolytic anaemia caused by severe hypophosphataemia in DKA have been reported (126). One factor that may have diminished the importance of hypophosphataemia is the use of smaller doses of insulin with consequently lesser falls in plasma phosphate.

Magnesium

Hypomagnesaemia is common in diabetes, especially during poor control (127) and during treatment of and recovery from DKA, when it may be associated with hypocalcaemia and hypophosphataemia (128). Replacement therapy is not generally recommended although it may occasionally be necessary. A case-report of an episode of DKA resistant to standard therapy until magnesium depletion was corrected (129) prompted the retort that magnesium supplements should be given to all juvenile diabetic patients (130).

Bicarbonate

Because of the possible complications of bicarbonate administration (local irritation, hypokalaemia, paradoxical worsening of CSF acidosis, rebound alkalosis and impaired oxyhaemoglobin dissociation) standard teaching has limited bicarbonate replacement therapy to patients with severe DKA and arterial pH<7.0 (1-3, 5, 6, 9, 10). However, even at this level, the benefits are not clear. A retrospective non-randomised study suggested that infusing bicarbonate did not improve the rate of clinical or biochemical recovery from severe DKA; and plasma glucose levels recovered less rapidly in the bicarbonate-treated group (131). A prospective, randomised study demonstrated a more rapid rise in pH and capillary blood bicarbonate in a group given 150 mmol sodium bicarbonate but no change in the rate of fall of blood glucose (132). There was a delay in the fall of blood lactate and ketone bodies to normal. Similar metabolic observations have been made in streptozotocin-diabetic rats with severe ketoacidosis (pH<6.9), although in this case blood glucose levels fell more rapidly with bicarbonate therapy. However, tissue studies suggested that this was due to stimulation of anaerobic glycolysis, particularly in liver (Cuthbert and Alberti, unpublished observations). Both these studies suggest that, metabolically at least, the use of bicarbonate is not advantageous. It has been suggested that although no biochemical benefit was seen in the study of Hale et al (132), the value of bicarbonate therapy in protecting against arrhythmias and in improving cardiac function remains unknown (133), an important point.

   In children, a study of mortality revealed no difference between those given bicarbonate and those not so treated (134).

Complications of diabetic ketoacidosis

Fluid overload

Despite the large water deficit, overenthusiastic resuscitation with 0.154 mol/l saline, especially in the presence of hypotension, not unnaturally may lead to fluid overload and pulmonary oedema, resulting in the suggestion that colloid rather than crystalloid infusions be given (135). However, it seems more relevant not to adhere rigidly to a set protocol but to modify therapy in the light of the patient's clinical response.

Adult respiratory distress syndrome

The adult respiratory distress syndrome (ARDS), characterised by the sudden onset of dyspnoea, profound and progressive hypoxaemia, decreasing lung compliance and diffuse pulmonary infiltrates on chest X-ray, has been reported with variable frequency during the treatment of DKA. Some authors claim never to have seen a case (136) whilst others recognise it as a distinct, albeit rare, complication (137).

Carroll and Matz reported 9 cases known to them and reviewed a further 9 reported in the literature (138). They found 7 cases in 281 episodes of uncontrolled diabetes (ketoacidosis or hyperglycaemic non-ketotic coma). No case had previous known pulmonary or cardiac disease. Mortality was high, both in their own (7 out of 9) and in reviewed cases (8 of 9). Particularly surprising was that 12 of the deaths occurred in patients less than 50 years of age, a group where mortality in those who did not develop ARDS was 3.5%. Hypotension, hypothermia and coma were indicative of increased risk of ARDS.

The mechanism of development of ARDS has been hotly debated (139). Based on 2 case-reports, Leonard has suggested that the main precipitant is rapidly decreasing plasma oncotic pressure induced by resuscitation with crystalloid fluids and decreased hepatic protein synthesis (140). Fein et al (141) have conducted a detailed study of 18 patients who were resuscitated with a mean of 7.7 litres 0.077 mol/l saline over 12 hours, with a net positive fluid balance of 4.5 litres. Serial measurements showed decreases in colloid oncotic arterial oxygen gradient. However, in a further case-report of 2 episodes of ARDS complicating DKA in one patient, transmural pulmonary capillary wedge pressure remained normal and the authors suggested that the primary defect was an alveolocapillary permeability defect induced by acidosis and hyperventilation (142). The possibility that the permeability defect might be due to specific diabetic microangiopathy was raised. Not mentioned was the fact that many of the cases reported were rehydrated with 0.077 mol/l saline, which would tend to lower plasma osmolality very rapidly. This was true of all the cases reported by Fein et al (141). These patients were also rehydrated rapidly, which would further exacerbate the problem.

Elucidation of the mechanism of ARDS is of prime importance with regard to preventive therapy. If the defect is simply one of falling oncotic pressure, infusion with colloid rather than crystalloid fluid may prevent its development (143). However, if an alveolar leak is the primary defect, resuscitation with colloid may aggravate the situation. Nonetheless, it is worth emphasizing that ARDS is a rare complication of treatment of DKA — except perhaps in the Bronx — and any preventive measure adopted should not prejudice other aspects of treatment.

Cerebral oedema

Cerebral oedema has long been recognised as a complication of therapy for DKA, especially in children. When clinical manifestations occur, the outcome is very poor. However, recent studies in children (144) and adults (141) have demonstrated that subclinical cerebral oedema, as indicated by temporary decrease in cerebroventricular size, is present in many patients during treatment of DKA. As with ARDS, the mechanism is disputed, but rapid infusion of crystalloid fluids has again been implicated (123). The authors of a brief case-report of death due to cerebral oedema in a 20-year-old female with DKA who had received only 1.2 l of 2.5% glucose in 5 hours speculated that relative insulin overdose may be important, even though the patient had received only 24 units of insulin in 5 hours (145).

Paradoxically a case of coma in DKA associated with internal hydrocephalus demonstrated by CAT scan has been reported (146). The authors suggested that a minor degree of brain swelling plus a congenital structural malformation of the brainstem ventricular drainage system resulted in ventricular dilation rather than contraction.

A feature common to the cases reported here (141, 144, 145) and to many of the cases reported previously in the literature is the infusion of 'free water' in the form of either hypotonic saline or glucose. This will inevitably lead a more rapid fall in plasma osmolality than with isotonic saline. This will enhance cellular uptake of water in the brain due perhaps to the osmotic effect of accumulated polyols or 'idiogenic' osmoles. It is also worth noting that cerebral oedema rarely occurs unless blood glucose levels fall below 15 mmol/l (for review, see Ref. 4). One may conclude that if isotonic saline is used for rehydration and infusion of glucose solutions is commenced when blood glucose levels reach 15 mmol/l, then cerebral oedema will rarely occur.

Mucormycosis

Mucormycosis is an opportunistic fungal infection of the nose, sinuses, orbit and brain associated with DKA, which is fulminant and usually rapidly fatal. Delay in diagnosis, because of unfamiliarity with the condition, may worsen the outlook (147, 148). Presenting features include persisting drowsiness despite correction of the metabolic abnormalities, facial pain, cellulitis, and varying eye and neurological signs. The reasons for the fulminant nature of the infection are unclear. Severe hyperglycaemia and ketoacidosis depress neutrophil chemotaxis (149). A further study has suggested that under acidotic conditions, the capacity of transferrin to bind iron is temporarily disrupted, abolishing an important host defense mechanism and allowing growth of the fungus (150).

Recommended therapy includes correction of the metabolic abnormalities, local excision and debridement of all necrotic tissue, adequate sinus and orbital drainage, and local and intravenous amphotericin B (151). Long-term therapy with ketoconazole is effective in amphotericin resistance (152).

Rhabdomyolysis

A recent prospective study has suggested that non-traumatic rhabdomyolysis during DKA may be commoner than previously realised (153). Hypermyoglobinaemia and increased muscle creatine kinase was found in 5 out of 12 patients. These patients had higher initial blood glucose values and serum osmolalities and decreased renal function compared to those without muscle breakdown. No patient had clinical evidence of rhabdomyolysis. Acute renal failure has been reported as a complication of rhabdomyolysis in DKA (154).

Other complications

Two cases of spontaneous pneumomediastinum which resolved rapidly have been reported (155). Hyperventilation *per se*, decreased surfactant activity, and increased intrathoracic pressure secondary to vomiting have been suggested as aetiological factors over the years (see Ref. 155).

Mortality

DKA remains a significant cause of death in diabetes, accounting for 10% of all diabetes-related deaths in the United States between 1970 and 1978 (156). Figures were slightly lower in 1980 (19). In an analysis of death certificate data, mortality from diabetes associated with ketosis or coma declined during the study period (1970-1978) from 1.4 to 0.9 per 100,000 total population per year or from 74.3 to 36.4 per 100,000 diabetics per year (156). Death rates were highest in non-whites and rose precipitously in all cases after the age of 65. These figures may be grossly underestimated, because a recent study from Minnesota has highlighted the inaccuracies of data derived from death certificates, diabetes not being mentioned in 62% of the 428 diabetic deaths between 1965 and 1974 (157). The average mortality from DKA has been estimated at 9-10% of all diabetic deaths or 57 per 100,000 diabetics per year (19). Of these deaths, 59% were in those aged more than 65 years and only 15% were judged to be due primarily to DKA.

Death rates from individual studies vary widely. Sheppard and Wright quoted rates of 5.4 and 6.2% for low- and high-dose insulin regimes respectively (30). Increasing age, initial blood glucose and urea and lower pH systolic blood pressure were all poor prognostic indicators. Death was attributed purely to metabolic factors in 7 out of 9 instances. Mortality in the Rhode Island study was 9% but was especially high in those over 55 years of age and in those admitted from nursing homes (17). No initial metabolic parameter correlated with outcome, although 7 of the 16 admitted in coma died. A Danish study gave death rates of 8.4% in 1943-1963 and 4.7% in 1960-1979, death from non-metabolic causes being excluded (18). For patients over 50 years of age, the rate increased to 9.4%. Death from all causes during DKA is, however, dramatically higher in the over-50s. Gale et al (158) reported a fatality rate of 43% in this age group compared with 3.4% in the under-50s. In a detailed U.K. review of deaths in the under-50s the majority were deemed retrospectively to be avoidable with errors by patients, by primary health care staff, and by hospital staff (159). Overall mortality has diminished greatly over the past 50 years: the death rate was 38% in a literature review covering 1930-1959, and 9% between 1960 and 1975 (see Ref. 19). This latter figure probably holds true now.

Up to October, 1982, 7 deaths from DKA whilst on CSII had been reported (27). Although the authors did not provide figures on injection therapy for comparison, the authors stated that the use of CSII was not associated with an excess mortality.

Pitfalls in diagnosis and management

Diabetic ketoacidosis without hyperglycaemia

Since the advent of home blood glucose monitoring, many patients manage during an intercurrent illness to keep in moderate metabolic control at home by frequent blood glucose testing, insulin dosage adjustment and adequate fluid intake. Two patients have been described who managed at home for several days before developing thirst, nausea and vomiting and being admitted with classical biochemical DKA (160). Neither had tested for ketonuria. This may be especially important for patients using CSII, where after disruption of insulin delivery, blood glucose values plateau at around 15 mmol/l after 4 hours whilst ketone body levels continue to rise (161).

Organophosphorous poisoning

A 3-year-old boy presented with sudden onset of coma and the biochemical features of DKA. However, the acute onset of coma with no prodromal illness plus the clinical signs of pinpoint pupils and tachycardia allowed the diagnosis of organophosphorous poisoning to be considered. Recovery was prompt after atropine administration (162). The mechanism underlying the biochemical changes is unclear.

Gastrointestinal symptoms

It has long been recognised that the abdominal pain, nausea and vomiting of DKA may simulate an acute intra-abdominal emergency (163). Conversely, an abdominal emergency may precipitate DKA, making the initial abdominal problem difficult to diagnose. In a recent case-report of DKA in a previously unknown diabetic, death was due to delay in diagnosis of a ruptured ectopic pregnancy (164). Barrett and Sherwin (165) recommend careful history and examination, judicious use of laboratory tests, early surgical consultation and intervention once therapy for DKA is underway if underlying abdominal pathology is suspected. Ketoacidosis can stimulate foetal contractions and cause foetal distress, adequate therapy for DKA reversing these problems (166). The management of DKA in pregnancy has recently been reviewed (167).

Serum amylase

A non-specific rise in serum amylase concentration commonly occurs in DKA, due to both the salivary and pancreatic forms (168), again complicating the diagnosis of intra-abdominal pathology.

Serum creatinine

Because of positive interference by acetoacetate, serum creatinine measured by alkaline picrate methods may be falsely elevated in DKA, leading to unnecessary investigation of 'abnormal' renal function (169). A mean discrepancy of 124 mol/l was reported in 50 ketoacidotic patients, two-thirds having serum creatinine levels within the normal range when measured by enzymatic methods but above normal by the picrate method (170). The elevation of creatinine was proportional to the level of acetoacetate. Similar considerations apply to urine creatinine measurement and may cause errors in determination of creatinine clearance (171).

Electrocardiography

The electrocardiogram (ECG) remains a valuable tool for monitoring plasma K^+ in DKA. A wide variety of abnormalities may be seen, reflecting abnormal levels of not only potassium, but also magnesium and calcium (172). Two cases of ST-segment elevation suggestive of acute myocardial infarction at presentation with DKA have been described (173). The changes resolved within 3 hours of initiation of treatment for DKA and there were no serum enzyme rises to substantiate the diagnosis of myocardial infarction. A similar event in a man with hypokalaemic metabolic acidosis, hypocalcaemia, hypophosphataemia and hypomagnesaemia has been attributed to hypomagnesaemia (174). It should be stressed that acidaemia also causes ECG abnormalities and in the early stages of the treatment of DKA the ECG should be used as a comparative guide to changes in plasma potassium, rather than as an indication of absolute levels.

Prevention

Delays in seeking and providing medical attention were thought to be major contributory factors to the deaths of 27 people in DKA previously unrecognised as diabetic in a U.K. survey (175). Of the total deaths in DKA, neglect of the diabetes by the patient was contributory in 40% and delay in diagnosis or in taking appropriate action by the family doctor in 36%. The management of 46% of those who died in hospital was criticised. Factors thought to have led to misdiagnosis of DKA in a developing country included failure to take a full history, failure to perform urinalysis, failure to recognise the classical but less well-known symptoms and concentration on the precipitating cause (176). More effective education of the general public, the diabetic patient and the medical profession is thus urgently required to prevent such deaths.

The Grady Memorial Hospital Diabetes Programme provides a comprehensive, intensive education programme and long-term primary follow-up care for its diabetic patients, most of whom come from inner city areas (177). Since its introduction, the incidence of DKA has fallen significantly and savings resulting from less hospitalisation have covered the cost of the education programme, plus a surplus of 3 million dollars. In those undergoing repeated episodes of DKA, emotional support and counselling may help to decrease the rate of DKA although not improving the overall diabetic control as judged by HbA_1 (32, 33). Psychological testing has revealed a group of patients apparently at higher risk of developing DKA whilst using CSII (178). These patients seemed to be looking for a medical solution to their diabetes and considered that they had little control over their disease. Testing for ketonuria when blood glucose is higher than 13 mmol/l is particularly important for those using CSII (179). Provision of detailed sick-day rules and encouragement to make early telephone contact with the diabetes team is vital to prevent DKA (1, 25).

Conclusions

Diabetic ketoacidosis remains a potentially lethal condition with an overall mortality of 5-10% in most specialist centres, the older patient contributing much of this mortality. The introduction of education teams is diminishing the incidence of DKA which must remain the most effective way of dealing with the condition. Advances in treatment have occurred in the last 15 years, notably with regard to insulin. It will be seen from the above, however, that more research into fluid and electrolyte therapy is needed, and more attention needs to be paid to complications of treatment, particularly thromboembolic phenomena, infection and abnormal fluid distribution. Hopefully, advances in these areas will be reported in subsequent volumes of *The Diabetes Annual*.

References

1. Schade DS, Eaton RP, Alberti KGMM, Johnston DG (1981): *Diabetic Coma: Ketoacidotic and Hyperosmolar*. University of New Mexico Press, Albuquerque.
2. Schade DS, Eaton RP (1983): Diabetic ketoacidosis — pathogenesis, prevention and therapy. *Clin. Endocrinol. Metab., 12*, 321.
3. Keller U (1986): Diabetic ketoacidosis: current views on pathogenesis and treatment. *Diabetologia, 29*, 71.
4. Halperin ML, Goldstein MB, Bear RA, Josse RG (1985): Diabetic comas. In: Arieff AI, DeFronzo RA (Eds), *Fluid, Electrolyte, and Acid-Base Disorders*, p. 933. Churchill-Livingstone, Edinburgh.
5. Vignati L, Asmal AC, Black WL et al (1985): Coma in diabetes. In: Marble A et al (Eds), *Joslin's Diabetes Mellitus*, p. 526. Lea and Febiger, Philadelphia.
6. Kandel G, Aberman A (1983): Selected developments in the understanding of diabetic ketoacidosis. *Can. Med. Assoc. J., 128*, 392.
7. Watkins PJ (1982): Diabetic emergencies. *Br. Med. J., 285*, 360.
8. Gill G (1983): The management of diabetic emergencies. *Postgrad. Doctor (Middle East), 6*, 516.
9. Griffith DNW, Yudkin JS (1986): Diabetic ketoacidosis. *Br. J. Hosp. Med., 35*, 82.
10. Johnston DG, Alberti KGMM (1980): Diabetic emergencies: practical aspects of the management of diabetic ketoacidosis and diabetes during surgery. *Clin. Endocrinol. Metab., 9*, 437.
11. Ehrlich RM (1982): Diabetes mellitus in childhood. *Clin. Endocrinol. Metab., 11*, 195.
12. Sperling MA (1984): Diabetic ketoacidosis. *Pediatr. Clin. North Am., 31*, 591.
13. Felts PW (1983): Ketoacidosis. *Med. Clin. North Am., 67*, 831.
14. Kreisberg RA (1983): Diabetic ketoacidosis, alcoholic ketosis, lactic acidosis and hyporeninemic hypoaldosteronism. In: Ellenberg M, Rifkin H (Eds), *Diabetes Mellitus*, p. 621. Medical Examination Publication Co., New York.
15. Foster DW, McGarry JD (1983): The metabolic derangements and treatment of diabetic ketoacidosis. *N. Engl. J. Med., 309*, 159.
16. Halperin ML, Bear RA, Hannaford MC et al (1981): Selected aspects of the pathophysiology of metabolic acidosis in diabetes mellitus. *Diabetes, 30*, 781.
17. Faich GA, Fishbein HA, Ellis SE (1983): The epidemiology of diabetic acidosis: a population-based study. *Am. J. Epidemiol., 117*, 551.
18. Ellemann K, Soerensen JN, Pedersen L et al (1984): Epidemiology and treatment of diabetic ketoacidosis in a community population. *Diabetes Care, 7*, 528.
19. Fishbein HA (1985): Diabetic ketoacidosis, hyperosmolar nonketotic coma, lactic acidosis and hypoglycemia. In: Harris MI, Hamman RF (Eds), *Diabetes in America (National Diabetes Group)*, p. XII-I. US Department of Health and Human Sciences.

20. Murphy CC, Faulkenberry EH, Rumpel JD (1985): The use of a County Hospital emergency room by diabetic patients. *Diabetes Care, 8,* 48.
21. Scott RS, Brown LJ, Clifford P (1985): Use of health services by diabetic persons. II. Hospital admissions. *Diabetes Care, 8,* 43.
22. Peden NR, Braaten JT, McKendry JBR (1984): Diabetic ketoacidosis during long-term treatment with continuous subcutaneous insulin infusion. *Diabetes Care, 7,* 1.
23. Mecklenburg RS, Benson EA, Benson Jr JW et al (1984): Acute complications associated with insulin infusion pump therapy. *J. Am. Med. Assoc., 252,* 3265.
24. Mecklenburg RS, Guinn TS, Sannar CA, Blumenstein BA (1986): Malfunction of continuous subcutaneous insulin infusion systems: a one-year prospective study of 127 patients. *Diabetes Care, 9,* 351.
25. Knight G, Jennings AM, Boulton AJM et al (1985): Severe hyperkalaemia and ketoacidosis during routine treatment with an insulin pump. *Br. Med. J., 291,* 371.
26. Bending JJ, Pickup JC, Keen H (1985): Frequency of diabetic ketoacidosis and hypoglycemic coma during routine treatment with continuous subcutaneous insulin infusion. *Am. J. Med., 79,* 685.
27. Teutsch SM, Herman WH, Dwyer DM, Lane JM (1984): Mortality among diabetic patients using continuous subcutaneous insulin-infusion pumps. *N. Engl. J. Med., 310,* 361.
28. DCCT Research Group (1986): Results of feasibility of the Diabetes Control and Complications Trial (DCCT): glycemic control, follow-up and complications of therapy. *Diabetes, 35, Suppl. 1,* 3A.
29. Davies AG, Price DA, Houlton CA et al (1984): Continuous subcutaneous insulin infusion in diabetes mellitus: a year's prospective trial. *Arch. Dis. Child., 59,* 11027.
30. Sheppard MC, Wright AD (1982): The effect on mortality of low-dose insulin therapy for diabetic ketoacidosis. *Diabetes Care, 5,* 111.
31. Tattersall R (1985): Brittle diabetes. *Br. Med. J., 291,* 555.
32. Orr DP, Golden MP, Myers G et al (1983): Characteristics of adolescents with poorly controlled diabetes referred to a tertiary care center. *Diabetes Care, 6,* 170.
33. White K, Kolman ML, Wexler P (1984): Unstable diabetes and unstable families: a psychosocial evaluation of diabetic children with recurrent ketoacidosis. *Pediatrics, 73,* 749.
34. Flexner CW, Weiner JP, Saudek CD et al (1984): Repeated hospitalization for diabetic ketoacidosis: the game of 'sartoris'. *Am. J. Med., 76,* 691.
35. Boulton AJM, Knight G, Drury J et al (1983): Diabetic ketoacidosis associated with outpatient treatment using continuous subcutaneous insulin infusion. *Postgrad. Med. J., 59,* 438.
36. Slater DN, Smith GT, Mundy K (1982): Diabetes mellitus with ketoacidosis presenting as Fournier's gangrene. *J. R. Soc. Med., 75,* 530.
37. O'Dell K, Shipp J (1983): Fournier's syndrome in a ketoacidotic diabetic patient after intrascrotal insulin injections because of impotence. *Diabetes Care, 6,* 601.
38. Mordes D, Kreutner K, Metzger W et al (1982): Dangers of intravenous ritodrine in diabetic patients. *J. Am. Med. Assoc., 248,* 973.
39. Robbins DS, Sims EAH (1984): Recurrent ketoacidosis in acquired, total lipodystrophy (lipoatrophic diabetes). *Diabetes Care, 7,* 381.
40. Ross JM, Murali MR, De Lara TC et al (1984): Anaphylaxis and immunologic insulin resistance in a diabetic woman with ketoacidosis. *Diabetes Care, 7,* 276.
41. Miles JM, Gerich JE (1983): Glucose and ketone body kinetics in diabetic ketoacidosis. *Clin. Endocrinol. Metab., 12,* 303.
42. Miles JM, Rizza RA, Haymond MW et al (1980): Effects of acute insulin deficiency in glucose and ketone body turnover in man: evidence for the primary overproduction of glucose and ketone bodies in the genesis of diabetic ketoacidosis. *Diabetes, 29,* 926.

43. Hcrs II-G, Van Schaflingen E (1982): Fructose 2,6-biphosphate 2 years after its discovery. *Biochem. J., 206*, 1.
44. El Maghrabi MR, Claus TH, Pilkis J et al (1982): Regulation of rat liver fructose 2,6-biphosphatase. *J. Biol. Chem., 257*, 7603.
45. El Maghrabi MR, Fox E, Pilkis J et al (1982): Cyclic AMP-dependent phosphorylation of rat liver 6-phosphofructo-2-kinase/fructose 2,6-biphosphatase. *Biochem. Biophys. Res. Commun., 106*, 794.
46. Neely P, El Maghrabi MR, Pilkis SJ et al (1981): Effect of diabetes, insulin, starvation and refeeding on the level of rat hepatic fructose 2,6-biphosphatase. *Diabetes, 30*, 1062.
47. Exton JH (1981): The effects of glucagon on hepatic glycogen metabolism and glycogenolysis. In: Unger RH, Orci L (Eds), *Glucagon: Physiology, Pathophysiology and Morphology of Pancreatic A Cells*, p. 195. Elsevier/North-Holland, Amsterdam.
48. Sumi S, Mineo I, Kono N et al (1984): Decreases in hepatic fructose 2,6-bisphosphate level and fructose-6-phosphate 2-kinase activity in diabetic mice: a close relationship to the development of ketosis. *Biochem. Biophys. Res. Commun., 120*, 103.
49. Malchoff CD, Pohl SL, Kaiser DL et al (1984): Determinants of glucose and ketoacid concentrations in acutely hyperglycemic diabetic patients. *Am. J. Med., 77*, 275.
50. Johnston DG, Alberti KGMM (1982): Hormone control of ketone body metabolism in the normal and diabetic state. *Clin. Endocrinol. Metab., 11*, 329.
51. McGarry JD, Robles-Valdes C, Foster DW (1975): Role of carnitine in hepatic ketogenesis. *Proc. Natl Acad. Sci. USA, 72*, 4385.
52. McGarry JD, Takabayashi Y, Foster DW (1978): The role of malonyl CoA in the coordination of fatty acid synthesis and oxidation in isolated rat hepatocytes. *J. Biol. Chem., 253*, 8294.
53. Cook G, King M, Veech R (1978): Ketogenesis and malonyl CoA content of isolated rat hepatocytes. *J. Biol. Chem., 253*, 2529.
54. Saggerson ED (1982): Does fasting decrease the inhibitory effect of malonyl CoA on hepatic B-oxidation? *Biochem. J., 208*, 525.
55. Cook GA, Stephens TW, Harris RA (1984): Altered sensitivity of carnitine palmitoyltransferase to inhibition by malonyl CoA in ketotic diabetic rats. *Biochem. J., 219*, 337.
56. Soltesz G, Melegh B, Sandor A (1983): The relationship between carnitine and ketone body levels in diabetic children. *Acta Paediatr. Scand., 72*, 511.
57. Scofield RF, Schumann WC, Kumaran K (1983): Ketone body production in diabetic ketosis by other than liver. *Metabolism, 32*, 1009.
58. Hall SEH, Wastney ME, Bolton TM et al (1984): Ketone body kinetics in humans: the effects of insulin dependent diabetes, obesity and starvation. *J. Lipid Res., 25*, 1184.
59. Fery F, Balasse EO (1985): Ketone body production and disposal in diabetic ketosis: a comparison with fasting ketosis. *Diabetes, 34*, 326.
60. Nosadini R, Avogaro A, Trevisan R et al (1985): Acetoacetate and 3-hydroxybutyrate kinetics in obese and insulin dependent diabetic humans. *Am. J. Physiol., 248*, R611.
61. Owen OE, Trapp VE, Skutches CL et al (1982): Acetone metabolism during diabetic ketoacidosis. *Diabetes, 31*, 242.
62. Hetenyi Jr G, Ferrarotto C (1985): Gluconeogenesis from acetone in starved rats. *Biochem. J., 231*, 151.
63. Reichard Jr GA, Skutches CL, Hoeldtke RD, Owen OE (1986): Acetone metabolism in humans during diabetic ketoacidosis. *Diabetes, 35*, 668.
64. Weidman SW, Ragland JB, Fisher JN et al (1982): Effects of insulin on plasma lipoproteins in diabetic ketoacidosis: evidence for a change in high density lipoprotein composition during treatment. *J. Lipid Res., 23*, 171.

65. Joven J, Rubies-Prat J, De la Figuera M et al (1985): High density lipoprotein changes during treatment of diabetic ketoacidosis. *Diabète Métab., 11,* 102.
66. Gerard A, Schooneman F, Guine JM et al (1982): Treatment by plasma exchange of a patient with hyperlipidemia and diabetic ketoacidosis with lesional pulmonary edema and acute pancreatitis. *Vox Sang., 43,* 147.
67. Bihari DJ (1986): Metabolic acidosis. *Br. J. Hosp. Med., 2,* 89.
68. Linter SPK, Ryan DW (1986): The anion gap. *Br. J. Hosp. Med., 2,* 79.
69. Adrogue HJ, Eknoyan G, Suki WK (1984): Diabetic ketoacidosis: role of the kidney in the acid-base homeostasis re-evaluated. *Kidney Int., 25,* 591.
70. Adrogue HJ, Wilson H, Boyd AE et al (1982): Plasma acid-base patterns in diabetic ketoacidosis. *N. Engl. J. Med., 307,* 1603.
71. Gamblin GT, Ashburn RW, Kemp DG, Beuttel SC (1986): Diabetic ketoacidosis presenting with a normal anion gap. *Am. J. Med., 80,* 758.
72. Hilton JG, Vandenbroucke AC, Josse RG et al (1984): The urine anion gap: the critical clue to resolve a diagnostic dilemma in a patient with ketoacidosis. *Diabetes Care, 7,* 486.
73. Cronin JW, Kroop SF, Diamond J et al (1984): Alkalemia in diabetic ketoacidosis. *Am. J. Med., 77,* 192.
74. Prando R, Odetti P, Deferrari G (1984): Metabolic alkalosis in diabetic ketosis: a case report. *Diabète Métab., 10,* 218.
75. Paton RC (1981): Haemostatic changes in diabetic coma. *Diabetologia, 21,* 172.
76. Campbell RR, Foster KJ, Stirling C et al (1986): Paradoxical platelet behaviour in diabetic ketoacidosis. *Diabetes Med., 3,* 161.
77. Janka HU, Mehnert H (1982): No rationale for antiplatelet drug treatment in diabetic ketoacidosis. *Diabetologia, 23,* 286.
78. Axelrod L, Levine L (1982): Plasma prostaglandin levels in rats with diabetes mellitus and diabetic ketoacidosis. *Diabetes, 31,* 994.
79. McRae JR, Day RP, Metz SA et al (1985): Prostaglandin E_2 metabolite levels during diabetic ketoacidosis. *Diabetes, 34,* 761.
80. Axelrod L, Shulman GI, Blackshear PJ et al (1986): Plasma level of 13,14-dihydro-15-keto-PGE_2 in patients with diabetic ketoacidosis and in normal fasting subjects. *Diabetes, 35,* 1004.
81. Axelrod L, Cornelius P (1984): Plasma prostaglandin levels and circulating fuel levels in rats with diabetic ketoacidosis: effects of cyclooxygenase inhibitors and of alpha and beta adrenergic blockade. *Prostaglandins, 28,* 333.
82. Evan-Wong L, Davidson RJ (1982): Raised Coulter mean corpuscular volume in diabetic ketoacidosis, and its underlying association with marked plasma hyperosmolarity. *J. Clin. Pathol., 36,* 334.
83. Bock HA, Fluckiger R, Berger W et al (1985): Real and artefactual erythrocyte swelling in hyperglycaemia. *Diabetologia, 28,* 335.
84. Harano Y, Suzuki M, Kojima H et al (1984): Development of paper-strip test for 3-hydroxybutyrate and its clinical application. *Diabetes Care, 7,* 481.
85. Narins RG, Jones ER, Stom MC et al (1982): Diagnostic strategies in disorders of fluid, electrolyte and acid base homeostasis. *Am. J. Med., 72,* 496.
86. Oster JR, Rietberg B, Taylor AL et al (1984): Can β-hydroxybutyrate be detected at the bedside by in vitro oxidation with hydrogen peroxide? *Diabetes Care, 7,* 80.
87. Carroll P, Matz R (1983): Uncontrolled diabetes mellitus in adults: experience in treating diabetic ketoacidosis and hyperosmolar nonketotic coma with low dose insulin and a uniform treatment regimen. *Diabetes Care, 6,* 579.
88. Kitabchi AE, Matteri R, Murphy MB (1982): Optimal insulin delivery in diabetic ketoacidosis (DKA) and hyperglycemic, hyperosmolar nonketotic coma (HONC). *Diabetes Care, 5, Suppl. 1,* 78.

89. Dieterlen Ph, Charlochel F, Desjeux JF et al (1982): Traitement de l'acidocétose diabétique sévère de l'enfant. *Sem. Hôp.*, *58*, 654.
90. Schwenk WF, Haymond MW (1983): Treatment of diabetic ketoacidosis in children and young adults. *Primary Care*, *10*, 663.
91. Debbabi A, Ghachem KB, Dougui N et al (1983): La perfusion d'insuline en continue dans le traitement du coma acidocétosique de l'enfant. *Pédiatrie*, *38*, 379.
92. Vanelli M, Bernasconi S, Rossi S et al (1982): Le traitement de l'acidocétose diabétique. *Arch. Fr. Pédiatr.*, *39*, 203.
93. Abdulkadir J, Mengistu M, Daniel S et al (1983): Low dose insulin in the management of diabetic ketoacidosis in a suboptimal clinical setting. *East Afr. Med. J.*, *60*, 160.
94. Pallangyo KJ, Yusufali AM, Salim SS et al (1984): Treatment of diabetic coma in a tropical environment. *Trop. Doct.*, *14*, 72.
95. Bachmann W, Walter H, Lotz N et al (1982): Efficiency of human insulin (recombinant DNA) in the treatment of diabetic ketoacidosis and severe nonketoacidotic hyperglycaemia. *Diabetes Care*, *5*, *Suppl. 2*, 161.
96. Barrett EJ, DeFronzo RA, Bevilacqua S et al (1982): Insulin resistance in diabetic ketoacidosis. *Diabetes*, *31*, 923.
97. Yasuda K, Kitabachi AE (1982): Increased insulin binding to erythrocytes in diabetic ketoacidosis: normalization with insulin therapy. *J. Clin. Endocrinol. Metab.*, *55*, 408.
98. Van Putten JPM, Wieringa Tj, Krans HMJ (1985): Low pH and ketoacids induce insulin receptor binding and postbinding alterations in cultured 3T3 adipocytes. *Diabetes*, *34*, 744.
99. Meinders AE, Koppeschaar HPF, Sindram EDA et al (1978): The influence of rehydration in uncontrolled insulin dependent diabetes mellitus. *Neth. J. Med.*, *21*, 3.
100. Owen OE, Licht JH, Sapir DG (1981): Renal function and effects of partial rehydration during diabetic ketoacidosis. *Diabetes*, *30*, 510.
101. Waldhäusl W, Kleinberger G, Korn A et al (1979): Severe hyperglycemia: effects of rehydration on endocrine derangements and blood glucose concentration. *Diabetes*, *28*, 577.
102. West ML, Marsden PA, Singer GG, Halperin ML (1986): Quantitative analysis of glucose loss during acute therapy for hyperglycaemic, hyperosmolar syndrome. *Diabetes Care*, *9*, 465.
103. Podolsky S, Emerson Jr K (1973): Potassium depletion in diabetic ketoacidosis. *Diabetes*, *22*, 299.
104. Ionescu-Tirgoviste C, Mincu I (1976): The study of potassium metabolism in terms of the gravity of ketoacidosis: comments with reference to 100 cases. *Rev. Roum. Méd.*, *13*, 227.
105. Moore RD (1983): Effects of insulin upon ion transport. *Biochim. Biophys. Acta*, *737*, 1.
106. Beigelman PM (1971): Severe diabetic ketoacidosis (diabetic 'coma'): 482 episodes in 257 patients — experience of three years. *Diabetes*, *20*, 490.
107. Van Gaal L, De Leeuw I, Bekaert J (1981): Serum potassium levels in untreated diabetic ketoacidosis. *Diabetologia*, *21*, 338A.
108. Knight G, Blair P, Parker B et al (1986): Potassium balance during insulin pump treatment and the effects on plasma potassium of an 8 hour disruption of CSII. *Diabetic Med.*, *3*, 348A.
109. Pickup JC (1986): Hyperkalaemia after interruption of CSII. *Diabetologia*, *29*, 823.
110. Editorial (1986): Hyperkalaemia in diabetic ketoacidosis. *Lancet*, *2*, 845.
111. Adrogue HJ, Madias NE (1981): Changes in plasma potassium concentration during acute acid-base disturbances. *Am. J. Med.*, *71*, 456.
112. Oster JR, Perez GO, Vaamonde CA (1978): Relationship between blood pH and potassium and phosphorus during acute metabolic acidosis. *Am. J. Physiol.*, *235*, F345.
113. Fulop M (1979): Serum potassium in lactic acidosis and ketoacidosis. *N. Engl. J. Med.*, *300*, 1087.

114. Adrogue HJ, Lederer ED, Suki WN, Eknoyan G (1986): Determinants of plasma potassium levels in diabetic ketoacidosis. *Medicine, 65,* 163.
115. Viberti GC (1978): Glucose-induced hyperkalaemia: a hazard for diabetics. *Lancet, 2,* 690.
116. Nicholis GL, Kahn T, Sanchez A, Gabrilove GA (1981): Glucose-induced hyperkalaemia in diabetic subjects. *Arch. Intern. Med., 141,* 49.
117. Cagiero E, Martina V, Massara F, Molinati GM (1983): Glucagon-induced increase in plasma potassium levels in type I (insulin-dependent) diabetic subjects. *Diabetologia, 24,* 85.
118. Paice B, Gray JMB, McBride D et al (1983): Hyperkalaemia in patients in hospital. *Br. Med. J., 286,* 1189.
119. Montoliu J, Revert L (1985): Lethal hyperkalemia associated with severe hyperglycemia in diabetic patients with renal failure. *Am. J. Kidney Dis., V,* 47.
120. Hayashi M, Senba S, Saito I et al (1984): Potassium homeostasis in chronic experimental diabetes mellitus in rats. *Acta Endocrinol., 105,* 239.
121. Hebden RA, Gardiner SM, Bennett T et al (1986): The influence of streptozotocin-induced diabetes mellitus on fluid and electrolyte handling in rats. *Clin. Sci., 70,* 111.
122. Alberti KGMM, Emerson PM, Darley JR et al (1973): 2,3-Diphosphoglycerate and tissue oxygenation in uncontrolled diabetes mellitus. *Lancet, 2,* 391.
123. Wilson HK, Keuer SP, Lea AS et al (1982): Phosphate therapy in diabetic ketoacidosis. *Arch. Intern. Med., 142,* 517.
124. Fisher JN, Kitabchi AE (1983): A randomized study of phosphate therapy in the treatment of diabetic ketoacidosis. *J. Clin. Endocrinol. Metab., 57,* 177.
125. Becker DJ, Brown DR, Steranka BH et al (1983): Phosphate replacement during treatment of diabetic ketosis: effects on calcium and phosphorus homeostasis. *Am. J. Dis. Child., 137,* 241.
126. Shilo S, Werner D, Hershko C (1985): Acute hemolytic anemia caused by severe hypophosphatemia in diabetic ketoacidosis. *Acta Haematol., 73,* 55.
127. Fujii S, Takemura T, Wada M et al (1982): Magnesium levels in plasma, erythrocyte and urine in patients with diabetes mellitus. *Horm. Metab. Res., 14,* 161.
128. Juan D (1982): Clinical review: the clinical importance of hypomagnesemia. *Surgery, 91,* 510.
129. Moles KW, McMullen JK (1982): Insulin resistance and hypomagnesaemia: case report. *Br. Med., J., 285,* 262.
130. Poston GJ (1982): Insulin resistance and hypomagnesaemia. *Br. Med. J., 285,* 575.
131. Lever E, Jaspan JB (1983): Sodium bicarbonate therapy in severe diabetic ketoacidosis. *Am. J. Med., 75,* 263.
132. Hale PJ, Crase J, Nattrass M (1984): Metabolic effects of bicarbonate in the treatment of diabetic ketoacidosis. *Br. Med. J., 289,* 1035.
133. Taylor KG (1985): Metabolic effects of bicarbonate in the treatment of diabetic ketoacidosis. *Br. Med. J., 290,* 68.
134. Marr TJ, Traisman HS, Traisman ES et al (1981): Juvenile ketoacidosis: the use of sodium bicarbonate in the treatment of diabetic children. *J. Kansas Med. Soc., 892,* 282.
135. Hillman KM (1983): Resuscitation in diabetic ketoacidosis. *Crit. Care Med., 11,* 53.
136. Axelrod L (1982): Crystalloid infusions in diabetes. *Lancet, 2,* 548.
137. Matz R, Carroll P (1982): Crystalloid infusions in diabetes. *Lancet, 2,* 549.
138. Carroll P, Matz R (1982): Adult respiratory distress syndrome complicating severe uncontrolled diabetes mellitus: report of 9 cases and a review of the literature. *Diabetes Care, 5,* 574.
139. Editorial (1982): Crystalloid infusions in diabetic ketoacidosis. *Lancet, 2,* 308.
140. Leonard RCF, Asplin C, McCormick CV et al (1983): Acute respiratory distress in diabetic ketoacidosis: possible contribution of low colloid osmotic pressure. *Br. Med. J., 286,* 760.

141. Fein IA, Rackow EC, Sprung CL et al (1982): Relation of colloid osmotic pressure to arterial hypoxemia and cerebral edema during crystalloid volume loading of patients with diabetic ketoacidosis. *Ann. Intern. Med., 96*, 570.

142. Brun-Buisson CJL, Bonnet F, Bergeret S et al (1985): Recurrent high-permeability pulmonary edema associated with diabetic ketoacidosis. *Crit. Care Med., 13*, 55.

143. Hillman KM (1982): Crystalloid infusions in diabetes. *Lancet, 2*, 548.

144. Krane EJ, Rockoff MA, Wallman JK et al (1985): Subclinical brain swelling in children during treatment of diabetic ketoacidosis. *N. Engl. J. Med., 312*, 1147.

145. Garre M, Boles JM, Garo B et al (1986): Cerebral oedema in diabetic ketoacidosis: do we use too much insulin? *Lancet, 1*, 220.

146. Hayes PC, Newton RW (1984): Reversible internal hydrocephalus complicating diabetic keto-acidosis. *Scot. Med. J., 29*, 195.

147. Cliff JL, Mhando P (1982): Cerebral mucormycosis: a case report. *East Afr. Med. J., 59*, 76.

148. Moss ALH (1983): Rhinocerebral mucormycosis. *Ann. Plast. Surg., 9*, 431.

149. Chinn RYW, Diamond RD (1982): Generation of chemotactic factor by *Rhizopus oryzae* in the presence and absence of serum: relationship to hyphal damage mediated by human neutrophils and effects of hyperglycemia and ketoacidosis. *Infect. Immun., 38*, 1123.

150. Artis WM, Fountain JA, Delcher HK et al (1982): A mechanism of susceptibility to mucormycosis in diabetic ketoacidosis: transferrin and iron availability. *Diabetes, 31*, 1109.

151. Kohn R, Hepler R (1986): Management of limited rhino-orbital mucormycosis without exenteration. *Ophthalmology, 92*, 1440.

152. Barnert J, Behr W, Reich H (1986): An amphotericin B-resistant case of rhinocerebral mucormycosis. *Infection, 13*, 134.

153. Moller-Petersen J, Andersen PT, Hjorne N et al (1986): Nontraumatic rhabdomyolysis during diabetic ketoacidosis. *Diabetologia, 29*, 229.

154. Pistor K, Graben N, Heber F et al (1984): Atraumatic rhabdomyolysis with reversible acute renal failure in a child with diabetic coma. *Monatsschr. Kinderheilkd., 132*, 51.

155. Goldszmidt D, Questiaux E, Bach CH (1984): Emphysème médiastinal au cours d'une acido-cétose diabétique. *Arch. Fr. Pédiatr., 41*, 131.

156. Holman RC, Herron CA, Sinnock P (1983): Epidemiologic characteristics of mortality from diabetes with acidosis or coma, United States, 1970-78. *Am. J. Publ. Health, 73*, 1169.

157. Ochi JW, Melton III J, Palumbo PJ et al (1985): A population-based study of diabetes mortality. *Diabetes Care, 8*, 224.

158. Gale EAM, Dornan TL, Tattersall RB (1981): Severely uncontrolled diabetes in the over fifties. *Diabetologia, 21*, 25.

159. Tunbridge WMG (1981): Deaths due to diabetic ketoacidosis. *Q. J. Med., 50*, 502.

160. Bell PM, Hadden DR (1983): Ketoacidosis without hyperglycemia during self-monitoring of diabetes. *Diabetes Care, 6*, 622.

161. Pickup JC, Viberti GC, Bilous RW et al (1982): Safety of continuous subcutaneous insulin infusion: metabolic deterioration and glycaemic autoregulation after deliberate cessation of infusion. *Diabetologia, 22*, 175.

162. Zadik Z, Blachar Y, Barak Y et al (1983): Organophosphate poisoning presenting as diabetic ketoacidosis. *Toxicology, 20*, 381.

163. McKittrick LS (1933): Abdominal symptoms with or without abdominal lesions in diabetic acidosis. *N. Engl. J. Med., 209*, 1033.

164. Glynn MJ, Elliot D (1984): Diabetic ketoacidosis and ruptured ectopic pregnancy: a fatal combination. *Br. Med. J., 288*, 1287.

165. Barrett EJ, Sherwin RS (1983): Gastrointestinal manifestations of diabetic ketoacidosis. *Yale J. Biol. Med., 56*, 175.

166. Rhodes RW, Ogburn Jr PL (1984): Treatment of severe diabetic ketoacidosis in the early third trimester in a patient with fetal distress. *J. Reprod. Med., 29,* 621.
167. Brumfield CG, Huddleston JF (1984): The management of diabetic ketoacidosis in pregnancy. *Clin. Obstet. Gynecol., 27,* 50.
168. Kjaergaard JJ, Salling N, Magid et al (1984): Serum amylase during recovery from diabetic ketoacidosis. *Diabète Métab., 10,* 25.
169. Assadi FK, John EG, Fornell L et al (1985): Falsely elevated serum creatinine concentration in ketoacidosis. *J. Pediatr., 107,* 562.
170. Gerard SK, Khayam-Bashi H (1985): Characterization of creatinine error in ketotic patients: a prospective comparison of alkaline picrate methods with an enzymatic method. *Am. J. Clin. Pathol., 84,* 659.
171. Blank DW, Nanji AA (1982): Ketone interference in estimation of urinary creatinine: effect on creatinine clearance in diabetic ketoacidosis. *Clin. Biochem., 15,* 279.
172. Chava NR (1984): ECG in diabetic ketoacidosis. *Arch. Intern. Med., 144,* 2379.
173. Fuller PJ, Colman PG, Harper RW et al (1982): Transient anterior electrocardiographic changes simulating acute anterior myocardial infarction in diabetic ketoacidosis. *Diabetes Care, 5,* 118.
174. Khardori R, Cohen B, Taylor D et al (1985): Electrocardiographic finding simulating acute myocardial infarction in a compound metabolic aberration. *Am. J. Med., 78,* 529.
175. Tunbridge WMG (1981): Factors contributing to deaths of diabetics under fifty years of age. *Lancet, 2,* 569.
176. Rwiza HT, Swai ABM, McLarty DG (1986): Failure to diagnose diabetic ketoacidosis in Tanzania. *Diabetic Med., 3,* 181.
177. Davidson JK (1983): The Grady Memorial Hospital Diabetes Programme. In: Mann JI, Pyorola K, Teuscher A (Eds), *Diabetes in Epidemiological Perspective,* p. 332. Churchill-Livingstone, Edinburgh.
178. Bradley C, Gamsu DS, Knight G et al (1986): Predicting risk of diabetic ketoacidosis in patients using continuous subcutaneous insulin infusion. *Br. Med. J., 293,* 242.
179. Marshall SM, Alberti KGMM, Home PD (1987): Continuous subcutaneous insulin infusion: problems encountered in clinical usage. In: Hotta N, Sakamotoa N, Alberti KGMM (Eds), *Trends in the Management of Diabetes.* Elsevier, Amsterdam. In press.

The Diabetes Annual/3
K.G.M.M. Alberti and L.P. Krall, editors
© 1987 Elsevier Science Publishers, B.V.

28   Exercise and diabetes

DAVID H. WASSERMAN AND MLADEN VRANIC

Understanding the hormonal and metabolic processes associated with exercise in diabetes is difficult, since factors involved in substrate metabolism, even during exercise in normal individuals, are not understood completely. Studies from Sweden, primarily in the 1970s, used the hepatic vein technique coupled with cross limb measurements and muscle biopsies to characterize aspects of substrate utilization during exercise in normal human subjects and insulin-dependent diabetic patients. Investigations conducted in animals and man in the late 1970s and the 1980s have focused on the hormonal and autonomic control mechanisms which may act to regulate metabolism such that the most optimal balance of substrates is utilized during muscular work. Despite the substantial progress made in recent years, many questions regarding control of exercise metabolism remain. An acute bout of exercise poses potential problems in insulin-dependent diabetes mellitus (IDDM) and the degree of insulinization adds a further degree of complexity to the therapeutic regimen. It is necessary to minimize the risks of exercise in this population so that the diabetic person who chooses to lead an active life can do so safely.

Exercise training is currently the subject of much interest as an adjuvant therapy, particularly in the treatment of non-insulin-dependent (NIDDM) diabetes. Habitual physical activity can be of value to both IDDM and NIDDM for its potential beneficial effects on cardiovascular disease risk factors.

This review will focus on substrate metabolism and the role of hormones that are thought to be metabolically important during an acute bout of exercise in normal human and diabetic subjects. Aspects of exercise training in diabetic populations will be discussed also. The emphasis will be placed on work published over the last 5 years and on selected older investigations which are needed to form a foundation for the understanding of the more recent work.

Physiology of exercise substrate metabolism

The capacity to store and mobilize fuel is essential in providing metabolic substrate in the postabsorptive state. For this purpose, carbohydrates are stored as glycogen in muscle and liver, and fatty acids as triglycerides, primarily in adipose tissue, but also in the muscle. To a lesser extent, amino acids may be used as fuel, particularly when the availability of other substrates becomes limited. The increased energy demand of muscular work necessitates an accelerated flow of these substrates from their storage sites to the energy-transducing machinery in working muscle. During the transition from rest to moderate-intensity exercise, the muscle shifts from using exclusively non-esterified 'free' fatty acids (FFA) to using a blend of FFA, extramuscular glucose, and glycogen. During the early stages of exercise, muscle glycogen is the chief source of energy for muscular contraction. With increasing exercise duration the contribution of circulating glucose and particularly of FFA becomes of increasing importance as muscle glycogen is gradually depleted (1). Also, with increasing duration of exercise the origin of the circulating glucose shifts from hepatic glycogenolysis to gluconeogenesis (1). With increasing exercise intensity the balance of substrates used shifts to greater oxidation of carbohydrates (2, 3). Specific aspects of substrate metabolism can be defined in terms of 3 functional aims (4):

Preserving glucose homeostasis

Exercise is generally characterized by euglycemia. Thus, there is an increase in hepatic glucose production during exercise which usually matches the increment in glucose uptake. Under certain conditions, however, blood glucose concentration may deviate from normal basal levels. Thus, during prolonged exercise, gradually diminishing carbohydrate stores often result in a fall in blood glucose levels (1). In contrast, during heavy exercise a rise in glycemia can ensue (2) as glucose production exceeds peripheral metabolism. The tendency for constant blood glucose levels despite large increases in glucose uptake is central to the understanding of glucoregulation during exercise.

Metabolizing the most efficient substrate

Metabolic efficiency During high-intensity work when adenosine triphosphate (ATP) hydrolysis is particularly rapid and oxygen availability may be limiting, carbohydrates are the preferred substrate. Generation of ATP from oxidation of glucose in the cytoplasm occurs more rapidly than from fat oxidation in the mitochondria (5). Furthermore, since glucose carbon atoms are already partly oxidized compared to the highly saturated carbon skeleton of fats, they require less oxygen for complete metabolism. Hence, when oxygen availability is limiting, such as during heavy exercise, glucose is the most efficient fuel.

Storage efficiency Low-intensity exercise which can potentially be sustained for long intervals is characterized by a preference for fat oxidation. Under these circumstances, speed and efficiency of energy transduction become secondary to fuel storage efficiency. Differences in the degree of saturation between fatty acids and glucose predict that twice as much energy can be gained from the oxidation of 1 gram of triglyceride as from 1 gram of glycogen. In addition, while glycogen is stored with water, fats are immiscible with water and are stored in pure form. Hence, the economy of fat storage makes this fuel the most efficient for long-duration muscular activity.

Delaying exhaustion

For exercise that is not limited by the cardiopulmonary system, muscle glycogen depletion appears to be a primary cause of muscular fatigue (6). Hence, prolonged exercise necessitates that intramuscular and extramuscular fat and extramuscular glucose be utilized as alternative substrates to delay the depletion of muscle glycogen, but without greatly perturbing homeostasis or sacrificing metabolic efficiency.

Role of hormones in control of substrate utilization

From the preceding it is clear that maximizing work capacity while minimizing alterations in glucose homeostasis requires not only a quantitative matching of glucose production to its accelerated uptake at the muscle, but also the maintenance of a specific balance of fat and carbohydrate utilization. Recent work indicates that the control of the optimal substrate balance during exercise is achieved largely by the combined action of insulin, glucagon, and the catecholamines (7-15). In addition to the factors mentioned, it is likely that other parameters such as blood flow shifts (7, 16), subtle changes in glycemia (17), or metabolic state (18-20) play a role in control of exercise fuel metabolism.

Hormonal responses to exercise

Exercise is characterized by diverse endocrine responses as well as increased adrenergic drive which are dependent on the duration and intensity of exercise (21). In general, exercise is characterized by a fall in insulin secretion (2, 22) and increases in glucagon (23), catecholamines (24), and cortisol (24), among others (21). Hormone levels may increase during exercise secondarily to an increase in adrenergic drive, a decrease in circulating glucose, or as a result of a decreased blood flow to the clearing organ (e.g. liver) (21). However, in general, the stimuli for the increase in adrenergic drive and the changes in hormone levels during exercise are, for the most part, unknown.

Glucagon-insulin interaction at the liver

Within the last several years, studies have demonstrated clearly an important role for the presence of glucagon (10, 12, 13, 25-27) and, more precisely, glucagon-insulin interactions (9, 12, 28) in regulation of hepatic glucose production during exercise and as a consequence, blood glucose. When glucagon secretion was suppressed during exercise with somatostatin, glucose production was attenuated by 3.9 mg/kg-min and as a result glucose levels fell by nearly 30 mg/100 ml (1.7 mM) (12). The fall in glucose levels elicited an excessive increase in epinephrine which partly restored glycemia by providing alternative substrates to glucose for muscle metabolism and possibly by stimulating hepatic glucose production. When glucagon was suppressed and euglycemia was maintained by exogenous glucose infusion, the full impact of glucagon suppression could be evidenced as compensatory mechanisms for the fall in glucose were eliminated. Under these circumstances, it could be determined that, in the dog, glucagon controls approximately 60% of the glucose released from the liver during exercise (12). In the resting state, glucagon also controls about 60% of the hepatic glucose production (29), but since the rate of glucose release is accelerated with muscular activity, the absolute effects of glucagon action are considerably greater during exercise (Fig. 1). It is particularly important that the strongest correlate to hepatic glucose production in the exercising dog does not appear to be glucagon *per se*, but instead the ratio of glucagon to insulin (9, 12). The importance of the presence of glucagon during exercise has also been demonstrated in human subjects (25) and in sheep (27) receiving somatostatin infusions and in rats administered glucagon antibodies (26).

Studies published within the last year (8, 15) extended the above work showing the importance of the presence of glucagon, by investigating whether changes in glucagon and insulin from basal levels are necessary to regulate hepatic glucose production in exercising human subjects. In these investigations, endogenous glucagon and insulin release was prevented by somatostatin infusion and the pancreatic hormones were replaced in a peripheral vein at matched rates which created normal arterial levels of these hormones and euglycemia. While with normal exercise glucagon increases and insulin decreases, in these studies the hormone levels were left unchanged. Despite the inability of the pancreatic hormones to adapt to muscular work, hepatic glucose production responded normally to exercise (8, 15). It is difficult to interpret these results because the normal entry site of the pancreatic hormones, into the portal vein, is largely inaccessible in human subjects and replacement must occur in a peripheral vein. Thus, the important porto-peripheral insulin gradient is lost and it is probable that the liver is actually hypoinsulinemic under these conditions. When an attempt was made to overcome this problem by replacing insulin at increased rates to create portal euinsulincmia (albeit

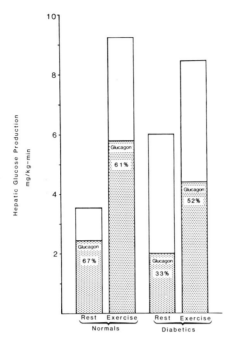

FIG. 1. *The role of glucagon in regulation of hepatic glucose production during rest and exercise in normal and alloxan-diabetic dogs. The shaded area represents the portion of the hepatic glucose production controlled by glucagon. Reproduced from Wasserman and Vranic (4), Diabetes/ Metabolism Reviews, by permission of John Wiley and Sons, Inc. Copyright © 1986, John Wiley and Sons, Inc.*

peripheral hyperinsulinemia), and euglycemia was maintained with glucose infusion, ^{13}C-glucose enrichment did not change. This indicated that hepatic glucose production did not increase from rest through exercise (15). From these latter studies it was concluded that a decrease in insulin and/or an increase in glucagon must occur for normal glucose kinetics during exercise.

Peripheral effects of insulin

Since insulin levels are reduced during exercise, it was suspected that insulin may not be important for the exercise-induced increment in glucose uptake. Indeed, in most instances (30-33), but not all (34), muscle contraction *per se* has been shown to stimulate glucose uptake in vitro even when no insulin is present. Nevertheless, it does not appear that results attained in vitro can be extrapolated completely to the whole organism where metabolic events antagonistic to glucose uptake occur (e.g. enhanced muscle FFA oxidation, increased muscle glycogenolysis, catecholamine action). In completely insulin-deprived (35, 36) or greatly underinsulinized (37) depancreatized dogs whole-body glucose clearance does not increase. When urinary excretion of glucose is subtracted from tracer-determined glucose disappearance during rest and exercise, a small, but still subnormal, increase in glucose clearance can be detected (35). Intraportal replacement of insulin during rest and exercise in depancreatized dogs returns glucose utilization to levels seen in normal dogs (37). It can be calculated from these studies that portal insulin replacement is responsible for 47% of the glucose cleared in depancreatized dogs (Fig. 2). It was concluded from this work that some insulin is essential for the normal exercise-induced increase in glucose metabolic clearance.

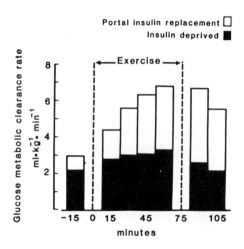

FIG. 2. *The role of insulin in control of glucose metabolic clearance during exercise in the depancreatized dog. Shaded area represents the level of glucose clearance in insulin-deprived depancreatized dogs and the open bar represents the additional increment in glucose clearance resulting from intraportal replacement of insulin to normal exercise levels. Reproduced from Wasserman and Vranic (4), Diabetes/Metabolism Reviews, by permission of John Wiley and Sons, Inc. Copyright © 1986, John Wiley and Sons, Inc.*

It appears that the metabolic and hemodynamic changes operative during exercise work to sensitize the tissues of the body to the reduced circulating insulin levels. Thus, the increased blood flow to the working muscles during exercise results in an increased delivery of fuel and insulin (7, 16). The ability of exercise to work synergistically with insulin was demonstrated by the substantial increase in glucose metabolism which occurred when a bout of exercise was superimposed on a hyperinsulinemic, euglycemic clamp (7). Leg glucose uptake increased with combined exercise and hyperinsulinemia to a greater extent then the sum of the two treatments performed independently of each other and this increase in glucose uptake paralleled the exercise-induced increment in leg blood flow. Support for increased insulin delivery to working muscle is the observation that exercising rats had an excessive accumulation of ^{3}H fragments in skeletal muscle following subcutaneous ^{3}H-insulin injection compared to resting controls (38). However, even in isolated rat muscle (39) or hindquarter (40-43) in which substrate and hormone availability can be regulated, or in the post-exercise state (44-46) when blood flow is slowly diverted from muscle, there is an increase in glucose tolerance and insulin sensitivity. Glycogen depletion which may occur with exercise is likely to be a key factor in the enhanced insulin sensitivity following muscular work (39-42, 44, 47). Whether the action of insulin is facilitated by an increase in binding to skeletal muscle is unclear. Binding of insulin to erythrocytes and monocytes has been shown to increase with moderate-intensity exercise (48, 49), while decreasing with heavy exercise (49). Only recently have studies examined insulin binding in skeletal muscle, the bulk of insulin-sensitive tissue.

Insulin binding to skeletal muscle after moderate-intensity exercise has been shown not to change in human subjects (50) and both to increase (51) and not change (52) in rats, while actually decreasing during high-intensity exercise in human subjects (50). Thus, it is not clear what role the changes in insulin binding to skeletal muscle play in regulating the enhanced insulin sensitivity seen with exercise. Post-receptor changes following exercise have not been investigated in skeletal muscle. However, insulin-stimulated generation of a pyruvate dehydrogenase activator that was shown to increase after exercise in rat liver and adipocyte membrane is likely to be due to some post-receptor event (53).

In addition to affecting glucose metabolism, insulin can also stimulate muscle amino acid uptake, a process enhanced by exercise (52). Furthermore, insulin has an antilipolytic effect on adipocytes, which may be minimized with the normal exercise-induced fall in levels of this hormone. Mild hyperinsulinemia has been shown to inhibit the normal exercise-induced increase in FFA levels (54). By regulating FFA release from adipose tissue, insulin may provide the muscle with alternate substrate to glucose and, thereby, indirectly affect muscular glucose uptake (55). This would effectively add a second level of control to insulin's direct effects on glucose metabolism.

Catecholamines

Role at the liver   The role of the catecholamines in regulation of hepatic glucose metabolism has been studied using β- and α-adrenergic receptor blockers, as well as by investigating the effects of adrenalectomy. Beta-blockade in normal rats (56), dogs (57), and human subjects (58) does not appear to affect hepatic glucose production during exercise. Furthermore, alpha-blockade (58) and combined alpha- and beta-blockade (8, 58) did not affect the increment in hepatic glucose production during normal exercise in human subjects. It was interesting, however, that when combined alpha- and beta-blockade was performed while changes in glucagon and insulin were prevented with somatostatin and peripheral hormone replacement, glucose production was markedly reduced (8). Thus, in the absence of the normal pancreatic response, an intact sympathochromaffin response was essential. To test whether this effect was due to the action of epinephrine, subjects adrenalectomized for treatment of Cushing's disease or bilateral pheochromocytoma were studied during exercise while changes in the pancreatic hormones were prevented as before (59). Under these circumstances, hepatic glucose production increased normally, leading the investigators to conclude that it was sympathetic release of norepinephrine that is most prominent in the counterregulatory hierarchy during exercise. Studies in the rat have been conflicting, demonstrating either no effect of adrenalectomy (60, 61) or a decrease (62, 63) in hepatic glycogenolysis. In contrast to the conclusions deduced indirectly from work in man (59), hepatic innervation was shown not to affect glucose turnover in the exercising rat. While data collected in the rat may not necessarily be comparable, technical problems preclude the direct assessment of hepatic innervation in human subjects and the diverse actions of the catecholamines make studies with adrenergic receptor blockers difficult to interpret.

Peripheral effects Muscle biopsies from human subjects studied during either beta-blockade (64) or epinephrine infusion (65) indicated that the catecholamines play a role in glycogen mobilization during dynamic exercise. This was supported by studies in the exercising dog in which tracer-determined glycogenolytic rate was shown to be significantly impaired with beta-blockade (57), resulting in diminished lactate levels (14, 57). The exercise-induced increase in plasma FFA levels in humans can be enhanced by alpha-blockade (58, 66) and inhibited by beta-blockade (66), presumably due to changes in lipolytic activity. With combined alpha- and beta-blockade, the beta-blocking effects predominate and the rise in FFA levels is abolished (8, 58). In this light, it is surprising that neither adrenalectomy (59) nor autonomic neuropathy (67) affects plasma FFA levels during exercise in human subjects. It is possible that with a deficit in either the adrenal glands or in sympathetic innervation the remaining system can compensate sufficiently.

Epinephrine inhibits insulin-mediated glucose uptake in skeletal muscle via β-adrenergic mechanisms (68). In dogs (57) and man (8, 58), propranolol tends to cause an excessive increase in glucose uptake during exercise. Oxidation of fat and glycogen in skeletal muscle initiated by an epinephrine-stimulated increase in mobilization of these fuel sources will result in the buildup of metabolic intermediates which can feedback to inhibit muscular glucose uptake (69). By preventing these processes, beta-blockade can stimulate muscle glucose uptake.

Metabolic factors in control of glucose uptake

The importance of factors within the working muscle *per se* are best illustrated by the excessive increments in glucose uptake seen in situations where oxygen availability is limited during exercise such as during anemia (20), when breathing a hypoxic gas mixture (18), or during severe work (2). Although catecholamines are greatly increased under these circumstances, glucose uptake is still exaggerated. In anemic dogs, glucose clearance was elevated 4-fold despite insulin levels which were similar and epinephrine levels which were 6-fold higher than exercising control dogs (20). In these studies the fall in plasma glucose was only moderate as the increment in glucose production was also exaggerated in anemic dogs relative to controls. These in vivo findings are consistent with work showing that tissue hypoxia can accelerate glucose uptake in rat skeletal muscle (19, 70). Thus, the increased metabolic demand for carbohydrates caused by tissue hypoxia clearly outweighs the peripheral counter-regulatory effects of the catecholamines. The precise mechanism by which metabolic rate controls glucose transport remains to be elucidated.

Hormonal and metabolic effects of acute exercise in diabetes

Due to the diverse actions of insulin, diabetes mellitus is characterized by abnormalities of carbohydrate, fat, and amino acid metabolism. The inability to regulate insulin secretion is clearly a deficit when trying to meet the enhanced metabolic requirements of muscular work. While, in general, the diabetic is able to meet the energy needs of exercise, it is often with less than the optimal balance of substrate usage. The metabolic response to exercise in the diabetic will vary with age, fitness, type of exercise, and nutritional status. In addition, the complications and metabolic abnormalities often characterizing the diabetic state can make exercise programs difficult. Due to a left-shifted oxygen dissociation curve as a result of high levels of glycosylated hemoglobin (71) and the high frequency of vascular disease in diabetics (72), oxygen delivery may be impaired, which may result in a change in hormonal and metabolic responses (18, 20). Furthermore, the development of neuropathies in patients with longstanding diabetes may hinder work tolerance (67).

Exercise in IDDM

Substrate utilization The most readily observable difference between inadequately controlled diabetic patients and normal subjects is the inability to regulate blood glucose levels, particularly when confronted by a metabolic challenge. Nevertheless, during exercise, increments in glucose fluxes are usually similar to those seen in normal subjects (13, 73). The mechanisms for the increase in glucose fluxes, however, in diabetic subjects are very different from those in healthy subjects. Thus, although the increase in glucose production is quantitatively similar in both populations, diabetic subjects rely more heavily on glucose derived from gluconeogenesis (73, 74). Total gluconeogenic precursor uptake by the splanchnic bed could account for up to 30% of the splanchnic glucose output after 40 min of exercise compared to just 11% in normal subjects, due to a greater delivery and fractional extraction of gluconeogenic substrate by the splanchnic bed (73).

Generally, glucose utilization also increases similarly in both normal and diabetic subjects, but whereas in normal subjects the increase in glucose utilization is due to an increase in glucose clearance, in inadequately controlled diabetic patients it is a result of an increased mass action effect due to the excessive hyperglycemia that is present (36, 37, 73, 75) coupled with a smaller increment in glucose clearance (35). In addition, a smaller percentage of the glucose taken up by muscle is completely oxidized in diabetic subjects (76), probably due to impaired pyruvate dehydrogenase activity (77). Increased FFA utilization appears to compensate, at least in part, for the reduction in energy production that results from the diminished capacity to oxidize glucose in diabetic subjects (73). From the data of Wahren et al (73), it can be estimated that during 40 min of moderate exercise FFA uptake can account for only up to 27% of the energy needs of the working leg in normal subjects, but as much as 33% and 56% in non-ketotic and ketotic diabetic subjects respectively. IDDM is also associated with a greater availability of ketone bodies for energy metabolism, the degree to which depends on the state of metabolic control (73-75, 78, 79). Splanchnic ketone body production is elevated during exercise in IDDM due to an increased splanchnic fractional extraction and a greater intrahepatic conversion of FFA to ketone bodies as assessed by ^{14}C-oleic acid infusion (79). Although the ketone bodies are still quantitatively unimportant as a fuel source, even in IDDM, the study of ketone body metabolism is critical to understanding the ketoacidosis in poorly controlled IDDM.

In addition to blood-borne substrate utilization, there are differences in intramuscular substrate utilization during exercise. When compared with normal subjects and well-controlled diabetic patients, diabetics exhibit a decrease in intramuscular glycogen storage and an increase in intramuscular fat storage when deprived of insulin for 24 hours (80). As predicted by the shift in intramuscular substrate stores, insulin-deficient diabetic subjects oxidize a greater amount of intramuscular fat and a diminished amount of intramuscular glycogen than normal subjects and well-controlled diabetic subjects (80). By using radioactively labeled palmitate and glucose in combination with gas exchange measurements, it was calculated that in the insulin-deficient depancreatized dog over twice as much intramuscular fat, but only about 60% of the muscle glycogen, is used (81).

Thus, in IDDM there is a general tendency to rely on fat metabolism to a greater degree than in normal subjects. This added reliance on fats appears to be a function of the state of metabolic control, such that a well-insulinized diabetic patient will respond to exercise in a manner more closely reflecting substrate metabolism in normal subjects than would a poorly controlled diabetic patient (73, 80). Although adequate insulinization is crucial for optimal substrate utilization during exercise in the IDDM patient it will be shown in the following section how insulin levels appropriate for resting conditions can result in relative overinsulinization and consequently, hypoglycemia, during exercise.

Importance of proper insulin administration to the metabolic response of acute exercise   The importance of proper insulin therapy in IDDM is illustrated by problems of metabolic regulation during exercise in patients in whom optimal insulinization has not been achieved. Patients with severe insulin-deficiency manifested by substantial hyperglycemia and ketosis can actually experience a worsened metabolic state during exercise (37, 78, 82). During studies in which IDDM patients were deprived of exogenous insulin for a prolonged period (18-48 h), ketosis and hyperglycemia resulted (78). When these subjects underwent a prolonged bout of exercise which would typically result in a decline in blood glucose in normal subjects and well-controlled diabetic patients, an exaggerated counterregulatory response ensued and paradoxically a further rise in blood glucose occurred (78). Studies in the depancreatized dog (36, 37) indicate that this rise in glucose with severe insulin-deficiency is due to an inadequate increase in glucose utilization. In addition, underinsulinization in the diabetic patient will lead to further increases in FFA and ketone body levels with exercise compared to normal subjects and well-controlled diabetic patients. Thus, exercise in the poorly controlled diabetic patient may contribute to the existing hyperglycemia, hyperlipidemia, and lead to ketoacidosis. The role of counterregulatory hormones in the deleterious effects of exercise in IDDM is discussed in a subsequent section.

Attaining optimal insulin therapy in the physically active IDDM patient is a two-sided problem. An adequate amount of insulin is essential during exercise in IDDM to avoid aggravating the metabolic state. However, hypoglycemia commonly occurs during and after exercise due to relative overinsulinization. Studies with labeled insulin preparations in rats (38) and in human subjects (83) have indicated that the absorption of insulin injected subcutaneously into the circulation can be accelerated during exercise. It has been proposed that insulin absorption kinetics from the subcutaneous depot can be dissipated (83) and the tendency toward hypoglycemia (83, 84) may be minimized by injecting away from the site of contraction. However, other studies have shown that this meas-

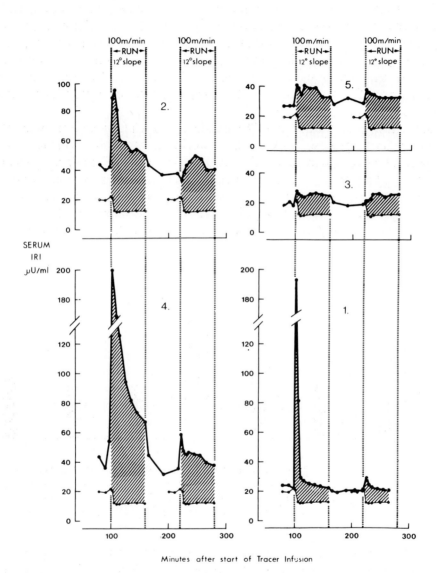

FIG. 3.   *Serum concentration of immunoreactive insulin (IRI) during rest and exercise in 5 de-pancreatized dogs 8-9 h after administration of food and insulin. Shaded areas designate the differences between individual IRI levels in each depancreatized dog (upper curves) and the mean levels of IRI in 5 normal dogs (lower curves). Numbers identify each dog. In each depancreatized dog, IRI increased during exercise and all exercise IRI values were higher than in normal dogs. Reproduced from Kawamori and Vranic (88) by courtesy of the Editors of Journal of Clinical Investigation; copyright The American Society for Clinical Investigation.*

ure alone is probably not a sufficient precaution in avoiding hypoglycemia (85, 86) since an exercise-induced fall in glucose has been shown to occur even when insulin mobilization from the injection site is not accelerated. The risk of hypo-glycemia during exercise may exist even when accelerated insulin absorption is not present simply because the physiological inhibition in insulin secretion is ab-sent. Deficient glucagon and epinephrine responses to hypoglycemia can further increase the vulnerability of diabetic patients to the hazards of exercise during relative overinsulinization (87).

Studies in depancreatized dog (88) and diabetic man (84) have given insight into the deficit in glucose kinetics which precipitates the fall in glucose levels following subcutaneous injection. Subcutaneous injection of long-acting insulin 8 hours prior to exercise in depancreatized dogs resulted in a substantial rise in circulating insulin which was in contrast to the physiological fall in insulin levels seen during exercise in normal dogs (88) (Fig. 3). Associated with this increase in insulin was a 100 mg/100 ml (5.7 mM) fall in plasma glucose after 60 min of

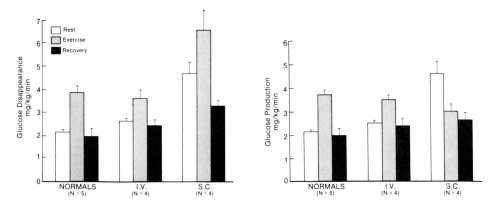

FIG. 4. *Glucose turnover: glucose disappearance (left panel) and glucose production (right panel) at rest, at 45 min exercise, and at 60 min recovery for normal control subjects insulin-infused (I.V.) and subcutaneous (S.C.) insulin-treated diabetic patients.Reproduced from Zinman et al (84) by courtesy of the Editors of Journal of Cinical Endocrinology and Metabolism.*

moderate-intensity exercise which was due to an 80% reduction in hepatic glu-cose production while glucose uptake was similar to that seen in normal dogs (88). The study of glucose kinetics during exercise in IDDM patients either in-fused intravenously with insulin or treated subcutaneously with intermediate-acting insulin prior to exercise has extended the results first obtained in the de-pancreatized dogs (84) (Fig. 4). As in the depancreatized dogs, plasma glucose concentration fell in the diabetic subjects. However, not only did hepatic glu-cose output fail to rise in the diabetic group, but it was actually suppressed by about 30%. An intravenous insulin infusion which creates normal peripheral insulin levels normalized the glucose fluxes and maintained glucose levels constant in the diabetic subjects.

Hypoglycemic episodes during or after exercise may be avoided by carbohydrate ingestion prior to, during, or after a bout of exercise (89). It has been shown for IDDM that glucose given orally during moderate-intensity exercise can be readily used, as long as adequate insulin is available (76). It should be noted, however, that an oral glucose load may be less available as an energy source during high-intensity exercise (90). Selection of the ideal food to avoid hypoglycemia is dependent on the type of exercise. For prolonged, moderate-intensity exercise a food with a slow absorption profile taken approximately 15 min before muscular work has been recommended (91). A reduction in insulin dosage can also be an important precaution when physical activity is planned (92, 93). Investigations have determined that diabetic subjects with fasting euglycemia can avoid hypoglycemia during prolonged exercise by reducing insulin treatment by 80%. On the other hand, IDDM subjects with fasting hyperglycemia were able to perform sustained exercise without encountering hypoglycemia with a less substantial reduction in insulin (50%) or by carbohydrate supplementation prior to exercise (92). Studies using open-loop intravenous insulin infusion have illustrated the importance of prudent insulin usage with exercise (93, 94). Failure to reduce the usual postprandial increase in insulin infusion back to basal rates at the onset of exercise consistently resulted in hypoglycemia (93). The exercise intensity is an important variable when assessing pre-exercise diet and insulin therapy (82, 95, 96). Heavy exercise appears to elicit more extreme adverse effects than moderate-intensity exercise of similar duration, whether it be the glucose-lowering action of relatively overinsulinized patients or the hyperglycemic effects of insulin-deficient patients (82, 96). General guidelines for diet and insulin administration for the physically active diabetic patient have been suggested (e.g. Ref. 97), but with the warning that a specific prescription cannot be applied to all cases.

The effect of exercise on glucose metabolism in IDDM can be summarized by the 3 potential scenarios shown in Figure 5: (a) during constant IV infusion of insulin, which presumably generates subnormal insulin concentrations in the portal vein, glucose homeostasis is preserved because glucose production and utilization are balanced as in normal subjects; (b) with insulin deficiency, exercise fails to stimulate glucose utilization, and hence the exercise-induced increase in hepatic glucose production leads to a rise in blood glucose levels; and (c) if exercise is performed following the subcutaneous injection of insulin, the continuous absorption of exogenous insulin into the circulation is maintained or may even be accelerated, inducing elevated plasma insulin levels. Due to the lack of the physiological fall of circulating insulin during exercise, glucose production rates are inhibited and, hence, the increased peripheral glucose uptake leads to a fall in blood glucose levels.

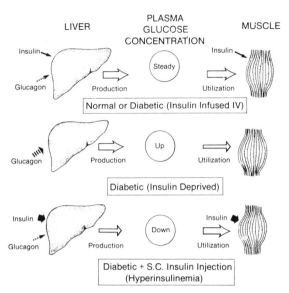

FIG. 5. *A hypothesis of the role of insulin in the regulation of glucose homeostasis in the normal and diabetic state. Different plasma concentrations of glucose result from changes in glucose production and utilization. Reproduced from Vranic et al (97) by courtesy of Thieme-Stratton, Inc.*

Counterregulatory hormones during exercise in IDDM   The deleterious response of underinsulinized diabetic patients to exercise is probably not exclusively due to diminished insulin levels *per se*, as exercise in these individuals is characterized by excessively increased glucagon (13, 73, 78, 79), growth hormone (78, 98), catecholamine (13, 79, 98), and cortisol (13, 78) responses, all of which can aggravate the diabetic state. Insulin therapy which improves metabolic control during rest and exercise can normalize the excessive counterregulatory response to exercise in diabetic patients (78, 98).

The alloxan-diabetic dog, deprived of exogenous insulin for 24 hours, has been used recently as a model to examine hormonal action on fuel metabolism during exercise in diabetes (13, 14). These dogs have hormonal and metabolic responses to exercise which are very similar to those seen in inadequately-controlled IDDM (13). Furthermore, many IDDM patients have reduced but still measurable basal insulin and C-peptide levels (99), which are similar to the residual basal insulin secretion seen in the alloxan-diabetic dog. This animal model was used in combination with somatostatin-induced glucagon suppression to study the role of glucagon during exercise in diabetes (13). As in normal dogs (12), alloxan-diabetic dogs are largely reliant on the presence of glucagon for normal hepatic glucose output during exercise. From these studies it was calculated that over 50% of the glucose released from the liver was dependent on glucagon (Fig. 1). To see if the increment in glucagon was crucial for the exercise-induced increase in hepatic glucose output with diabetes, depancreatized dogs were studied during exercise with an intraportal insulin infusion designed to create normal exercising insulin levels (37). Depancreatized dogs were used to assess the role of basal glucagon, since these animals have normal resting glucagon levels from an extrapancreatic source (100) which is unresponsive to exercise (37). In light of the findings in alloxan-diabetic dogs, it is interesting that in depancreatized dogs basal glucagon, without the normal exercise-induced increase, was found to be sufficient to stimulate hepatic glucose production (37). Thus, it is possible that the presence of glucagon, but not necessarily the exercise-induced increment of this hormone, is critical for the increase in hepatic glucose output in depancreatized dogs. Elevated glucagon concentrations may also play a role in ketogenesis by the liver (101) in diabetes. Exercise in IDDM has been associated with strong positive correlations between splanchnic ketone body output and plasma glucagon concentrations (74, 79); however, a causal relationship has not been established.

The role of the catecholamines in exercise metabolism has been investigated using adrenergic blockade in well-controlled IDDM (58), as well as in poorly controlled alloxan-diabetic dogs (14). Since both β- and α-adrenergic effects of the catecholamines are important in maintaining basal hepatic glucose output in IDDM (58, 102), it was thought that through these mechanisms catecholamines may be important in control of this variable during exercise. In well-maintained, insulin-infused diabetic patients (basal plasma glucose of 144 mg/100 ml: 8 mM) with normal increments in counterregulatory hormones, β-adrenergic blockade did not appear to affect hepatic glucose output (58). However, this is difficult to interpret because even in the absence of beta-blockade the subjects did not have an appreciable increase in glucose output in response to exercise. Nevertheless, hepatic glucose production during exercise in alloxan-diabetic dogs in poor metabolic control and with excessive counterregulatory hormone levels was also unaffected by beta-blockade (14). In contrast, in insulin-infused diabetic subjects α-adrenergic blockade actually stimulated hepatic glucose output excessively during exercise (58). The effect of combined blockade has not been studied during exercise in IDDM, thus it is not clear whether α- or β-adrenergic activity predominates.

Although it is not certain whether catecholamines are primary regulators of glucose release from the liver during exercise in diabetes, they have potent peripheral effects. Beta-blockade markedly decreased FFA levels in exercising alloxan-diabetic dogs deprived of exogenous insulin (14) and prevented the exercise-induced increment in FFA concentration in insulin-infused human diabetics (58). On the other hand, alpha-blockade in insulin-infused diabetic subjects caused a twofold increase in the FFA increment with exercise (58). Moreover, beta-blockade prevented the rise in lactate in alloxan-diabetic dogs (14), offering indirect evidence that muscle glycogenolysis may be impaired (57). Alloxan-diabetic dogs offer a unique opportunity to define further the importance of the catecholamines in regulating glucose uptake. These animals have basal insulin levels that are reduced by about 70% compared to normal dogs, and that remain constant through exercise (14). The marked suppression of insulin release during exercise in normal dogs (12), coupled with the constant insulin concentration from rest through exercise in diabetic dogs, creates similar insulin levels in both groups during exercise. However, the exercise-induced increment in glucose clearance in diabetic dogs is only 28% of the response observed in normal dogs (14). This is not entirely surprising since diabetic dogs are chronically exposed to lower insulin levels and therefore normal concentrations during exercise (56) are not necessarily associated with normal glucose metabolism. The importance of the catecholamines in control of glucose uptake during exercise in diabetes is shown in Figure 6, which illustrates that after 90 min of exercise with beta-blockade in diabetic dogs glucose clearance was returned to 93% of that seen in normal dogs. Thus, with a reduction in insulin action, total suppression of β-adrenergic activity can normalize glucose uptake by the muscle.

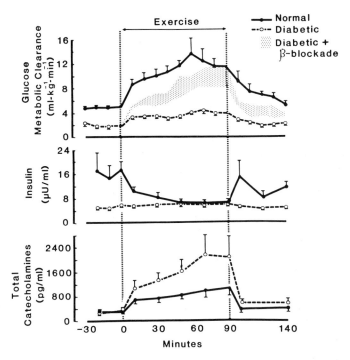

FIG. 6.   *Effect of exercise on glucose metabolic clearance rate, immunoreactive insulin, and total catecholamines in normal (n=5, solid line) and alloxan-diabetic (n=6, dashed line) dogs. Stipled area in top panel represents the effect of exercise with beta-blockade in alloxan-diabetic dogs (n=6). Reproduced from Wasserman and Vranic (4), Diabetes/Metabolism Reviews, by permission of John Wiley and Sons, Inc. Copyright © 1986, John Wiley and Sons, Inc.*

Although normal subjects may have a tendency to show many of the same qualitative changes as do diabetics, it is important to note that the effects of adrenergic-blockade on exercise metabolism seen in IDDM patients differ markedly in magnitude from those seen in normal subjects (58). It is not clear whether these differences are due to a change in catecholamine sensitivity *per se*, or whether they are due to other inherent abnormalities which may be present in diabetes.

Response to acute exercise in NIDDM

Although NIDDM is the predominant form of diabetes, the metabolic response to exercise in this population has not received a corresponding degree of attention. While hyperglycemia in IDDM is due to insulin deficiency, NIDDM is characterized by hyperglycemia which reflects insulin resistance and a defect in the first phase of insulin release. Insulin resistance can be due to receptor and/or post-receptor defects. NIDDM is often but not consistently characterized by obesity and hyperinsulinemia and treatment consists of a prescribed diet, oral hypoglycemic agents, and/or insulin. Interpretation of the effects of exercise in NIDDM must take into account all the above features.

The effects of an acute bout of exercise have been investigated in obese NIDDM patients with postabsorptive plasma glucose levels in excess of 200 mg/100 ml (11.1 mM) and normal basal insulin levels (a state of glycemic control not uncommon in NIDDM), and in obese, non-diabetic controls (103). Diabetic patients were maintained on diet therapy alone or with diet and sulfonylurea therapy (chlorpropamide). Moderate-intensity exercise for 45 min resulted in decreased hyperglycemia in both diabetic groups, while obese controls remained euglycemic. The fall in glucose with exercise in diabetic subjects was due to an attenuation of the normal rise in hepatic glucose production in the face of a normal increase in glucose utilization (Fig. 7). This was possibly due to the failure of insulin levels to fall during exercise in the diabetic groups. In addition, the hyperglycemia present in these patients may impair the response of hepatic glucose production to exercise. These findings are consistent with those for plasma glucose and insulin responses to 3 hours of moderate-intensity exercise in NIDDM patients with moderate fasting hyperglycemia and hyperinsulinemia (104). As before, exercise in diabetic subjects resulted in an excessive fall in plasma glucose compared to normal controls, but the more prolonged exercise duration uncovered a decrease in the elevated plasma insulin levels. Nevertheless, diabetic subjects were still hyperinsulinemic relative to controls, which may explain the exaggerated fall in glucose. The potential importance of acute exercise as an adjuvant therapy in NIDDM is demonstrated by its glucose-lowering effect which may acutely improve insulin resistance.

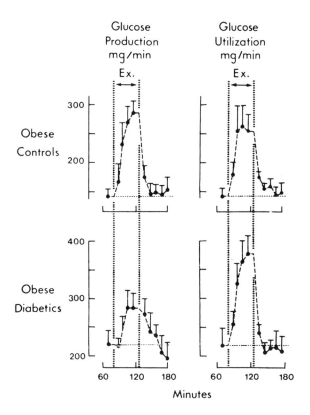

FIG. 7. *Glucose production and utilization in 7 obese controls (upper panel) and 10 obese NIDDM patients (lower panel) during rest, exercise (60% Vo_{2max}) and recovery. Mean and SE are shown. Reproduced from Minuk et al (103) by courtesy of the American Physiological Society.*

In contrast to IDDM, NIDDM patients are not at major risk of developing hypoglycemia during exercise. NIDDM patients on diet therapy alone should be able to exercise with no more caution than the individual with normal glucose tolerance provided there are no major vascular complications. There may be a tendency for hypoglycemia during prolonged exercise when oral hypoglycemic agents are used because of their ability to enhance insulin action. However, more work is necessary to ascertain more precisely the metabolic response to exercise as a function of the therapeutic regimen.

Physical training

Regular physical activity results in adaptations to the physiological and biochemical systems involved in the exercise response and physical inactivity reverses these adaptations (for review, see Ref. 105). From the perspective of the diabetic patient, there are two aspects of exercise training that take on particular relevance: (a) Will training improve glycemic control in IDDM or NIDDM? (b) Can training impede the progression of atherogenic complications resulting from diabetes?

In this section, the former question will be addressed by evaluating the effects of exercise training on carbohydrate metabolism in normal subjects and diabetic populations. The potential role of exercise training in retarding the cardiovascular complications of diabetes will then be assessed.

Effects on glucoregulation

Normal human subjects It was first recognized in the early 1970s that insulin sensitivity is increased in physically active individuals relative to sedentary controls (106, 107). Athletes or exercise-trained subjects have normal or even increased glucose tolerance, while fasting and glucose-stimulated insulin levels are lower than normal (107-109). Hyperinsulinemic, euglycemic clamp experiments have demonstrated that submaximal insulin-stimulated glucose disposal is increased in aerobically trained athletes (110, 111). Supporting these findings is the demonstration that maximal aerobic capacity is correlated significantly to insulin-stimulated glucose uptake in a heterogenous group of non-diabetic subjects (112). These results were substantiated by the demonstration that oxidation of an exogenous glucose load was increased during exercise after a 6-week training period even though insulin levels were not higher after training than before (113). The effect of aerobic training on the increase in insulin sensitivity may be lost within 10 days after cessation of training (45, 114). Insulin sensitivity exhibits significant positive and negative correlations to % muscle mass and % body fat of an individual, respectively (111). This relationship may relate to the greater degree of physical activity and the higher oxidative capacity in those individuals with less % fat and greater % muscle mass. These effects of training are probably specific to aerobic exercise. Strength training results in a net increase in submaximal insulin-stimulated glucose disposal (111) and glucose tolerance (115), but this increase is proportional to the increased muscle mass and probably does not represent an increase in insulin sensitivity *per se* (111, 115).

Different tissues adapt to aerobic exercise training in response to their specific function during a particular type of exercise. Skeletal muscle will adjust its metabolic profile so as to enhance the ability to use fuel and oxygen. In skeletal muscle, there are increased mitochondrial enzyme concentrations, capillary recruitment, and an increased tendency for fat usage in response to habitual exercise (105). Skeletal muscles of trained rats are more insulin-sensitive than those from sedentary controls due mainly to an increased rate of glucose oxidation (116-118). Euglycemic clamps performed over a range of insulin infusions combined with bolus administration of ^{3}H-2-deoxyglucose demonstrated an increase in maximal insulin-stimulated estimates of glucose metabolism in soleus and red gastrocnemius and a decreased sensitivity in soleus, gastrocnemius, extensor digitorum longus, and diaphragm in exercise-trained rats compared to sedentary controls (118)(Fig. 8). An increased insulin sensitivity was originally shown to occur without an increase in insulin binding to skeletal muscle (116). However, more recent studies in the rat have been

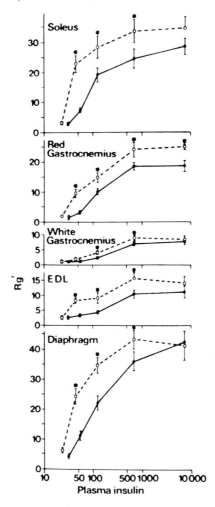

FIG. 8. *The effect of exercise-training on Rg' (μmol [100 g·min]$^{-1}$), an index of glucose metabolism, in soleus, red and white gastrocnemius, extensor digitorum longus (EDL) and diaphragm. Each value is the mean ± SEM of 5-7 observations; •, control animals; ○, exercise-trained animals. *Significantly different from control at same plasma insulin concentration (P<0.05). Reproduced from James et al (120) by courtesy of the American Physiological Society.*

conflicting showing both no effect (119), as in the earlier study, and an increase (120) in insulin binding to skeletal muscle preparations in response to training. An increase in skeletal muscle insulin sensitivity with training could be also seen with the increased insulin-stimulated glucose uptake in isolated perfused hindquarters (121) and hindlimb (122) of exercise-trained rats.

While exercise-training may increase overall insulin sensitivity and glucose tolerance, it does not appear that the liver contributes to this effect, since perfused livers from trained rats clear even less glucose than those from control rats (122). Furthermore, insulin-stimulated incorporation of ^{14}C-glucose into liver glycogen and fat was unaffected by training in the rat (118). Also exercise-training which increased insulin binding to skeletal muscle did not increase insulin binding to liver (120). Thus, liver does not appear to be a primary site for the increased glucose tolerance with training.

Regular physical activity increases insulin-stimulated glucose uptake (119, 123-125), oxidation (123, 125), and incorporation into fatty acids (119, 125) in rat adipocytes. These observations are consistent with the demonstration that trained rats have a greater number of glucose transporters in fat cells than do controls (126). The increase in insulin action in adipocytes of trained rats occurs in the absence of any changes in insulin binding (125, 127), implicating a modification in a post-binding event. In addition to changes in glucose metabolism, catecholamine-stimulated lipolysis is increased in adipocytes of trained rats compared to untrained controls (125, 128). It is interesting that the increased sensitivity to insulin and the catecholamines will lead to adaptations in adipocyte fat metabolism with opposing actions, one effect enhancing fat storage and the other enhancing fat mobilization. It is likely that the adaptation which prevails is dependent on the metabolic state of the organism at any particular time (e.g. activity level, nutritional status).

IDDM Physical training has been recommended for IDDM based on the observations that a bout of exercise can lower blood glucose and that exercise-training can reduce insulin requirements (97). This is important since insulin resistance also occurs in IDDM (129). In the last few years studies have demonstrated that insulin sensitivity can be increased following training in diabetic subjects using conventional (130) or pump insulin therapy (131). When diabetics were exposed to 6 weeks of exercise-training which increased their maximum oxygen uptake by 8%, glucose uptake in response to a hyperinsulinemic, euglycemic clamp was increased by 60% (131).

As in non-diabetic human subjects, IDDM is characterized by an increase in metabolic enzyme activities with training. It has been suggested that the improved insulin sensitivity following training may be due to the increase in enzyme activities which are normally deficient in diabetic skeletal muscle (130, 132, 133). Streptozotocin-diabetic rats have deficits in cytoplasmic and mitochondrial enzyme activities in both slow- and fast-twitch muscle fibers which are increased markedly by training (132-134). In IDDM patients, training programs have been shown to increase skeletal muscle citrate synthase and succinate dehydrogenase activities in parallel with an increase in insulin sensitivity (130). Whether the relationship between training-induced changes in enzyme activity and insulin sensitivity in diabetic or normal subjects is causal is unknown. Studies in streptozotocin-diabetic rat indicate that the ability to adapt to chronic exercise may depend on the severity of the diabetic state. Mildly diabetic rats respond to exercise-training by increasing insulin sensitivity (135), while severely diabetic rats do not show this change (136).

Despite the improved insulin sensitivity and increased muscular metabolic capacity, substantial evidence that glycemic control is improved is lacking. Recent studies (130, 137-139) have not demonstrated an improvement in glycosylated hemoglobin levels, glycosuria, or fasting plasma glucose concentrations following an exercise-training program which resulted in significant increments in maximum oxidative capacity. Even with daily exercise training for 5 months no change in glycemic control could be observed (138). In one study, exercise-training when combined with a program of intensified insulin therapy did result in improved glucose control (140); however, the effects of intensified insulin therapy cannot be differentiated from training effects alone. Further work is needed to determine whether physical activity under optimal conditions can, indeed, improve metabolic control in IDDM.

NIDDM Physical training is certainly a potential adjuvant therapy in NIDDM, in which insulin resistance predominates. In a recent epidemiological study of Indian and Melanesian men in Fiji, it was concluded that in this population the prevalence of diabetes is more than twice as high in sedentary individuals than in the active (141). Studies in NIDDM have shown that exercise-training can cause an increase in glucose tolerance (142-146) and lower basal (146, 147) and glucose-stimulated insulin levels (142). Insulin sensitivity, as assessed by glucose disposal during hyperinsulinemic, euglycemic clamps, improves with exercise-training (104, 142, 146, 147). An exercise-training and diet program was shown to increase the total glucose disposal rate during an insulin clamp in NIDDM by approximately 27% due primarily to an accelerated rate of non-oxidative carbohydrate disposal (147). Diet therapy alone did not affect total glucose disposal rate. Basal and insulin-suppressed hepatic glucose output was also reduced by diet and training, but no more than the diet program alone (147).

Obesity can result in insulin resistance, leading to augmented basal and glucose-stimulated insulin levels and a reduction in insulin-mediated glucose uptake as assessed by hyperinsulinemic, euglycemic clamps (129). Exercise-training programs have demonstrated an improvement in insulin sensitivity in obese subjects without concurrent weight loss or change in body composition (106, 142). Before and after training, glucose tolerance tests were normal in obese subjects; however, indices of insulin release were decreased (105, 142). Since weight reduction by itself can also improve insulin sensitivity, it is likely that exercise-training, which results in loss of body fat, will be most effective (107).

The obese Zucker rat has been used as a model to examine the effects of training in insulin-resistant states (116, 125, 148). These rats trained for 8 weeks did not exhibit a change in resting plasma insulin or glucose levels, but showed a greater drop in glucose in response to insulin injections (148). Moreover, 6-8 weeks of training in obese Zucker rats resulted in an improved rate of glucose disappearance and decreased plasma insulin response following an intravenous glucose load (116). Surprisingly, however, the site of training adaptations appears to be in adipose tissue and not muscle. Soleus strips from trained obese Zucker rats did not show a greater insulin binding or an increased rate of glucose metabolism compared to sedentary rats (116). On the other hand, adipocytes from trained obese Zucker rats have an increased rate of insulin-stimulated glucose utilization due to accelerated glucose transport, oxidation, and incorporation into triglyceride in comparison with non-exercised controls (125).

In contrast to its effects in IDDM, glycemic control appears to be improved by exercise-training in NIDDM. Glycosylated hemoglobin (145, 146) and fasting plasma glucose levels (143, 145-147) are reduced following an exercise-training program (Fig. 9). It has been suggested that these improvements may be due to the accumulative effects of single exercise bouts as opposed to long-

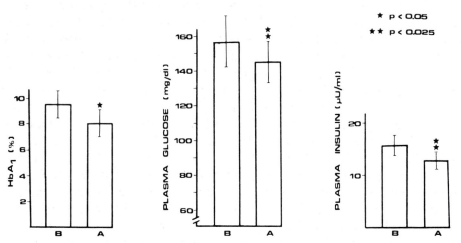

FIG. 9.   *Concentrations of glycosylated hemoglobin, fasting plasma glucose, and fasting plasma insulin before (B) and after (A) 6-wk physical training in 5 NIDDM patients. Glucose and insulin values are the mean of 3 consecutive days' determinations. Data are expressed as mean ± SEM. Reproduced from Trovati et al (146) by permission of the American Diabetes Association, Inc.*

term adaptations from exercise-training (145). This conclusion was based on the demonstration that the effects of a 6-week training program on fasting plasma glucose levels and glucose tolerance are significantly reduced from 12 to 72 hours after the last exercise session.

Effect on the atherogenic complications of diabetes

It is well established that exercise-training, or a change in lifestyle which accompanies exercise-training, decreases risk factors for cardiovascular disease in normal populations (for review, see Ref. 149). Whether regular physical activity actually reduces mortality from cardiovascular disease is contentious. Epidemiological studies illustrate the possible relevance of these decreased risk factors by showing a decreased prevalence of cardiovascular disease in active compared to inactive individuals (150). In-depth discussion of this topic with respect to normal human subjects is beyond the scope of this Chapter.

Considering the potentially beneficial effects of regular physical activity on cardiovascular disease and the evidence that diabetic subjects are at major risk of developing cardiovascular impairments, training may have potential value in alleviating some diabetic complications. Glucose intolerance, hyperinsulinemia, and insulin resistance have been proposed as atherogenic agents (151) and can be present in both IDDM and NIDDM. Furthermore, from the above discussion it should be clear there is evidence that all these atherogenic risk factors can be minimized by training.

Hyperlipidemia and disorders in lipoprotein metabolism are major risk factors for cardiovascular disease and they occur with higher frequency in IDDM and particularly in NIDDM (72) (see also Chapter 25). There is an increased prevalence of hyperlipidemia and diminished HDL cholesterol in diabetic patients which may be a function of the degree of metabolic control (72, 152). Regular exercise in normal human subjects affects favorably the lipoprotein profile (153). Diabetic patients also appear to show adaptations in lipid metabolism. Recent studies in IDDM (130, 132, 138) have shown that exercise-training increases the ratio of HDL cholesterol to total cholesterol. One study investigating the effect of training in NIDDM did not observe these favorable changes (154). However, the exercise program may not have been rigorous enough to cause adaptive changes (1 exercise session per week for 10 weeks). Other studies have revealed a tendency for training to reduce circulating triglyceride levels in NIDDM (144, 145), an effect which appears to be readily reversed by inactivity (145). Hypertension, which markedly increases the frequency of vascular disease, occurs with greater frequency in diabetic than in normal subjects (72). Epidemiological studies indicate that active individuals have lower systolic and diastolic blood pressures than sedentary controls matched for age (155). In support of this, 8-10 months of exercise-training with self-monitored glucose determinations and self-adjusted insulin therapy has been shown to cause a decrease in muscle capillary basement thickening and an improvement in arterial pulse volume recordings in IDDM (140).

Obesity irrespective of insulin insensitivity, is a risk factor for cardiovascular disease. The association of obesity with atherosclerosis may be, at least in part, related to the increased frequency of hypertension and lipoprotein disorders in this syndrome. Weight loss in the obese may diminish the magnitude of these atherogenic risk factors (156). Thus, the increase in energy expenditure with regular physical exercise in many individuals can improve caloric balance leading to weight loss and, consequently, lower blood pressure and improve lipid profile.

In short, there is evidence that the potentially beneficial effects of exercise on cardiovascular disease in normal human subjects also applies to diabetic patients. Hence, from the standpoint of minimizing complications from diabetes, habitual exercise may be of value.

Conclusions

In normal subjects, the appropriate hormonal and neural response to exercise provides the most optimal balance of substrate fluxes to the working muscles. The importance of proper hormonal regulation of substrate metabolism during exercise is seen clearly in diabetic patients in whom the normal endocrine response is lost. With a single bout of exercise the IDDM patient can experience either a worsening of the diabetic state or profound hypoglycemia depending on the degree of insulinization. On the other hand, it seems that NIDDM patients can generally exercise without concern for a deleterious metabolic response. Exercise-training appears to improve glycemic control in NIDDM, but this has not been consistently demonstrated in IDDM. Epidemiological investigation, as well as studies conducted in the laboratory, indicate that exercise-training may be valuable in minimizing risk factors for cardiovascular disease, many of which are more prevalent in diabetic patients. For the above reasons, an exercise prescription may be of considerable therapeutic value in NIDDM. In contrast, there is some concern about physical training as an adjuvant therapy in IDDM because of the risks involved, as well as the added therapeutic complexities. Nevertheless, understanding the metabolic response to exercise is critical so that diabetic patients who wish to participate in physical activity can do so safely. A safe exercise program for the diabetic patient can best be designed if metabolic regulation is understood. This underscores the need for continued research in the areas of neural and hormonal control of metabolism during exercise.

References

1. Ahlborg G, Felig P, Hagenfeldt L et al (1974): Substrate turnover during prolonged exercise in man. *J. Clin. Invest., 53,* 1080.
2. Wahren J, Felig P, Ahlborg G et al (1971): Glucose metabolism during leg exercise in man. *J. Clin. Invest., 50,* 2715.
3. Saltin B, Karlsson J (1971): Glycogen usage during work of varied intensity. In: Pernow B, Saltin B (Eds), *Muscle Metabolism during Exercise,* p.289 Plenum Press, London.
4. Wasserman DH, Vranic M (1986): Interaction bertween insulin and counterregulatory hormones in control of substrate utilization in health and diabetes during exercise. *Diabetes/ Metab. Rev., 1,* 359.
5. McGilvery RW (1975): The use of fuels for muscular work. In: Howald H, Poortsman J (Eds), *Metabolic Adaptations to Prolonged Physical Exercise,* p.12. Birkhauser, Basel.
6. Hermansen L, Hultman E, Saltin B (1967): Muscle glycogen during prolonged severe exercise. *Acta Physiol. Scand., 71,* 129.
7. DeFronzo RA, Ferrannini E, Sato Y et al (1981): Synergistic interaction between exercise and insulin on peripheral glucose uptake. *J. Clin. Invest., 68,* 1468.
8. Hoelzer D, Dalsky G, Clutter W et al (1986): Glucoregulation during exercise: hypoglycemia is prevented by redundant glucoregulatory systems during exercise: sympathochromaffin activation, and changes in hormone secretion. *J. Clin. Invest., 77,* 212.
9. Issekutz B (1980): The role of hypoinsulinemia in exercise metabolism. *Diabetes, 29,* 629.
10. Issekutz B, Vranic M (1980): Significance of glucagon in the control of glucose production during exercise. *Am. J. Physiol., 238,* E13.
11. Jenkins AB, Furler SM, Chisholm DJ et al (1986): Regulation of hepatic glucose output during exercise by circulating glucose and insulin in humans. *Am. J. Physiol., 250,* R411.
12. Wasserman DH, Lickley HLA, Vranic M (1984): Interactions between glucagon and other counterregulatory hormones during normoglycemic and hypoglycemic exercise. *J. Clin. Invest., 74,* 1404.
13. Wasserman DH, Lickley HLA, Vranic M (1985): Important role of glucagon during exercise and diabetes. *J. Appl. Physiol., 59,* 1272.
14. Wasserman DH, Lickley HLA, Vranic M (1985): Role of beta-adrenergic mechanisms during exercise in poorly-controlled insulin deficient diabetes. *J. Appl. Physiol., 59,* 1282.
15. Wolfe RR, Nadel ER, Shaw JHF et al (1986): Role of changes in insulin and glucagon in glucose homeostasis in exercise. *J. Clin Invest., 77,* 900.
16. Schultz TA, Lewis SB, Westbie DK et al (1977): Glucose delivery: a modulator of glucose uptake in contracting skeletal muscle. *Am. J. Physiol., 233,* E514.
17. Jenkins AB, Chisholm DJ, James DE et al (1985): Exercise induced hepatic glucose output is precisely sensitive to the rate of systemic glucose supply. *Metabolism, 34,* 431.
18. Cooper DM, Wasserman DH, Vranic M et al (1986): Glucose turnover in response to exercise during high- and low-FiO$_2$ breathing in humans. *Am. J. Physiol., 14,* E209.
19. Idstrom JP, Subramanian VH, Chance B et al (1985): Oxygen dependence of energy metabolism in contracting and recovering rat skeletal muscle. *Am. J. Physiol., 248,* H40.
20. Wasserman DH, Lickley HLA, Vranic M (1985): Effect of hematocrit reduction on hormonal and metabolic responses to exercise. *J. Appl. Physiol., 58,* 1257.
21. Galbo H (1983): *Hormonal and Metabolic Adaptation to Exercise.* Thieme, New York.
22. Cochran B, Marbach EP, Poucher R et al (1966): Effect of acute muscular exercise on serum immunoreactive insulin concentration. *Diabetes, 15,* 838.
23. Bottger I, Schlein EM, Faloona GR et al (1972): The effect of exercise on glucagon secretion. *J. Clin. Endocrinol. Metab., 35,* 117.
24. Hartley LH, Mason JW, Hogan RP et al (1972): Multiple hormonal responses to graded

exercise in relation to physical training. *J. Appl. Physiol., 33*, 602.

25. Chalmers RJ, Bloom SR, Duncan G et al (1979): The effect of somatostatin on metabolic and hormonal changes during and after exercise. *Clin. Endocrinol., 10*, 451.
26. Richter EA, Galbo H, Holst JJ et al (1981): Significance of glucagon for insulin secretion and hepatic glycogenolysis during exercise in rats. *Horm. Metab. Res., 13*, 323.
27. Brockman RP (1979): Effect of somatostatin on plasma glucagon and insulin and glucose turnover in exercising sheep. *J. Appl. Physiol., 47*, 273.
28. Wasserman DH, Vranic M (1986): Interaction between insulin, glucagon, and catecholamines in the regulation of glucose production and uptake during exercise: physiology and diabetes. In: Saltin B (Ed.), *Biochemistry of Exercise VI*, p. 167. International Series on Sports Sciences, Copenhagen.
29. Cherrington AD, Liljenquist JE, Shulman GI (1979): Importance of hypoglycemia-induced glucose production during isolated glucagon deficiency. *Am. J. Physiol., 236*, E263.
30. Garthwaite SM, Holloszy JO (1982): Increased permeability to sugar following muscle contraction. *J. Biol. Chem., 257*, 5008.
31. Holloszy JO, Narahara HT (1965): Studies of tissue permeability. X. Changes in permeability to 3-methylglucose associated with contraction of isolated frog muscle. *J. Biol. Chem., 240*, 3493.
32. Nesher R, Karl IE, Kipnis DM (1985): Dissociation of the effect(s) of insulin and contraction on glucose transport in rat epitrochlearis muscle. *Am. J. Physiol., 249*, C226.
33. Wallberg-Henriksson H, Holloszy JO (1984): Contractile activity increases glucose uptake by muscle in severely diabetic rats. *J. Appl. Physiol., 57*, 1045.
34. Berger M, Hagg S, Ruderman NB (1975): Glucose metabolism in perfused skeletal muscle: interaction of insulin and exercise on glucose uptake. *Biochem. J., 146*, 231.
35. Bjorkman O, Miles P, Wasserman DH et al (1986): Muscle glucose uptake during exercise in total insulin deficiency: effect of beta-adrenergic blockade. *Diabetes, 35, Suppl. 1*, 29A.
36. Vranic M, Wrenshall GA (1969): Exercise, insulin, and glucose turnover in dogs. *Endocrinology, 85*, 165.
37. Vranic M, Kawamori R, Pek S et al (1976): The essentiality of insulin and the role of glucagon in regulating glucose utilization and production during strenuous exercise in dogs. *J. Clin. Invest., 57*, 245.
38. Berger M, Halban PA, Assal JP et al (1978): Mobilization of subcutaneously injected tritiated insulin in rats: effects of muscular exercise. *Diabetologia, 15*, 133.
39. Davis TA, Klahr S, Tegtmeyer ED et al (1986): Glucose metabolism in epitrochlearis muscle of acutely exercised and trained rats. *Am. J. Physiol., 250*, E137.
40. Garetto LP, Richter EA, Goodman MN et al (1984): Enhanced muscle glucose metabolism after exercise in the rat: the two phases. *Am. J. Physiol., 246*, E471.
41. Richter EA, Garetto LP, Goodman MN et al (1982): Muscle glucose metabolism following exercise in the rat: increased sensitivity to insulin. *J. Clin. Invest., 69*, 785.
42. Richter EA, Garetto LP, Goodman MN et al (1984): Enhanced muscle glucose metabolism following exercise: modulation by local factors. *Am. J. Physiol., 246*, E476.
43. Zorzano A, Balon TW, Goodman MN et al (1986): Additive effects of prior exercise and insulin on glucose and AIB uptake by rat muscle. *Am. J. Physiol., 251*, E21.
44. Bogardus C, Thuillez P, Ravussin E et al (1983): Effect of muscle glycogen depletion on in vivo insulin action in man. *J. Clin. Invest., 72*, 1605.
45. Heath GW, Gavin JR, Hinderlites JR et al (1983): Effects of exercise and lack of exercise on glucose tolerance and insulin sensitivity. *J. Appl. Physiol., 55*, 512.
46. Maehlum S, Felig P, Wahren J (1978): Splanchnic glucose and muscle glycogen metabolism after glucose feeding during postexercise recovery. *Am. J. Physiol., 235*, E255.
47. Devlin JT, Horton ES (1985): Effects of prior high-intensity exercise on glucose metabolism in normal and insulin-resistant men. *Diabetes. 34*, 973.

48. Pedersen O, Beck-Nielsen H, Heding L (1980): Increased insulin receptors after exercise in patients with insulin-dependent diabetes mellitus. *N. Engl. J. Med., 302,* 886.
49. Michel G, Vocke T, Fiehn W et al (1984): Bidirectional alteration on insulin receptor affinity by different forms of physical exercise. *Am. J. Physiol., 246,* E153.
50. Bonen A, Tan MH, Clune P et al (1985): Effects of exercise on insulin binding to human muscle. *Am. J. Physiol., 248,* E403.
51. Webster B, Vigna SR, Paquette T (1986): Acute exercise, epinephrine, and diabetes enhance insulin binding to skeletal muscle. *Am. J. Physiol., 250,* E186.
52. Zorzano A, Balon TW, Garetto LP et al (1985): Muscle alpha aminoisobutyric acid transport after exercise: enhanced stimulation by insulin. *Am. J. Physiol., 248,* E546.
53. Begum N, Terjung R, Tepperman H et al (1986): Effect of acute exercise on insulin generation of pyruvate dehydrogenase activator by rat liver and adipocyte plasma membranes. *Diabetes, 35,* 785.
54. Martin MJ, Horwitz DL, Nattrass JF et al (1981): Effects of mild hyperinsulinemia on the metabolic response to exercise. *Metabolism, 30,* 688.
55. Randle PJ, Hales CN, Garland PB et al (1963): The glucose fatty-acid cycle: its role in insulin sensitivity and the metabolic disturbances of diabetes mellitus. *Lancet, 1,* 7285.
56. Juhlin-Dannfeldt AC, Terblanche SE, Fell RD et al (1982): Effect of beta-adrenergic receptor blockade on glycogenolysis during exercise. *J. Appl. Physiol., 53,* 549.
57. Issekutz B (1978): Role of beta-adrenergic receptors in mobilization of energy sources in exercising dogs. *J. Appl. Physiol., 44,* 869.
58. Simonson DC, Koivisto V, Sherwin RS et al (1984): Adrenergic blockade alters glucose kinetics during exercise in insulin-dependent diabetics. *J. Clin. Invest., 73,* 1648.
59. Hoelzer DR, Dalsky GP, Schwartz NS et al (1986): Epinephrine is not critical to prevention of hypoglycemia during exercise in humans. *Am. J. Physiol., 251,* E104.
60. Arnall DA, Marker JC, Conlee RK et al (1986): Effect of infusing epinephrine on liver and muscle glycogenolysis during exercise in rats. *Am. J. Physiol., 250,* E641.
61. Carlson KI, Marker JC, Arnall DA et al (1985): Epinephrine is unessential for stimulation of liver glycogenolysis during exercise. *J. Appl. Physiol., 58,* 544.
62. Richter EA, Galbo H, Sonne B et al (1980): Adrenal medullary control of muscular and hepatic glycogenolysis and of pancreatic hormonal secretion in exercising rats. *Acta Physiol. Scand., 108,* 235.
63. Sonne B, Mikines KJ, Richter EA et al (1985): Role of liver nerves and adrenal medulla in glucose turnover in running rats. *J. Appl. Physiol., 59,* 1640.
64. Chasiostis D, Sahlin K, Hultman E (1982): Regulation of glycogenolysis in human muscle at rest and during exercise. *J. Appl. Physiol., 53,* 708.
65. Jansson E, Hjemdahl P, Kaijser L et al (1986): Epinephrine-induced changes in muscle carbohydrate metabolism during exercise in male subjects. *J. Appl. Physiol., 60,* 1466.
66. Galbo H, Christensen NJ, Holst JJ (1977): Catecholamines and pancreatic hormones during autonomic blockade in exercising man. *Acta Physiol. Scand., 101,* 428.
67. Hilsted J, Galbo H, Christensen NJ (1980): Impaired responses of catecholamines, growth hormone, and cortisol to graded exercise in diabetic autonomic neuropathy. *Diabetes, 29,* 257.
68. Chiasson JL, Shikama H, Chu DTW et al (1981): Inhibitory effect of epinephrine on insulin-stimulated glucose uptake by rat skeletal muscle. *J. Clin. Invest., 68,* 706.
69. Newsholme EA, Start C (1973): *Regulation in metabolism.* Wiley, Toronto.
70. Randle PJ, Smith GH (1958): Regulation of glucose uptake by muscle. I. The effects of insulin, anaerobiosis and cell poisons on the uptake of glucose and release of potassium by isolated rat diaphragm. *Biochem. J., 70,* 490.
71. Ditzel J (1976): Oxygen transport impairment in diabetes. *Diabetes, 24, Suppl. 1,* 832.

72. Nikkila EA (1984): Plasma lipid and lipoprotein abnormalities in diabetes. In: Jarrett RJ (Ed.), *Diabetes and Heart Disease*, p. 133. Elsevier, Amsterdam.
73. Wahren J, Hagenfeldt L, Felig P (1975): Splanchnic and leg exchange of glucose, amino acids, and free fatty acids during exercise in diabetes mellitus. *J. Clin. Invest., 55,* 1303.
74. Sestoft L, Trap-Jensen J, Lyngsoe J et al (1977): Regulation of gluconeogenesis during rest and exercise in diabetic subjects and normal men. *Clin. Sci. Mol. Med., 53,* 411.
75. Lyngsoe J, Clausen JP, Trap-Jensen J et al (1978): Exchange of metabolites in the leg of exercising juvenile diabetic subjects. *Clin. Sci. Mol. Med., 55,* 73.
76. Krzentowski G, Pirnay F, Pallikarakis N et al (1981): Glucose utilization in normal and diabetic subjects: the role of insulin. *Diabetes, 30,* 983.
77. Hagg SA, Taylor SI, Ruderman NB (1976): Glucose metabolism in perfused skeletal muscle: pyruvate dehydrogenase activity in starvation, diabetes and exercise. *Biochem. J., 158,* 203.
78. Berger M, Berchtold P, Cuppers HJ et al (1977): Metabolic and hormonal effects of muscular exercise in juvenile type diabetics. *Diabetologia, 13,* 355.
79. Wahren J, Sato Y, Ostman J et al (1984): Turnover and splanchnic metabolism of free fatty acids and ketones in insulin-dependent diabetics during exercise. *J. Clin. Invest., 73,* 1367.
80. Standl E, Lotz N, Dexel TH et al (1980): Muscle triglycerides in diabetic subjects. *Diabetologia, 18,* 463.
81. Issekutz B, Paul P (1968): Intramuscular energy sources in exercising normal and pancreatized dogs. *Am. J. Physiol., 215,* 197.
82. Zander E, Bruns W, Wulfert P et al (1983): Muscular exercise in type 1-diabetics. I. Different metabolic reactions during heavy muscular work in dependence on actual insulin availability. *Exp. Clin. Endocrinol., 82,* 78.
83. Koivisto V, Felig P (1978): Effects of leg exercise on insulin absorption in diabetic patients. *N. Engl. J. Med., 298,* 77.
84. Zinman B, Murray FT, Vranic M et al (1977): Glucoregulation during moderate exercise in insulin treated diabetics. *J. Clin. Endocrinol. Metab., 45,* 641.
85. Kemmer FW, Berchtold P, Berger M et al (1979): Exercise induced fall of blood glucose in insulin treated diabetics unrelated to alteration of insulin mobilization. *Diabetes, 28,* 1131.
86. Susstrunk H, Morrell B, Ziegler WH et al (1982): Insulin absorption from the abdomen and the thigh in healthy subjects during rest and exercise: blood glucose, plasma insulin, growth hormone, adrenaline, and noradrenaline levels. *Diabetologia, 22,* 171.
87. Gerich JE (1986): Glucose counterregulation. In: Alberti KGMM, Krall LP (Eds), *The Diabetes Annual/2*, p. 248. Elsevier, Amsterdam.
88. Kawamori R, Vranic M (1977): Mechanism of exercise-induced hypoglycemia in depancreatized dogs maintained on long-acting insulin. *J. Clin. Invest., 59,* 331.
89. Lefebvre PJ, Pirnay F, Pallikarakis N et al (1986): Metabolic availability of carbohydrates ingested during, before, or after muscular exercise. *Diabetes/Metab. Rev., 1,* 483.
90. Pirnay F, Crielaard JM, Pallikarakis N et al (1982): Fate of exogenous glucose during exercise of different intensities. *J. Appl. Physiol., 53,* 1620.
91. Nathan DM, Madnek SF, Delahanty L (1985): Programming pre-exercise snacks to prevent post-exercise hypoglycemia in intensively treated insulin-dependent diabetics. *Ann. Intern. Med., 1-2,* 483.
92. Kemmer FW, Berger M (1986): Therapy and better quality of life: the dichotomous role of exercise in diabetes mellitus. *Diabetes/Metab. Rev., 2,* 53.
93. Poussier P, Zinman B, Marliss EB et al (1983): Open loop intravenous insulin waveforms for postprandial exercise in type 1 diabetics. *Diabetes Care, 66,* 129.
94. Nelson JD, Poussier P, Marliss EB et al (1982): The metabolic responses of normal and insulin infused diabetics to postprandial exercise. *Am. J. Physiol., 242,* E309.

95. Hubinger A, Ridderskamp I, Lehmann E et al (1985): Metabolic response to different forms of physical exercise in type I diabetics and the duration of the glucose lowering effect. *Eur. J. Clin. Invest., 15,* 197.

96. Zander E, Schulz B, Chlup R et al (1985): Muscular exercise in type 1-diabetics. II. Hormonal and metabolic responses to moderate exercise. *Exp. Clin. Endocrinol., 85,* 95.

97. Vranic M, Lickley HLA, Davidson JK (1986): Exercise and stress in diabetes mellitus. In: Davidson JK (Ed.), *Clinical Diabetes Mellitus,* Ch. 15, p. 172. Thieme-Stratton, New York.

98. Tamborlane WV, Sherwin RS, Koivisto V et al (1979): Normalization of the growth hormone and catecholamine response to exercise in juvenile-onset diabetic subjects treated with a portable insulin infusion pump. *Diabetes, 28,* 785.

99. Kuzuya H, Blix PM, Horwitz DL et al (1977): Determination of free and total insulin and C-peptide in insulin-treated diabetics. *Diabetes, 26,* 22.

100. Vranic M, Pek S, Kawamori R (1974): Increased 'glucagon immunoreactivity' in plasma of totally depancreatized dogs. *Diabetes, 23,* 905.

101. Liljenquist JE, Bomboy JD, Lewis SB et al (1974): Effect of glucagon on lipolysis and ketogenesis in normal and diabetic man. *J. Clin. Invest., 53,* 190.

102. Sherwin RS, Shamoon H, Hendler R et al (1980): Epinephrine and the regulation of glucose metabolism: effect of diabetes and hormonal interactions. *Metabolism, 29,* 1146.

103. Minuk HL, Vranic M, Marliss EB et al (1981): Glucoregulatory and metabolic response to exercise in obese noninsulin-dependent diabetes. *Am. J. Physiol., 240,* E458.

104. Koivisto V, DeFronzo R (1984): Exercise in the treatment of type II diabetes. *Acta Endocrinol., 262, Suppl.,* 107.

105. Holloszy JO, Coyle EF (1984): Adaptations of skeletal muscle to endurance exercise and their metabolic consequences. *J. Appl. Physiol., 56,* 831.

106. Bjorntorp P, deFounge K, Sjostrom L et al (1970): The effect of physical training on insulin production in obesity. *Metabolism, 19,* 631.

107. Bjorntorp P, Fahlen M, Grimby G et al (1972): Carbohydrate and lipid metabolism in middle aged physically well-trained men. *Metabolism, 21,* 631.

108. Lohmann D, Liebold F, Heilmann W et al (1978): Diminished insulin response in highly trained athletes. *Metabolism, 27,* 521.

109. Seals DR, Hagberg JM, Allen WK et al (1984): Glucose tolerance in young and older athletes and sedentary men. *J. Appl. Physiol., 56,* 1521.

110. Sato Y, Iguchi A, Sakamoto N (1983): Biochemical determination of training effects using insulin clamp technique. *Horm. Metab. Res., 16,* 483.

111. Yki-Jarvinen H, Koivisto V (1983): Effects of body composition on insulin sensitivity. *Diabetes, 32,* 965.

112. Rosenthal M, Haskell WL, Solomon R et al (1983): Demonstration of a relationship between level of physical training and insulin-stimulated glucose utilization in normal humans. *Diabetes, 32,* 408.

113. Krzentowski G, Pirnay F, Luyckx AS et al (1984): Effect of physical training on utilization of a glucose load given orally during exercise. *Am. J. Physiol., 246,* E412.

114. Burstein R, Polychronakos C, Toews CJ et al (1985): Acute reversal of the enhanced insulin action in trained athletes: association with insulin receptor changes. *Diabetes, 34,* 756.

115. Miller WJ, Sherman WM, Ivy JL (1984): Effect of strength training on glucose tolerance and post-glucose insulin response. *Med. Sci. Sport Exerc., 16,* 539.

116. Crettaz M, Horton ES, Wardzala LJ et al (1983): Physical training of Zucker rats: lack of alleviation of muscle insulin resistance. *Am. J. Physiol., 244,* E414.

117. Espinal J, Dohm GL, Newsholme EA (1983): Sensitivity to insulin of glycolysis and glycogen synthesis of isolated soleus-muscle strips from sedentary, exercised and exercise-trained rats. *Biochem. J., 212,* 453.

118. James DE, Kraegan EW, Chisholm DJ (1985): Effects of exercise training on in vivo insulin action in individual tissues of the rat. *J. Clin. Invest., 76*, 657.
119. Grimditch GK, Barnard RJ, Kaplan SA et al (1986): Effect of training on insulin binding to rat skeletal muscle sarcolemmal vesicles. *Am. J. Physiol., 250*, E570.
120. Bonen A, Clune PA, Tan MH (1986): Chronic exercise increases insulin binding in muscles but not liver. *Am. J. Physiol., 251*, E196.
121. Berger M, Kemmer FW, Becker K et al (1979): Effect of physical training on glucose tolerance and of glucose metabolism of muscle in anaesthetized rats. *Diabetologia, 16*, 179.
122. Mondon C, Dolkas CB, Reaven G (1980): Site of enhanced insulin activity in exercise-trained rats. *Am. J. Physiol., 239*, E169.
123. Craig BW, Hammons GT, Garthwaite SM et al (1981): Adaptation of fat cells to exercise: response of glucose uptake and oxidation to insulin. *J. Appl. Physiol., 51*, 1981.
124. Vinten J, Galbo H (1983): Effect of physical training on transport and metabolism of glucose in adipocytes. *Am. J. Physiol., 244*, E129.
125. Wardzala LJ, Horton ED, Crettaz M et al (1982): Physical training of lean and genetically obese Zucker rats: effect on fat cell metabolism. *Am. J. Physiol., 243*, E418.
126. Vinten J, Norgaard Petersen L, Sonne B et al (1985): Effect of physical training on glucose transporters in fat cell fractions. *Biochim. Biophys. Acta, 841*, 223.
127. Wirth A, Holm G, Nilsson B et al (1980): Insulin kinetics and insulin binding to adipocytes in physically trained and food restricted rats. *Am. J. Physiol., 238*, E108.
128. Bukowiecki L, Lupien D, Follea N et al (1980): Mechanism of enhanced lipolysis in adipose tissue of exercise-trained rats. *Am. J. Physiol., 239*. E422.
129. DeFronzo R, Simonson DC, Ferrannini E (1982): Hepatic and peripheral insulin resistance: a common feature of type II (non-insulin-dependent) and type I (insulin-dependent) diabetes mellitus. *Diabetologia, 23*, 313.
130. Wallberg-Henriksson H, Gunnarson R, Henriksson J et al (1982): Increased peripheral insulin sensitivity and muscle mitochondrial enzymes but unchanged blood glucose control in type 1 diabetics after physical training. *Diabetes, 31*, 1044.
131. Yki-Jarvinen H, DeFronzo R, Koivisto V (1984): Normalization of insulin sensitivity in type I diabetic subjects by physical training during insulin pump therapy. *Diabetes Care, 7*, 520.
132. Ianuzzo CD, Noble EG, Hamilton N, Dabrowski B (1984): Effects of streptozotocin diabetes, insulin treatment, and training on the diaphragm. *J. Appl. Physiol., 52*, 1471.
133. Noble EG, Ianuzzo CD (1985): Influence of training on skeletal muscle enzymatic adaptations in normal and diabetic rats. *Am. J. Physiol., 249*, E360.
134. Narimiya M, Chang H, Azhar S et al (1984): Amelioration of streptozotocin-induced diabetes in the rat by exercise-training: role of muscle glycogenolytic and glycolytic enzyme activity. *Horm. Metab. Res., 16*, 67.
135. Tancrede G, Rousseau-Migneron S, Nadeau A (1982): Beneficial effects of physical training in rats with a mild streptozotocin-induced diabetes mellitus. *Diabetes, 31*, 406.
136. Vallerand AL, Lupien J, Deshaies Y et al (1986): Intensive exercise training does not improve intravenous glucose tolerance in severely diabetic rats. *Horm. Metab. Res., 18*, 79.
137. Landt KW, Campaigne BN, James FW et al (1985): Effects of exercise training on insulin sensitivity in adolescents with type 1 diabetes. *Diabetes Care, 8*, 461.
138. Wallberg-Henriksson H, Gunnarson R, Rossner S et al (1986): Long-term physical training in female type I (insulin-dependent) diabetic patients: absence of significant effect on glycemic control and lipoprotein levels. *Diabetologia, 29*, 53.
139. Zinman B, Zuniga-Guajardo S, Kelly D (1984): Comparison of the acute and long-term effects of exercise on glucose control in type 1 diabetes. *Diabetes Care, 7*, 515.
140. Peterson CM, Jones RL, Esterly JA et al (1980): Changes in basement membrane thicken-

ing and pulse volume concomitant with improved glucose control and exercise in patients with insulin-dependent diabetes mellitus. *Diabetes Care, 3,* 586.

141. Taylor R, Ram P, Zimmet P et al (1984): Physical activity and prevalence of diabetes in Melanesian and Indian men in Fiji. *Diabetologia, 27,* 578.
142. Krotkiewski M, Lonnroth P, Mandroukas K et al (1985): The effects of physical training on insulin secretion and effectiveness and on glucose metabolism in obesity and type II (non-insulin-dependent) diabetes mellitus. *Diabetologia, 28,* 881.
143. Reitman JS, Vasquez B, Klimes I et al (1984): Improvement of glucose homeostasis after exercise training in non-insulin-dependent diabetes. *Diabetes Care, 7,* 434.
144. Ruderman NB, Ganda OP, Johansen K (1979): Effects of physical training on glucose tolerance and plasma lipids in maturity onset diabetes mellitus. *Diabetes, 28, Suppl.,* 89.
145. Schneider SH, Amorosa LF, Khachadurian AK et al (1984): Studies on the mechanism of improved glucose control during regular exercise in type II (non-insulin-dependent) diabetes. *Diabetologia, 26,* 355.
146. Trovati M, Carta Q, Cavalot F et al (1984): Influence of physical training on blood glucose control, glucose tolerance, insulin secretion, and insulin action in non-insulin-dependent diabetic patients. *Diabetes Care, 7,* 416.
147. Bogardus C, Ravussin E, Robbins DC et al (1984): Effects of physical training and diet therapy on carbohydrate metabolism in patients with glucose intolerance and non-insulin-dependent diabetes mellitus. *Diabetes, 33,* 311.
148. Wallberg JL, Upton D, Stern JS (1984): Exercise training improves insulin sensitivity in the obese Zucker rat. *Metabolism, 33,* 1075.
149. Schneider SH, Vitug A, Ruderman NB (1986): Atherosclerosis and physical activity. *Diabetes/Metab. Rev., 1,* 514.
150. Paffenbarger RS (1980): Exercise as a protection against heart attack. *N. Engl. J. Med., 302,* 1026.
151. Pyorala K (1979): Relationship of glucose tolerance and plasma insulin to the incidence of coronary heart disease: results from two population studies in Finland. *Diabetes Care, 2,* 131.
152. Lopes-Virella MF, Wohltmann HJ, Loadholt CB et al (1981): Plasma lipids and lipoproteins in young insulin-dependent diabetic patients: relationship with control. *Diabetologia, 21,* 216.
153. Wood P, Haskell W, Blan S et al (1983): Increased exercise level and plasma lipoprotein concentration: a one year prolonged study on sedentary middle aged men. *Metabolism, 32,* 31.
154. Kaplan RM, Wilson DK, Hartwell SL et al (1985): Prospective evaluation of HDL cholesterol changes after diet and physical conditioning programs for patients with type II diabetes mellitus. *Diabetes Care, 8,* 343.
155. Montoye H, Metzner H, Keller J et al (1972): Habitual physical activity and blood pressure. *Med. Sci. Sports Exerc., 4,* 175.
156. Gordon T, Castelli WP, Hjortland MC et al (1977): High density lipoprotein as a protective factor against coronary heart disease: the Framingham study. *Am. J. Med., 62,* 707.

The Diabetes Annual/3
K.G.M.M. Alberti and L.P. Krall, editors
© 1987 Elsevier Science Publishers, B.V.

29   Glucose sensors for the management of diabetes mellitus

MARCO F. CARDOSI AND ANTHONY P.F. TURNER*

Introduction

The need to develop cheap, accurate and reliable glucose sensors for monitoring diabetes has been the principal driving force behind research into enzyme electrodes and other biosensors since their inception 25 years ago (1). These sensing elements have been envisaged as the key component in 4 types of device:

The hypoglycaemia alarm

The greatest fear of the insulin-dependent diabetic patient is hypoglycaemia. Unpredictable hypoglycaemic attacks can be caused by factors such as erratic absorption of insulin from subcutaneous tissue, exercise, missed meals and inappropriate insulin injection regimes. In addition to this, many patients lack the symptoms of hypoglycaemia such as sweating and fail to recognise that their blood glucose concentration is dangerously low (2). Nocturnal hypoglycaemia is a particular concern since the patient fears that the attacks will be longer and more severe if hypoglycaemia fails to interrupt sleep. Moreover, the patient is unable to monitor his/her metabolic status by capillary blood analysis during this period. An audible alarm triggered by an implanted glucose sensor could alert the patient to his/her condition during the daytime and in the event of nocturnal hypoglycaemia wake the patient so that the appropriate action could be taken.

Home blood glucose monitoring

The various techniques and their merits for home blood glucose monitoring (HBGM) have been reviewed elsewhere *(The Diabetes Annual/1-3)*. An alternative approach to HBGM might be an implantable glucose sensor which gives

---

*A.P.F.T. is a Senior Research Fellow of the British Diabetic Association.

a continuous readout of the levels of blood glucose. Furthermore, facilities could be made available for recording the daily profiles of glucose levels for later playback and assessment by the clinician.

In vitro blood glucose analyser

The current generation of bench-top analysers for blood, serum and plasma glucose measurement are both bulky and expensive (approx. £ 2000-4000). These instruments are therefore not ideally suited to situations where only a few samples require analysis, e.g. in the general practitioner's office, in the outpatient clinic or in the emergency and general accident departments. The use of cheap, disposable 'one-shot' glucose sensors would prove most useful in these cases.

Closed-loop insulin delivery system

Continuous monitoring in vivo of blood sugar levels would enable feedback control to an insulin-infusion pump which could be either external or implanted. With a closed-loop system it is hoped to achieve more stable normoglycaemic control in patients than is present possible with open-loop insulin-infusion devices (3, 4).

General considerations for a glucose biosensor

Since most clinical information in diabetes concerns blood glucose levels, it would be of most interest to be able to sense glucose in this milieu. Chronic access to blood vessels would presumably require either a device connected to the blood (but situated under the skin, with a resealable diaphragm for removal of blood), insertion of the probe or the creation of an arteriovenous shunt or fistula. Long-term implantation within the vascular system, however, is likely to lead to thrombosis and infection. A more acceptable alternative is to implant sensors subcutaneously, but then the relationship between blood and tissue glucose concentrations must be considered. Diffusion of glucose to the sensor might be additionally hampered by fouling or encapsulation. Interfering chemicals such as ascorbete or paracetamol present a particular problem in vivo where they cannot easily be compensated for or removed by conventional protocols. In addition, serum proteases may degrade the enzyme component of the sensors. Because of these types of problems no practical long-term in vivo glucose biosensors have yet appeared.

A more favoured alternative to performing the glucose assay in vivo is to withdraw the blood from the body and carry out an determination ex vivo.

Using this regime, the physical and chemical conditions under which the assay is carried out can be controlled in a more precise and favourable manner.

The glucose biosensor

A glucose biosensor is a device which converts the specific recognition of glucose into an electronic signal, the amplitude of which is related to the concentration of the analyte in the test solution. In general terms, the sensor consists of a biological component, usually an enzyme, held in close proximity to a suitable transducer. In this configuration, the biological element serves a dual purpose. It confers selectivity upon the device and it produces or consumes a species which can be readily detected by the transducer. The intimate contact between the biological component and the surface of the transducer ensures both a rapid response and high sensitivity.

The transducer in a biosensor converts the changing physicochemical parameters associated with the interaction of the biocatalyst with its substrate into a processable signal. As a rule, the transducer should accommodate the following desirable features: (a) it must be highly specific for the change which is to be measured; (b) the response should be fast and the signal produced should be amenable to some form of manipulation such as amplification, storage and display; (c) the transducer should be amenable to both miniaturisation and mass production.

The transducers which have been incorporated into glucose sensors can be coveniently catagorised into 3 main types: thermometric, optical and electrochemical. Arguably the most successful and certainly the most documented of these has been the electrochemical device.

Thermometric glucose sensors

Most enzyme-catalysed reactions are exothermic and the heat generated during the catalytic turnover of substrate to product can be measured and related to the amount of substrate converted. Enzyme thermistors have been constructed to measure glucose concentrations using either hexokinase or glucose oxidase. These devices retain a flow through design and incorporate a bulky heat exchanger so that their use in vivo is not a practical proposition. Mosbach and co-workers have suggested, however, that they may be used in the bedside monitoring of glucose and be incorporated into an artificial pancreas (5).

More recently, Scheller et al (6) developed a high-sensitivity enzyme thermistor for the determination of glucose by using substrate recycling. To achieve this, the enzymes, glucose oxidase, glucose dehydrogenase and catalase, were co-immobilised onto the same reactor column. When substrate recycling was activated by the addition of NADH, a 3-fold signal amplification was observed compared to the response from immobilised glucose oxidase alone.

Optical glucose sensors

In 1979, Schultz and Sims (7) described an optical glucose sensor based on the detection of fluorescein-labelled dextran (dextran*) using a single optical fibre. When the dextran was exposed to concanavalin A and glucose, a competitive reaction occurred:

$$concanavalin\ A + glucose = concanavalin\ A\text{-}glucose$$
$$concanavalin\ A + dextran^* = concanavalin\ A\text{-}dextran^*$$

The amount of free dextran which caused the fluorescence was therefore related to the concentration of glucose in the sample. A probe was constructed by enclosing the reactants in a dialysis hollow fibre permeable to glucose. Light was delivered to the reaction chamber and any fluorescence monitored via an optical fibre. Only the free labelled dextran could enter the exciting light path to produce a signal. The probe responded linearly to glucose up to 10 mM.

Optical glucose sensors based on the flavoprotein glucose oxidase have also been described. Glucose oxidase catalyses the reaction:

$$glucose + O_2 + H_2O = gluconic\ acid + H_2O_2.$$

The hydrogen peroxide produced in this reaction can, under certain conditions, react with organic molecules to produce chemiluminescence. Bostick and Hercules (8) reported an optical sensor for blood glucose based on the induced chemiluminescence of luminol. In the presence of certain metals, generally metal ions possessing oxidation states requiring a one-electron transfer, peroxide reacts with luminol in basic media to form an excited aminophthalate anion which returns to ground state by the emission of a photon (9). In their system, the hydrogen peroxide generated from an immobilised glucose oxidase column was reacted with a mixture of ferricyanide and luminol in a continuous flow apparatus to produce chemiluminescence (8). The sensor gave a linear response between 10^{-8} and 10^{-4} M glucose and was found to correlate well with standard methods of glucose analysis. Following the removal of uric acid, the chemiluminescent technique was applied to the analysis of glucose in urine. A similar approach has also been described by Auses et al (10). In this case the chemiluminescent response arising from the interaction of luminol with basic ferricyanide was integrated over the first 5 minutes of the reaction. This resulted in a linear response for glucose over the entire range of ordinary clinical interest.

The determination of catalytically generated hydrogen peroxide has also been coupled to other chemiluminescent systems. Seitz and co-workers (11), for example, evaluated the use of 2,4,6-trichlorophenyl oxalate (TCPO) in their glucose sensors. In this particular case, chemiluminescence involves energy transfer from an excited intermediate to a fluorophor in solution such as rhodamine B. This reaction is summarised in Figure 1. The advantages offered by this technique over the luminol reaction were lower levels of background and a freedom uric acid interference, thereby facilitating glucose monitoring in urine.

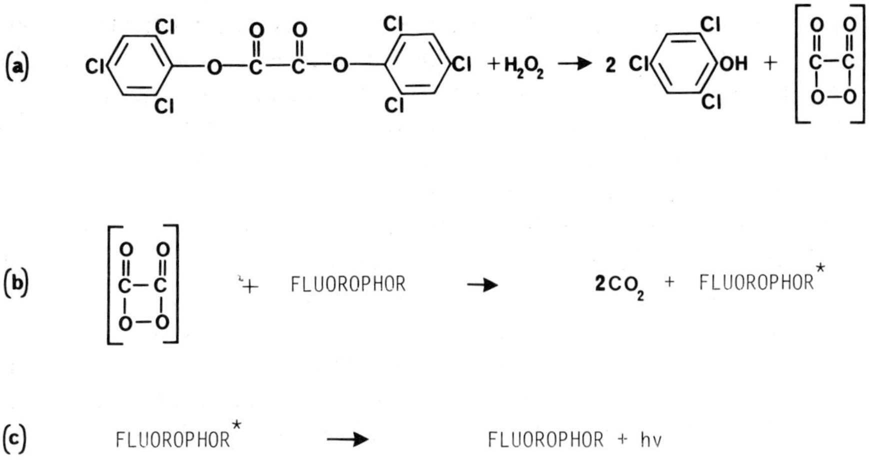

FIG. 1. *Peroxyoxalate chemiluminescence. The first step (a) in the chemiluminescent reaction involves the production of a key chemical intermediate containing the necessary excitation energy. The second step (b) involves the conversion of this chemical energy into electronic excitation energy. The final step (c) is the emission of light energy as the excited molecule returns to its ground electronic state.*

Electrochemical glucose sensors

Electrochemical glucose sensors can be divided into two groups: those which incorporate a potentiometric sensing element and those which utilise an amperometric indicator electrode.

In the potentiometric approach, the sensor head acts like a battery generating a potential difference which is measured relative to an inert reference electrode. The magnitude of the potential difference is related in a logarithmic fashion to the concentration of glucose in the solution. In the case of an amperometric sensor, a voltage is applied between a working and a reference electrode with the result that the imposed potential encourages electron transfer (redox) reactions to take place, causing a net current to flow in the external circuit. The magnitude of the current is directly related to the concentration of analyte in the test sample.

The vast majority of amperometric glucose biosensors reported to date exploit the reaction catalysed by the enzyme, glucose oxidase:

$$glucose + O_2 + H_2O = gluconic\ acid + H_2O_2.$$

This reaction has usually been followed either by monitoring the comsumption of oxygen with a Clark-type oxygen electrode or by oxidising the hydrogen peroxide produced during the reaction at a platinum working electrode poised at 600 mV versus the Ag/AgCl reference electrode. The rate at which hydrogen peroxide is produced or the rate at which oxygen is consumed during the catalytic oxidation of glucose to gluconic acid is related to the concentration of glucose in the original sample. In a classic paper dealing with the continuous monitoring of chemical substances in blood (1), Clark and Lyons proposed the first designs for a glucose biosensor. One suggestion was that a thin layer of soluble glucose oxidase may be retained at the surface of an oxygen electrode using a dialysis membrane. Glucose and oxygen would diffuse into the enzyme layer from the bulk solution and the resultant depletion of oxygen in the vicinity of the working electrode would provide a measure of the glucose concentration.

The first definitive example of an immobilised enzyme biosensor was reported by Updike and Hicks in 1967 (12). In their device, glucose oxidase was occluded at the surface of an oxygen electrode within a polyacrylamide gel matrix. A second electrode containing denatured enzyme was also included in the construction. This served as a blank, compensating for extraneous fluctuations in dissolved oxygen tensions and background oxidations at the working electrode.

In 1970, Clark patented a device based on measuring catalytically produced hydrogen peroxide at a platinum indicator electrode (13). This approach was subsequently commercialised by the Yellow Springs Instrument Company (Yellow Springs, Ohio). Glucose oxidase was entrapped between two membranes and the hydrogen peroxide produced was determined amperometrically at a platinum electrode poised at 700 mV versus the saturated calomel reference electrode (SCE). An outer polycarbonate membrane served to exclude large molecules and to produce a diffusion-limited system with consequent advantages in linearity and stability (14). A cellulose acetate membrane separated the enzyme from the surface of the working electrode and prevented the access of molecules such as ascorbate and urate, which would otherwise be oxidised at the platinum surface and produce artificially high signals. A 14:1 dilution of sample was recommended in order to reduce the concentration of potentially interfering substances to a manageable level and to ensure that the measurement was not limited by the availability of dissolved oxygen.

In 1973, Cuilbault and Lubrano (15) described a similar glucose sensor consisting of a thin film of glucose oxidase held in place over a platinum electrode by cellophane. Analysis of the kinetic response of the electrode instead of the steady-state reading was used to reduce the time of measurement from 1 minute to 12 seconds. The electrodes were relatively stable showing approximately 0.1% change in the slope of the calibration curve per day over a period of 10 months. High sensitivity is possible with this configuration; glucose has been measured down to 10 nM using amperometric detection of hydrogen peroxide, with electrochemical interference being compensated for by a non-enzymatic electrode (16).

It is important that variations in the dissolved oxygen tension of the sample should not affect the reading obtained from a glucose sensor, particularly if the sensor is to be used for monitoring in vivo where any dilution step would be impractical. One possible solution to this problem is to generate molecular oxygen in situ by the controlled electrolysis of water. This principle has been employed by Enfors (17) to produce an oxygen-insensitive probe, albeit for fermentation control that could in theory be extended to glucose monitoring in vivo.

Another approach is to use membranes in the construction of the probe which restrict the diffusion of glucose while at the same time allowing relatively free passage to oxygen. In this configuration the reaction becomes glucose-limited over a wide range of analyte concentrations (18-22). Mullen et al (23), for example, described an enzyme electrode suitable for extracorporeal glucose determination in unstirred whole blood. The sensor comprised a hydrogen-peroxide-detecting electrode over which was placed a membrane laminate incorporating glucose oxidase. The external membrane, porous polycarbonate, was pretreated with methyl-trichlorosilane, yielding a device with a linear dependence on glucose up to 50 mM, a response time of 30-90 seconds and a decreased dependence on dissolved oxygen (the electrode responded linearly to glucose up to 30 mM at a dissolved oxygen partial pressure of 20 mmHg). A further advantage afforded by the silane treatment was an improvement compatibility of the resulting outer membrane with blood (24).

A third approach to overcoming the problem of fluctuating oxygen tension is to replace oxygen, the natural redox partner of the enzyme, by an alternative electron sink resulting in a mediated enzyme electrode. In 1970, Williams et al (25) described an enzyme electrode in which oxygen was replaced by benzoquinone in the glucose-oxidase-catalysed reaction. The resulting reaction scheme was as follows:

$$glucose + H_2O + benzoquinone = gluconic\ acid + hydroquinone.$$

The hydroquinone produced in the above step was measured amperometrically by oxidation at a platinum electrode poised at a potential of 400 mV versus the SCE:

$$hydroquinone = benzoquinone + 2H^+ + 2e^-.$$

The enzyme was retained at the surface of the electrode in a porous gel matrix covered with a dialysis membrane. A second non-enzymic electrode was used to compensate for background currents produced by the non-specific oxidation of other electroactive species present in the sample. The sensor took 3-10 minutes to reach steady state and gave a linear response up to approximately 5 mM glucose.

Recently, a similar sensor has been described by Japanese workers (26) in which glucose oxidase was immobilised onto the surface of a *p*-benzoquinone carbon paste electrode by coating the enzyme-loaded surface with a nitrocellulose film. This electrode was found to be stable for more than a week and relatively insensitive to the levels of dissolved oxygen. The response produced by the electrode was linearly dependent on the concentration of glucose up to 30 mM. The electrode was operated at a potential of 500 mV versus the SCE.

Glucose sensors based on glassy carbon electrodes modified by redox polymers containing *p*-quinone groups have also been described in the literature. Cenas et al (27) reported electrodes modified with redox polymers (Fig. 2)

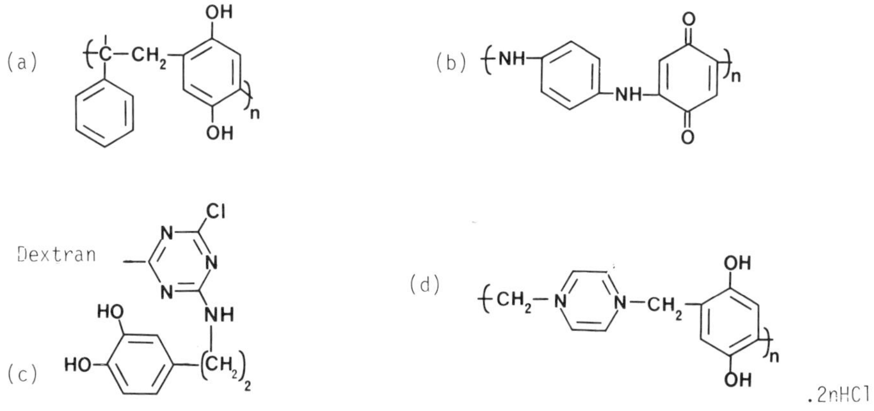

FIG. 2. *Types of redox polymers used to modify carbon electrodes: (a) styrene-hydroquinone copolymer; (b) p-phenylenediamine-benzoquinone copolymer; (c) dopamine-modified dextran; (d) hydroquinone-piperazine copolymer.*

which were efficient electrocatalytic surfaces for the oxidation of reduced glucose oxidase. The electrocatalytic currents, at pH 7, were generated at the peak potentials of the surface modifiers (50 = 500 mV *vs* Ag/AgCl). The electrodes were only stable for a period of 4-5 days, the instability being attributed to loss of electrocatalytic activity by the redox polymer.

Other mediator compounds such as 2,6-dichlorophenolindophenol (28), hexacyanoferrate (III) (29) and ferrocene monocarboxylate (30) have been used to couple the glucose oxidase reaction electrochemically in homogeneous solution. A glucose sensor in which the hexacyanoferrate (II)/(III) couple was retained at a carbon electrode surface by a protonated (pH 1-4) polyvinyl-pyridine polyelectrolyte film has also been reported (27). Jonsson and Gorton (31) described an amperometric glucose sensor based on glucose oxidase immobilised onto graphite which has been previously treated with *N*-methyl-phenazine (NMP). These electrodes responded linearly to glucose over the concentration range 0.5-15 μM. The immobilised enzyme was found to be stable for several months, but the mediator had to be renewed on a daily basis.

The ideal mediator should react rapidly with the reduced enzyme and exhibit good electrochemistry at a practical electrode. It should be amenable to simple immobilisation, stable in both the reduced and oxidised form, and unreactive towards oxygen. In order to avoid the problem of interference in real samples, the oxidation potential of the mediators should be low and independent of pH. Finally, especially for clinical applications, the mediator should be safe to handle and non-toxic. In 1984 Cass et al (30) demonstrated that ferrocene (Fig. 3)

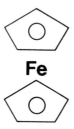

FIG. 3.   *Dicyclopentadienyl iron (ferrocene).*

and some of its derivatives met these criteria and could be incorporated into enzyme electrodes. Glucose sensors have been constructed by covalently coupling glucose oxidase to carbon foil, which had been previously modified with 1,1′-dimethylferrocene. The reaction sequence in the enzyme electrode may be summarised as follows:

$$glucose + 2\,ferricinium^+ + H_2O = gluconic\ acid + 2\,ferrocene.$$

The reduced couple is then reoxidised by polarising the electrode (160 mV *vs* the SCE) and allowing current to flow:

$$2\,ferrocene = 2\,ferricinium^+ + 2e^-.$$

These electrodes exhibited a linear range for glucose up to 30 mM whilst retaining rapid response times (60-90 s to 95% of the steady-state response). Good correlations were obtained with standard methods when the electrodes were used to measure blood glucose concentrations. Potential interferences were minimised by virtue of the low operating potential and the inclusion of a perm-selective membrane in the sensor head. Finally, the electrodes showed essentially no difference in the response when the analysis was performed under aerobic or anaerobic conditions, although high oxygen concentrations did reduce the signal.

Lange and Chambers (32) constructed a glucose probe by immobilising glucose oxidase and ferrocene into cross-linked polyacrylamide gels. The electrodes were easily constructed and gave current responses proportional to glucose concentrations up to 30 mM. The electrodes showed good stability when stored at 0°C in the dry state. Only a 3% decrease in the limiting current was observed for an electrode stored under these conditions for 120 hours. The electrodes did, however, require a period of 'break-in' before the maximum electrocatalytic current was obtained, presumably due to hydration of the polyacrylamide gel. The electrodes were less stable under aqueous conditions. The authors suggest that this was due to the gel matrix swelling and thereby losing electrical contact with the underlying graphite matrix. This phenomenon was found to be very pH-dependent and effectively limited the working range to pH 7-9.

Recent work in our laboratory has revealed another class of organic compounds, the tetrathiafulvalenes (TTF) (Fig. 4), which also satisfy the required

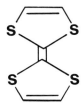

FIG. 4. $\triangle^{2,2'}$-*Bi-1,3-dithiole (tetrathiafulvalene)*.

properties of a good mediator (33). Glucose sensors incorporating TTF were prepared in essentially the same way as the afore-mentioned ferrocene probes. Operational characteristics of these sensors include low working potentials (220 mV *vs* Ag/AgCl), linear calibration curves up to 25 mM, rapid response times and improved oxygen interference characteristics.

Amperometric glucose sensors have been reported consisting of glucose oxidase incorporated into electrodes constructed from organometallic complexes such as those formed from a donor molecule like 7,7′,8,8′-tetra-cyanoquinodimethane (TCNQ) and an acceptor such as TTF or NMP. These donor-acceptor complexes are metallic at room temperature with a conductivity of 500 $(\Omega \cdot cm)^{-1}$ for the $TTF^+ \cdot TCNQ^-$ salt and 200 $(\Omega \cdot cm)^{-1}$ for the $NMP^+ \cdot TCNQ^-$ complex (34). Kulys and co-workers (35, 36) have reported efficient coupling to the redox centre of glucose oxidase to $NMP^+ \cdot TCNQ^-$ and $NMA^+ \cdot TCNQ^-$ (NMA = *N*-methylacridinium). The construction of these sensors was relatively simple. Either powdered enzyme was mixed with finely divided samples of the charge transfer salts and pressed into a disc (10^5 lb $\cdot$ in^{-2}) or an aliquot of glucose oxidase was entrapped at the surface of the electrode behind a membrane. Electrodes in which the glucose oxidase was adsorbed onto $NMA^+ \cdot TCNQ^-$ or $TTF^+ \cdot TCNQ^-$ were found to respond to glucose at potentials higher than 100 mV versus Ag/AgCl. These electrodes exhibited a good linear range for glucose and remarkable stability, retaining their activity for more than 100 days (36). Kulys et al (37) have also reported a bienzyme glucose electrode based on the enzymes, glucose oxidase and peroxidase. The enzymes were co-immobilised onto an organic metal electrode, yielding probes which were both stable and free from interference in real plasma samples.

Albery and co-workers (38, 39) have also investigated the use of organic metal electrodes as suitable charge-transfer surfaces from glucose oxidase. The best materials in their hands were the $TCNQ^+$ salts of NMP^+, NMP^+ and quinolinium (Q^+). Albery and co-workers also found the system to be stable. After a period of 28 days continuous operation the response of a typical electrode was found to have decreased only by 20% (39 and references therein).

Amperometric glucose sensors based on other enzymes

Although glucose oxidase is an extremely versatile enzyme, there are other glucose-utilising enzymes which may be successfully incorporated into a biosensor. Marko-Varga et al (40) have described a glucose sensor based on the enzyme, glucose dehydrogenase (D-glucose:NAD^+, 1-oxidoreductase). The sensor was prepared by absorbing Meldola blue (N,N'-dimethyl-7-amino-1,2-benzophenoxazinium) as well as glucose dehydrogenase onto the surface of a carbon electrode. The nicotinamide coenzyme was reduced in the catalytic cycle and reoxidised amperometrically at 0 mV versus Ag/AgCl (in this configuration the Meldola-blue-modified carbon acts as an efficient electrocatalytic surface for the regeneration of NAD^+ from reduced coenzyme (41)). Linear calibration curves were obtained in the range 5 µM — 2 mM glucose with the highest sensitivity being achieved at pH 6.

The value of replacing glucose oxidase with a glucose-utilising enzyme that has no cofactor requirements has been detailed in the literature (42-44). One such candidate is the NAD^+-independent quinoprotein, glucose dehydrogenase (43, 44). This enzyme has no soluble cofactor requirement and does not use oxygen as a cosubstrate. It does however catalyse substrate-dependent reduction of artificial electron acceptors (45). Mullen et al (46) described a glucose sensor incorporating glucose dehydrogenase (GDH) using phenazine ethosulphate (PES) or 2,6-dichlorophenolindophenol (DCPIP) as the mediators. With PES a linear response for up to 0.8 mM glucose was obtained with response times of 3-5 minutes. With DCPIP as the mediator longer response times were obtained (> 30 min), but the measurement was reduced to 30 seconds by monitoring the first-order differential of the response. This also allowed temporal separation of the enzyme-mediated signal from electrochemical interferenc. D'Costa and co-workers have described a glucose sensor based on GDH incorporating 1,1'-dimethylferrocene as the mediator. These electrodes responded in a non-linear fashion to glucose between 0.5 and 4 mM. The range was extended to 15 mM by varying the immobilisation procedure. The electrodes had a rapid response time (90 s to 100% of the signal) and were found to be stable over a period of 24 hours continuous use. No oxygen interference was detected using ferrocene as the mediator (47).

As a final example, glucose-selective electrodes have been described utilising whole organisms (48, 49). Although these electrodes would not be suitable for monitoring in vivo, they could in principle be used for extracorporeal glucose monitoring.

Examples of potentiometric glucose probes are more limited than their amperometric counterparts. Sensors which rely on potentiometric electrodes as the transducing element suffer from two distinct disadvantages. Firstly, accurate information about the concentration of analyte will only be obtained if there is a local thermodynamic equilibrium at the electrode surface. This requires the electrode kinetics to be rapid with a standard electrochemical rate constant greater than 10^{-2} cm·s^{-1}. This seriously limits the number of systems that can be used as indicator electrodes. The second disadvantage arises from the exponential dependence of the analyte concentration (c) on the electrode potential (E):

$$ln(c) = constant + nEF/RT,$$

where n is the valency of the ion, F the faraday unit, R the gas constant and T the absolute temperature. Small errors in E can give quite substantial errors in c. Thus, when $n=1$ an error in E of 10 mV leads to a 19% error in the value of c (38). Despite these serious operational disadvantages, potentiometric glucose sensors have been described in the literature, although it is generally accepted that at present the amperometric approach offers the more practical solution.

In 1973, Nagy et al (50) reported a glucose sensor utilising the iodide-ion-selective electrode as the indicator electrode. In this configuration, catalytically generated hydrogen peroxide (from the action of glucose oxidase on glucose) was reacted with potassium iodide to liberate free iodine:

$$H_2O_2 + 2KI + 2H^+ = 2H_2O_2 + I_2 + 2K^+.$$

The decrease in the concentration of iodide was used to indicate the concentration of glucose in the solution. The assay did however suffer from the lack of specificity of the ion-selective electrode (ISE), which responded to thiocyanate, sulphide, cyanide, and silver (1). In addition, species such as uric acid, ascorbic acid and ferrous ions were found to compete with iodide for peroxide.

The original paper by Clark and Lyons (I) contained a suggestion for an alternative glucose probe based on the pH-sensitive glass electrode. In this design, glucose oxidase was retained by cuprophane membranes at the electrode surface. The increase in hydrogen ion concentration resulting from the glucose oxidase reaction gave a measure of the glucose concentration. Nillson et al (51) demonstrated this principle and detected glucose down to 1 mM. The assay was, however, very susceptible to the initial pH, temperature and buffering capacity of the solution.

In 1982, Siddiqi (52) described a more practical glucose sensor based on the fluoride ISE. In this particular scheme an organofluorine compound was reacted with hydrogen peroxide, produced by the glucose oxidase reaction, in the presence of horseradish peroxidase, to generate free F^-. The resultant increase in the fluoride ion concentration was measured by the ISE. The rate of appearance of F^- was used to estimate the amount of glucose in the solution. This technique was applied quite successfully to the determination of glucose in real samples.

Wingard et al (53) described a sensor consisting of glucose oxidase and catalase co-immobilised onto the surface of a platinum disc. By measuring the potential that developed at the enzyme electrode relative to a blank, a linear relationship between current and concentration was obtained up to 8.3 mM glucose. The authors found that the potentiometric response to glucose by these electrodes could be altered depending on the electrochemical and/or thermal pretreatments imposed on the platinum surface (54).

Wilkins and Wilkins (55) described a coated wire electrode for glucose incorporating a quaternary ammonium salt, an insoluble glucose salt and polyvinyl chloride. The electrode responded both amperometrically and potentiometrically to glucose, but the mechanism of the response remains unclear.

Extracorporeal glucose sensors

Although the ultimate aim of glucose biosensor research is to produce stable, miniaturized probes suitable for continuous monitoring in vivo, the majority of sensors which have been successfully applied to diabetes management and research to date are those based on an ex vivo design. Fogt et al (56), for example, described an online glucose analyser based on the amperometric detection of hydrogen peroxide, which was incorporated in a computerised feedback control system allowing the dynamic control of blood glucose levels. This instrument, the Biostator, is a non-portable bedside machine which draws blood from a peripheral vein and then measures the blood glucose level. The on-board computer calculates, according to pre-set algorithms, the amount of glucose or insulin to be infused into another vein in order to maintain normoglycaemia.

Ljunggren (57) described an ex vivo microcircuit capable of continuous monitoring of blood glucose. The device utilised immobilised glucose oxidase and a pseudo-flow injection technique. To enable continuous blood sampling, the blood was first diluted 1:1 with anticoagulant in a double lumen catheter. The diluted blood was then passed through a dialyser and the dialysate pumped via a diverter through the dioreactor column and then onto a modified Clark-type electrode. On-line calibration was achieved by altering the flow path so that calibrant flowed through the enzyme column. Continuous blood monitoring via a catheter connected into an ear vein was carried out for a period of 5 hours in piglets. Non-diabetic subjects showed normal glucose variations after food intake, whereas diabetic piglets showed drastic increases in blood glucose levels when fed, followed by a rapid decay after insulin infusion.

In vivo glucose sensors

Although there is still no commercially available in vivo glucose sensor, work in this area continues apace. The major objectives in this field are to produce sensors of adequate stability, fast response times and with clinically relevant linear ranges. Advances in immobilisation, membrane chemistry and membrane design have already indicated the way forward. Perhaps the greatest challenge is that of biocompatibility and tissue rejection. Adsorption of proteins, platelets and other blood components to the sensor head affect mass transfer and result in unpredictable changes in the response. Consequently, frequent recalibration is required which greatly limits the long-term use of such electrodes (58). Additional demands are imposed by the need for safety; electrodes need to be sterilisable, mechanically robust and fabricated from non-toxic materials. It is also important that there is no direct contact between tissue and the immobilised components of the sensor.

Shichiri et al (20-22, 59) have reported a needle electrode consisting of a fine platinum wire with a bulbous tip. After polishing the tip with fine-sand paper, a stainless steel tube coated with silver (the cathode) was placed around the platinum anode. The electrode was then dipped into a suspension of glucose oxidase and heparin in 50% acetone and 50% ethanol containing 2.5% cellulose diacetate. The electrode was allowed to dry and was stabilised by dipping in 1% gluteraldehyde solution. After a period of 12 hours the sensor was dipped into 4% polyurethane in 10% dimethylformamide and 90% tetrahydrofuran. The resultant sensor was 2 cm in length and 0.4-1 nm in diameter. Although the currents produced by the sensor were in the nA range, electrical noise was not found to be a problem. The sensor output was directly proportional to glucose concentrations up to 28 mM with response times of around 16-25 seconds. These electrodes were incorporated in a wearable closed-loop system consisting of the sensor, a microcomputer and a two syringe driving system. The device succeeded in controlling glycaemia in depancreatised dogs for a period of 3 days. When these sensors were inserted into the subcutaneous tissue of the forearms or abdomen of volunteer diabetic subjects, glycaemic control was reported in the subjects by infusing insulin either intravenously or subcutaneously in response to the implanted glucose sensor.

Similar electrodes have been described by Churchouse et al (60) consisting of 4 insulated platinum wires (25-125 μm) housed in stainless steel tubing (0.2-1 mm o.d.). By careful optimisation of the various dip coating procedures these workers were able to produce electrodes which were extremely selective in blood and which had a linear range extending to 20-30 mM glucose. An important design modification was the inclusion of a continuous non-cellulosic underlying membrane which ensured the high selectivity. Preliminary experiments in animals indicated their suitability for short-term monitoring in vivo.

Abel et al (61) described a modified Clark electrode suitable for implantation and connection to a glucose control infusion system. The response from the sensor was linear up to 40 mM glucose, although the response times were slow. Glucose concentrations up to 15 mM were reliably measured in subcutaneous tissue even when the Po_2 was as low as 2-5 kPa.

Gough et al (62) have described an implantable glucose sensor coupled to a telemetry system which, when implanted in mongrel dogs, was capable of continuous blood glucose monitoring for periods of months. Furthermore, they reported that over this period the implant's operation was not limited by enzyme inactivation or sensor bio-incompatibility. The sensor itself had a cylindrical oxygen probe that was electrochemically active on its curved surface. Surrounding the oxygen sensor was a concentric hydrophilic gel containing the enzymes, glucose oxidase and catalase. A hydrophobic, oxygen-permeable silicone rubber tube that was impermeable to glucose was placed adjacent to the enzyme layer. The enzyme gel was exposed to the sample medium at one end. This particular design allowed both glucose and oxygen to diffuse into the immobilised enzyme layer through the exposed anular end but only oxygen to diffuse radially into the gel through the silicone membrane. This gave rise to a two-dimensional supply of oxygen (radial and axial) but only a one-dimensional supply of glucose (axial). This novel design ensured that the sensor could operate even at low oxygen tensions. It has also been shown that sufficient gaseous oxygen can be supplied to the electrode from an implanted Silastic drum. This also results in an integral glucose sensor which is glucose-dependent and essentially Po_2-independent (63).

Miniature mediated glucose sensors suitable for implantation have also been reported. Claremont et al (64, 65), for example, described miniature glucose oxidase/1,1'-dimethylferrocene sensors which were implanted into the subcutaneous tissue of non-diabetic pigs. Tissue glucose levels were found to be lower than blood values. Following an intravenous infusion of glucose the tissue levels were found to increase at virtually the same time as blood glucose, but the rate of rise was much slower in the tissues. After administration of insulin the tissue glucose fell more slowly than the blood glucose levels.

Matthews et al (66) have described a ferrocene-mediated glucose oxidase sensor based on a 25-gauge needle covered with a membrane. The needles were inserted subcutaneously into the abdomens of normal subjects. The current time curves obtained from the needles showed good agreement with blood glucose levels measured by a Yellow Springs Instrument. The response was found to be unimpaired over a period of 4.5 hours' continuous monitoring.

A number of mathematical models relating to the behaviour of glucose probes in vivo are now being described in the literature (67-69). Parameters which are being modelled include response times, diffusion of substrates to the electrode surface, and the relationship between maximum current output versus enzyme loadings. This approach coupled with those outlined above may result in a probe which is both biocompatible and self-correcting, thus providing a feasible route to the long-awaited in vivo sensor. In the interim period, however, recent developments in glucose biosensor research will result in new commercial products for the testing of blood samples. These devices may well offer improved performance over currently available methods, but one undoubted benefit to the diabetic patient from this increased competition amongst manufacturers will be lower cost per test and more convenient devices.

References

1. Clark LC, Lyons C (1962): Electrode system for continuous monitoring in cardiovascular surgery. *Ann. NY Acad. Sci., 102,* 29.
2. Turner APF, Pickup JC (1985): Diabetes mellitus: biosensors for research and management. *Biosensors, 1,* 85.
3. Schade DS, Eaton RP, Edwards WS et al (1982): A remotely controlled programmable insulin delivery system: successful short-term implantation in man. *J. Med. Soc., 247,* 1848.
4. Irsigler K, Kritz H, Lovett R (Eds) (1983): *Diabetes Treatment with Implantable Insulin Infusion Systems.* Urban and Schwarzenberg, Munich.
5. Mosbach K, Mandenius CF, Danielsson B (1983): New biosensor devices. In: *Biotech 83,* pp. 665-678. Online Publications, Northwood, U.K.
6. Scheller F, Siegbahn N, Danielsson B, Mosbach K, (1985): High sensitivity enzyme thermistor determination of L-lactate by substrate recycling. *Anal. Chem., 57,* 1740.
7. Schultz JS, Sims G, (1979): Affinity sensors for individual metabolites. *Biotechnol. Bioeng. Symp., 9,* 65.

8. Bostick DT, Hercules DM (1975): Quantitative determination of blood glucose using enzyme induced chemiluminescene of luminol. *Anal. Chem., 47,* 447.
9. Seitz WR, Hercules DM (1973): Peroxide induced chemiluminescence of luminol. In: Cormier MJ, Hercules DM, Lee J (Eds), *Chemiluminescence and Bioluminescence.* Plenum Press, New York.
10. Auses JP, Cook SL, Maloy JT (1975): Chemiluminescent enzyme method for glucose. *Anal. Chem., 47,* 244.
11. Williams DC, Huff GF, Seitz RW (1976): Evaluation of peroxyoxalate chemiluminescence for determination of enzyme generated peroxide. *Anal. Chem., 48,* 1003.
12. Updike JW, Hicks JP (1967): The enzyme electrode. *Nature (London), 214,* 986.
13. Clark LC (1970): Membrane polarographic electrode system and method for electrochemical compensation. U.S. Patent No. 3 539 455.
14. Mell LD, Maloy JT (1975): A model for the amperometric enzyme electrode obtained through digital simulation and applied on the immobilised glucose system. *Anal. Chem., 47,* 299.
15. Guilbault GG, Lubrano GJ (1973): An enzyme electrode for the amperometric determination of glucose. *Anal. Chim. Acta, 64,* 439.
16. Thevenot DR, Coulet PR, Sternberg R, Gautheron DC (1978): A highly sensitive glucose electrode using a glucose oxidase collagen film. *Bioelectrochem. Bioenerg., 5,* 548.
17. Enfors SO (1981): Oxygen-stabilised enzyme electrode for D-glucose analysis in fermentation broths. *Enzyme Microbiol. Technol., 3,* 29.
18. Clark LC, Duggan CA (1982): Implanted electroenzymatic glucose sensors. *Diabetes Care, 5,* 174.
19. Romette JL, Froment B, Thomas D (1979): Glucose oxidase electrode: measurement of glucose in samples exhibiting high variability in oxygen content. *Clin. Chim. Acta, 95,* 249.
20. Schichiri M, Kawamori RM, Yamasaki Y et al (1982): Wearable artificial endocrine pancreas with needle type glucose sensor. *Lancet, 2,* 1129.
21. Schichiri M, Kawamori RM, Goriya Y et al (1983): Glycaemic control in pancreatectomized dogs with a wearable artificial pancreas. *Diabetologia, 24,* 179.
22. Schichiri M, Kawamori RM, Hakui et al (1984): The development of wearable-type artificial endocrine pancreas and its usefulness in glycaemic control of human diabetes mellitus. *Biomed. Biochim. Acta, 43,* 561.
23. Mullen WH, Keedy FH, Churchouse SJ, Vadgama PM (1986): Glucose enzyme electrode with extended linearity: application to undiluted blood measurements. *Anal. Chim. Acta, 183,* 59.
24. Hanning I, Vadgama AK, Covingtin AK, Alberti KGMM (1986): Improved blood compatibility at a glucose enzyme electrode used for extracorporeal monitoring. *Anal. Lett., 19,* 461.
25. Williams DL, Doig AR, Korosi A (1970): Electrochemical enzymatic analysis of blood glucose and lactate. *Anal. Chem., 42,* 118.
26. Ikeda T, Katasho I, Kamei M, Senda M (1983): Electrocatalysis with a glucose oxidase immobilized graphite electrode. *Agric. Biol. Chem., 48,* 1969.
27. Cenas NK, Pocius AK, Kulys JJ (1983): Electron exchange between flavin and heme containing enzymes and electrodes modified by rendox polymers. *Bioelectrochem. Bioenerg., 11,* 61..
28. Mindt W, Racine P, Schleapfer P (1973): Sensoren für Lactat und Glucose. *Ber. Busenges. Phys. Chem., 77,* 804.
29. Mahenc J, Aussaresses H (1979): Electrode à enzyme spécifique du glucose basée sur la détection ampérométrique de l'héxacyanoferrate (III). *CR Acad. Sci. Paris, 289,* 357.
30. Cass AEG, Davis G, Francis GD et al (1984): Ferrocene mediated enzyme electrode for the amperometric determination of glucose. *Anal. Chem., 56,* 667.

31. Jonsson G, Gorton L (1985): An amperometric glucose sensor made by modification of a graphite electrode surface with immobilized glucose oxidase and adsorbed mediator. *Biosensors, 1*, 355.
32. Lange M, Chambers JQ (1985): Amperometric determination of glucose with a ferrocene mediated glucose oxidase/polyacrylamide gel electrode. *Anal. Chim. Acta, 175*, 89.
33. Hendry SP, Cardosi MF, Turner APF (1986): An amperometric enzyme electrode for glucose based on tetrathiafulvalene modified carbon electrodes. *Biosensors*, submitted for publication.
34. Bryce MR, Murphy LC (1984): Organic metals. *Nature (London) 309*, 119.
35. Kulys JJ, Samalius AS, Svirmickas GJS (1980): Electron exchange between the enzyme active centre and organic metal. *FEBS Lett., 114*, 7.
36. Kulys JJ (1986): Enzyme electrodes based on organic metals. *Biosensors, 2*, 3.
37. Kulys JJ, Pesliakiene MV, Samalius AS (1981): The development of bienzyme glucose electrodes. *Biolectrochem. Bioenerg., 8*, 81.
38. Albery WJ, Craston DH, Hagett BGD (1985): The development of novel biosensors. *World Biotech. Rep., 1*, 392.
39. Albery WJ, Craston DH (1986): Amperometric enzyme electrodes: theory and experiment. In: Turner APP, Karube I, Wilson GS (Eds), *Biosensors: Fundamentals and Applications*, pp. 182-212. Oxford University Press, Oxford.
40. Marko-Varga G, Appelqvist R, Gorton L (1986): A glucose sensor based on glucose dehydrogenase adsorbed on a modified carbon electrode. *Anal. Chim. Acta, 179*, 317.
41. Gorton L (1986): Chemically modified electrodes for the electrocatalytic oxidation of nicotinamide coenzymes. *J. Chem. Soc. Faraday Trans. I, 82*, 1245.
42. D'Costa EJ, Turner APF, Higgins IJ (1985): Quinoprotein glucose dehydrogenase based glucose sensor. In: Mosbach K (Ed.), *Proceedings, VIII International Conference on Enzyme Engineering, Helsingør, 1985*, p. 197. Plenum Press, New York.
43. D'Costa EJ, Duine JA, Dokter P et al (1984): Kinetics of a microbial quinoprotein glucose dehydrogenase. *Soc. Gen. Microbiol., 11*, M11.
44. Turner APF (1983): Applications of direct electron transfer bioelectrochemistry in sensors and fuel cells. In: *Biotech 83*, pp. 643-654. Online Publications, Northwood, U.K.
45. Duine JA, Frank J (1981): Quinoproteins: a novel class of dehydrogenases. *Trends Biochem, Sci, 6*, 278.
46. Mullen WH, Churchouse SJ, Vadgama PM (1985): Enzyme electrode for glucose based on the quinoprotein glucose dehydrogenase. *Analyst, 110*, 925.
47. D'Costa EJ, Higgins IJ, Turner APF (1986): Quinoprotein glucose dehydrogenase and its application in an amperometric glucose sensor. *Biosensors, 2*, 71.
48. Karube I, Suzuki S (1984): Amperometric and potentiometric determinations with immobilized cells and microorganisms. *Ion Sel. Electrode Rev., 6*, 15.
49. Karube I, Mitsuda S, Suzuki S (1979): Glucose sensors using immobilised whole cells of *Pseudomonas fluorescens. Eur J. Appl. Microbiol. Biotechnol., 7*, 343.
50. Nagy G, Von Storp LH, Guilbault GG (1973): Glucose enzyme electrode based on the use of an iodide membrane (sensor). *Anal. Chim. Acta, 66*, 443.
51. Nilsson H, Akerlund AC, Mosbach K (1973): Determination of glucose, urea and penicillin using enzyme-pH electrodes. *Biochim. Biophys. Acta, 320*, 529.
52. Siddiqi IW (1982): An electrochemical assay system for peroxidase and peroxidase-coupled reactions based on a fluoride ion-selective electrode. *Clin. Chem., 28*, 1962.
53. Wingard LB, Schiller JG, Wolfson SK et al (1979): Immobilized enzyme electrodes for the potentiometric measurement of glucose concentrations: immobilisation techniques and materials. *J. Biomed. Mater. Res., 13*, 921.

54. Castner JF, Wingard LB (1984): Alterations in the potentiometric response of glucose oxidase platinum electrodes resulting from electrochemical or thermal pretreaments of a metal surface. *Anal. Chem., 51,* 2891.
55. Wilkins E, Wilkins MG (1983): Implantable glucose sensor. *J. Biomed. Eng., 5,* 309.
56. Fogt EJ, Dodd LM, Jenning EM, Clemens AH (1978): Development and evaluation of a glucose analyzer for a glucose controlled insulin infusion system (Biostator). *Clin. Chem., 24,* 1366.
57. Ljunggren L (1986): Methods for continuous monitoring of glucose and urea in blood. In: Aucoutourier JL, Cauhape JS, Destriau M et al (Eds), *Proceedings, 2nd International Meeting on Chemical Sensors, Bordeaux, 1986,* pp. 527-530. Imprimerie Biscaye, Bordeaux.
58. Vadgama P (1981): Enzyme electrodes as practical biosensors. *J. Med. Eng., 5,* 293.
59. Shichiri M, Asakawa N, Yamasaki Y et al (1986): Telemetry glucose monitoring device with needle type glucose sensor: a useful tool for blood glucose monitoring in diabetic individuals, *Diabetes Care, 9,* 289.
60. Churchouse S, Mullen W, Bettersby C, Vadgama P (1986): Design and use of needle glucose electrodes. In: *Proceedings, 2nd Assisi International Symposium on Advance Models for the Therapy of Insulin Dependent Diabetes, 1986.* Raven Press, New York. In press.
61. Abel P, Muller A, Fischer U (1984): Experience with an implantable glucose sensor as a prerequisite of an artificial beta cell. *Biomed. Biochim. Acta, 43,* 577.
62. Gough DA, Armour JC, Biermann E et al (1986): An implantable glucose sensor. In: Aucoutourier JL, Cauhape JS, Destriau M (Eds), *Proceedings, 2nd International Meeting on Chemical Sensors, Bordeaux, 1986,* pp. 566-567. Imprimerie Biscaye, Bordeaux.
63. Clark LC, Noyes LK, Spokane RB et al (1985): Design and long-term performance of surgically implanted electroenzymatic glucose sensors. *Ann. NY Acad. Sci.,* in press.
64. Claremont DJ, Penton C, Pickup JC (1986): Potentially-implantable, ferrocene-mediated glucose sensor. *J. Biomed. Eng., 8,* 272.
65. Claremont DJ, Sambrook IE, Penton C, Pickup JC (1986): Subcutaneous implantation of a ferrocene-mediated glucose sensor in pigs. *Diabetologia,* in press.
66. Matthews DR, Brown E, Beck T et al (1986): A transcutaneous 25 guage amperometric glucose-sensing needle, and its use in man. *Diabetic Med.,* in press.
67. Conway PJ, Gough DA (1986): Long term in vitro operation of enzyme electrode-based glucose sensors. In: Aucoutourier JL, Cauhape JS, Destriau M (Eds), *Proceedings, 2nd International Meeting on Chemical Sensors, Bordeaux, 1986,* pp. 547-549. Imprimerie Biscaye, Bordeaux.
68. El Degheidy MM, Wilkins ES (1986): Optimization of an implantable coated wire glucose sensor. *J. Biomed. Eng., 8,* 121.
69. Furler SM, Kreagen EW, Smallwood RH, Chisolm DM (1985): Blood glucose control by intermittent loop closure in the basal mode: computer simulation studies with a diabetic model. *Diabetes Care, 8,* 553.

The Diabetes Annual/3
K.G.M.M. Alberti and L.P. Krall, editors
© 1987 Elsevier Science Publishers, B.V.

30 Organising and evaluating diabetes care

D.W. BEAVEN AND R.S. SCOTT

Planning for diabetes services

The aims of a diabetes service should be to reduce or prevent the health and social consequences of the disorder. There will be limitations in meeting these goals, but the services available for diabetic subjects should by organised in such a way as to allow effective health care to be provided for all those with diabetes mellitus. Since the previous reviews in *The Diabetes Annual* (1, 2) there have been further articles which have identified deficiencies of diabetes care and which have examined the need for reorganisation if the goals for effective health care are to be developed. Assal et al (3) have pointed out, however, that the quality of diabetes care has remained poor despite the many advances made in the last 20 years. They have attributed this to widespread failure to acknowledge the impact of diabetes education: the recommendations introduced over 50 years ago have still not been incorporated in some diabetes services in spite of their proven benefits. Improved health care would undoubtedly follow if strategies combining biomedical, psychosocial and educational advances were incorporated in the health services for diabetes mellitus.

As indicated in our review in *The Diabetes Annual/2* (2), the adoption of health care models in the reorganisation of diabetes services does depend upon adequate epidemiological data. Some authors have used information on the health impact of the disorder to modify the service. Connell (4) reported that problems with access to care and with service deficiencies contributed to high mortality amongst diabetic patients. This author suggested that there would be an improved health outcome if these service deficiencies were identified by appropriate studies of hospitalisation patterns and therapeutic approaches. In this particular study, conducted in Washington State, U.S.A., the author found that suboptimal medical care was associated with high hospital admission rates for diabetes, with poor therapeutic and diagnostic discrimination between those with mild and those with severe metabolic problems.

An alternative approach to data collection which can be applied to planning of health services is to use the epidemiological approach. Mather and Keen (5) undertook a house-to-house enquiry for known diabetes mellitus in Southall, West London. Prevalence rate for Asians in this population was 3.8 times higher than that for Europeans; for patients between the ages of 20 and 64 years it was at least 5 times higher. Prevalence rates were 12% in Asians aged 60-69 years. Clearly, such data are critical to the planning of care for diabetic patients in any health district, and will obviously influence the way in which resources should be allocated. Similar approaches in Singapore have been used by Cheah et al (6). These authors have identified prevalence differences amongst populations in this multiracial community, with Indians having higher rates (6.07%) than Malays (2.43%) and Chinese (1.55%). This study and further surveys by Omar et al (7) from South Africa and Merriman and Ross in Malaysia (8) emphasised that epidemiological factors unique to the community, such as ethnicity (i.e. Indian), must be accommodated within the local diabetes services.

Epidemiological approaches can also be applied to identification of the population at risk for complications. However, to date, the much-needed studies reporting reduced complication rates and decreased mortality resulting from improvements to a health care system are few (2). Lawrence et al (9) suggest that patients at high risk of proliferative diabetic retinopathy may be able to be identified at a first clinic visit. These authors presented a multifactorial model identifying frequency of hyperglycaemia, refractive index, HLA phenotype and patients' self-testing techniques to establish increased risk. Such approaches for other complications of diabetes such as amputation and nephropathy may prove very useful in identifying high-risk groups in the community. This would, in turn, allow an increase of resources to be applied. Given the very high cost of tertiary care which results from poorly treated diabetes through its complications, such approaches have obvious merit.

Accommodating patients' attitudes

Patients' attitudes may be critical to the success of any health service plan for chronic disorders such as diabetes mellitus (10, 11). In particular, a paper by McLaughlin and Sliepcevich (10) describes models for the development of a self-care behaviour inventory which could be useful for such disorders as multiple sclerosis, arthritis, epilepsy and diabetes. Interactions with the family greatly influence behaviour and compliance. Schafer and colleagues have used a family behaviour check-list to identify individuals with non-supportive family behaviour (12). Harrison and Linn (13) suggested that improved attitudes towards health care may be a means of directly influencing the control of the disease itself. Like other authors studying health beliefs recently (14, 15), they have found that these were better predictors of metabolic control than physiological measures of compliance.

It is apparent from these articles that the planning of a diabetes service needs to be considerably broadened beyond that currently available in most centres.

The report on facilities available in diabetic clinics in the United Kingdom by Spathis, based on a survey conducted on behalf of the Medical Advisory Committee of the British Diabetic Association, gives cause for concern at the level of deficit when contrasted with a minimum recommended system (16). The recommendations proposed would be considered by many to be most conservative. As more is learned about the factors which relate to complications, susceptibility, non-compliance and poor control, it is apparent to many professionals that plans for different facilities and approaches will need to be incorporated within diabetes services if improved health outcomes are to be effected. The excellent article by Holmes (17) provides the physician with great insight into the psychological and social components of the disorder which are inadequately accommodated in most diabetes services.

In every diabetes service there will be a conflict of interest between the various sections of the service: preventive education, early detection programmes, diabetes education, diabetes management service and patient investigation and treatment. All too often the costly demands of poorly treated or untreated diabetes dominate over primary care or prevention, community education and early interventionist strategies.

Organisation of diabetes services

The importance of education in the diabetes service organisation has been stressed already (3). In the study by Hoskins et al (18) phone contact was used extensively for communication between the specialist unit and patients. This low-cost approach to improving metabolic control amongst diabetics has important social and economic benefits from the aspect of avoiding repeated hospitalisation.

A number of papers have examined the organisation of medical care within tertiary institutions. Kosecoff and colleagues evaluated 15 internal medicine group practices within university teaching hospitals (19). They found that quality of care standards were not uniformly met. The type of medical care provided was traditional and facilities for education were not available.

Morrison and Richards (20) undertook a retrospective study at the University Hospital of the West Indies. Of patients being seen for the first time, most had had their disorder for at least 10 years by which stage complications had already been established. This study highlighted the need for reorganisation of the health care system so that early intervention programmes could be undertaken. From the University Hospital in Groningen, Van Ballegooie (21) reported the outcome since 1980 following planned changes to their diabetes services. This service, in its reorganised form, had adopted the principles widely promoted by other units, that of a multidisciplinary clinic utilising dietitian, nurse educator, podiatrist and laboratory services as well as other specialist medical resources. The importance of this multidisciplinary approach in the reorganisation of a diabetes service has been detailed in *The Diabetes Annual/2* by Beaven and Scott (2) and Assal and Aufseesser-Stein (22).

Changes to a more effective health system can often be quite simple. Barnett reported a good study on the feasibility and effects of changeover from a traditional to more modern methods of diabetic management in insulin-dependent diabetic subjects attending a standard British hospital outpatient department (23). He arranged for patients to switch from urine-testing to self-measurement of blood glucose, to use a high-fibre diet and to commence insulin regimes using 2 injections a day. Helped only by a diabetes education nurse, the new management techniques were accepted by 80% of patients and were found easy to apply and proved effective. This paper suggests that these changes should by now have been effected in outpatient services in all westernised countries even with a minimal diabetes service. The changes could likewise be introduced in many clinics of Third World countries.

It is salutary to note the article by Wylie-Rosett et al (24) reporting the health care standards in a 1000-bed chronic care institution in the United States. They used techniques of chart audit, staff interviews and education to improve standards. Following these interventions, they noted substantial alterations in care with acceptable standards being met in the following areas: diabetes diagnosis according to National Diabetes Data Group criteria, urine testing, capillary blood testing, rotation of insulin injection site, assessment of patients for adherence to regimen, assessment of patients' skills and knowledge and interdisciplinary coordination of care.

These two studies highlight the fact that current resources within institutions may well be adequate, but with appropriate reorganisation, great improvement in health care standards, as they relate to diabetes management, can be introduced.

The special problem of case recording for individuals with chronic diseases such as diabetes mellitus has been previously described (2) and the potential use of computerised systems is being increasingly explored by a number of units. Mahler and Greenwood (25) have described a simple method for managing the records of a diabetic clinic in a district general hospital in the United Kingdom. They considered this inexpensive system suitable for smaller hospitals as it could be applied to patient and clinical management and also to research projects. These authors found that the system simplified the management of the clinic and could be easily used by inexperienced staff.

Evaluating health care

To measure attitudes and understanding about diabetes, questionnaires have been widely used. Mellor and colleagues employed a questionnaire survey of diabetes care in general practice in Leicestershire, U.K. (26). In Prague, Pav and Sperl (27) undertook a study of 269 patients from different diabetic clinics. Information obtained on diet and organisation of dietary practices in relation to work and family circumstances were used to form conclusions on replanning of a dietary service for diabetics. However, for an area known to be so fundamental to good diabetes care, there are all too few studies of any substances attempting evaluation of dietary practices in different communities.

Wing et al (28) have reported that behaviour modification coupled with nutrition education was important for sustaining weight loss and adherence to dietary programmes. These data of course are not new, having been shown in previous years by other workers (1, 2).

The outcome of controlled diabetes educational programmes aimed at improving short-term parameters have once again been reported by a number of groups; these are similar in style and conclusions to those reported in previous years (29-31). Beyond those referenced in *The Diabetes Annual/2*, relating to reduction of hospitalisation rates, there have been no further excellent studies attempting to show benefits in the longer term through diminished complication rates.

Two articles relating to educational methods are, however, worthy of attention. Damoiseaux et al (32) from Geneva have analysed the type of questions that health education personnel ask their patients. Using an educational specialist, they analysed the potential use of these questions, their number, their type and their function. They suggested that a change in the style of questioning could encourage the thinking process and promote problem-solving. Pichert et al (33) reported that nearly two-thirds of patient time was spent on assessment and only 20% actually spent on patient education or instruction. These messages have important implications for all diabetes education programmes.

The availability of biochemical procedures for evaluating glycaemic control have greatly facilitated the ability of the clinician to interpret responses to diet or educational interventionist programmes. The position paper by the Health and Public Policy Committee of the American College of Physicians sums up, in an accurate manner, factors affecting assays for glycosylated haemoglobin and the clinical usefulness of these measurements (34). Self-measurement of blood glucose is now well established as a technique with which to achieve behaviour modification and improve compliance with treatment regimens. Of more recent advent are meters with inbuilt memory chips capable of storing glucose determinations. Experience with their use as an educational tool is still very limited (35, 36). A recent article by Mazze et al (36) reported that subjects using these meters maintained accurate and reliable record-keeping throughout a 6-week study period. This contrasts with the findings of a previous report by these authors (37) when patients were unaware of the memory function of the meters in which recording problems were great. Notwithstanding this improved performance, alterations in glycaemic control were not found (see also Chapter 13). An article by Wing et al (38) has again emphasised the widespread problem of compliance with respect to self-measurement of blood glucose. They emphasised the need for planned behavioural strategies to correct this.

Complications and mortality from diabetes mellitus

Complication rates and death rates from diabetes mellitus would appear useful as long-term markers to establish the efficacy of a health delivery system. It is therefore of interest to note the article by Hadden et al (39) reporting the natural history of diabetes mellitus presenting between the ages of 40 and 69 years. These authors found that 80% of their patients were able to be managed by diet alone for a 6-year period. During this treatment period, the mortality from all causes in these subjects was no different from that of the general population of Northern Ireland. Beischer and Pfeiffer (40) have reviewed the life expectancy of patients using insulin, aged 15-74 years, in the Federal Republic of Germany. This useful study comes from an area where diabetes care has reached a high standard. They found that their current life expectancy was two-thirds that of the general population, irrespective of age of onset. In this respect, this paper contrasts with that from Ireland (39). They also documented substantial morbidity from eye and renal damage. For diabetic subjects in the adult age group up to 74 years, the mortality rate for all vascular diseases was 2½ times greater for men and 3½ times greater for women: this confirmed earlier studies showing high vascular mortality of female diabetic patients. The study also examined morbidity from the disorder. After 30 years of treatment for IDDM, 33% of the patients were blind and 24% had renal failure. Whether the newer treatment approaches used over the last few years offer reduced morbidity and improved mortality rates for diabetic patients remains to be established. These represent studies of considerable importance.

Mihara et al (41) also provide useful data in a 7-year follow-up study on the mortality of Japanese diabetic patients. The leading cause of death amongst insulin-dependent subjects was acute cardiac failure. In people with either non-insulin-dependent diabetes mellitus or impaired glucose tolerance, the major cause of death was, surprisingly, that of malignancy. Amongst non-insulin-dependent subjects there was a statistically significant excess of deaths from diabetes mellitus itself, ischaemic heart disease and malignant neoplasms compared with the general population. This valuable report is the first concerning mortality amongst Japanese diabetic patients who have been divided into classes of impaired glucose tolerance, non-insulin-dependent diabetes mellitus and insulin dependency.

There is indirect evidence for improved outcomes from newer, and hopefully better, treatment approaches. An article by Hjortrup et al (42) found that the postoperative morbidity in carefully managed diabetic individuals was not significantly greater than that for non-diabetic subjects when matched according to operative procedure, sex, age, complicating cardiovascular disease and weight.

Use of health resources by people with diabetes

The greatest cost relating to diabetes care is that of hospitalisation. Williams (43) has reported hospital admissions for 1981 in East Anglia, U.K. He found that 1.6% of hospital bed days were attributed to diabetes mellitus as the principal cause for admission. Overall, 5.6% of beds were occupied by diabetic patients on an average day. These statistics are very similar to those reported by Scott and colleagues from New Zealand (44). This latter paper, however, found that admission rates for insulin-treated subjects were lower for individuals who participate in education programmes than for those who had not taken the opportunity to participate.

Murphy et al (45) have reported the use of county hospital emergency rooms by diabetic subjects. Usage was characterised by excessive numbers of visits relating to diabetes complications. Approximately 20% of visits to hospital were considered to be attributable to preventable complications of diabetes. The authors concluded that improved access to primary health care facilities and educational services could assist in reducing the requirement for a visit to, and admission from, the hospital emergency rooms.

Fulop (46) reported on recurrent admissions for diabetic ketoacidosis at the Bronx Municipal Hospital Center. In recent years the number of patients with frequent recurrences has declined and currently most patients in this category have been young men. No obvious explanation for these changes, such as education of the women, was offered by the authors.

A number of studies have been reported in previous years showing the potential benefits of educational strategies in altering hospitalisation and re-hospitalisation patterns for individuals with chronic disorders (12). A recent article by Bartlett has added to these by describing the economic impact of education on patients with diabetes and asthma (47). This author found the main benefits of education to be reduction in use of emergency services, decrease in re-hospitalisation, reduction in length of stay and reduction in mortality rates. Reduced use of hospital resources has also been observed in the management of pregnancy amongst insulin-dependent diabetic subject (48). In common with many other centres, Heller et al (48) undertake management of pregnancy and insulin-dependent diabetes mellitus with the aid of home blood-glucose monitoring, avoiding the necessity for routine admissions prior to delivery. They again found such strategies a safe and effective way of managing pregnant diabetic women as outpatients.

Hopper and Schechtman (49) have made positive suggestions as to the potential usefulness of a number of activities by health educators which could reduce hospitalisation rates. These authors studied 161 low-income, predominantly black and female diabetic clinic patients. They suggested that education should be aimed at re-focusing health beliefs and behavioural training to increase practical dietary skills. They emphasised that the structural characteristics of their clinics needed to be modified to accommodate patient needs. A common strategy amongst conventional diabetes clinics is to arrange for more frequent follow-up of individuals who are perceived as having poor control or complications. However, it was emphasised in the article by Matzen et al (50) that the frequency of attendance at outpatient clinics does not bear any relationship to the quality of control. These authors emphasised the need for other tutorial and counselling approaches in the management of those with disordered control.

The implications of these studies reporting health and economic benefits amongst individuals participating in educational programmes have great significance for third-party reimbursements. Recently in Maine, U.S.A. (51), costs associated with the delivery and prevention-orientated education programme have been recoverable under third-party reimbursement, this representing a significant change in philosophy for hospital and third-party carriers.

Barriers to health care

In the review in *The Diabetes Annual/2,* a number of papers were described which had addressed the problem of access to the health care system (2). Contributing to this were inadequate records and very incomplete systems for follow-up. Whereas these problems in the health service are potentially remedial by improved administration, there are other identifiable barriers to good health care which rest with the patients themselves. In the last year, a number of articles have concentrated on this (52-58). Participation in educational programmes and concern to accept self-management approaches appears to be very dependent upon the individual's health locus of control and level of social support (52, 58). Patient self-sufficiency or physician-patient shared care appear to be dependent upon both cultural and educational backgrounds.

Consideration of these psychosocial aspects is obviously essential in any situation where there is poor diabetic control, recurrent hospitalisation or non-participation in teaching treatment programmes. Clearly, more research is needed, but these psychosocial factors may prove to be as important a barrier to health care as those which exist through poor planning of the health service and disorganisation within the service.

Conclusions

Very few studies reporting new initiatives with diabetes services and outcome measurements have been reported over the period 1985-1986. Health care costs relating to diabetes mellitus are posing increasing concern to health administrators in many countries throughout the world. In the last year various papers have, once again, hinted at potential ways of improving the access of patients to health care systems, of the worth of soundly based education and intervention programmes, and of the likely benefit of these programmes in reducing their requirement for much more costly hospitalisation. In the final analysis the long-term benefits will depend upon studies showing that these same strategies have importance in reducing chronic complications of the disorder.

At this time when well-known sociologists are addressing the concept of the economics of social care and cost-benefit analysis (59) it is important that all concerned with diabetes care must examine their service to see if its organisation is meeting the community's needs as it relates to diabetes mellitus.

References

1. Beaven DW (1985): Organization of diabetic care. In: Alberti KGMM, Krall LP (Eds), *The Diabetes Annual/1*, p. 363. Elsevier, Amsterdam.
2. Beaven DW, Scott RS (1986): The organisation of diabetes care. In: Alberti KGMM, Krall LP (Eds), *The Diabetes Annual/2*, p. 39. Elsevier, Amsterdam.
3. Assal JP, Muhlhauser I, Pernet A et al (1985): Patient education as the basis for diabetes care in clinical practice and research. *Diabetologia, 28*, 602.
4. Connell FA (1985): Epidemiologic approaches to the identification of problems in diabetes care. *Diabetes Care, 1*, 82.
5. Mather HM, Keen H (1985): The Southall Diabetes Survey: prevalence of known diabetes in Asians and Europeans. *Br. Med. J., 291*, 1081.
6. Cheah JS, Yeo PPB, Thai AC et al (1985): Epidemiology of diabetes mellitus in Singapore: comparison with other Asian countries. *Ann. Acad. Med. Singapore, 14*, 232.
7. Omar MAK, Seedat MA, Dyer RB et al (1985): The prevalence of diabetes mellitus in a large group of South African Indians. *S. Afr. Med. J., 67*, 924.
8. Merriman A, Ross I (1985): Findings among 100 type 2 diabetics in a clinic in Penang, Malaysia, 1983-84. *Ann. Acad. Med. Singapore, 14*, 277.
9. Lawrence I, Rand MD, Andrzej S et al (1985): Multiple factors in the prediction of risk of proliferative diabetic retinopathy. *N. Engl. J. Med., 313*, 1433.

10. McLaughlin J, Sliepcevich M (1985): The self-care behavior inventory: a model for behavioral instrument development. *Patient Educ. Couns., 7,* 289.
11. Menkinbrant J, De Bock C (1985): Integration of health education with medical care. *Bull. Educ. Patient Mal., 4,* 7.
12. Schafer LC, McCaul KD, Glasgow RE (1986): Supportive and nonsupportive family behaviors: relationships to adherence and metabolic control in persons with type I diabetes. *Diabetes Care, 9,* 179.
13. Harris R, Linn MW (1985): Health beliefs, compliance, and control of diabetes mellitus. *South. Med. J., 78,* 162.
14. Newbrough JR, Simpkins CG, Maurer H (1985): A family development approach to studying factors in the management and control of childhood diabetes. *Diabetes Care, 8,* 83.
15. Retting BA, Shrauger DG, Recker RR et al (1986): A randomized study of the effects of a home diabetes education program. *Diabetes Care, 9,* 173.
16. Spathis GS (1986): Facilities in diabetic clinics in the UK: shortcomings and recommendations. *Diabetic Med., 3,* 131.
17. Holmes DM (1986): The person and diabetes in psychosocial context. *Diabetes Care, 9,* 194.
18. Hoskins P, Alford J, Fowler P et al (1985): Outpatient stabilization programme — an innovative approach in the management of diabetes. *Diabetes Res., 2,* 85.
19. Kosecoff J, Fink A, Brook RH et al (1985): General medical care and the education of internists in university hospitals: an evaluation of the teaching hospital general medicine group practice program. *Ann. Intern. Med., 102,* 250.
20. Morrison EY, Richards R (1985): Clinical profile of diabetes mellitus in Jamaica (phasic insulin dependence). *West Indian Med. J., 34,* 94.
21. Van Ballegooie E (1985): The organization of diabetes care. *Tijdschr. Ned. Ver. Chem., 10,* 25.
22. Assal JP, Aufseesser-Stein M (1986): Patient education in diabetes therapy. In: Alberti KGMM, Krall LP (Eds), *The Diabetes Annual/2,* p. 156. Elsevier, Amsterdam.
23. Barnett AH (1985): Diabetic control and the effect of changing a diabetic clinic to modern management. *Diabetic Med., 2,* 57.
24. Wylie-Rosett J, Villeneuve M, Mazze R (1985): Professional education in a long-term-care facility: program development in diabetes. *Diabetes Care, 8,* 481.
25. Mahler RF, Greenwood RM (1984): A simple diabetic clinic information and audit system. *Diabetic Med., 1,* 301.
26. Mellor JG, Samanta A, Blandford RL, Burden AC (1985): Questionnaire survey of diabetic care in general practice in Leicestershire. *Health Trends, 17,* 61.
27. Pav J, Sperl M (1985): Medical and social problems in the care of diabetics: results of a survey comprising 269 patients. *Vnitr. Lek., 31,* 585.
28. Wing RR, Epstein LH, Nowalk MP et al (1985): Behavior change, weight loss, and physiological improvements in type II diabetic patients. *J. Consult. Clin. Psychol., 53,* 111.
29. Mazzuca SA, Moorman NH, Wheeler ML et al (1986): The Diabetes Education Study: a controlled trial of the effects of diabetes patient education. *Diabetes Care, 9,* 1.
30. Adamson TE, Gullion DS (1986): Assessment of diabetes continuing medical education. *Diabetes Care, 9,* 11.
31. Paulozzi LJ, Norman JE, McMahon P, Connell FA (1984): Outcome of a diabetes education program. *Public Health Rep., 99,* 575.
32. Damoiseaux P, Lacroix A, Assal JP (1985): Teaching of diabetic subjects: appraisal of the questions that are asked of patients by health auxiliaries and of the usefulness of a pedagogical analysis. *Diabète Métabol., 11,* 9.
33. Pichert JW, Hanson SL, Pechmann CA (1985): A system for assessing use of patients' time. *Eval. Health Prof., 8,* 39.

34. Health and Public Policy Committee, American College of Physicians, Philadelphia, Pennsylvania (1984): Glycosylated hemoglobin assays in management and diagnosis of diabetes mellitus. *Ann. Intern. Med.*, *101*, 710.
35. Zimmet P, Gerstman M, Raper LR et al (1984): Computerized assessment of self-monitored blood glucose results using a glucometer reflectance photometer with memory and microcomputer. *Diab. Res. Clin. Pract.*, *1*, 55.
36. Mazze RS, Pasmantier R, Murphy JA, Shamoon H (1985): Self-monitoring of capillary blood glucose: changing the performance of individuals with diabetes. *Diabetes Care*, *8*, 207.
37. Mazze RS, Shamoon H, Pasmantier R et al (1984): Reliability of blood glucose monitoring by patients with diabetes mellitus. *Am J. Med.*, *77*, 211.
38. Wing RR, Epstein LH, Nowalk MP et al (1985): Compliance to self-monitoring of blood glucose: a marked-item technique compared with self-report. *Diabetes Care*, *8*, 456.
39. Hadden DR, Blair ALT, Wilson EA et al (1986): Natural history of diabetes presenting age 40-69 years: a prospective study of the influence of intensive dietary therapy. *Q. J. Med.*, *59*, 579.
40. Beischer W, Pfeiffer EF (1985): Remarks on the prognosis of diabetes mellitus. I. Previous prognosis and new possibilities of metabolic monitoring and therapy. *Fortschr. Med.*, *103*, 501.
41. Mihara T, Ohashi H, Hirata Y (1986): Mortality of Japanese diabetics in a seven-year follow-up study. *Diabetes Res. Clin. Pract.*, *2*, 139.
42. Hjortrup A, Sorensen C, Dyremose E et al (1985): Influence of diabetes mellitus on operative risk. *Br. J. Surg.*, *72*, 783.
43. Williams DRR (1985): Hospital admissions of diabetic patients: information from hospital activity analysis. *Diabetes Med.*, *2*, 27.
44. Scott RS, Brown LJ, Clifford (1985): Use of health services by diabetic persons. II. Hospital admissions. *Diabetes Care*, *8*, 43.
45. Murphy CC, Faulkenberry EH, Rumpel JD, Wheeler FC (1985): The use of a county hospital emergency room by diabetic patients. *Diabetes Care*, *8*, 48.
46. Fulop M (1985): Recurrent diabetic ketoacidosis. *Am. J. Med.*, *78*, 54.
47. Bartlett E (1985): Economic impact of education of patients: significant results. *Bull. Educ. Patient Mal.*, *4*, 16.
48. Heller SR, Lowe LM, Johnson IR et al (1984): Seven years experience of home management in pregnancy in women with insulin-dependent diabetes. *Diabetic Med.*, *1*, 199.
49. Hopper SV, Schechtman KB (1985): Factors associated with diabetic control and utilization patterns in a low-income, older adult population. *Patient Educ. Couns.*, *7*, 275.
50. Matzen LE, Larsen JB, Froland A (1985): Glycosylated hemoglobin Asub 1 used in quality-control of diabetes care: a cross-sectional study in an outpatient clinic. *Diabetes Res.*, *2*, 243.
51. Schwartz R, Zaremba M, Ra K (1985): Third-party coverage for diabetes education program. *Qual. Rev. Bull.*, *11*, 213.
52. Schlenk EA, Hart LK (1984): Relationship between health locus of control, health value, and social support and compliance of persons with diabetes mellitus. *Daibetes Care*, *7*, 566.
53. Back M, Otto S, Zorkenstein H, Huber HP (1984): Psychologic aspects of metabolic regulation in juvenile diabetics. *Z. Klin. Psychol.*, *13*, 263.
54. Bobrow ES, AvRuskin TW, Siller J (1985): Mother-daughter interaction and adherence to diabetes regimens. *Diabetes Care*, *8*, 146.
55. Magy VT, Wolfe GR (1984): Cognitive predictors of compliance in chronic disease patients. *Med. Care*, *22*, 912.
56. Anderson RM (1986): The personal meaning of having diabetes: implications for patient behaviour and education or kicking the bucket theory. *Diabetic Med.*, *3*, 85.

57. Etzwiler DD (1984): Identification and management of psychosocial aspects of diabetes. *Acta Paediatr. Jpn.*, *26*, 442.
58. Kaplan RM, Chadwick MW, Schimmel LE (1985): Social learning intervention to promote metabolic control in type I diabetes mellitus: pilot experiment results. *Diabetes Care*, *8*, 152.
59. Knapp MRJ (1984): *The Economics of Social Care*. Studies in Social Policy, Macmillan, London.

Subject Index